AAOS Comprehensive Orthopaedic Review 2

Study Questions

AAOS
American Academy of Orthopaedic Surgeons

AAOS Comprehensive Orthopaedic Review 2

Study Questions

Edited by
Martin I. Boyer, MD, MSc, FRCS(C)
Carol B. and Jerome T. Loeb Professor
Department of Orthopedic Surgery
Washington University School of Medicine
St. Louis, Missouri

AAOS
American Academy of Orthopaedic Surgeons

AAOS

AMERICAN ACADEMY OF ORTHOPAEDIC SURGEONS

Staff

Ellen C. Moore, *Chief Education Officer*

Hans Koelsch, PhD, *Director, Department of Publications*

Lisa Claxton Moore, *Senior Manager, Book Program*

Steven Kellert, *Senior Editor*

Michelle Wild, *Associate Senior Editor*

Mary Steermann Bishop, *Senior Manager, Production and Content Management*

Courtney Astle, *Editorial Production Manager*

Abram Fassler, *Publishing Systems Manager*

Suzanne O'Reilly, *Graphic Designer*

Susan Morritz Baim, *Production Coordinator*

Karen Danca, *Permissions Coordinator*

Charlie Baldwin, *Production Database Associate*

Hollie Muir, *Production Database Associate*

Emily Nickel, *Page Production Assistant*

Published 2014 by the
American Academy of Orthopaedic Surgeons
6300 North River Road
Rosemont, IL 60018

Library of Congress Control Number:
2014938528
ISBN
978-0-89203-845-9

Printed in the USA

Bone and Joint Initiative USA

Acknowledgments

Editorial Board
AAOS Comprehensive Orthopaedic Review, ed 2
Study Questions

Martin I. Boyer, MD *(Editor and Orthopaedic Oncology/Systemic Disease)*
Carol B. and Jerome T. Loeb Professor
Department of Orthopedics
Washington University in St. Louis
St. Louis, Missouri

Lisa Berglund, MD *(Pediatrics)*
Assistant Professor of Orthopaedic Surgery
Department of Pediatric Orthopaedic Surgery
Children's Mercy Hospital
Kansas City, Missouri

Jacob M. Buchowski, MD, MS *(Spine)*
Associate Professor
Department of Orthopedic Surgery
Washington University School of Medicine
St. Louis, Missouri

D. Nicole Deal, MD *(Hand and Wrist)*
Assistant Professor
Department of Orthopaedic Surgery
University of Virginia
Charlottesville, Virginia

Michael J. Gardner, MD *(Trauma)*
Associate Professor
Department of Orthopedic Surgery
Washington University School of Medicine
St. Louis, Missouri

Jonathan N. Grauer, MD *(Basic Science)*
Associate Professor
Department of Orthopaedics and Rehabilitation
Yale University School of Medicine
New Haven, Connecticut

Jay D. Keener, MD *(Shoulder and Elbow)*
Assistant Professor
Department of Orthopedic Surgery
Washington University School of Medicine
St. Louis, Missouri

Ryan M. Nunley, MD *(Preservation, Arthroplasty, and Salvage Surgery of the Hip and Knee)*
Assistant Professor of Orthopedics
Department of Orthopaedic Surgery
Washington University School of Medicine
St. Louis, Missouri

Kurt P. Spindler, MD *(Sports Injuries of the Knee and Sports Medicine)*
Professor of Orthopaedics
Director of Sports Medicine
Department of Orthopaedic Surgery and Rehabilitation
Vanderbilt University Medical Center
Nashville, Tennessee

Andrew Brian Thomson, MD *(Foot and Ankle)*
Director, Division of Foot and Ankle Surgery
Department of Orthopaedics and Rehabilitation
Vanderbilt University
Nashville, Tennessee

Many of the questions in this book were originally prepared for inclusion in the following AAOS examinations:

2006 Foot and Ankle Self-Assessment Examination

2006 Musculoskeletal Trauma Self-Assessment Examination

2006 Orthopaedic Basic Science Self-Assessment Examination

2006 Adult Spine Self-Assessment Examination

2007 Adult Reconstructive Surgery of the Hip and Knee Self-Assessment Examination

2007 Pediatric Orthopaedic Self-Assessment Examination

2007 Sports Medicine Self-Assessment Examination

2008 Anatomy-Imaging Self-Assessment Examination

2008 Musculoskeletal Tumors and Diseases Self-Assessment Examination

2008 Upper Extremity Self-Assessment Examination

Preface

To accurately evaluate gaps in knowledge, self-assessment by means of learning from study questions has been an integral part of examination preparation for many students. By reviewing and answering study questions, assumptions made during rote or didactic learning can be tested and corrections made.

It is my hope that the questions provided in this book will assist students in obtaining the knowledge needed for passing the Orthopaedic Board Examination.

On behalf of the section editors of this text, I wish you all the best of luck in your studies and written examinations.

Martin I. Boyer, MD
Carol B. and Jerome T. Loeb Professor
Department of Orthopedic Surgery
Washington University in St. Louis
St. Louis, Missouri

Table of Contents

Basic Science

Q-1: A 74-year-old man reports progressive left hip pain with weight-bearing activities. A radiograph is shown in Figure 1. What is the most likely underlying diagnosis?

1. Infection
2. Lymphoma
3. Paget disease
4. Massive bone infarct
5. Old pelvic trauma

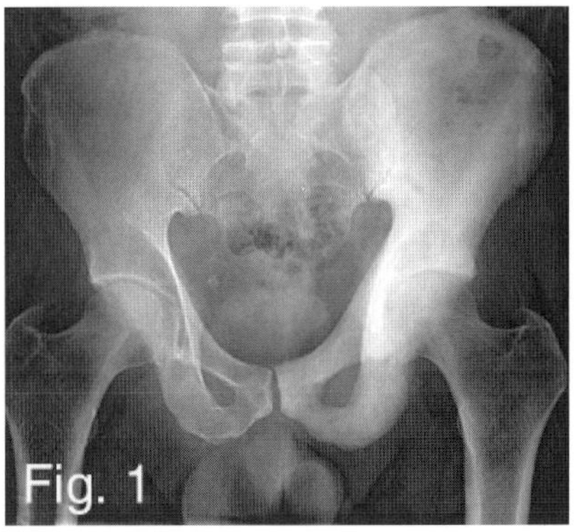
Fig. 1

Q-2: You are interested in learning a new technique for minimally invasive total knee arthroplasty. The Keyhole Genuflex system seems appealing to you because the instrumentation comes with wireless controls. Which of the following represents an acceptable arrangement?

1. The local Keyhole representative has invited you and your spouse out to dinner at a local restaurant to discuss your interest in their new minimally invasive total knee system, the Keyhole Genuflex knee.
2. Keyhole has offered to pay your tuition to attend a CME course sponsored by the American Association of Hip and Knee Surgeons where both the Genuflex and the competing Styph total knee are discussed and demonstrated.
3. Keyhole will pay your expenses to attend a workshop, in Phoenix at their company headquarters, to learn how to implant the Genuflex knee and to see how the implant is manufactured and tested.
4. Keyhole will pay you $500 for each knee that you implant if you switch from your current total knee system.
5. After you have implanted 25 Genuflex knees, Keyhole will list you on their website as a consultant, pay you a consulting fee of $5,000 per year, and invite you to a golf tournament for their consultants at a resort.

Q-3: A 20-year-old woman with a history of subtotal meniscectomy has a painful knee. What associated condition is a contraindication to proceeding with a meniscal allograft?

1. Grade I posterior cruciate ligament tear
2. Grade II medial collateral ligament tear
3. Lateral meniscal tear
4. 5° of genu varum
5. 5 × 5–mm patellar chondral lesion

Q-4: Figures 2A through 2C show the radiograph and MRI scans of a 16-year-old patient who has a painful hip. Examination reveals a significant limp, limited abduction and internal rotation, and severe pain with internal rotation and adduction. A photomicrograph from a biopsy specimen is shown in Figure 2D. What is the deposited pigment observed in this condition?

1. Hemoglobin
2. Myoglobin
3. Melanin
4. Copper
5. Hemosiderin

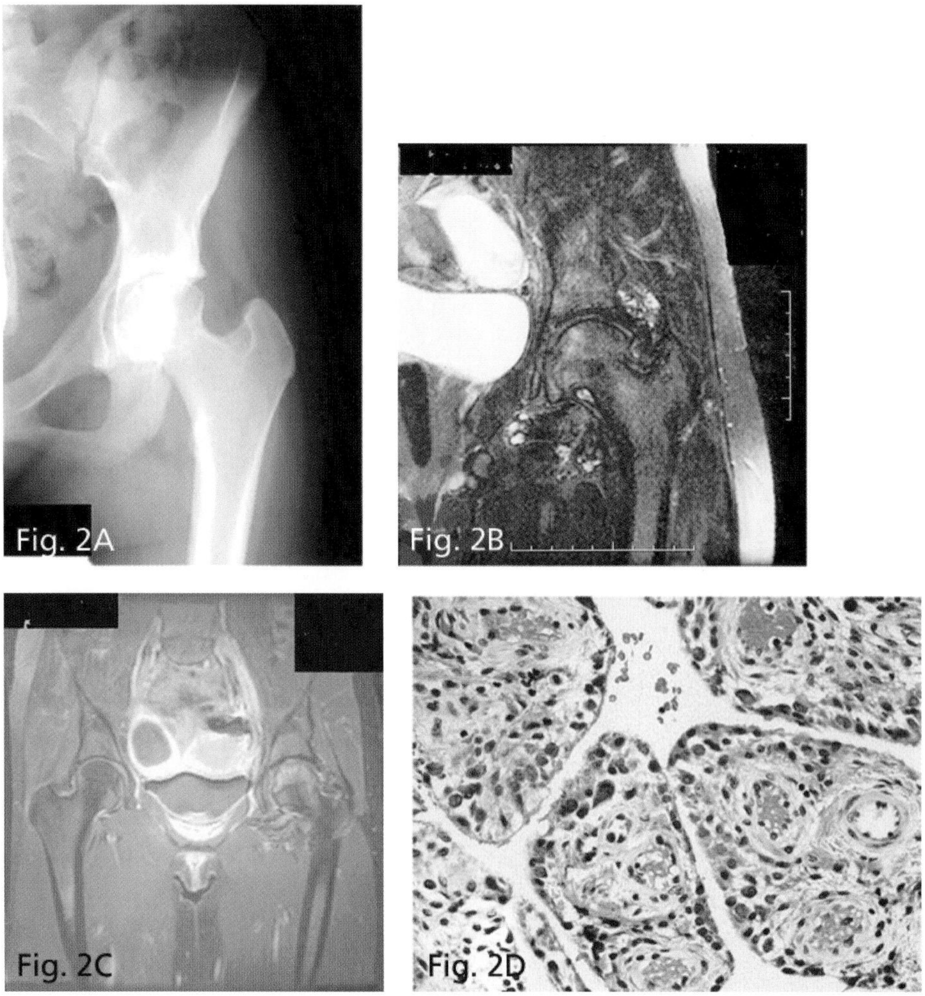

Q-5: Titanium and its alloys are unsuitable candidates for which of the following implant applications?

1. Fracture plates
2. Femoral heads in a hip prosthesis
3. Bone screws
4. Intramedullary nails
5. Porous coatings for bone ingrowth

Q-6: A 30-year-old man reports pain and weakness in his right arm. Examination reveals grade 4 strength in wrist flexion and elbow extension, decreased sensation over the middle finger, and decreased triceps reflex. These symptoms are most compatible with impingement on what spinal nerve root?

1. C5
2. C6
3. C7
4. C8
5. T1

Q-7: Why is tendon considered an anisotropic material?

1. Young modulus is greater than that of bone.
2. Young modulus is greater than that of ligament.
3. Mechanical properties change with preconditioning.
4. Intrinsic mechanical properties vary depending on the direction of loading.
5. Intrinsic mechanical properties vary depending on the rate of loading.

Q-8: Which of the following changes to heart rate, blood pressure, and bulbocavernosus reflex are typical of spinal shock?

1. Tachycardia, hypertension, intact bulbocavernosus reflex
2. Tachycardia, hypotension, intact bulbocavernosus reflex
3. Tachycardia, hypotension, absent bulbocavernosus reflex
4. Bradycardia, hypotension, absent bulbocavernosus reflex
5. Bradycardia, hyperthermia, intact bulbocavernosus reflex

Q-9: What is the primary intracellular signaling mediator for bone morphogenetic protein (BMP) activity?

1. Interleukin-1 (IL-1)
2. Runx2
3. NFK-B
4. SMADs
5. P53

Q-10: Which of the following properties primarily provides the excellent corrosion resistance of metallic alloys such as stainless steel and cobalt-chromium-molybdenum?

1. High surface hardness
2. High levels of nickel
3. Adherent oxide layer
4. Low galvanic potential
5. Metallic carbides

Q-11: Immobilization of human tendons leads to what changes in structure and/or function?

1. Decrease in tensile strength
2. Decrease in the likelihood of rupture
3. Increase in cellularity
4. Increase in aggrecan
5. Increase in collagen fibril diameter

Q-12: Human menisci are made up predominantly of what collagen type?

1. I
2. II
3. III
4. V
5. VI

Q-13: What changes in muscle physiology would be expected in an athlete who begins a rigorous aerobic program for an upcoming marathon?

1. Hypertrophy of type I muscle fibers
2. Reduced fatigue resistance
3. Decreased capillary density
4. Decreased VO_2 max
5. Decreased mitochondrial density per muscle cell

Q-14: A 16-year-old girl has had anterior leg pain and a mass for the past 8 months. Figures 3A and 3B show a radiograph and a hematoxylin and cosin stained histologic specimen. Which of the following disorders is believed to be a precursor of this lesion?

1. Nonossifying fibroma
2. Fibrous dysplasia
3. Unicameral bone cyst
4. Osteogenesis imperfecta
5. Osteofibrous dysplasia

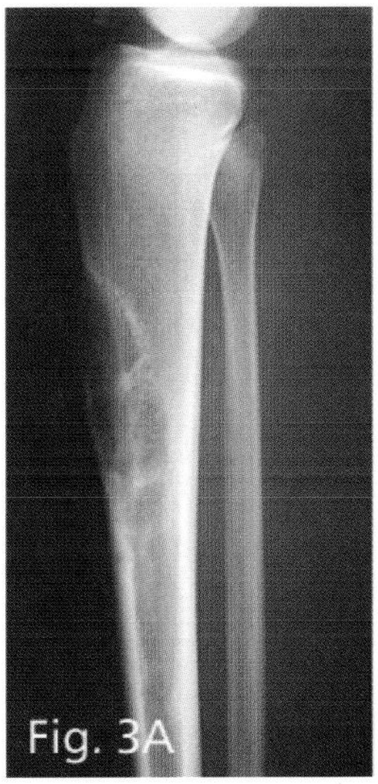

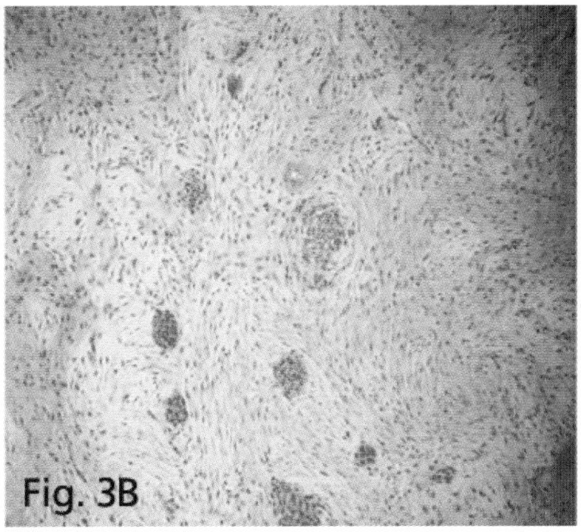

Q-15: Acetaminophen is an antipyretic medication. It exerts its pharmacologic effects by inhibiting which of the following enzymes?

1. Cyclooxygenase-2
2. Interleukin-1 beta (IL-1 β)
3. Tumor necrosis factor-alpha (TNF-α)
4. 5-Hydroxytryptamine
5. Matrix metalloproteinases

Q-16: Nutritional rickets is associated with which of the following changes in chemical blood level?

1. Low vitamin D levels
2. High to normal calcium levels
3. High phosphate levels
4. Decreased parathyroid hormone (PTH)
5. Decreased alkaline phosphatase levels

Q-17: What assay most directly assesses gene expression at the posttranslational level?

1. Real-time polymerase chain reaction (PCR)
2. Standard PCR
3. Northern blot
4. Western blot
5. Microarray expression profile analysis

Q-18: What is the relative amount of type II collagen synthesis in disease-free adult articular cartilage compared to that in developing teenagers?

1. Less than 5%
2. 25%
3. 50%
4. 75%
5. 90%

Q-19: What gene is expressed the earliest during the differentiation of a chondrocyte during endochondral ossification?

1. Aggrecan
2. *Sox*-9
3. Collagen type II
4. Collagen type IV
5. Collagen type XI

Q-20: The vascular supply to the medial meniscus comes primarily from what artery?

1. Lateral genicular
2. Lateral branch of the superior genicular
3. Medial branch of the superior genicular
4. Medial branch of the inferior genicular
5. Medial genicular

Q-21: What term best describes the process involved when a growth factor produced by an osteoblast stimulates the differentiation of an adjacent undifferentiated mesenchymal cell during fracture repair?

1. Mechanical
2. Autocrine
3. Paracrine
4. Endocrine
5. Systemic

Q-22: What additional percentage of energy expenditure above baseline is required for ambulation after an above-the-knee amputation?

1. 0%
2. 5%
3. 20%
4. 65%
5. 90%

Q-23: Ceramic bone substitutes have which of the following properties?

1. There is vascular ingrowth and subsequent graft resorption with host bone ingrowth.
2. Their interconnectivity is similar to that of cancellous bone.
3. They are brittle with significant tensile strength.
4. They are resorbed at a fairly constant rate.
5. Because of their strength, rigid stabilization of the surrounding bone is not necessary.

Q-24: Human tendons are made up primarily of what collagen type (~95%)?

1. I
2. II
3. III
4. IV
5. V

Q-25: The therapeutic effect of etanercept in the treatment of rheumatoid arthritis is primarily mediated through

1. antagonism of tumor necrosis factor-alpha (TNF-α).
2. antagonism of matrix metalloproteinases.
3. inhibition of cyclooxygenase-2 (COX-2).
4. stimulation of interleukin-1 (IL-1).
5. stimulation of tissue inhibitors of metalloproteinases.

Q-26: A 21-year-old woman has a nontraumatic rupture of the Achilles tendon. Which of the following commonly prescribed medications has been associated with this condition?

1. Ibuprofen
2. Fluoroquinolones
3. Bisphosphonates
4. Metoprolol
5. Simvistatin

Q-27: Bioabsorbable polymers are used in a wide range of orthopaedic devices, including anchors, staples, pins, plates, and screws. What is the primary drawback for bioabsorbable implants?

1. High cost
2. Increased rates of infection
3. High elastic modulus
4. Brittleness
5. Foreign body reaction

Q-28: What ligament is the primary restraint to applied valgus loading of the knee?

1. Posteromedial capsule
2. Posterior cruciate ligament (PCL)
3. Superficial medial collateral ligament (MCL)
4. Deep MCL
5. Medial meniscus

Q-29: What region of the thoracic curve is most dangerous for pedicle screw insertion while performing a posterior fusion for adolescent idiopathic scoliosis?

1. Concave side at the stable vertebra
2. Concave side at the apex of the curve
3. Convex side at the stable vertebra
4. Convex side at the apex of the curve
5. Thoracolumbar junction

Q-30: What mechanism is associated with the spontaneous resorption of herniated nucleus pulposus?

1. Macrophage infiltration and phagocytosis
2. Granuloma formation
3. Antibody-mediated destruction
4. Complement cascade activation
5. Major histocompatibility complex-mediated pathways

Q-31: Clinical evidence suggests that grafts for replacing a torn anterior cruciate ligament often stretch after surgery. What is the most probable mechanism for this behavior?

1. Gross failure at the attachment sites
2. Fatigue failure of the ligament tissue
3. Creep of the graft material
4. Water absorption by the graft material
5. Elastic stretch of collagen fibers

Q-32: Which of the following clinical disorders is the result of a mutation in fibroblast growth factor recepter 3 (FGFR3)?

1. Cleidocranial dysplasia
2. Schmid metaphyseal chondrodysplasia
3. Achondroplasia
4. Fibrous dysplasia
5. Camptomelic dysplasia

Q-33: What is the main mechanism for nutrition of the adult disk?

1. Capillary network from the adjacent segmental arteries
2. Capillary network from the arterioles in the vertebral body
3. Diffusion through the anulus fibrosus
4. Diffusion through pores in the end plates
5. Diffusion through nerves in the dorsal root ganglion

Q-34: A knockout mouse for the vitamin D receptor has which of the following phenotypes?

1. Osteopetrosis
2. Renal failure
3. Rickets
4. Jansen-type metaphyseal dysplasia
5. Compensatory hyperparathyroidism and no skeletal phenotype

Q-35: Intramembranous ossification during fracture repair is characterized by absence of which of the following elements?

1. Alkaline phosphatase
2. Osteonectin
3. Osteopontin
4. Collagen type I expression
5. Collagen type II expression

Q-36: Patients with rheumatoid arthritis may exhibit an increase in viral load for which of the following viruses?

1. HIV
2. Papilloma virus
3. Epstein-Barr virus (EBV)
4. Hepatitis C virus (HCV)
5. Hepatitis B virus (HBV)

Q-37: Osteopenia is defined by the World Health Organization (WHO) as a bone mineral density (BMD) that is

1. within 1 standard deviation of age-matched normals.
2. within 1 and 2.5 standard deviations below age-matched normals.
3. within 1 standard deviation of young normals.
4. within 1 and 2.5 standard deviations below young normals.
5. more than 2.5 standard deviations below age-matched normals.

Q-38: Which of the following best describes the mechanism of action of gentamycin?

1. Inhibits cell wall synthesis by inhibiting peptidyl traspeptidase
2. Increases cell membrane permeability
3. Binds to the 30S ribosome subunit interfering with protein synthesis
4. Inhibits DNA gyrase
5. Forms oxygen radicals leading to loss of helical structure and breakage of DNA strands

Q-39: What type of muscle contraction occurs while the muscle is lengthening?

1. Isometric
2. Isotonic
3. Concentric
4. Isokinetic
5. Eccentric

Q-40: Osteoclasts originate from which of the following cell types?

1. Fibroblasts
2. Monocytes
3. Megakaryocytes
4. Plasma cells
5. Osteoprogenitor cells

Q-41: A study is being designed to compare the effectiveness of an antibiotic. The choice of the number of patients (the sample size) depends on several factors. What type of calculation assesses the potential of the study to successfully address the effectiveness of the antibiotic?

1. Regression analysis
2. Power analysis
3. Correlation analysis
4. Nonparametric analysis
5. Analysis of variance

Q-42: What is the most common cause of mechanical failure of an orthopaedic biomaterial during clinical use?

1. Fatigue
2. Tension
3. Compression
4. Shear
5. Torsion

Q-43: Which of the following body positions is associated with the highest intradiskal pressure?

1. Standing, bending forward
2. Standing, bending back
3. Sitting, bending forward
4. Sitting, bending back
5. Supine, lateral decubitus

Q-44: Stiffness relates the amount of load applied to a structure like a long bone or an intramedullary nail to the amount of resulting deformation that occurs in the structure. What is the most important material property affecting the axial and bending stiffness of a structure?

1. Elastic modulus
2. Ductility
3. Ultimate stress
4. Yield stress
5. Toughness

Q-45: Osteoclasts are primarily responsible for bone resorption of malignancy. Which of the following stimulates osteoclast formation?

1. Receptor activator of nuclear factor-κB ligand gene (NF-κB ligand)
2. Osteoprotegerin (OPG)
3. Interleukin-5 (IL-5)
4. Matrix metalloproteinase-2 (MMP-2)
5. Collagen type I

Q-46: Collagen orientation is parallel to the joint surface in what articular cartilage zone?

1. Diagonal
2. Middle
3. Deep
4. Superficial
5. Calcified

Q-47: Which of the following agents increases the risk for a nonunion following a posterior spinal fusion?

1. Ibuprofen
2. Intranasal calcitonin
3. Simvastatin
4. Gentamycin
5. Tamoxifen

Q-48: A study was conducted in 500 patients to measure the effectiveness of a new growth factor in reducing healing time of distal radial fractures. The authors reported that average healing time was reduced from 9.2 to 8.9 weeks ($P < 0.0001$). Because the difference was highly statistically significant, they recommended routine clinical use of this drug despite its high cost. A more appropriate interpretation of these results is that they are

1. clinically significant.
2. statistically significant but perhaps not clinically significant.
3. statistically and clinically significant.
4. not statistically or clinically significant.
5. nonconclusive.

Q-49: What type of multiple lesions is associated with Maffucci syndrome?

1. Nonossifying fibromas
2. Enchondromas
3. Langerhans cell histiocytosis
4. Osteochondromas
5. Giant cell tumors

Q-50: Joint contact pressure in normal or artificial joints can best be minimized by what mechanism?

1. Increasing joint force and contact area
2. Increasing joint force and decreasing contact area
3. Decreasing joint force and contact area
4. Decreasing joint force and increasing contact area
5. Decreasing joint force only

A-1: A 74-year-old man reports progressive left hip pain with weight-bearing activities. A radiograph is shown in Figure 1. What is the most likely underlying diagnosis?

1. Infection
2. Lymphoma
3. Paget disease
4. Massive bone infarct
5. Old pelvic trauma

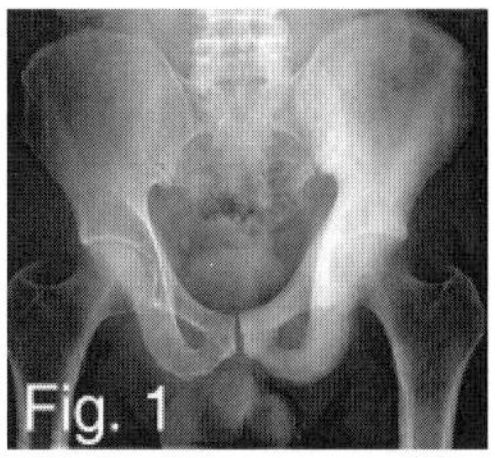

PREFERRED RESPONSE: 3

DISCUSSION: The radiograph shows enlargement of the bone, coarse trabeculation, a blastic appearance, and thickening of the cortex, revealing the classic appearance of Paget disease in the sclerotic phase, the most common presentation. While lymphoma may present as a blastic lesion, it will not have the same enlargement, coarse trabeculation of bone, and the significant sclerosis seen here.

REFERENCES: Friedlaender GE, Katz LD, Flynn SD: Paget's disease and Paget's sarcoma, in Menendez LR, ed: *Orthopaedic Knowledge Update: Musculoskeletal Tumors*. Rosemont, IL, American Academy of Orthopaedic Surgeons, 2002, pp 211-215.

Resnick D, ed: *Diagnosis of Bone and Joint Disorders*. Philadelphia, PA, WB Saunders, 2002, pp 1947-2000.

A-2: You are interested in learning a new technique for minimally invasive total knee arthroplasty. The Keyhole Genuflex system seems appealing to you because the instrumentation comes with wireless controls. Which of the following represents an acceptable arrangement?

1. The local Keyhole representative has invited you and your spouse out to dinner at a local restaurant to discuss your interest in their new minimally invasive total knee system, the Keyhole Genuflex knee.
2. Keyhole has offered to pay your tuition to attend a CME course sponsored by the American Association of Hip and Knee Surgeons where both the Genuflex and the competing Styph total knee are discussed and demonstrated.
3. Keyhole will pay your expenses to attend a workshop, in Phoenix at their company headquarters, to learn how to implant the Genuflex knee and to see how the implant is manufactured and tested.
4. Keyhole will pay you $500 for each knee that you implant if you switch from your current total knee system.
5. After you have implanted 25 Genuflex knees, Keyhole will list you on their website as a consultant, pay you a consulting fee of $5,000 per year, and invite you to a golf tournament for their consultants at a resort.

PREFERRED RESPONSE: 3

DISCUSSION: Both the American Academy of Orthopaedic Surgeons (AAOS) and AdvaMed, the medical device manufacturer's trade organization, have written guidelines that address potential conflicts of interest regarding interactions between physicians and manufacturer's representatives when it comes to patients' best interest. The AAOS thinks that the orthopaedic profession exists for the primary purpose of caring for the patient and that the physician-patient relationship is the central focus of all ethical concerns. When an orthopaedic surgeon receives anything of significant value from industry, a potential conflict of interest exists. The AAOS believes that it is acceptable for industry to provide financial and

(continued on next page)

(A-2: *continued*)

other support to orthopaedic surgeons if such support has significant educational value and has the purpose of improving patient care. All dealings between orthopaedic surgeons and industry should benefit the patient and be able to withstand public scrutiny. A gift of any kind from industry should in no way influence the orthopaedic surgeon in determining the most appropriate treatment for his or her patient. Orthopaedic surgeons should not accept gifts or other financial support with conditions attached. Subsidies by industry to underwrite the costs of educational events where CME credits are provided can contribute to the improvement of patient care and are acceptable. A corporate subsidy received by the conference's sponsor is acceptable; however, direct industry reimbursement for an orthopaedic surgeon to attend a CME educational event is not appropriate. Special circumstances may arise in which orthopaedic surgeons may be required to learn new surgical techniques demonstrated by an expert or to review new implants or other devices on-site. In these circumstances, reimbursement for expenses may be appropriate.

REFERENCES: AAOS Standard of Professionalism -Orthopaedist -Industry Conflict of Interest (Adopted 4/18/07), Mandatory Standard numbers 6, 9, 12-15. http://www3.aaos.org/member/profcomp/SOPConflictsIndustry.pdf.

The Orthopaedic Surgeon's Relationship with Industry, in Guide to the Ethical Practice of Orthopaedic Surgery, ed 7. Rosemont, IL, American Academy of Orthopaedic Surgeons, 2007. http://www.aaos.org/about/papers/ethics/1204eth.asp.

AdvaMed Code of Ethics on Interactions with Health Care Professionals, 2005. http://www.advamed.org/MemberPortal/searchresults.htm?query=Advamed%20Code%20of%20Ethics%20on%20Interactions%20with%20Health%20Care%20Professionals%202005.

A-3: A 20-year-old woman with a history of subtotal meniscectomy has a painful knee. What associated condition is a contraindication to proceeding with a meniscal allograft?

1. Grade I posterior cruciate ligament tear
2. Grade II medial collateral ligament tear
3. Lateral meniscal tear
4. 5° of genu varum
5. 5 × 5–mm patellar chondral lesion

PREFERRED RESPONSE: 4

DISCUSSION: Patients with substantial joint malalignment place increased stresses on the allograft, and this malalignment must be corrected to decrease the likelihood of meniscal allograft failure. None of the other options would lead to failure of the allograft.

REFERENCE: Bush-Joseph C, Carter TR, Miller MD, Rokito AS, Stuart MJ: Knee and leg: Soft-tissue trauma, in Koval KJ, ed: *Orthopaedic Knowledge Update*, ed 7. Rosemont, IL, American Academy of Orthopaedic Surgeons, 2002, p 499.

A-4: Figures 2A through 2C show the radiograph and MRI scans of a 16-year-old patient who has a painful hip. Examination reveals a significant limp, limited abduction and internal rotation, and severe pain with internal rotation and adduction. A photomicrograph from a biopsy specimen is shown in Figure 2D. What is the deposited pigment observed in this condition?

1. Hemoglobin
2. Myoglobin
3. Melanin
4. Copper
5. Hemosiderin

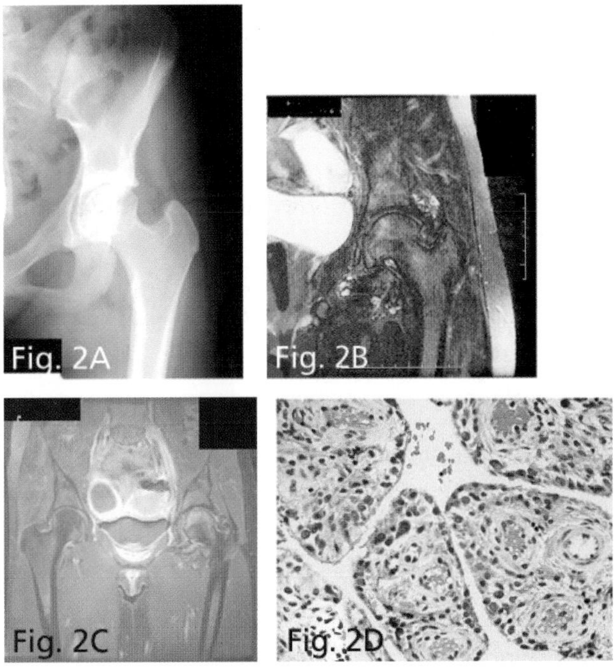
Fig. 2A Fig. 2B Fig. 2C Fig. 2D

PREFERRED RESPONSE: 5

DISCUSSION: Pigmented villonodular synovitis (PVNS) is a synovial proliferative disorder that remains difficult to diagnose. The most common clinical features are mechanical pain and limited joint motion. On radiographs, the classic finding is often a large lesion, associated with multiple lucencies. Other findings may include a normal radiographic appearance, loss of joint space, osteonecrosis of the femoral head, or acetabular protrusion. MRI is the imaging modality of choice and will show the characteristic findings of a joint effusion, synovial proliferation, and bulging of the hip. The synovial lining has a low signal on T1- and T2-weighted images, secondary to hemosiderin deposition. Copper deposition occurs in patients with Wilson disease, which mainly affects the liver.

REFERENCES: Bhimani MA, Wenz JF, Frassica FJ: Pigmented villonodular synovitis: Keys to early diagnosis. *Clin Orthop* 2001;386:197-202.

Cotten A, Flipo RM, Chastanet P, et al: Pigmented villonodular synovitis of the hip: Review of radiographic features in 58 patients. *Skeletal Radiol* 1995;24:1-6.

Basic Science: Answers

A-5: Titanium and its alloys are unsuitable candidates for which of the following implant applications?

1. Fracture plates
2. Femoral heads in a hip prosthesis
3. Bone screws
4. Intramedullary nails
5. Porous coatings for bone ingrowth

PREFERRED RESPONSE: 2

DISCUSSION: Titanium alloy is highly biocompatible, has higher strength than stainless steel, and is highly resistant to corrosion. It is particularly suited for use in fracture plates, bone screws, and intramedullary nails because of its low modulus of elasticity (low stiffness), which can reduce stress shielding. It is also widely used for porous-ingrowth coatings. However, clinical experience has shown that titanium alloy bearing surfaces such as a femoral ball are highly susceptible to severe metallic wear, particularly in the presence of third-body abrasive particles (such as polymethyl methacrylate fragments, bone chips, or metal debris).

REFERENCES: McKellop HA, Sarmiento A, Schwinn CP, et al: In vivo wear of titanium-alloy hip prostheses. *J Bone Joint Surg Am* 1990;72:512-517.

Salvati EA, Betts F, Doty SB: Particulate metallic debris in cemented total hip arthroplasty. *Clin Orthop* 1993;293: 160-173.

Evans BG, Salvati EA, Huo MH, et al: The rationale for cemented total hip arthroplasty. *Orthop Clin North Am* 1993;24:599-610.

A-6: A 30-year-old man reports pain and weakness in his right arm. Examination reveals grade 4 strength in wrist flexion and elbow extension, decreased sensation over the middle finger, and decreased triceps reflex. These symptoms are most compatible with impingement on what spinal nerve root?

1. C5
2. C6
3. C7
4. C8
5. T1

PREFERRED RESPONSE: 3

DISCUSSION: Motor impulses to the triceps, wrist flexion and elbow extension, and sensation to the middle finger are associated most commonly with the C7 root.

REFERENCES: Hoppenfeld S: *Physical Examination of the Spine and Extremities*. Upper Saddle River, NJ, Prentice Hall, 1976, p 125.

Lauerman WC, Goldsmith ME: Spine, in Miller MD, ed: *Review of Orthopaedics*, ed 3. Philadelphia, PA, WB Saunders, 2000, pp 353-378.

A-7: Why is tendon considered an anisotropic material?

1. Young modulus is greater than that of bone.
2. Young modulus is greater than that of ligament.
3. Mechanical properties change with preconditioning.
4. Intrinsic mechanical properties vary depending on the direction of loading.
5. Intrinsic mechanical properties vary depending on the rate of loading.

PREFERRED RESPONSE: 4

DISCUSSION: Anisotropic materials have mechanical properties that vary based on the direction of loading. The relative values of Young modulus for tendon, ligament, and bone are not relevant to isotropy. The mechanical properties of tendon do change with preconditioning, but this change is related to viscoelasticity. The intrinsic mechanical properties of tendon do vary with the rate of loading, but this variance is related to viscoelasticity.

REFERENCES: Mow VC, Flatow EL, Ateshian GA: Biomechanics, in Buckwalter JA, Einhorn TA, Simon SR, eds: *Orthopaedic Basic Science: Biology and Biomechanics of the Musculoskeletal System*, ed 2. Rosemont, IL, American Academy of Orthopaedic Surgeons, 2000, pp 134-180.

Lu L, Kaufman KR, Yaszemski MJ: Biomechanics, in Einhorn TA, O'Keefe RJ, Buckwalter JA, eds: *Orthopaedic Basic Science: Foundations of Clinical Practice*, ed 3. Rosemont, IL, American Academy of Orthopaedic Surgeons, 2006, pp 49-64

A-8: Which of the following changes to heart rate, blood pressure, and bulbocavernosus reflex are typical of spinal shock?

1. Tachycardia, hypertension, intact bulbocavernosus reflex
2. Tachycardia, hypotension, intact bulbocavernosus reflex
3. Tachycardia, hypotension, absent bulbocavernosus reflex
4. Bradycardia, hypotension, absent bulbocavernosus reflex
5. Bradycardia, hyperthermia, intact bulbocavernosus reflex

PREFERRED RESPONSE: 4

DISCUSSION: The term spinal shock applies to all phenomena surrounding physiologic or anatomic transection of the spinal cord that results in temporary loss or depression of all or most spinal reflex activity below the level of the injury. Hypotension and bradycardia caused by loss of sympathetic tone is a possible complication, depending on the level of the lesion. The mechanism of injury that causes spinal shock is usually traumatic in origin and occurs immediately, but spinal shock has been described with mechanisms of injury that progress over several hours. Spinal cord reflex arcs immediately above the level of injury also may be depressed severely on the basis of the Schiff-Sherrington phenomenon. The end of the spinal shock phase of spinal cord injury is signaled by the return of elicitable abnormal cutaneospinal or muscle spindle reflex arcs. Autonomic reflex arcs involving relay to secondary ganglionic neurons outside the spinal cord may be affected variably during spinal shock, and their return after spinal shock abates is variable. The returning spinal cord reflex arcs below the level of injury are irrevocably altered and are the substrate on which rehabilitation efforts are based.

REFERENCE: Ditunno JF, Little JW, Tessler A, et al: Spinal shock revisited: A four-phase model. *Spinal Cord* 2004;42:383-395.

A-9: What is the primary intracellular signaling mediator for bone morphogenetic protein (BMP) activity?

1. Interleukin-1 (IL-1)
2. Runx2
3. NFK-B
4. SMADs
5. P53

PREFERRED RESPONSE: 4

DISCUSSION: BMPs signal through the activation of a transmembrane serine/threonine kinase receptor that leads to the activation of intracellular signaling molecules called SMADs. There are currently eight known SMADs, and the activation of different SMADs within a cell leads to different cellular responses. The other mediators are not believed to be directly involved with BMP signaling.

REFERENCES: Lieberman J, Daluiski A, Einhorn TA: The role of growth factors in the repair of bone: Biology and clinical applications. *J Bone Joint Surg Am* 2002;84:1032-1044.

Li J, Sandell LJ: Transcriptional regulation of cartilage-specific genes, in Rosier RN, Evans C, eds: *Molecular Biology in Orthoapedics*, Rosemont, IL, American Academy of Orthopaedic Surgeons, 2002, pp 21-24.

Zuscik MJ, Drissi MH, Reynolds PR, et al: Molecular and cell biology in orthopaedics, in Einhorn TA, O'Keefe RJ, Buckwalter JA, eds: *Orthopaedic Basic Science: Foundations of Clinical Practice*, ed 3. Rosemont, IL, American Academy of Orthopaedic Surgeons, 2006, pp3-23.

A-10: Which of the following properties primarily provides the excellent corrosion resistance of metallic alloys such as stainless steel and cobalt-chromium-molybdenum?

1. High surface hardness
2. High levels of nickel
3. Adherent oxide layer
4. Low galvanic potential
5. Metallic carbides

PREFERRED RESPONSE: 3

DISCUSSION: All of the metals and metallic alloys used in orthopaedic surgery obtain their corrosion resistance from an adherent oxide layer. For stainless steel and cobalt alloy, the addition of chromium as an alloying element ensures the formation of a chromium oxide passive layer that forms on the surface and separates the bulk material from the corrosive body environment. Titanium alloy achieves the same result without chromium by forming an adherent passive layer of titanium oxide. Although these layers can indeed be hard, hardness does not in and of itself provide corrosion resistance. Adding nickel to both metallic alloys adds to strength but does not influence corrosion resistance appreciably. Galvanic potential can influence corrosion but does so by differences in potential between two contacting materials; for example, stainless steel and cobalt alloy have substantially different potentials, and if they were in contact within an aqueous environment, corrosion would commence with the stainless steel becoming the sacrificial anode. Metallic carbides are important in strengthening the alloys but have no role in providing corrosion resistance.

(continued on next page)

(A-10: *continued*)

REFERENCES: Williams DF, Williams RL: Degradative effects of the biological environment on metal and ceramics, in Ratner BD, Hoffman AS, Shoen FJ, et al, eds: *Biomaterials Science*. San Diego, CA, Academic Press, 1996, pp 260-265.

Wright TM, Li S: Biomaterials, in Buckwalter JA, Einhorn TA, Simon SR, eds: *Orthopaedic Basic Science: Biology and Biomechanics of the Musculoskeletal System*, ed 2. Rosemont, IL, American Academy of Orthopaedic Surgeons, 2000, pp 190-193.

Wright TM, Maher SA: Biomaterials, in Einhorn TA, O'Keefe RJ, Buckwalter JA, eds: *Orthopaedic Basic Science: Foundations of Clinical Practice*, ed 3. Rosemont, IL, American Academy of Orthopaedic Surgeons, 2006, pp 65-85.

A-11: Immobilization of human tendons leads to what changes in structure and/or function?

1. Decrease in tensile strength
2. Decrease in the likelihood of rupture
3. Increase in cellularity
4. Increase in aggrecan
5. Increase in collagen fibril diameter

PREFERRED RESPONSE: 1

DISCUSSION: Recent in vivo and in vitro experiments demonstrate that immobilization of tendon decreases its tensile strength, stiffness, and total weight. Microscopically, there is a decrease in cellularity, overall collagen organization, and collagen fibril diameter.

REFERENCE: Garrett WE, Speer KP, Kirkendall DT, eds: *Principles & Practice of Orthopaedic Sports Medicine*. Philadelphia, PA, Lippincott Williams & Wilkins, 2000, p 687.

A-12: Human menisci are made up predominantly of what collagen type?

1. I
2. II
3. III
4. V
5. VI

PREFERRED RESPONSE: 1

DISCUSSION: Type I collagen accounts for more than 90% of the total collagen content. Other minor collagens present include types II, III, V, and VI.

REFERENCES: Mow VC, Arnoczky SP, Jackson DW, eds: *Knee Meniscus: Basic and Clinical Foundations*. New York, NY, Raven Press, 1992, p 41.

Kawamura S, Rodeo SA: Form and function of the meniscus, in Einhorn TA, O'Keefe RJ, Buckwalter JA, eds: *Orthopaedic Basic Science: Foundations of Clinical Practice*, ed 3. Rosemont, IL, American Academy of Orthopaedic Surgeons, 2006, pp 175-189

A-13: What changes in muscle physiology would be expected in an athlete who begins a rigorous aerobic program for an upcoming marathon?

1. Hypertrophy of type I muscle fibers
2. Reduced fatigue resistance
3. Decreased capillary density
4. Decreased VO_2 max
5. Decreased mitochondrial density per muscle cell

PREFERRED RESPONSE: 1

DISCUSSION: Muscle fibers can be categorized grossly into two types. Type I muscle, also known as slow-twitch muscle, is responsible for aerobic, oxidative muscle metabolism. It has a much lower strength and speed of contraction than fast-twitch type II muscle but is significantly more fatigue resistant. With training for endurance sports, the type I muscle undergoes adaptive changes to the increased stress. Increases in capillary density, oxidative capacity, mitochondrial density, and subsequent fatigue resistance are all observed changes. Hypertrophy of type IIb muscle is seen in strength training.

REFERENCES: Garrett WE Jr, Best TM: Anatomy, physiology, and mechanics of skeletal muscle, in Simon SR, ed: *Orthopaedic Basic Science*. Rosemont, IL, American Academy of Orthopaedic Surgeons, 1994, pp 89-125.

Thayer R, Collins J, Noble EG, et al: A decade of aerobic endurance training: Histological evidence for fibre type transformation. *J Sports Med Phys Fitness* 2000;40:284-289.

A-14: A 16-year-old girl has had anterior leg pain and a mass for the past 8 months. Figures 3A and 3B show a radiograph and a hematoxylin and eosin stained histologic specimen. Which of the following disorders is believed to be a precursor of this lesion?

1. Nonossifying fibroma
2. Fibrous dysplasia
3. Unicameral bone cyst
4. Osteogenesis imperfecta
5. Osteofibrous dysplasia

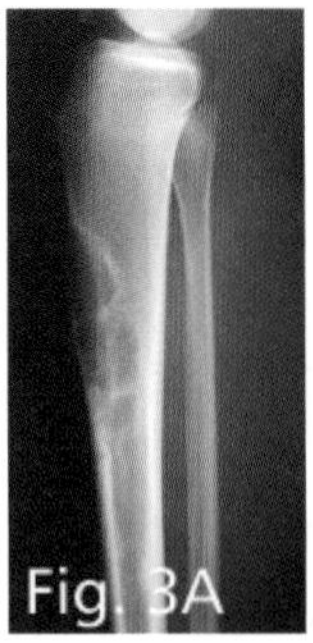

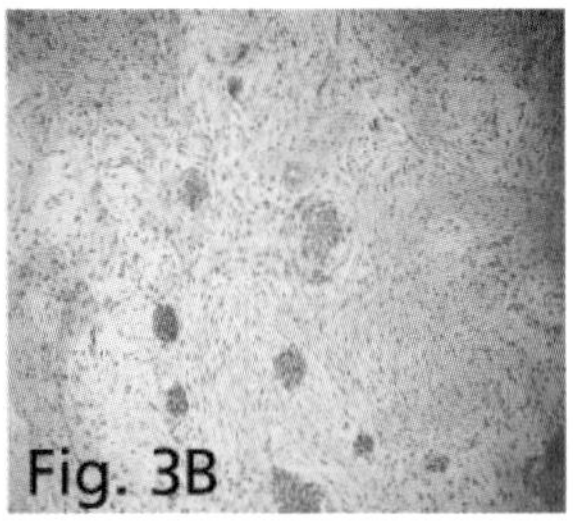

PREFERRED RESPONSE: 5

DISCUSSION: The radiograph and pathology are consistent with adamantinoma. Although the mechanism underlying adamantinoma has not been identified, it is believed to be closely related to osteofibrous dysplasia, which may represent a precursor. The other diagnoses are not known to give rise to adamantinoma.

REFERENCE: Springfield DS, Rosenberg AE, Mankin HJ, et al: Relationship between osteofibrous dysplasia and adamantinoma. *Clin Orthop* 1994;309:234-244.

A-15: Acetaminophen is an antipyretic medication. It exerts its pharmacologic effects by inhibiting which of the following enzymes?

1. Cyclooxygenase-2
2. Interleukin-1 beta (IL-1β)
3. Tumor necrosis factor-alpha (TNF-α)
4. 5-Hydroxytryptamine (5-HT)
5. Matrix metalloproteinases

PREFERRED RESPONSE: 2

DISCUSSION: Acetaminophen inhibits prostaglandin E2 production via IL-1β, without affecting cyclooxygenase-2 enzymatic activity. The therapeutic concentrations of acetaminophen induce an inhibition of IL-1β–dependent nuclear factor of kappa B nuclear translocation. The selectivity of this effect suggests the existence of an acetaminophen-specific activity at the transcriptional level that may be one of the mechanisms through which the drug exerts its pharmacologic effects. Acetaminophen does not affect any of the other enzymes named above.

REFERENCE: Mancini F, Landolfi C, Muzio M, et al: Acetaminophen down-regulates interleukin-1beta-induced nuclear factor-kappaB nuclear translocation in a human astrocytic cell line. *Neurosci Lett* 2003;353:79-82.

A-16: Nutritional rickets is associated with which of the following changes in chemical blood level?

1. Low vitamin D levels
2. High to normal calcium levels
3. High phosphate levels
4. Decreased parathyroid hormone (PTH)
5. Decreased alkaline phosphatase levels

PREFERRED RESPONSE: 1

DISCUSSION: Nutritional rickets is associated with decreased dietary intake of vitamin D, resulting in low levels of vitamin D that result in decreased intestinal absorption of calcium and low to normal serologic levels of calcium. To boost serum calcium levels, there is a compensatory increase in PTH and bone resorption, leading to increased alkaline phosphatase levels.

REFERENCES: Brinker MR: Cellular and molecular biology, immunology, and genetics in orthopaedics, in Miller MD, ed: *Review of Orthopaedics*, ed 3. Philadelphia, PA, WB Saunders, 2001, pp 81-94.

Pettifor J: Nutritional and drug-induced rickets and osteomalacia, in Farrus MJ, ed: *Primer on the Metabolic Bone Diseases and Disorders of Mineral Metabolism*, ed 5. Philadelphia, PA, Lippincott Williams and Wilkins, 2003, pp 399-466.

Einhorn TA: Metabolic bone disease, in Einhorn TA, O'Keefe RJ, Buckwalter JA, eds: *Orthopaedic Basic Science: Foundations of Clinical Practice*, ed 3. Rosemont, IL, American Academy of Orthopaedic Surgeons, 2006, pp 415-426.

A-17: What assay most directly assesses gene expression at the posttranslational level?

1. Real-time polymerase chain reaction (PCR)
2. Standard PCR
3. Northern blot
4. Western blot
5. Microarray expression profile analysis

PREFERRED RESPONSE: 4

DISCUSSION: Gene expression at the posttranslational level refers to proteins, as opposed to DNA or RNA. The only assay listed that targets protein expression directly is the Western blot. Standard PCR is amplification of targeted DNA segments, regardless of whether or not they are actively expressed. Real-time PCR, Northern blot, and microarray expression profile analysis all quantify RNA as a means to determine posttranscriptional gene expression.

REFERENCES: Brinker MR: Cellular and molecular biology, immunology, and genetics in orthopaedics, in Miller MD, ed: *Review of Orthopaedics*, ed 3. Philadelphia, PA, WB Saunders, 2001, pp 81-94.

Rosier RN, Reynolds, PR, O'Keefe RJ: Molecular and cell biology in orthopaedics, in Buckwalter JA, Einhorn TA, Simon SR, eds: *Orthopaedic Basic Science: Biology and Biomechanics of the Musculoskeletal System*, ed 2. Rosemont, IL, American Academy of Orthopaedic Surgeons, 2000, pp 19-76.

A-18: What is the relative amount of type II collagen synthesis in disease-free adult articular cartilage compared to that in developing teenagers?

1. Less than 5%
2. 25%
3. 50%
4. 75%
5. 90%

PREFERRED RESPONSE: 1

DISCUSSION: Adult articular cartilage has less than 5% of the synthesis rate of type II collagen than that seen in developing teenagers. Both synthesis and degradation of type II collagen in normal adult articular cartilage is very low compared to that in children. In osteoarthrosis, both synthesis and degradation are increased, but the collagen does not properly incorporate into the matrix.

REFERENCES: Lippiello L, Hall D, Mankin HJ: Collagen synthesis in normal and osteoarthritic human cartilage. *J Clin Invest* 1977;59:593-600.

Nelson F, Dahlberg L, Laverty S, et al: Evidence for altered synthesis of type II collagen in patients with osteoarthritis. *J Clin Invest* 1998;102:2115-2125.

A-19: What gene is expressed the earliest during the differentiation of a chondrocyte during endochondral ossification?

1. Aggrecan
2. *Sox*-9
3. Collagen type II
4. Collagen type IV
5. Collagen type XI

PREFERRED RESPONSE: 2
DISCUSSION: Transcription factors regulate the activation or repression of cartilage-specific genes. *Sox*-9, considered a major regulator of chondrogenesis, regulates several cartilage-specific genes during endochondral ossification, including genes for collagen types II, IV, and XI and aggrecan.

REFERENCES: Li J, Sandell LJ: Transcriptional regulation of cartilage-specific genes, in Rosier RN, Evans C, eds: *Molecular Biology in Orthoapedics*, Rosemont, IL, American Academy of Orthopaedic Surgeons, 2002, pp 21-24.

Sandell LJ: Genes and gene expression. *Clin Orthop* 2000;379:S9-S16.

A-20: The vascular supply to the medial meniscus comes primarily from what artery?

1. Lateral genicular
2. Lateral branch of the superior genicular
3. Medial branch of the superior genicular
4. Medial branch of the inferior genicular
5. Medial genicular

PREFERRED RESPONSE: 4

DISCUSSION: The vascular supply to the medial and lateral menisci originates predominantly from the medial and lateral genicular arteries. The popliteal artery splits into the superior genicular, which splits into medial and lateral branches supplying the patellar cartilage and the posterior cruciate ligament. The middle genicular artery also supplies the anterior curciate ligament, posterior cruciate ligament, and collateral ligaments. The inferior genicular splits into medial and lateral branches and supplies the menisci and other knee ligaments. Despite propagation of incorrect terminology, there is no superior or lateral genicular artery.

REFERENCE: Mow VC, Arnoczky SP, Jackson DW, eds: *Knee Meniscus: Basic and Clinical Foundations*. New York, NY, Raven Press, 1992, p 4.

A-21: What term best describes the process involved when a growth factor produced by an osteoblast stimulates the differentiation of an adjacent undifferentiated mesenchymal cell during fracture repair?

1. Mechanical
2. Autocrine
3. Paracrine
4. Endocrine
5. Systemic

PREFERRED RESPONSE: 3

DISCUSSION: Growth factors are proteins secreted by cells that can act on target cells to produce certain biologic actions. These actions can be described as autocrine, paracrine, and endocrine. Autocrine actions are those in which the growth factor influences an adjacent cell of its origin or identical phenotype. Paracrine actions are those in which the protein influences an adjacent cell that is different in its origin or phenotype. Endocrine actions are those in which the factor influences a cell located at a distant anatomic site.

REFERENCES: Lieberman J, Daluiski A, Einhorn TA: The role of growth factors in the repair of bone: Biology and clinical applications. *J Bone Joint Surg Am* 2002;84:1032-1044.

Zuscik MJ, Drissi MH, Reynolds PR, et al: Molecular and cell biology in orthopaedics, in Einhorn TA, O'Keefe RJ, Buckwalter JA, eds: *Orthopaedic Basic Science: Foundations of Clinical Practice*, ed 3. Rosemont, IL, American Academy of Orthopaedic Surgeons, 2006, pp 3-23.

A-22: What additional percentage of energy expenditure above baseline is required for ambulation after an above-the-knee amputation?

1. 0%
2. 5%
3. 20%
4. 65%
5. 90%

PREFERRED RESPONSE: 4

DISCUSSION: Patients with an above-the-knee amputation have a 65% increase in energy expenditure. A patient with a transtibial amputation requires 25% more energy above baseline values; however, bilateral transtibial amputations are associated with a 40% increase in energy expenditure.

REFERENCES: Otis JC, Lane JM, Kroll MA: Energy cost during gait in osteosarcoma patients after resection and knee replacement and after above-the-knee amputation. *J Bone Joint Surg Am* 1985;67:606-611.

Pinzur MS, Gold J, Schwartz D, et al: Energy demands for walking in dysvascular amputees as related to the level of amputation. *Orthopedics* 1992;15:1033-1036.

A-23: Ceramic bone substitutes have which of the following properties?

1. There is vascular ingrowth and subsequent graft resorption with host bone ingrowth.
2. Their interconnectivity is similar to that of cancellous bone.
3. They are brittle with significant tensile strength.
4. They are resorbed at a fairly constant rate.
5. Because of their strength, rigid stabilization of the surrounding bone is not necessary.

PREFERRED RESPONSE: 1

DISCUSSION: Ceramics have the following properties: They are resorbed at varying rates, and the chemical composition of the ceramic significantly affects the rate of resorption. For example, tricalcium phosphate (TCP) undergoes biologic resorption 10 to 20 times faster than hydroxyapatite. The partial conversion of TCP to hydroxyapatite once it is in the body significantly reduces the rate of resorption. Some segments of hydroxyapatite can remain in place in the body for 7 to 10 years. In clinical trials, TCP more readily remodels because of its porosity, but it is weaker. The success of converted corals as a bone graft substitute relies on a complex sequence of events of vascular ingrowth, differentiation of osteoprogenitor cells, bone remodeling, and graft resorption occurring together with host bone ingrowth into and on the porous coralline microstructure or voids left behind during resorption.

REFERENCES: Lane JM, Bostrom MP: Bone grafting and new composite biosynthetic graft materials. *Instr Course Lect* 1998;47:525-534.

Walsh WR, Chapman-Sheath PJ, Cain S, et al: A resorbable porous ceramic composite bone graft substitute in a rabbit metaphyseal defect model. *J Orthop Res* 2003;21:655-661.

Wright TM, Maher SA: Biomaterials, in Einhorn TA, O'Keefe RJ, Buckwalter JA, eds: *Orthopaedic Basic Science: Foundations of Clinical Practice*, ed 3. Rosemont, IL, American Academy of Orthopaedic Surgeons, 2006, pp 65-85.

A-24: Human tendons are made up primarily of what collagen type (~95%)?

1. I
2. II
3. III
4. IV
5. V

PREFERRED RESPONSE: 1

DISCUSSION: Tendons are dense, primarily collagenous tissues that attach muscle to bone. Collagen content of the dry weight is slightly greater than that found in ligaments and is predominantly type I. Type III collagen makes up the remaining ~5% of total collagen content.

REFERENCES: Kasser JR, ed: *Orthopaedic Knowledge Update*, ed 5. Rosemont, IL, American Academy of Orthopaedic Surgeons, 1996, pp 10-12.

Garrett WE, Speer KP, Kirkendall DT, eds: *Principles & Practice of Orthopaedic Sports Medicine*. Philadelphia, PA, Lippincott Williams & Wilkins, 2000, pp 21-37.

Frank CB, Shrive NG, Lo IK, et al: Form and function of tendon and ligament, in Einhorn TA, O'Keefe RJ, Buckwalter JA, eds: *Orthopaedic Basic Science: Foundations of Clinical Practice*, ed 3. Rosemont, IL, American Academy of Orthopaedic Surgeons, 2006, pp 191-222.

A-25: The therapeutic effect of etanercept in the treatment of rheumatoid arthritis is primarily mediated through

1. antagonism of tumor necrosis factor-alpha (TNF-α).
2. antagonism of matrix metalloproteinases.
3. inhibition of cyclooxygenase-2 (COX-2).
4. stimulation of interleukin-1 (IL-1).
5. stimulation of tissue inhibitors of metalloproteinases.

PREFERRED RESPONSE: 1

DISCUSSION: Etanercept is a fusion protein that combines the ligand-binding domain of the TNF-α receptor to the Fc portion of human immunoglobulin G. Protein serves as a competitive inhibitor of TNF-α signaling. COX-2 is the target of NSAIDs, including newer formulations that are more COX-2–specific. The remaining responses are not direct targets of etanercept.

REFERENCES: Weinblatt ME, Kremer JM, Bankhurst AD, et al: A trial of etanercept, a recombinant tumor necrosis factor receptor: Fc fusion protein, in patients with rheumatoid arthritis receiving methotrexate. *N Engl J Med* 1999;340:253-259.

Recklies AD, Poole AR, Banerjee S, et al: Pathophysiologic aspects of inflammation in diarthrodial joints, in Buckwalter JA, Einhorn TA, Simon SR, eds: *Orthopaedic Basic Science: Biology and Biomechanics of the Musculoskeletal System*, ed 2. Rosemont, IL, American Academy of Orthopaedic Surgeons, 2000, pp 489-530.

A-26: A 21-year-old woman has a nontraumatic rupture of the Achilles tendon. Which of the following commonly prescribed medications has been associated with this condition?

1. Ibuprofen
2. Fluoroquinolones
3. Bisphosphonates
4. Metoprolol
5. Simvistatin

PREFERRED RESPONSE: 2

DISCUSSION: Fluoroquinolones have been associated with increased rates of tendinitis, with special predilection for the Achilles tendon. Tenocytes in the Achilles tendon have exhibited degenerative changes when viewed microscopically after fluoroquinolone administration. Recent clinical studies have shown an increased relative risk of Achilles tendon rupture of 3.7. The other drugs listed have no known increase in tendon rupture rates nor tendinitis.

REFERENCES: van der Linden PD, van de Lei J, Nab HW, et al: Achilles tendinitis associated with fluoroquinolones. *Br J Clin Pharmacol* 1999;48:433-437.

Bernard-Beaubois K, Hecquet C, Hayem G, et al: In vitro study of cytotoxicity of quinolones on rabbit tenocytes. Cell Biol Toxicol 1998;14:283-292.

Maffulli N: Rupture of the Achilles tendon. *J Bone Joint Surg Am* 1999;81:1019-1036.

A-27: Bioabsorbable polymers are used in a wide range of orthopaedic devices, including anchors, staples, pins, plates, and screws. What is the primary drawback for bioabsorbable implants?

1. High cost
2. Increased rates of infection
3. High elastic modulus
4. Brittleness
5. Foreign body reaction

PREFERRED RESPONSE: 5

DISCUSSION: A number of bioabsorbable polymers are used in orthopaedic applications, and all have in common reports of foreign body reactions, which occur in more than 50% of patients in some series. In general, the high cost of these polymers is offset by the elimination of a second surgery to remove the implant. Bioabsorbable polymers are low strength in comparison to metallic alloys but of sufficient strength for many orthopaedic applications. The elastic modulus is not as high as many other orthopaedic biomaterials, making them suitable for applications where lower stiffness is an asset.

REFERENCES: Ambrose CG, Clanton TO: Bioabsorbable implants: Review of clinical experience in orthopedic surgery. *Ann Biomed Eng* 2004;32:171-177.

Bergsma JE, de Bruijn WC, Rozema FR, et al: Late degradation tissue response to poly (L-lactide) bone plates and screws. *Biomaterials* 1995;16:25-31.

A-28: What ligament is the primary restraint to applied valgus loading of the knee?

1. Posteromedial capsule
2. Posterior cruciate ligament (PCL)
3. Superficial medial collateral ligament (MCL)
4. Deep MCL
5. Medial meniscus

PREFERRED RESPONSE: 3

DISCUSSION: The superficial portion of the MCL contributes 57% and 78% of medial stability at 5° and 25° of knee flexion, respectively. The deep MCL and posteromedial capsule act as secondary restraints at full knee extension. The anterior cruciate ligament and PCL also provide secondary resistance to valgus loads.

REFERENCE: Garrett WE, Speer KP, Kirkendall DT, eds: *Principles & Practice of Orthopaedic Sports Medicine.* Philadelphia, PA, Lippincott Williams & Wilkins, 2000, p 767.

A-29: What region of the thoracic curve is most dangerous for pedicle screw insertion while performing a posterior fusion for adolescent idiopathic scoliosis?

1. Concave side at the stable vertebra
2. Concave side at the apex of the curve
3. Convex side at the stable vertebra
4. Convex side at the apex of the curve
5. Thoracolumbar junction

PREFERRED RESPONSE: 2

DISCUSSION: Morphologic and anatomic studies confirm the pedicle is smaller on the concave side of thoracic curves. The dura is also closer to the pedicle on the concave side of the curves.

REFERENCES: Liljenqvist U, Allkemper T, Hackenberg L, et al: Analysis of vertebral morphology in idiopathic scoliosis with use of magnetic resonance imaging and multiplanar reconstruction. *J Bone Joint Surg Am* 2002;84:359-368.

Parent S, Labelle H, Skalli W, et al: Thoracic pedicle morphometry in vertebrae from scoliotic spines. *Spine (Phila Pa 1976)* 2004;29:239-248.

A-30: What mechanism is associated with the spontaneous resorption of herniated nucleus pulposus?

1. Macrophage infiltration and phagocytosis
2. Granuloma formation
3. Antibody-mediated destruction
4. Complement cascade activation
5. Major histocompatibility complex-mediated pathways

PREFERRED RESPONSE: 1

DISCUSSION: Nonsurgical modalities remain the mainstay for treatment of herniated disks. Spontaneous resorption of herniated disks frequently is detected by MRI. Marked infiltration by macrophages and neovascularization are observed on histologic examination of herniated disks, and the resorption is believed to be related to this process. Many cytokines such as vascular endothelial growth factor, tumor necrosis factor-α, and matrix metalloproteinases have been implicated in this process, but none has been found to be singularly responsible.

REFERENCES: Haro H, Kato T, Kamori H, et al: Vascular endothelial growth factor (VEGF)-induced angiogenesis in herniated disc resorption. *J Orthop Res* 2002;20:409-415.

Doita M, Kanatani T, Ozaki T, et al: Influence of macrophage infiltration of herniated disc tissue on the production of matrix metalloproteinases leading to disc resorption. *Spine (Phila Pa 1976)* 2001;26:1522-1527.

A-31: Clinical evidence suggests that grafts for replacing a torn anterior cruciate ligament often stretch after surgery. What is the most probable mechanism for this behavior?

1. Gross failure at the attachment sites
2. Fatigue failure of the ligament tissue
3. Creep of the graft material
4. Water absorption by the graft material
5. Elastic stretch of collagen fibers

PREFERRED RESPONSE: 3

DISCUSSION: The stretching of the graft occurs over time as the graft is loaded. Time-dependent deformation under load is called creep and is common in viscoelastic materials such as ligament tissue. Creep can occur under both static and cyclic load conditions; time-dependent deformation will occur as long as load is applied to the tissue. Similarly, when a graft is initially tensioned to a given deformation at surgery, the load generated in the graft will decrease over time; this behavior is called stress relaxation and also is indicative of a viscoelastic material. Water content may affect the viscoelastic properties by changing the friction between collagen fibers, but studies have shown little difference in water content between grafts and normal ligaments. Fatigue failures may manifest themselves through damage to the ligament tissue, but this would require higher loads than are routinely experienced by grafts. Elastic stretch is recoverable and, therefore, does not contribute to a permanent stretch. Similarly, gross failure at the attachment would not cause a stretch, but rather a catastrophic instantaneous instability.

REFERENCES: Boorman RS, Thornton GM, Shrive NG, et al: Ligament grafts become more susceptible to creep within days after surgery. *Acta Orthop Scand* 2002;73:568-574.

Woo SL-Y, An K-N, Frank CB, et al: Anatomy, biology, and biomechanics of tendon and ligament, in Buckwalter JA, Einhorn TA, Simon SR, eds: *Orthopaedic Basic Science: Biology and Biomechanics of the Musculoskeletal System*, ed 2. Rosemont, IL, American Academy of Orthopaedic Surgeons, 2000, pp 596-609.

Lu L, Kaufman KR, Yaszemski MJ: Biomechanics, in Einhorn TA, O'Keefe RJ, Buckwalter JA, eds: *Orthopaedic Basic Science: Foundations of Clinical Practice*, ed 3. Rosemont, IL, American Academy of Orthopaedic Surgeons, 2006, pp49-64.

A-32: Which of the following clinical disorders is the result of a mutation in fibroblast growth factor recepter 3 (FGFR3)?

1. Cleidocranial dysplasia
2. Schmid metaphyseal chondrodysplasia
3. Achondroplasia
4. Fibrous dysplasia
5. Camptomelic dysplasia

PREFERRED RESPONSE: 3

DISCUSSION: Camptomelic dysplasia is caused by a heterozygous loss of function of the *Sox9* gene. The alternatives have genetic causes, but are not linked to *Sox9*. Cleidocranial dysplasia is related to a defect in *Cbfa-1* (*Osf-2*, *Runx2*). Schmid metaphyseal chondrodysplasia is related to type X collagen. Fibrous dysplasia is related to a defect in the alpha subunit of stimulatory guanine-nucleotide-binding

(continued on next page)

(A-32: *continued*)

protein (Gs). Achondroplasia is related to a defect in fibroblast growth factor receptor 3.

REFERENCES: Wagner T, Wirth J, Meyer J, et al: Autosomal sex reversal and camptomelic dysplasia are caused by mutations in and around the SRY-related gene SOX9. *Cell* 1994;79:1111-1120.

Dietz FR, Murray JC: Update on the genetic basis of disorders with orthopaedic manifestations, in Buckwalter JA, Einhorn TA, Simon SR, eds: *Orthopaedic Basic Science: Biology and Biomechanics of the Musculoskeletal System*, ed 2. Rosemont, IL, American Academy of Orthopaedic Surgeons, 2000, pp 111-131.

Dietz FR, Murray JC: Genetic basis of disorders with orthopaedic manifestations, in Einhorn TA, O'Keefe RJ, Buckwalter JA, eds: *Orthopaedic Basic Science: Foundations of Clinical Practice*, ed 3. Rosemont, IL, American Academy of Orthopaedic Surgeons, 2006, pp 25-47.

A-33: What is the main mechanism for nutrition of the adult disk?

1. Capillary network from the adjacent segmental arteries
2. Capillary network from the arterioles in the vertebral body
3. Diffusion through the anulus fibrosus
4. Diffusion through pores in the end plates
5. Diffusion through nerves in the dorsal root ganglion

PREFERRED RESPONSE: 4

DISCUSSION: Disk nutrition occurs via diffusion through pores in the end plates. The disk has no direct blood supply, and the anulus fibrosus is not porous to allow diffusion. The dorsal root ganglion does not provide blood supply to the disk.

REFERENCES: Biyani A, Andersson GB: Low back pain: Pathophysiology and management. *J Am Acad Orthop Surg* 2004;12:106-115.

Urban JG, Holm S, Maroudas A, et al: Nutrition of the intervertebral disc: Effect of fluid flow on solute transport. *Clin Orthop* 1982;170:296-302.

Park AE, Boden SD: Form and function of the intervertebral disk, in Einhorn TA, O'Keefe RJ, Buckwalter JA, eds: *Orthopaedic Basic Science: Foundations of Clinical Practice*, ed 3. Rosemont, IL, American Academy of Orthopaedic Surgeons, 2006, pp 259-264.

A-34: A knockout mouse for the vitamin D receptor has which of the following phenotypes?

1. Osteopetrosis
2. Renal failure
3. Rickets
4. Jansen-type metaphyseal dysplasia
5. Compensatory hyperparathyroidism and no skeletal phenotype

PREFERRED RESPONSE: 3

DISCUSSION: A knockout mouse to the vitamin D receptor would cause loss of vitamin D function, resulting in rickets. Renal failure would not occur; although vitamin D is converted from 25 (OH) D to

(continued on next page)

(A-34: *continued*)

1,25 (OH) D in the kidney, the active hormone acts on the gut and bone. Osteopetrosis can be seen as the phenotype for the c-fos knockout mouse; the Jansen-type metaphyseal dysplasia phenotype results from overactivation of the parathyroid hormone (PTH)/receptor protein receptor. Although compensatory hyperparathyroidism would occur, excessive PTH would not be able to rescue the skeletal loss and instead phosphaturia and phosphatasia would result.

REFERENCES: Glowacki J, Hurwitz S, Thornhill TS, et al: Osteoporosis and vitamin-D deficiency among postmenopausal women with osteoarthritis undergoing total hip arthroplasty. *J Bone Joint Surg Am* 2003;85:2371-2377.

Rosier RN, Reynolds PR, O'Keefe RJ: Molecular and cell biology in orthopaedics, in Buckwalter JA, Einhorn TA, Simon SR, eds: *Orthopaedic Basic Science: Biology and Biomechanics of the Musculoskeletal System*, ed 2. Rosemont, IL, American Academy of Orthopaedic Surgeons, 2000, p 51.

A-35: Intramembranous ossification during fracture repair is characterized by absence of which of the following elements?

1. Alkaline phosphatase
2. Osteonectin
3. Osteopontin
4. Collagen type I expression
5. Collagen type II expression

PREFERRED RESPONSE: 5

DISCUSSION: Intramembranous ossification occurs through the direct formation of bone without the formation of a cartilaginous intermediate. Clinically, both intramembranous and endochondral ossification occur simultaneously during fracture healing; however, the latter is characterized by the differentiation and maturation of chondrocytes, vascular invasion of a hypertrophic cartilage matrix, and bone formation. Collagens type II and X are cartilage specific and would be characteristic of endochondral ossification, not intramembranous ossification.

REFERENCES: Li J, Sandell LJ: Transcriptional regulation of cartilage-specific genes, in Rosier RN, Evans C, eds: *Molecular Biology in Orthoapedics*, Rosemont, IL, American Academy of Orthopaedic Surgeons, 2002, pp 21-24.

Buckwalter JA, Einhorn TA, Bolander ME: Healing of the musculoskeletal tissues, in Rockwood CA Jr, Green DP, Bucholz RW, et al, eds: *Rockwood and Green's Fractures in Adults*, ed 4. Philadelphia, PA, Lippincott-Raven, 1996, pp 261-276.

A-36: Patients with rheumatoid arthritis may exhibit an increase in viral load for which of the following viruses?

1. HIV
2. Papilloma virus
3. Epstein-Barr virus (EBV)
4. Hepatitis C virus (HCV)
5. Hepatitis B virus (HBV)

PREFERRED RESPONSE: 3

DISCUSSION: Rheumatoid arthritis (RA) is a complex multisystem disorder. It has been suggested that patients with RA have an impaired capacity to control infection with EBV. EBV has oncogenic potential and is implicated in the development of some lymphomas. Recent publications provide evidence for an altered EBV-host balance in patients with RA who have a relatively high EBV load. Large epidemiologic studies confirm that lymphoma is more likely to develop in patients with RA than in the general population. The overall risk of development of lymphoma has not risen with the increased use of methotrexate or biologic agents. Histologic analysis reveals that most lymphomas in patients with RA are diffuse large B cell lymphomas, a form of non-Hodgkin lymphoma. EBV is detected in a proportion of these. Patients with RA do not have prevalence for infection with any of the other mentioned viruses.

REFERENCES: Callan MF: Epstein-Barr virus, arthritis, and the development of lymphoma in arthritis patients. *Curr Opin Rheumatol* 2004;16:399-405.

Baecklund E, Sundstrom C, Ekbom A, et al: Lymphoma subtypes in patients with rheumatoid arthritis: Increased proportion of diffuse large B cell lymphoma. *Arthritis Rheum* 2003;48:1543-1550.

A-37: Osteopenia is defined by the World Health Organization (WHO) as a bone mineral density (BMD) that is

1. within 1 standard deviation of age-matched normals.
2. within 1 and 2.5 standard deviations below age-matched normals.
3. within 1 standard deviation of young normals.
4. within 1 and 2.5 standard deviations below young normals.
5. more than 2.5 standard deviations below age-matched normals.

PREFERRED RESPONSE: 4

DISCUSSION: Osteopenia, decreased bone mass without fracture risk as defined by the WHO criteria for diagnosis of osteoporosis, is when a woman's T-score is within -1 to -2.5 SD. The T-score represents a comparison to young normals or optimum peak density. The Z-score represents a comparison of BMD to age-matched normals. Measurements of bone mineral density (BMD) at various skeletal sites help in predicting fracture risk. Hip BMD best predicts fracture of the hip, as well as fractures at other sites.

REFERENCE: Kanis JA, Johnell O, Oden A, et al: Risk of hip fracture according to the World Health Organization criteria for osteopenia and osteoporosis. *Bone* 2000;27:585-590.

A-38: Which of the following best describes the mechanism of action of gentamycin?

1. Inhibits cell wall synthesis by inhibiting peptidyl traspeptidase
2. Increases cell membrane permeability
3. Binds to the 30S ribosome subunit interfering with protein synthesis
4. Inhibits DNA gyrase
5. Forms oxygen radicals leading to loss of helical structure and breakage of DNA strands

PREFERRED RESPONSE: 3

DISCUSSION: Gentamycin and the aminoglycosides (streptomycin, tobramycin, amikacin, and neomycin) work by binding to the 30S ribosome subunit, leading to the misreading of mRNA. This misreading results in the synthesis of abnormal peptides that accumulate intracellularly and eventually lead to cell death. These antibiotics are bactericidal. Cephalosporins, vancomycin, and penicillins interfere with cell wall synthesis by inhibiting the transpeptidase enzyme. Polymyxin, nystatin, and amphotericin increase cell membrane permeability by disrupting the functional integrity of the cell membrane. The quinolones inhibit the enzyme, DNA gyrase. Metronidazole forms oxygen radicals that are toxic to anaerobic organisms because they lack the protective enzymes, superoxide dismutase and catalase.

REFERENCE: Morris CA, Einhorn TA: Principles of orthopaedic pharmacology, in Buckwalter JA, Einhorn TA, Simon SR, eds: *Orthopaedic Basic Science: Biology and Biomechanics of the Musculoskeletal System*, ed 2. Rosemont, IL, American Academy of Orthopaedic Surgeons, 2000, pp 217-236.

A-39: What type of muscle contraction occurs while the muscle is lengthening?

1. Isometric
2. Isotonic
3. Concentric
4. Isokinetic
5. Eccentric

PREFERRED RESPONSE: 5

DISCUSSION: A muscle that lengthens as it is activated is an eccentric contraction. Isometric contraction involves no change in length. Concentric contraction occurs while the muscle is shortening. In isotonic contraction, the force remains constant through the contraction range. Isokinetic muscle contraction occurs at a constant rate of angular change of the involved joint.

REFERENCES: Garrett WE, Speer KP, Kirkendall DT, eds: *Principles & Practice of Orthopaedic Sports Medicine*. Philadelphia, PA, Lippincott Williams & Wilkins, 2000, pp 12-13.

Lieber RL: Form and function of skeletal muscle, in Einhorn TA, O'Keefe RJ, Buckwalter JA, eds: *Orthopaedic Basic Science: Foundations of Clinical Practice*, ed 3. Rosemont, IL, American Academy of Orthopaedic Surgeons, 2006, pp 223-243.

A-40: Osteoclasts originate from which of the following cell types?

1. Fibroblasts
2. Monocytes
3. Megakaryocytes
4. Plasma cells
5. Osteoprogenitor cells

PREFERRED RESPONSE: 2

DISCUSSION: Osteoclasts originate from the monocyte/macrophage lineage. Fibroblasts and osteoprogenitor cells originate from mesenchymal stem cells and do not form osteoclasts. Plasma cells reside in the bone marrow and are derivatives of the hematopoietic system. Megakaryocytes are also in the bone marrow and synthesize platelets.

REFERENCES: Zaidi M, Blair HC, Moonga BS, et al: Osteoclastogenesis, bone resorption, and osteoclast-based therapeutics. *J Bone Miner Res* 2003;18:599-609.

Brinker MR: Bone (Section 1), in Miller M, ed: *Review of Orthopaedics*, ed 2. Philadelphia, PA, WB Saunders, 1996, pp 1-35.

Zuscik MJ, Drissi MH, Reynolds PR, et al: Molecular and cell biology in orthopaedics, in Einhorn TA, O'Keefe RJ, Buckwalter JA, eds: *Orthopaedic Basic Science: Foundations of Clinical Practice*, ed 3. Rosemont, IL, American Academy of Orthopaedic Surgeons, 2006, pp 3-23.

A-41: A study is being designed to compare the effectiveness of an antibiotic. The choice of the number of patients (the sample size) depends on several factors. What type of calculation assesses the potential of the study to successfully address the effectiveness of the antibiotic?

1. Regression analysis
2. Power analysis
3. Correlation analysis
4. Nonparametric analysis
5. Analysis of variance

PREFERRED RESPONSE: 2

DISCUSSION: Power analysis is used to determine the minimum number of specimens (sample size) such that, if a difference is found that is large enough to be clinically important, the associated level of statistical reliability will be high enough (ie, the P-value will be small enough) for the investigators to conclude that the difference observed in the study also holds in general. For the statistician to do a power analysis, the investigators must first decide on the minimum difference that they consider to be clinically important, for example, a reduction of 3% in the rate of infection. It is important to recognize that the choice of what constitutes the minimum difference in the rate of infection that is clinically (medically) important cannot and should not be done by the statistician. Rather, this is a clinical-medical issue and must be done by the physician researcher based on a comprehensive assessment of the medical risks and benefits. The power analysis also requires an estimate of the variance in the data, which may be based on previous similar studies, if available. A statistician can then calculate the minimum sample size (number of patients) required such that, if a clinically important difference does, in fact, exist between

(continued on next page)

(A-42: *continued*)

the full populations, there is a reasonable probability or power (typically 80% to 90%) that a difference this large also will occur between the sample populations at the desired level of statistical significance (usually, but not necessarily, $P < 0.05$). The other answers refer to types of analyses that are usually conducted after the data are collected.

REFERENCE: Ebramzadeh E, McKellop H, Dorey F, et al: Challenging the validity of conclusions based on P-values alone: A critique of contemporary clinical research design and methods. *Instr Course Lect* 1994;43:587-600.

A-42: What is the most common cause of mechanical failure of an orthopaedic biomaterial during clinical use?

1. Fatigue
2. Tension
3. Compression
4. Shear
5. Torsion

PREFERRED RESPONSE: 1

DISCUSSION: In most orthopaedic applications, the materials are strong enough to withstand a single cycle of loading in vivo. However, these loads may be large enough to initiate a small crack in the implant that can grow slowly over thousands or millions of cycles, eventually leading to gross failure. Such fatigue failure has occurred with virtually every type of implant, including stainless steel fracture plates and screws, bone cement in joint arthroplasty, and polyethylene inserts in total knee arthroplasty.

REFERENCES: Lewis G: Fatigue testing and performance of acrylic bone-cement materials: State-of-the-art review. *J Biomed Mater Res Br* 2003;66:457-486.

Stolk J, Verdonschot N, Huiskes R: Stair climbing is more detrimental to the cement in hip replacement than walking. *Clin Orthop* 2002;405:294-305.

Wright TM, Maher SA: Biomaterials, in Einhorn TA, O'Keefe RJ, Buckwalter JA, eds: *Orthopaedic Basic Science: Foundations of Clinical Practice*, ed 3. Rosemont, IL, American Academy of Orthopaedic Surgeons, 2006, pp 65-85.

A-43: Which of the following body positions is associated with the highest intradiskal pressure?

1. Standing, bending forward
2. Standing, bending back
3. Sitting, bending forward
4. Sitting, bending back
5. Supine, lateral decubitus

(continued on next page)

(A-43: *continued*)

PREFERRED RESPONSE: 3

DISCUSSION: Intradiskal pressure is lowest when the patient is in the supine position. Sitting is associated with higher intradiskal pressures than standing. Flexion also increases intradiskal pressure. The combination of flexion and sitting produces the highest intradiskal pressure. Nachemson and Morris found that intradiskal pressure increases as position changes from lying supine, lying prone, standing, leaning forward, sitting, and sitting leaning forward. Twisting or straining in positions of relatively high intradiskal pressure may predispose patients to herniation of the intervertebral disk. Patients with a herniated disk may also notice their pain worsens with activities that increase the disk pressure, including the positions mentioned, or activities that increase intra-abdominal pressure (coughing, sneezing, straining).

REFERENCES: Nachemson A, Morris JM: In vivo measurements of intradiscal pressure. *J Bone Joint Surg Am* 1964;46:1077-1092.

Buckwalter JA, Mow VC, Boden SD, Eyre DR, Weidenbaum M: Intervertebral disk structure, composition, and mechanical function, in Buckwalter JA, Einhorn TA, Simon SR, eds: *Orthopaedic Basic Science: Biology and Biomechanics of the Musculoskeletal System*, ed 2. Rosemont, IL, American Academy of Orthopaedic Surgeons, 2000, pp 547-556.

A-44: Stiffness relates the amount of load applied to a structure like a long bone or an intramedullary nail to the amount of resulting deformation that occurs in the structure. What is the most important material property affecting the axial and bending stiffness of a structure?

1. Elastic modulus
2. Ductility
3. Ultimate stress
4. Yield stress
5. Toughness

PREFERRED RESPONSE: 1

DISCUSSION: The amount of deformation resulting in response to an applied load depends on the stress distribution that the load creates in the structure and the stress versus strain behavior of the material that makes up the structure. Axial and bending loads create stress distributions that involve normal stresses and normal strains. Although all five responses are indeed material properties, only one, elastic modulus, relates normal stresses to normal strains. In fact, axial and bending stiffness are directly proportional to modulus, so that a nail made from stainless steel will have nearly twice the stiffness of a nail made from titanium alloy (because their respective elastic moduli differ by about a factor of two).

REFERENCES: Hayes WC, Bouxsein ML: Analysis of muscle and joint loads, in Mow VC, Hayes WC, eds: *Basic Orthopaedic Biomechanics*, ed 2. New York, NY, Lippincott-Raven, 1997, pp 74-82.

Mow VC, Flatow EL, Ateshian GR: Biomechanics, in Buckwalter JA, Einhorn TA, Simon SR, eds: *Orthopaedic Basic Science: Biology and Biomechanics of the Musculoskeletal System*, ed 2. Rosemont, IL, American Academy of Orthopaedic Surgeons, 2000, pp 159-165.

Wright TM, Maher SA: Biomaterials, in Einhorn TA, O'Keefe RJ, Buckwalter JA, eds: *Orthopaedic Basic Science: Foundations of Clinical Practice*, ed 3. Rosemont, IL, American Academy of Orthopaedic Surgeons, 2006, pp 65-85.

A-45: Osteoclasts are primarily responsible for bone resorption of malignancy. Which of the following stimulates osteoclast formation?

1. RANKL gene (NF-kB ligand)
2. Osteoprotegerin (OPG)
3. Interleukin-5 (IL-5)
4. Matrix metalloproteinase-2 (MMP-2)
5. Collagen type I

PREFERRED RESPONSE: 1

DISCUSSION: Bone destruction is primarily mediated by osteoclastic bone resorption, and cancer cells stimulate the formation and activation of osteoclasts next to metastatic foci. Increasing evidence suggests that RANKL is the ultimate extracellular mediator that stimulates osteoclast differentiation into mature osteoclasts. In contrast, OPG inhibits osteoclast development. IL-8 but not IL-5 is known to play a role in osteoclastogenesis. MMP-2 and collagen type I do not have a direct role in osteoclastogenesis.

REFERENCES: Kitazawa S, Kitazawa R: RANK ligand is a prerequisite for cancer-associated osteolytic lesions. *J Pathol* 2002;198:228-236.

Einhorn TA: Metabolic bone disease, in Einhorn TA, O'Keefe RJ, Buckwalter JA, eds: *Orthopaedic Basic Science: Foundations of Clinical Practice*, ed 3. Rosemont, IL, American Academy of Orthopaedic Surgeons, 2006, pp 415-426.

A-46: Collagen orientation is parallel to the joint surface in what articular cartilage zone?

1. Diagonal
2. Middle
3. Deep
4. Superficial
5. Calcified

PREFERRED RESPONSE: 4

DISCUSSION: The collagen orientation changes from parallel in the superficial zone to a more random pattern in the middle zone and finally to perpendicular in the calcified zone.

REFERENCES: Bush-Joseph C, Carter TR, Miller MD, Rokito AS, Stuart MJ: Knee and leg: Soft-tissue trauma, in Koval KJ, ed: *Orthopaedic Knowledge Update*, ed 7. Rosemont, IL, American Academy of Orthopaedic Surgeons, 2002, pp 498-499.

Mankin HJ, Grodzinsky AJ, Buckwalter JA: Articular cartilage and osteoarthritis, in Einhorn TA, O'Keefe RJ, Buckwalter JA, eds: *Orthopaedic Basic Science: Foundations of Clinical Practice*, ed 3. Rosemont, IL, American Academy of Orthopaedic Surgeons, 2006, pp 161-174.

A-47: Which of the following agents increases the risk for a nonunion following a posterior spinal fusion?

1. Ibuprofen
2. Intranasal calcitonin
3. Simvastatin
4. Gentamycin
5. Tamoxifen

PREFERRED RESPONSE: 1

DISCUSSION: NSAIDs have been shown to increase the risk of pseudarthrosis. In a controlled rabbit study, nonunions were reported with the use of toradol and indomethacin. NSAIDs are commonly used medications with the potential to diminish osteogenesis. Studies clearly have demonstrated inhibition of spinal fusion following the postoperative administration of several NSAIDs, including ibuprofen. Cigarette smoking is another potent inhibitor of spinal fusion.

REFERENCES: Glassman SD, Rose SM, Dimar JR, et al: The effect of postoperative nonsteroidal anti-inflammatory drug administration on spinal fusion. *Spine (Phila Pa 1976)*1998;23:834-838.

Martin GJ Jr, Boden SD, Titus L: Recombinant human bone morphogenetic protein-2 overcomes the inhibitory effect of ketorolac, a nonsteroidal anti-inflammatory drug (NSAID), on posterolateral lumbar intertransverse process spine fusion. *Spine (Phila Pa 1976)*1999;24:2188-2193.

A-48: A study was conducted in 500 patients to measure the effectiveness of a new growth factor in reducing healing time of distal radial fractures. The authors reported that average healing time was reduced from 9.2 to 8.9 weeks ($P < 0.0001$). Because the difference was highly statistically significant, they recommended routine clinical use of this drug despite its high cost. A more appropriate interpretation of these results is that they are

1. clinically significant.
2. statistically significant but perhaps not clinically significant.
3. statistically and clinically significant.
4. not statistically or clinically significant.
5. nonconclusive.

PREFERRED RESPONSE: 2

DISCUSSION: The results are statistically significant (at the arbitrary level of $P < 0.05$). That is, they indicate a probability of only 1/10,000 that the observation that the drug is effective in reducing healing time by 0.3 weeks occurred by chance selection of the study subjects. However, because the statistical power of a study increases with the number of subjects included (sample size), a difference that is trivial clinically can occur with a very high level of statistical significance (a very small P-value) if enough patients are included in the study. Because of this, the P-value alone, no matter how small, does not establish clinical significance or importance. Rather, the clinical significance of the observed difference must be assessed taking into consideration the medical importance of the difference if it is, in fact, true in the general population. In this example, the reduction in healing time of only a few days is probably clinically unimportant, particularly if the use of the new growth factor is expensive, complex, and/or has substantial side effects.

(continued on next page)

(A-48: *continued*)

REFERENCE: Ebramzadeh E, McKellop H, Dorey F, et al: Challenging the validity of conclusions based on P-values alone: A critique of contemporary clinical research design and methods. *Instr Course Lect* 1994;43:587-600.

A-49: What type of multiple lesions is associated with Maffucci syndrome?

1. Nonossifying fibromas
2. Enchondromas
3. Langerhans cell histiocytosis
4. Osteochondromas
5. Giant cell tumors

PREFERRED RESPONSE: 2

DISCUSSION: Maffucci syndrome is a form of enchondromatosis associated with subcutaneous and deep hemangiomas. Similar to Ollier disease, the risk of malignant transformation of the enchondromas is much higher than that of a solitary enchondroma. Multifocal nonossifying fibromas associated with other clinical findings such as mental retardation and café-au-lait spots is known as Jaffe-Campanacci syndrome. There are two types of multifocal forms of histiocytosis: Letterer-Siwe and Hand-Schüller-Christian disease.

REFERENCES: Schwartz HS, Zimmerman NB, Simon MA, et al: The malignant potential of enchondromatosis. *J Bone Joint Surg Am* 1987;69:269-274.

Frassica F: Orthopaedic pathology, in Miller M, ed: *Review of Orthopaedics*, ed 2. Philadelphia, PA, WB Saunders, 1996, pp 292-335.

Yuan J, Fuchs B, Scully SP: Molecular basis of cancer, in Einhorn TA, O'Keefe RJ, Buckwalter JA, eds: Orthopaedic Basic Science: Foundations of Clinical Practice, ed 3. Rosemont, IL, American Academy of Orthopaedic Surgeons, 2006, pp 379-393.

A-50: Joint contact pressure in normal or artificial joints can best be minimized by what mechanism?

1. Increasing joint force and contact area
2. Increasing joint force and decreasing contact area
3. Decreasing joint force and contact area
4. Decreasing joint force and increasing contact area
5. Decreasing joint force only

PREFERRED RESPONSE: 4

DISCUSSION: Joint contact pressure is a stress and as such is defined as the load transferred across the joint divided by the contact area between the joint surfaces (the area over which the joint load is distributed). Therefore, any mechanism that decreases the load across the joint (for example, a walking aid) will decrease the stress. Similarly, any mechanism that increases the area over which the load is distributed (for example, using a more conforming set of articular surfaces in a knee joint arthroplasty)

(continued on next page)

(A-50: *continued*)

will also decrease the stress. Other mechanisms that influence joint contact pressure include the elastic modulus of the materials (cartilage in the case of natural joints and polyethylene in joint arthroplasty) and the thickness of the structures through which the joint loads pass.

REFERENCES: Bartel DL, Bicknell VL, Wright TM: The effect of conformity, thickness, and material on stresses in UHMWPE components for total joint replacement. *J Bone Joint Surg Am* 1986;68:1041-1051.

Wright TM: Biomechanics of total knee design, in Pellicci PM, Tria AJ Jr, Garvin KL, eds: *Orthopaedic Knowledge Update: Hip and Knee Reconstruction*, ed 2. Rosemont, IL, American Academy of Orthopaedic Surgeons, 2000, pp 265-274.

Trauma

Q-1: In patients with displaced radial neck fractures treated with open reduction and internal fixation with a plate and screws, the plate must be limited to what surface of the radius to avoid impingement on the proximal ulna?

1. 2 cm distal to the articular surface of the radial head
2. 1 cm distal to the articular surface of the radial head
3. Within a 90° arc or safe zone
4. Within a 120° arc or safe zone
5. Within a 180° arc or safe zone

Q-2: When harvesting an iliac crest bone graft from the posterior approach, what anatomic structure is at greatest risk for injury if a Cobb elevator is directed too caudal?

1. Sciatic nerve
2. Cluneal nerves
3. Inferior gluteal artery
4. Superior gluteal artery
5. Sacroiliac joint

Q-3: A 36-year-old woman sustained a tarsometatarsal joint fracture-dislocation in a motor vehicle accident. The patient is treated with open reduction and internal fixation. What is the most common complication?

1. Posttraumatic arthritis
2. Infection
3. Fixation failure
4. Malunion
5. Nonunion

Q-4: What is the most appropriate indication for replantation in an otherwise healthy 35-year-old man?

1. Isolated transverse amputation of the thumb through the middle of the nail bed
2. Isolated transverse amputation of the index finger through the proximal phalanx
3. Isolated transverse amputation of the ring finger through the proximal phalanx
4. Isolated transverse amputation of the hand at the level of the wrist
5. Forearm amputation with a 10-hour warm ischemia time

Q-5: A 46-year-old man fell 20 feet and sustained the injury shown in Figure 1. The injury is closed; however, the soft tissues are swollen and ecchymotic with blisters. The most appropriate initial management should consist of

1. a long leg cast.
2. a short leg cast.
3. immediate open reduction and internal fixation.
4. a temporizing spanning external fixator.
5. primary ankle fusion.

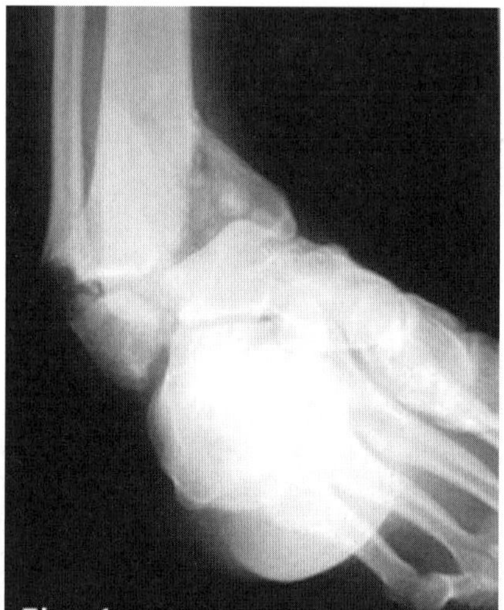
Fig. 1

Q-6: A collegiate golfer sustained a hook of the hamate fracture. After 12 weeks of splinting and therapy, the hand is still symptomatic. What is the most appropriate management to allow return to competitive activity?

1. Continued observation
2. Open reduction and internal fixation of the fracture
3. Excision of the hook of the hamate
4. Carpal tunnel release
5. Guyon canal release

Q-7: A 20-year-old man sustained a closed tibial fracture and is treated with a reamed intramedullary nail. What is the most common complication associated with this treatment?

1. Nonunion
2. Malunion
3. Infection
4. Knee pain
5. Compartment syndrome

Q-8: What is the most likely complication following treatment of the humeral shaft fracture shown in Figure 2?

1. Nonunion
2. Shoulder pain
3. Infection
4. Elbow injury
5. Radial nerve injury

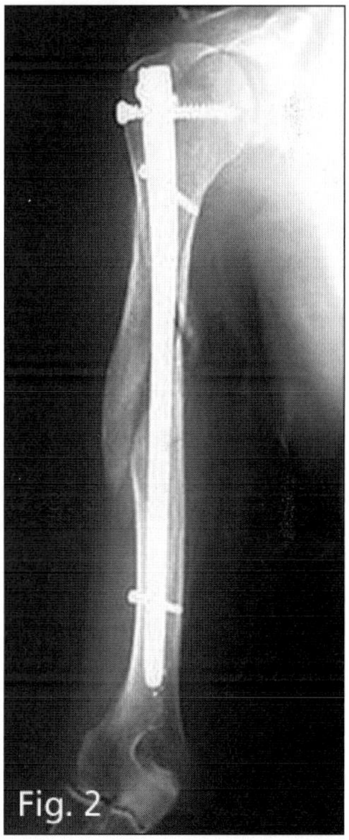

Fig. 2

Q-9: A 16-year-old girl sustained the injury shown in Figure 3A. CT scans are shown in Figures 3B through 3D. The results of treatment of this injury have been shown to correlate most with which of the following factors?

1. Surgical approach
2. Location of the transverse fracture
3. Timing of surgery
4. Accuracy of reduction
5. Use of skeletal traction

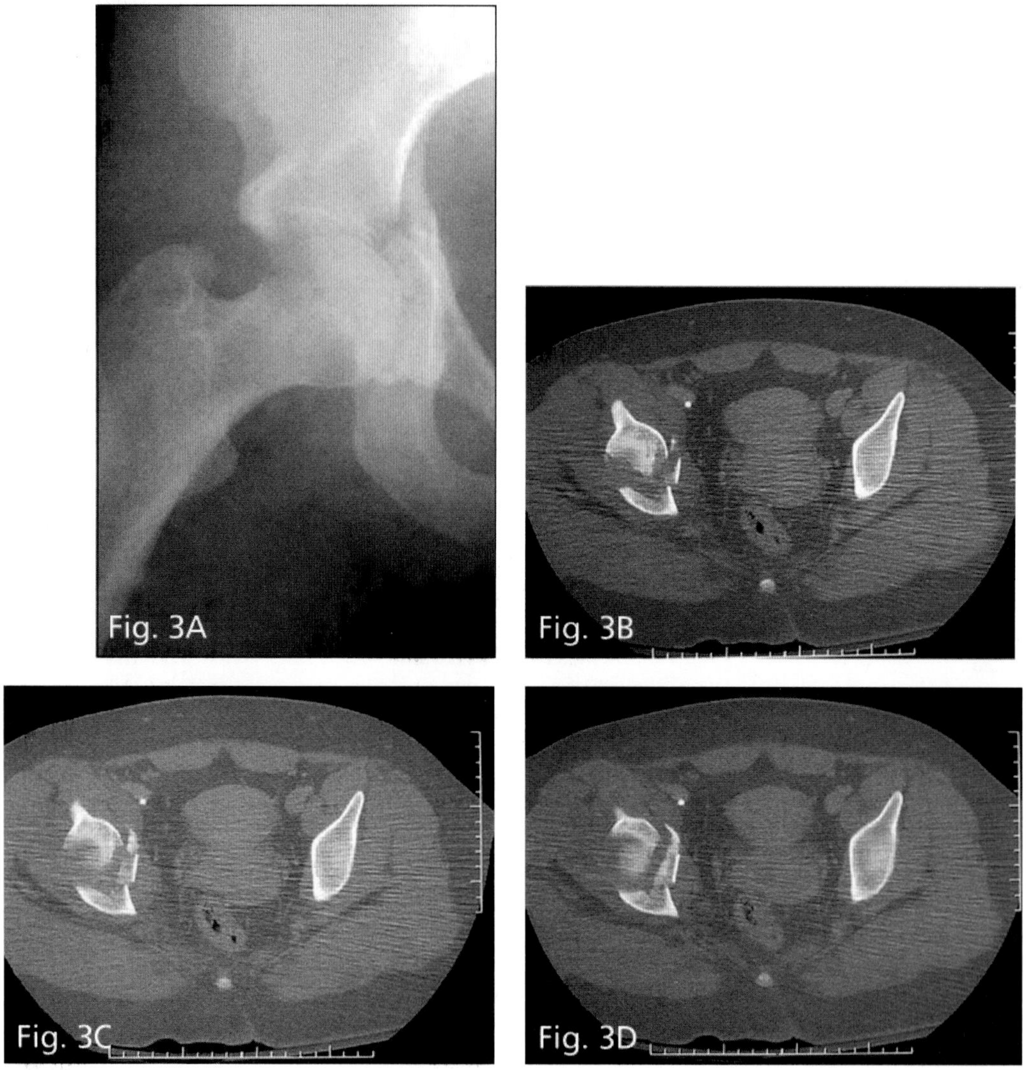

Q-10: An active 49-year-old woman who sustained a diaphyseal fracture of the clavicle 8 months ago now reports persistent shoulder pain with daily activities. An AP radiograph is shown in Figure 4. Management should consist of

1. external electrical stimulation.
2. external ultrasound stimulation.
3. implanted electrical stimulation.
4. closed reduction and percutaneous fixation.
5. open reduction and internal fixation with bone graft.

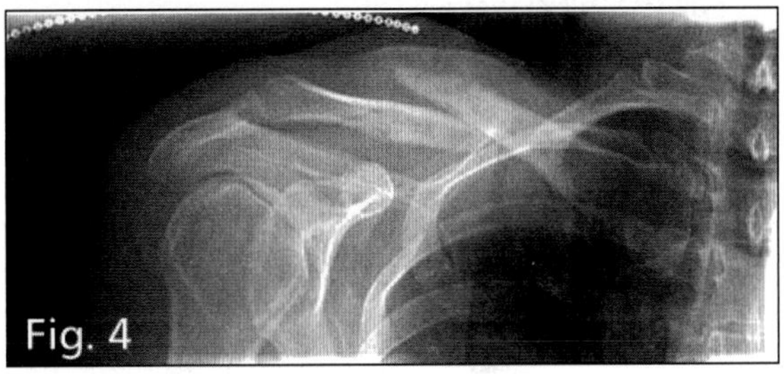
Fig. 4

Q-11: Examination of a 25-year-old man who was injured in a motor vehicle accident reveals a fracture-dislocation of C5-6 with a Frankel B spinal cord injury. He also has a closed right femoral shaft fracture and a grade II open ipsilateral midshaft tibial fracture. Assessment of his vital signs reveals a pulse rate of 45/min, blood pressure of 80/45 mm Hg, and respirations of 25/min. A general surgeon has assessed the abdomen, and peritoneal lavage results are negative. His clinical presentation is most consistent with what type of shock?

1. Neurogenic
2. Hemorrhagic
3. Spinal
4. Septic
5. Hypovolemic

Q-12: A 32-year-old woman sustained an injury to her left upper extremity in a motor vehicle accident. Examination reveals a 2-cm wound in the midportion of the dorsal surface of the upper arm and deformities at the elbow and forearm; there are no other injuries. Her vital signs are stable, and she has a base deficit of -1 and a lactate level of less than 2. Radiographs are shown in Figures 5A and 5B. In addition to urgent débridement of the humeral shaft fracture, management should include

1. closed management of the medial condyle and humeral shaft fractures and open reduction and internal fixation of the both-bones forearm fracture.
2. closed management of the humeral shaft fracture and open reduction and internal fixation of the medial condyle and the both-bones forearm fractures.
3. open reduction and internal fixation of the humeral shaft, medial condyle, and the both-bones forearm fractures.
4. open reduction and internal fixation of the medial condyle and both-bones forearm fractures, and external fixation of the humeral shaft fracture.
5. delayed stabilization of all fractures after the open wound has healed.

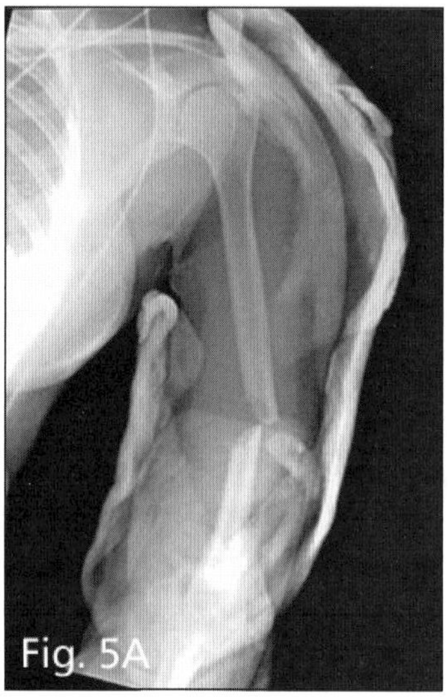
Fig. 5A

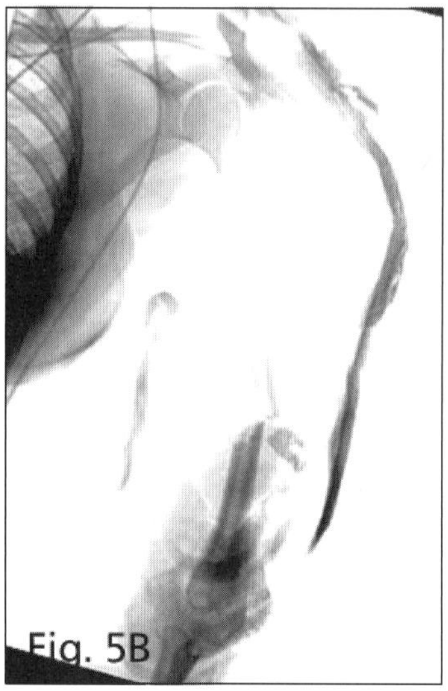
Fig. 5B

Q-13: A patient sustained the injuries shown in the radiographs and clinical photograph seen in Figures 6A through 6C. The neurovascular examination is normal. The first step in emergent management of the extremity injuries should consist of

1. application of a femoral traction pin.
2. intramedullary nailing of the femur and tibia.
3. surgical irrigation and débridement.
4. external fixation of the femoral fracture.
5. reduction of the femoral head.

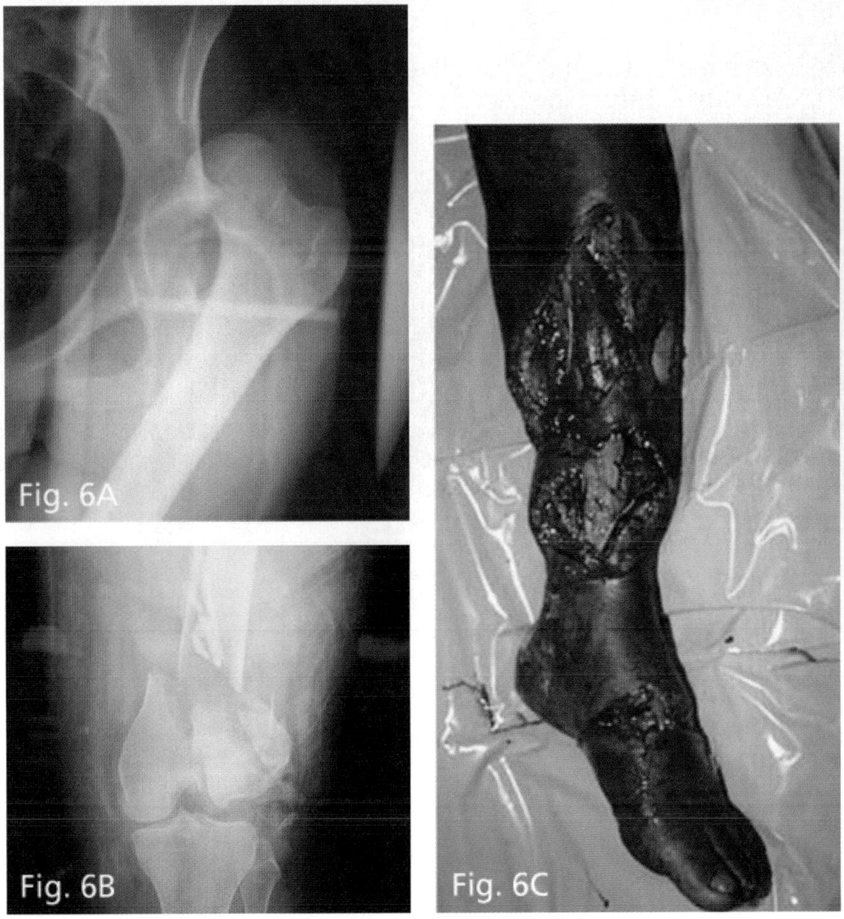

Fig. 6A

Fig. 6B

Fig. 6C

Q-14: A 25-year-old patient sustains the injury shown in Figures 7A through 7C after falling off a curb. Initial management should consist of

1. weight bearing as tolerated in a hard-soled shoe.
2. weight bearing as tolerated in an ankle lacer.
3. weight bearing as tolerated in a short leg cast.
4. no weight bearing in a hard-soled shoe.
5. no weight bearing in a short leg cast.

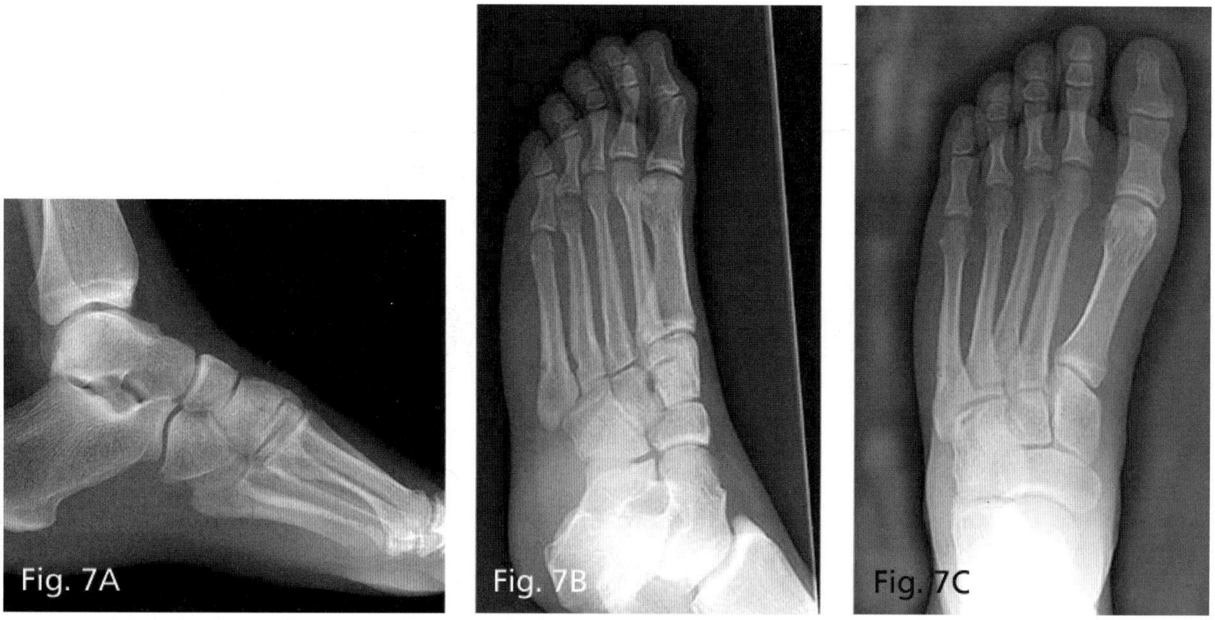

Q-15: What structure is most often injured in a volar proximal interphalangeal joint dislocation?

1. Sagittal bands
2. Central slip
3. Lumbrical
4. Juncturae tendinum
5. Terminal extensor tendon

Q-16: What patient factor is predictive of better outcomes for surgical management of a displaced calcaneal fracture compared to nonsurgical management?

1. Young man injured at the work site
2. Young woman injured during recreational activities
3. Heavy smoker
4. Patient older than 50 years
5. Patient with bilateral fractures

Q-17: Figures 8A and 8B show the initial radiographs of an 18-year-old man who fell while snowboarding. Figures 8C and 8D show the radiographs obtained following closed reduction. Examination reveals that the elbow is stable with range of motion. Management should now consist of

1. immediate return to unrestricted activity.
2. a posterior long arm splint for 7 to 10 days, followed by elbow range-of-motion exercises.
3. a long arm cast for 4 weeks.
4. immediate surgical repair of the collateral ligaments.
5. immediate surgical repair of the collateral ligaments and placement of a hinged external fixator.

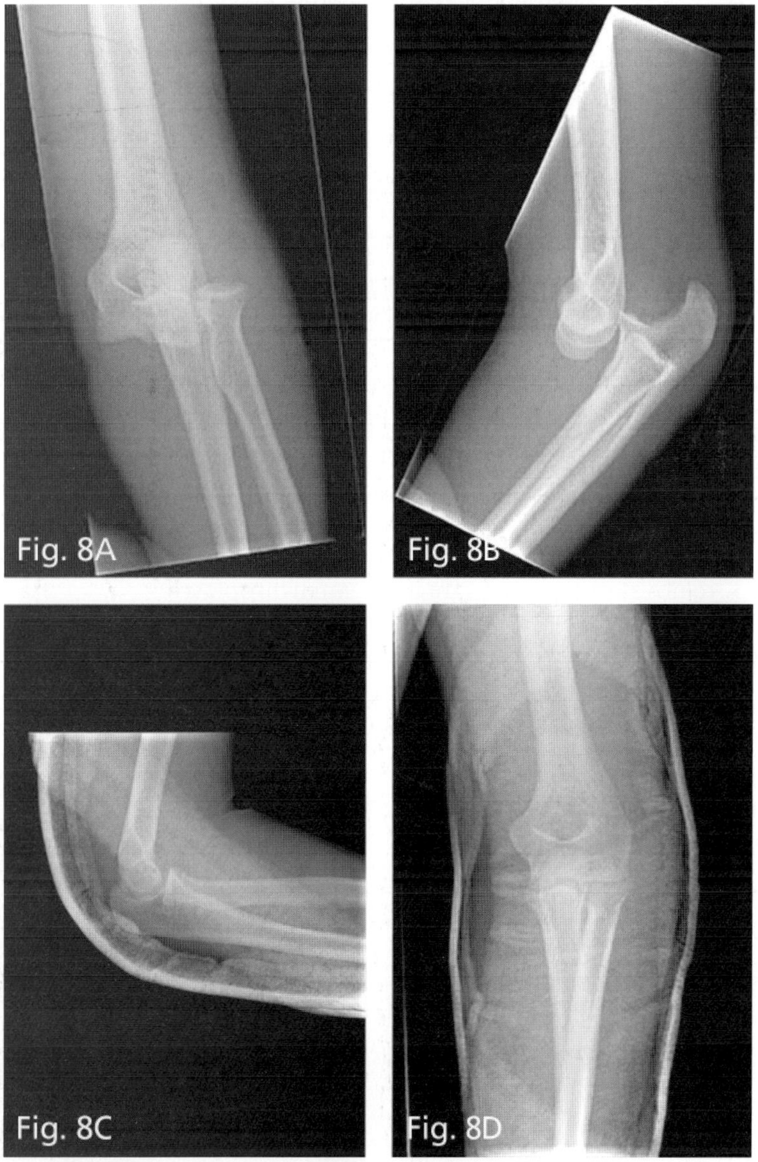

Fig. 8A Fig. 8B Fig. 8C Fig. 8D

Q-18: Which of the following is an advantage of unreamed nailing of the tibia compared to reamed nailing?

1. Less surgical time
2. Lower risk of nonunion
3. Lower rate of malunion
4. Faster time to union
5. Less secondary procedures to achieve union

Q-19: An otherwise healthy 35-year-old woman reports dorsal wrist pain and has trouble extending her thumb after sustaining a minimally displaced fracture of the distal radius 3 months ago. What is the most appropriate next step in management?

1. Neurophysiologic test to evaluate the posterior interosseous nerve
2. Transfer of the extensor indicis proprius to the extensor pollicis longus tendon
3. Interphalangeal joint arthrodesis of the thumb
4. Extension splinting of the thumb
5. Fine-cut CT of the distal radius to evaluate Lister tubercle

Q-20: Figure 9A is a radiograph from a 34-year-old woman who sustained a basicervical fracture of the femoral neck. The fracture was treated with a compression screw and side plate. Seven months post-operatively, she continues to have significant hip pain and cannot bear full weight on her hip. A recent radiograph is shown in Figure 9B. Management should now consist of

1. continued non-weight-bearing and a bone stimulator.
2. removal of the hardware, bone grafting of the femoral neck, and refixation.
3. removal of the hardware and hemiarthroplasty.
4. removal of the hardware and total hip arthroplasty.
5. removal of the hardware and a valgus osteotomy.

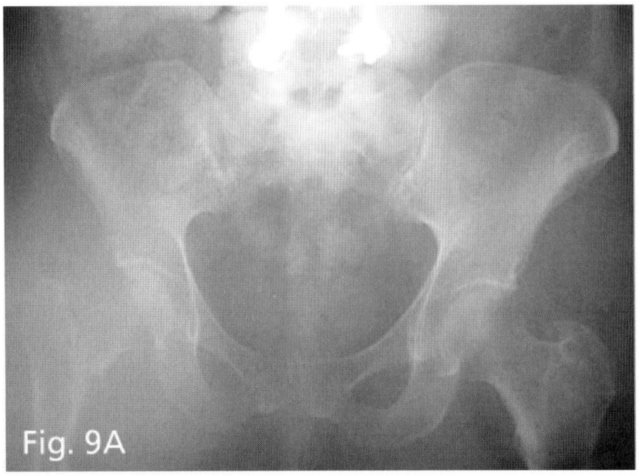

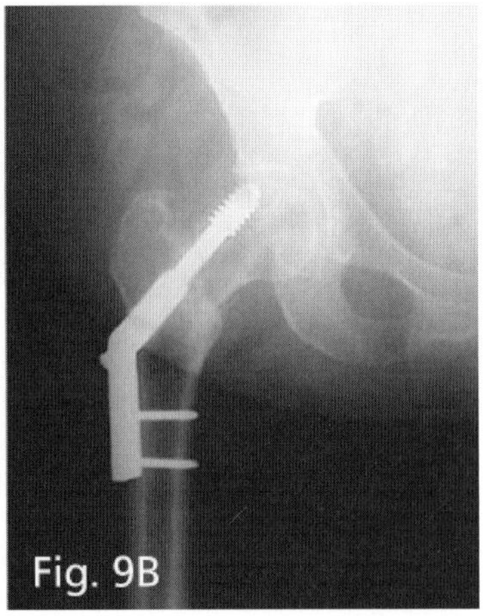

Q-21: An 18-year-old man was in a motor vehicle accident and sustained a closed head injury, right displaced scapular body and glenoid fractures, a right proximal humeral fracture, fractures of ribs one through three, facial fractures, and bilateral pubic rami fractures with minimal displacement. He has a systolic blood pressure of 80/40 mm Hg despite fluid resuscitation. A radiograph is shown in Figure 10. Spiral CT does not identify any thoracic or abdominal injuries. What is the most appropriate next step in management?

1. Pelvic angiography
2. Intracranial pressure monitoring
3. Pelvic external fixation
4. Evaluation of peripheral pulses
5. Urgent open stabilization of the clavicular and humeral fractures

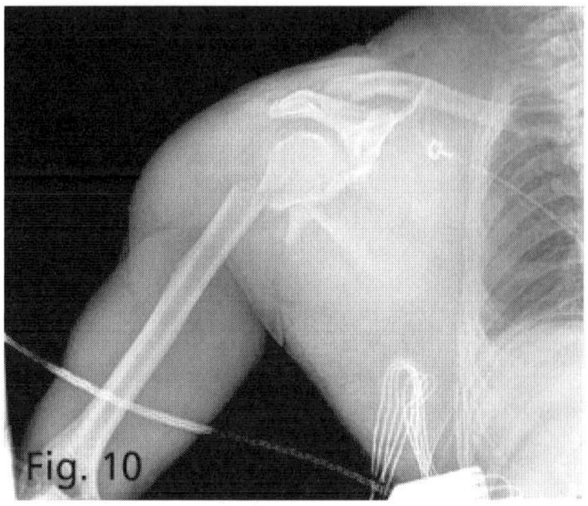
Fig. 10

Q-22: What is the major difference in outcome following open reduction and internal fixation (ORIF) of the tibial plafond at 2 to 5 days versus 10 to 20 days?

1. Improved ankle range of motion
2. Increased risk of wound complications
3. Decreased ankle pain
4. Decreased risk of nerve injuries
5. Decreased risk of development of traumatic arthritis

Q-23: Figure 11 shows the radiograph of a 45-year-old woman who has a painful nonunion. Treatment should consist of

1. revision internal fixation with a longer side plate and bone grafting.
2. open reduction and internal fixation with a 95° fixed angle device and bone grafting.
3. hardware removal and retrograde intramedullary nailing.
4. placement of an implantable bone stimulator.
5. proximal femoral resection and total hip arthroplasty.

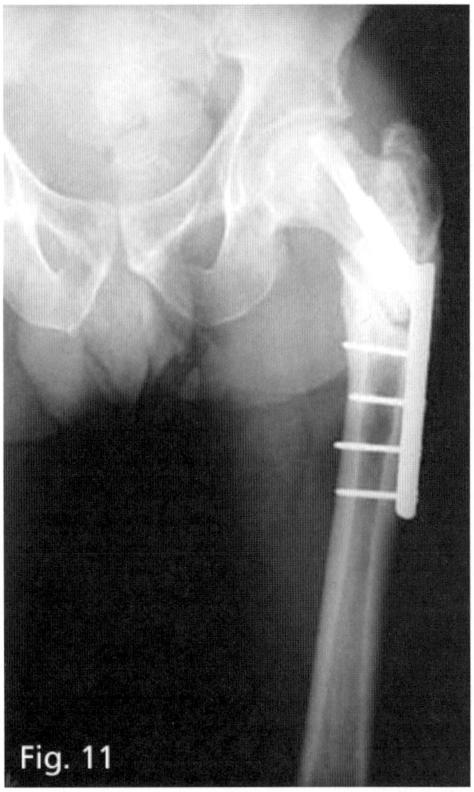
Fig. 11

Q-24: What is the treatment of choice for the injury shown in Figures 12A through 12C?

1. Closed reduction and a short arm cast
2. Splinting in a functional position and early motion
3. Closed or open reduction and internal fixation with Kirschner wires
4. Open reduction and internal fixation with minifragment screws
5. Primary arthrodeses of the carpometacarpal joints

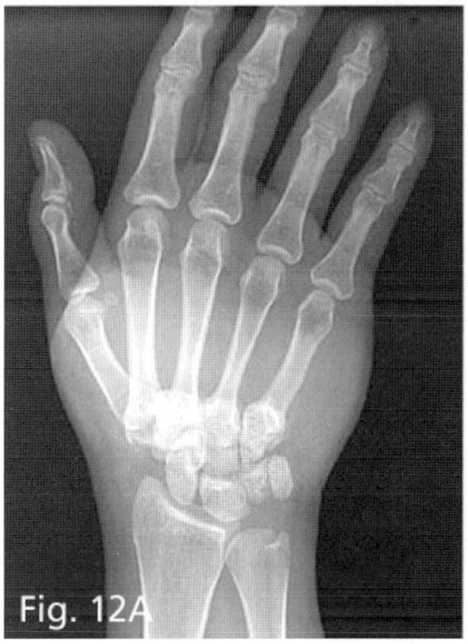
Fig. 12A

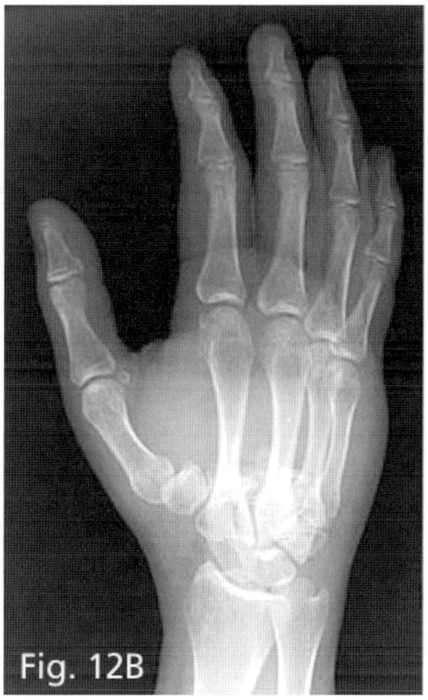
Fig. 12B

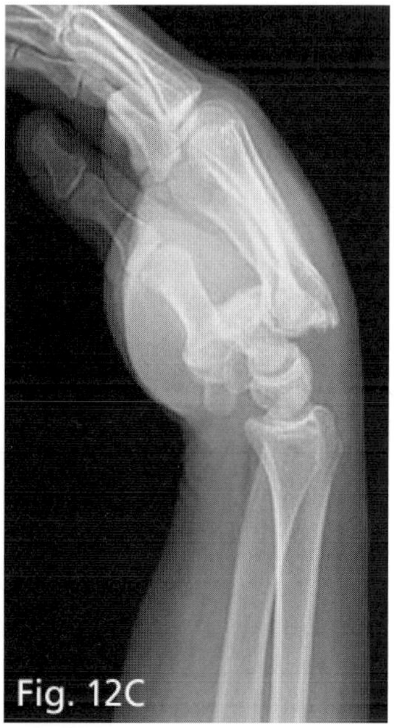
Fig. 12C

Q-25: A 55-year-old woman fell and sustained an elbow dislocation with a coronoid fracture and a radial head fracture. The elbow is reduced and splinted. What is the most common early complication?

1. Brachial artery intimal tear
2. Recurrent dislocation
3. Forearm compartment syndrome
4. Posterior interosseous nerve injury
5. Ulnar nerve palsy

Q-26: A 25-year-old man sustained the closed injury shown in Figures 13A and 13B. Examination reveals that this is an isolated injury, and the patient is hemodynamically stable. Treatment should consist of

1. multiple flexible intramedullary nails.
2. unreamed intramedullary nailing with static interlocking.
3. unreamed intramedullary nailing with dynamic interlocking.
4. reamed intramedullary nailing with static interlocking.
5. reamed intramedullary nailing with dynamic interlocking.

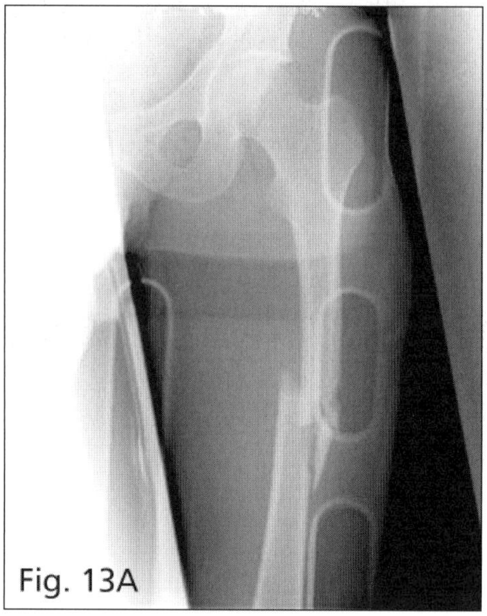
Fig. 13A

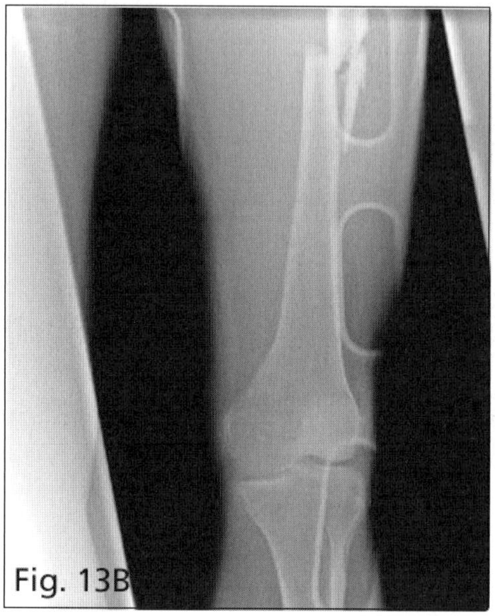
Fig. 13B

Q-27: Figure 14 shows the radiograph of an elderly man who fell on his right arm. What is the most important determinate of a good outcome following this injury?

1. Early open reduction and internal fixation
2. Initiation of physical therapy and passive motion within 2 weeks of the injury
3. Fracture involvement of the greater tuberosity
4. Immobilization with a sling and swathe for 4 weeks
5. Age younger than 70 years

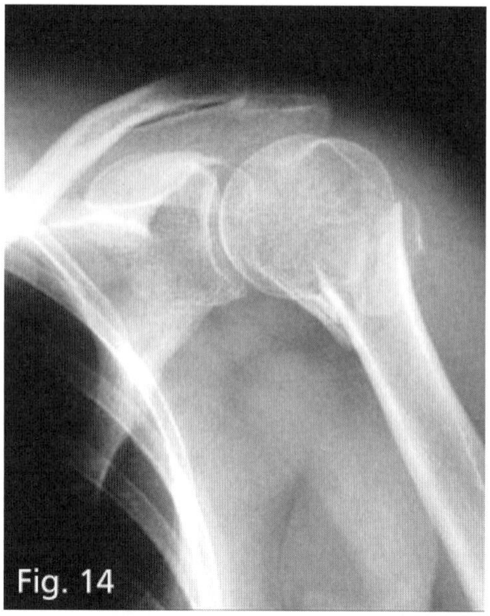
Fig. 14

Q-28: A 40-year-old man was involved in a motor vehicle accident and sustained the pelvic injury seen in Figures 15A and 15B. Definitive management of the injury should consist of reduction by

1. skeletal traction, and bed rest.
2. anterior external fixation.
3. internal fixation of the symphysis pubis.
4. internal fixation of the symphysis pubis with supplemental external fixation.
5. internal fixation of the symphysis pubis and sacral fracture.

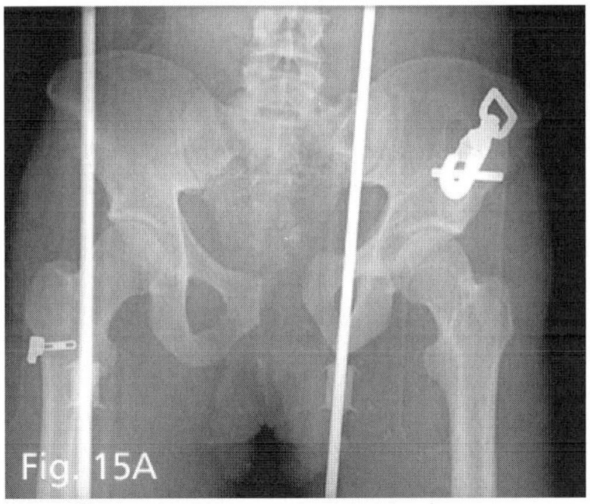
Fig. 15A

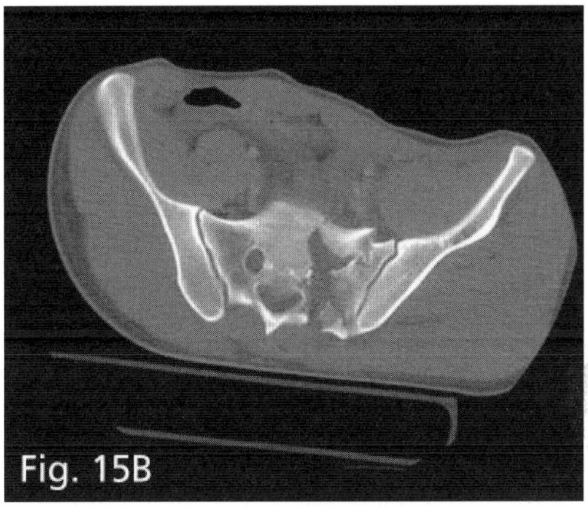
Fig. 15B

Q-29: A 35-year-old patient sustained a bimalleolar ankle fracture. What is the most reliable method of predicting a tear of the interosseous membrane?

1. Level of the fibular fracture
2. Lauge-Hansen fracture class
3. Intraoperative stress testing
4. Widening of the medial clear space
5. Talar dislocation

Q-30: A distal radius fracture in an elderly man is strongly predictive for what subsequent injury?

1. Another distal radius fracture
2. Insufficiency fracture of the spine
3. Insufficiency fracture of the pelvis
4. Hip fracture
5. Proximal humerus fracture

Q-31: What measure of physiologic status best evaluates whether an injured patient is fully resuscitated and best predicts that perioperative complications will be minimized following definitive stabilization of long bone fractures?

1. Urine output greater than 100 mL/h
2. Cardiac output greater than 2
3. Serum lactate level less than 2.5 mmol/L
4. Systolic blood pressure greater than 100 mm Hg
5. Hemoglobin level greater than 10 g/dL

Q-32: In the treatment of ankle fractures, the superficial peroneal nerve is most commonly injured by

1. a posterior-lateral approach.
2. a lateral approach.
3. a medial approach.
4. an anterior-medial approach.
5. rigid cast immobilization.

Q-33: A 54-year-old man sustained a small superficial abrasion over the left acromioclavicular joint after falling from his bicycle. Examination reveals no other physical findings. Radiographs show a displaced fracture of the lateral end of the clavicle distal to a line drawn vertically to the coracoid process. Management should consist of

1. open reduction and plate fixation.
2. a figure-of-8 bandage for 4 to 6 weeks.
3. a sling for comfort, followed by physical therapy when pain free.
4. excision of the outer end of the clavicle.
5. a tension band and Kirschner wires.

Q-34: A 47-year-old man sustained a degloving injury over the pretibial surface and anterior ankle region in a motor vehicle accident. After débridement and irrigation, there is inadequate tissue for closure of the exposed anterior tibial tendon and tibia. Prior to definitive soft-tissue coverage, management should consist of

1. immediate split-thickness skin grafting.
2. immediate xenograft application.
3. a vacuum-assisted closure device.
4. dressing changes with sulfasalazine cream.
5. a cross-leg flap.

Q-35: The humeral nonunion shown in Figure 16 is most likely to unite when using what method of treatment?

1. Intramedullary nail
2. Pulsed electromagnetic fields
3. Compression plate
4. Intramedullary nail and bone graft
5. Compression plate and bone graft

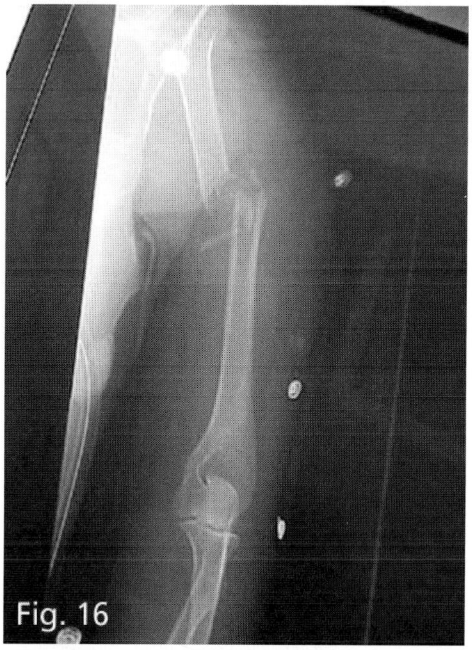

Fig. 16

Q-36: An adult with a distal humeral fracture underwent open reduction and internal fixation. What is the most common postoperative complication?

1. Loss of elbow range of motion
2. Nonunion
3. Malunion
4. Infection
5. Ulnar nerve dysfunction

Q-37: The radiographs and CT scan seen in Figures 17A through 17D reveal what type of acetabular fracture pattern?

1. Transverse
2. Transverse with posterior wall
3. Both column
4. Posterior wall anterior hemitransverse
5. T-type

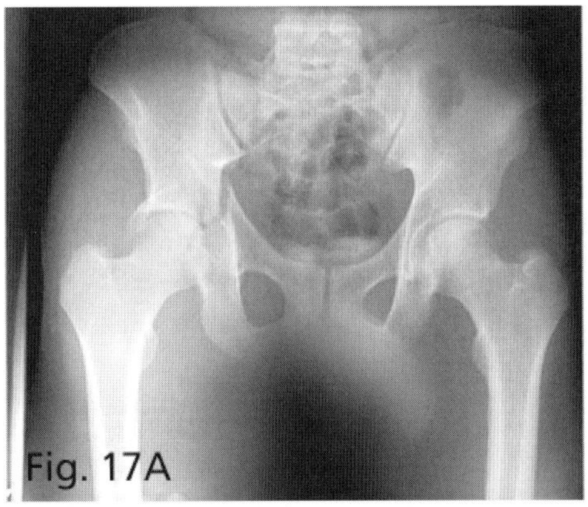
Fig. 17A

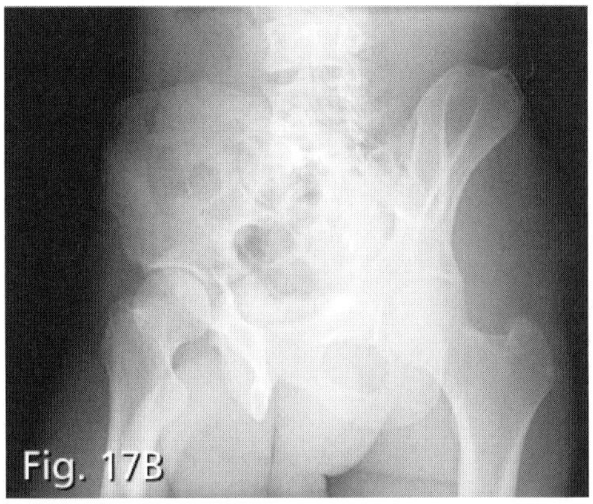
Fig. 17B

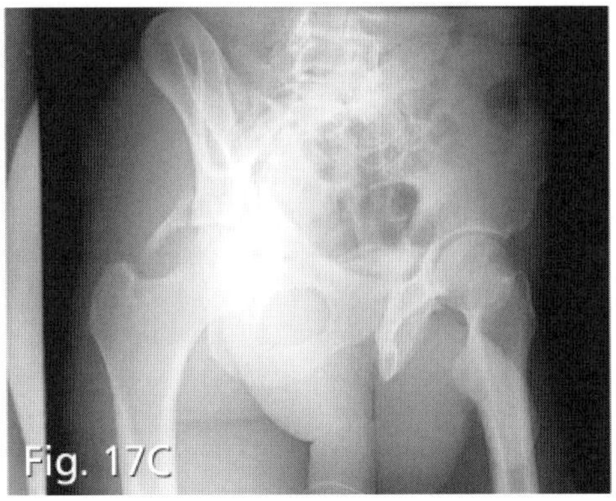
Fig. 17C

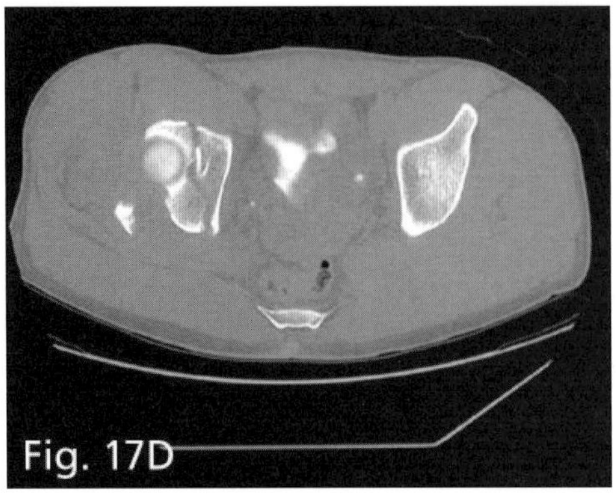
Fig. 17D

Q-38: A 26-year-old man sustained an isolated injury to his left hip joint in a motor vehicle accident. Closed reduction was performed, and the postreduction radiograph is shown in Figure 18. Management should now consist of

1. emergent open reduction and fixation of the fracture.
2. skeletal traction and expedient open reduction and fixation of the fracture.
3. skeletal traction for 6 weeks, followed by physical therapy.
4. crutches and no weight bearing for 6 weeks.
5. bed rest for 1 week and follow-up radiographs to determine if the fragment has moved.

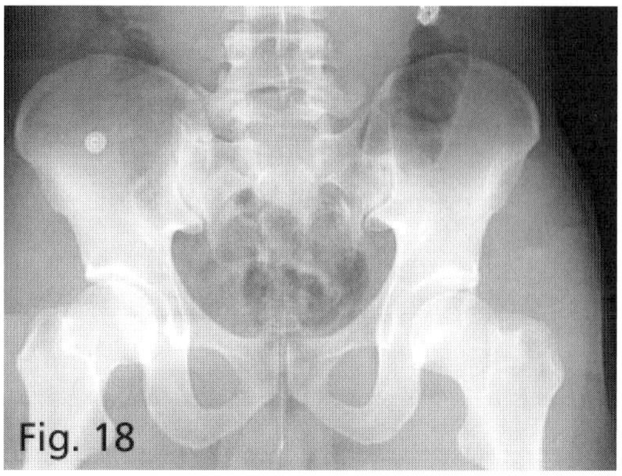
Fig. 18

Q-39: A 35-year-old man is brought to the emergency department following a motorcycle accident. He is breathing spontaneously and has a systolic blood pressure of 80 mm Hg, a pulse rate of 120/min, and a temperature of 98.6° F (37° C). Examination suggests an unstable pelvic fracture; AP radiographs confirm an open book injury with vertical displacement on the left side. Ultrasound evaluation of the abdomen is negative. Despite administration of 4 L of normal saline solution, he still has a systolic pressure of 90 mm Hg and a pulse rate of 110. Urine output has been about 20 mL since arrival 35 minutes ago. What is the best next course of action?

1. Continued resuscitation with fluids and blood
2. Ongoing resuscitation and pelvic angiography
3. Application of an external fixator in the emergency department
4. A pelvic binder and continued resuscitation
5. A pelvic binder, skeletal traction, and continued resuscitation

Q-40: A healthy 25-year-old man sustains a grade IIIB open tibial fracture. Following appropriate débridement, irrigation, and stabilization with an external fixator, the soft-tissue injury is shown in Figure 19. What is the most appropriate definitive soft-tissue coverage procedure?

1. Split-thickness skin graft
2. Full-thickness skin graft
3. Soleus rotation flap
4. Medial gastrocnemius rotation flap
5. Free latissimus dorsi flap with microvascular anastomosis

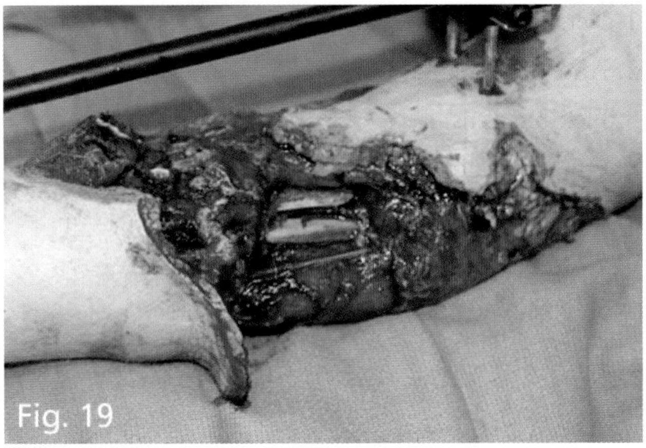

Fig. 19

Q-41: A 25-year-old woman undergoes surgical treatment of a displaced proximal humeral fracture via a deltopectoral approach. At the first postoperative visit, she reports a tingling numbness along the anterolateral aspect of the forearm. What structure is most likely injured?

1. Medial cord of the brachial plexus
2. Radial nerve
3. Median nerve
4. Axillary nerve
5. Musculocutaneous nerve

Q-42: A 32-year-old man sustained a fracture of his upper arm in a motor vehicle accident. Radiographs are shown in Figure 20. Because of other associated injuries, surgical stabilization is chosen. What technique will result in the fewest complications and the best outcome?

1. Retrograde locked intramedullary nail
2. Antegrade reamed locked intramedullary nail
3. Flexible nails
4. Open reduction and plate fixation
5. External fixation

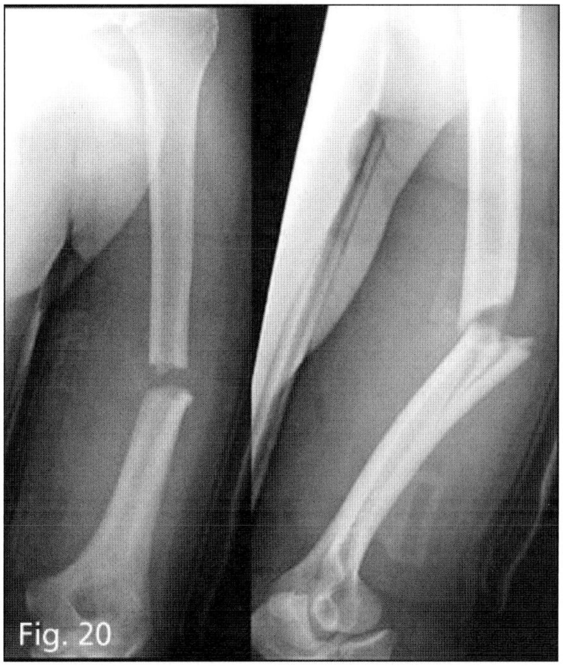

Fig. 20

Q-43: During a posterior approach to the glenoid with retraction as shown in Figure 21, care should be taken during superior retraction to avoid injury to which of the following structures?

1. Axillary artery
2. Axillary nerve
3. Branch of the circumflex scapular artery
4. Profunda brachii artery
5. Suprascapular nerve and artery

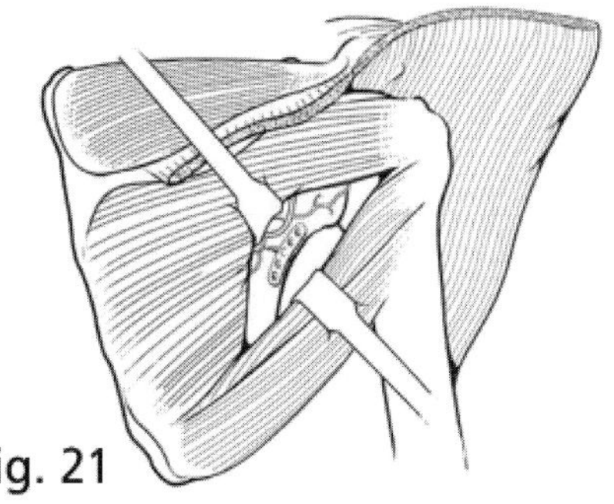

Fig. 21

Q-44: A 42-year-old woman sustained a closed, displaced talar neck fracture in a motor vehicle accident. Which of the following is an avoidable complication of surgical treatment?

1. Posttraumatic arthritis of the subtalar joint
2. Posttraumatic arthritis of the ankle joint
3. Malunion of the talus
4. Osteonecrosis of the talus
5. Complex regional pain syndrome

Q-45: Figures 22A and 22B show the radiographs of a 48-year-old woman who smokes cigarettes and sustained a segmental femoral shaft fracture in a motor vehicle accident 9 months ago. Initial management consisted of stabilization with a reamed statically locked intramedullary nail. She now reports lower leg pain that increases with activity. In addition to advising the patient to quit smoking, management should include

1. ultrasonic stimulation for 3 months.
2. removal of the nail and plate fixation.
3. continued observation.
4. removal of the distal locking screws to dynamize the nail.
5. exchange reamed nailing with bone graft.

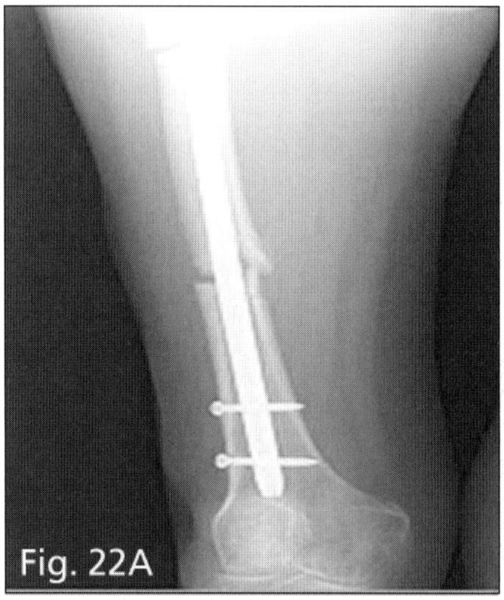

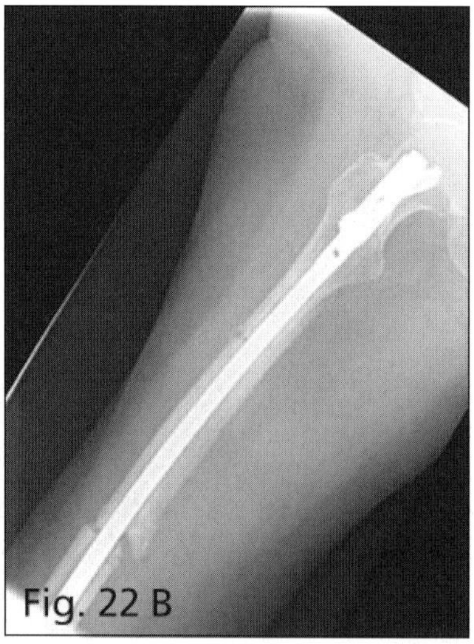

Q-46: A 34-year-old man sustained a tibial fracture in a motorcycle accident. What perioperative variable is associated with the greatest relative risk for reoperation to achieve bone union?

1. Sex
2. Delay in initial surgical treatment
3. Use of NSAIDs
4. Smoking
5. Cortical contact of ≤ 50%

Q-47: A 17-year-old boy sustained a 5-mm laceration on the lateral aspect of the hindfoot while working on a farm. Examination in the emergency department revealed no fractures. Twenty-four hours later, he returns to the emergency department with increasing foot pain. A thin, brown drainage is seen emanating from the wound. He has a temperature of 102.0° F (38.9° C), a pulse rate of 120, and a blood pressure of 80/40 mm Hg. Examination of the foot reveals diffuse swelling, ecchymosis, tenderness, and crepitus with palpation. Current radiographs are shown in Figures 23A and 23B. Management should now consist of

1. intravenous antibiotics.
2. hyperbaric oxygen therapy and intravenous antibiotics.
3. surgical débridement, primary wound closure, and intravenous antibiotics.
4. surgical débridement, closure of the wound over drains, and intravenous antibiotics.
5. surgical débridement, leaving the wound open, and intravenous antibiotics.

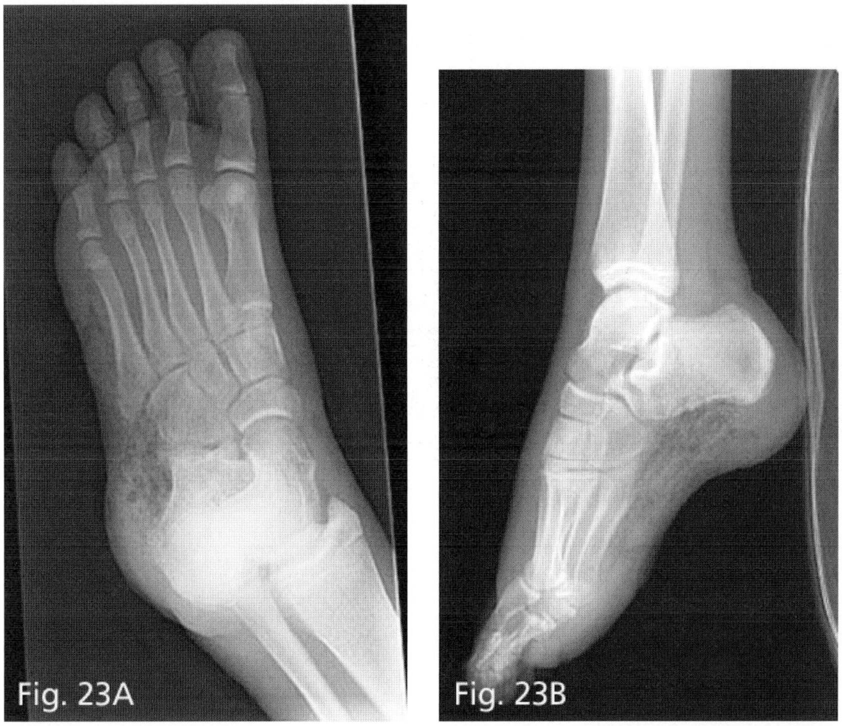

Q-48: A healthy, active, independent 74-year-old woman fell and sustained the elbow injury shown in Figures 24A and 24B. Management should consist of

1. a sling and early elbow range-of-motion exercises.
2. a long arm cast for 6 weeks.
3. open reduction and internal fixation.
4. total elbow arthroplasty.
5. elbow arthrodesis.

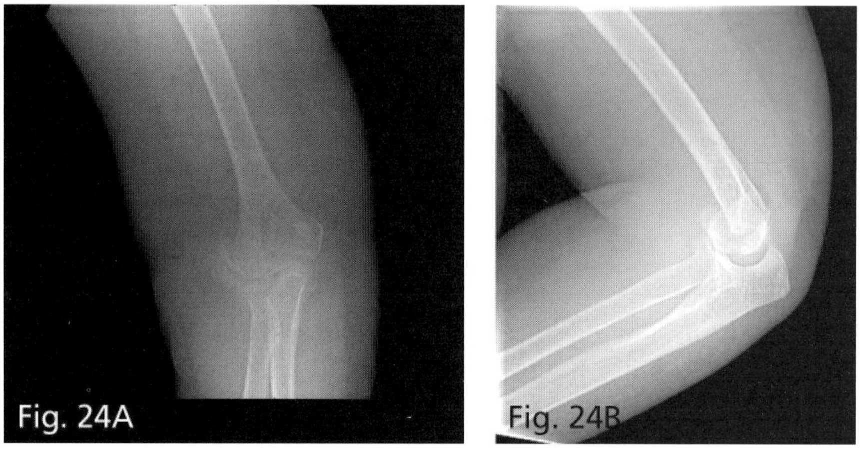

Fig. 24A Fig. 24B

Q-49: A 25-year-old man is brought to the emergency department following a motor vehicle accident. Extrication time was 2 hours, and in the field he had a systolic blood pressure by palpation of 90 mm Hg. Intravenous therapy was started, and on arrival to the emergency department his systolic blood pressure is 90 mm Hg with a pulse rate of 130. Examination reveals a flail chest and a femoral diaphyseal fracture. Ultrasound of the abdomen is positive. The trauma surgeons take him to the operating room for an exploratory laparotomy. At the conclusion of the procedure, systolic pressure is 100 mm Hg with a pulse rate of 110. Oxygen saturation is 90% on 100% oxygen, and the patient's temperature is 95.0° F (35° C). What is the recommended treatment of the femoral fracture at this time?

1. Reamed intramedullary nail
2. Unreamed intramedullary nail
3. Percutaneous plate fixation
4. Skeletal traction
5. External fixation

Q-50: A 26-year-old man was thrown from a car and sustained the injury seen in Figures 25A and 25B. Nonsurgical management of this injury is recommended. Which of the following factors increases the risk of nonunion?

1. Male sex
2. Diaphyseal location
3. Comminuted displaced fracture
4. Young age
5. Associated injuries

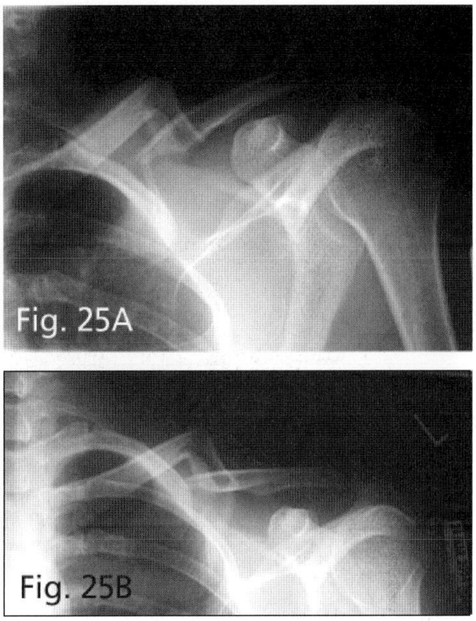

A-1: In patients with displaced radial neck fractures treated with open reduction and internal fixation with a plate and screws, the plate must be limited to what surface of the radius to avoid impingement on the proximal ulna?

1. 2 cm distal to the articular surface of the radial head
2. 1 cm distal to the articular surface of the radial head
3. Within a 90° arc or safe zone
4. Within a 120° arc or safe zone
5. Within a 180° arc or safe zone

PREFERRED RESPONSE: 3

DISCUSSION: The radial head is covered by cartilage on 360° of its circumference. However, with the normal range of forearm rotation of 160° to 180°, there is a consistent area that is nonarticulating. This area is found by palpation of the radial styloid and Lister tubercle. The hardware should be kept within a 90° arc on the radial head subtended by these two structures.

REFERENCES: Smith GR, Hotchkiss RN: Radial head and neck fractures: Anatomic guidelines for proper placement of internal fixation. *J Shoulder Elbow Surg* 1996;5:113-117.

Caputo AE, Mazzocca AD, Santoro VM: The nonarticulating portion of the radial head: Anatomic and clinical correlations for internal fixation. *J Hand Surg Am* 1998;23:1082-1090.

A-2: When harvesting an iliac crest bone graft from the posterior approach, what anatomic structure is at greatest risk for injury if a Cobb elevator is directed too caudal?

1. Sciatic nerve
2. Cluneal nerves
3. Inferior gluteal artery
4. Superior gluteal artery
5. Sacroiliac joint

PREFERRED RESPONSE: 4

DISCUSSION: If a Cobb elevator is directed caudally while stripping the periosteum over the iliac wing, it will encounter the sciatic notch. Although this puts the sciatic nerve at risk, the first structure encountered is the superior gluteal artery. Because it is tethered at the superior edge of the notch, it is very vulnerable to injury and can then retract inside the pelvis, making it difficult to obtain hemostasis. The inferior gluteal artery exits the sciatic notch below the piriformis and is more protected. The cluneal nerves are at risk only if the incision extends too anteriorly, and the sacroiliac joint can be entered while harvesting the graft.

REFERENCES: Banwart JC, Asher MA, Hassanein RS: Iliac crest bone graft harvest donor site morbidity: A statistical evaluation. *Spine (Phila Pa 1976)* 1995;20:1055-1060.

Shin AY, Moran ME, Wenger DR: Superior gluteal artery injury secondary to posterior iliac crest bone graft harvesting: A surgical technique to control hemorrhage. *Spine (Phila Pa 1976)* 1996;21:1371-1374.

A-3: A 36-year-old woman sustained a tarsometatarsal joint fracture-dislocation in a motor vehicle accident. The patient is treated with open reduction and internal fixation. What is the most common complication?

1. Posttraumatic arthritis
2. Infection
3. Fixation failure
4. Malunion
5. Nonunion

PREFERRED RESPONSE: 1

DISCUSSION: The most common complication associated with tarsometatarsal joint injury is posttraumatic arthritis. In one series, symptomatic arthritis developed in 25% of the patients and half of those went on to fusion. In another series, 26% had painful arthritis. Initial treatment should consist of shoe modification, inserts, and anti-inflammatory drugs. Fusion is reserved for failure of nonsurgical management. Hardware failure may occur, but it is clinically unimportant.

REFERENCES: Kuo RS, Tejwani NC, DiGiovanni CW, et al: Outcome after open reduction and internal fixation of Lisfranc joint injuries. *J Bone Joint Surg Am* 2000;82:1609-1618.

Arntz CT, Veith RG, Hansen ST Jr: Fractures and fracture-dislocations of the tarsometatarsal joint. *J Bone Joint Surg Am* 1988;70:173-181.

Thompson MC, Mormino MA: Injury to the tarsometatarsal joint complex. *J Am Acad Orthop Surg* 2003;11:260-267.

A-4: What is the most appropriate indication for replantation in an otherwise healthy 35-year-old man?

1. Isolated transverse amputation of the thumb through the middle of the nail bed
2. Isolated transverse amputation of the index finger through the proximal phalanx
3. Isolated transverse amputation of the ring finger through the proximal phalanx
4. Isolated transverse amputation of the hand at the level of the wrist
5. Forearm amputation with a 10-hour warm ischemia time

PREFERRED RESPONSE: 4

DISCUSSION: Vascular anastomoses are exceedingly difficult with amputations distal to the nail fold because the digital vessels bifurcate or trifurcate at this level, and little functional benefit is gained compared to other means of soft-tissue coverage. Single-digit amputations, other than the thumb, are a relative contraindication for replantation. Replantations at the level of the proximal phalanx lead to poor motion of the proximal interphalangeal joint. In a healthy, active adult, an amputation through the wrist is an appropriate situation to proceed with a replantation. A transverse forearm amputation is a good indication with a warm ischemia time of less than 6 hours.

REFERENCES: Urbaniak JR: Replantation, in Green DP, Hotchkiss RN, eds: *Operative Hand Surgery*, ed 3. New York, NY, Churchill Livingstone, 1993, p 1085.

Boulas HJ: Amputations of the fingers and hand: Indications for replantation. *J Am Acad Orthop Surg* 1998;6:100-105.

A-5: A 46-year-old man fell 20 feet and sustained the injury shown in Figure 1. The injury is closed; however, the soft tissues are swollen and ecchymotic with blisters. The most appropriate initial management should consist of

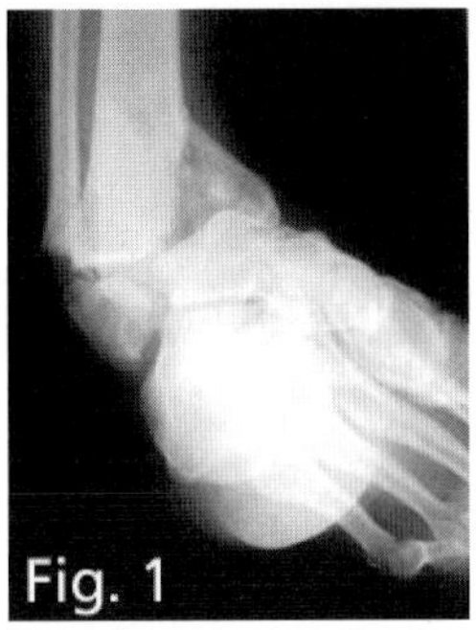

1. a long leg cast.
2. a short leg cast.
3. immediate open reduction and internal fixation.
4. a temporizing spanning external fixator.
5. primary ankle fusion.

PREFERRED RESPONSE: 4

DISCUSSION: Although this is a fracture of the medial and lateral malleoli, the degree of displacement and comminution of the medial dome indicate that this injury is similar to a pilon fracture. Initial management should consistent of stabilization to allow for soft-tissue healing. The use of temporizing spanning external fixation should be the initial step, followed by limited or more extensive open reduction and internal fixation when the soft-tissue status will allow. Initial placement in either a short or long leg cast does not provide the needed stability and does not allow for care and monitoring of soft tissues. In addition, maintaining reduction of the talus may be very difficult. Immediate open reduction and internal fixation through an injured soft-tissue envelope adds the risk of difficulties with incision healing and a higher risk of deep infection. In the acute setting, a primary ankle fusion through this soft-tissue envelope is not indicated.

REFERENCES: Marsh JL, Bonar S, Nepola JV, et al: Use of an articulated external fixator for fractures of the tibial plafond. *J Bone Joint Surg Am* 1995;77:1498-1509.

Wyrsch B, McFerran MA, McAndrew M, et al: Operative treatment of fractures of the tibial plafond: A randomized, prospective study. *J Bone Joint Surg Am* 1996;78:1646-1657.

Thordarson DB: Complications after treatment of tibial pilon fractures: Prevention and management strategies. *J Am Acad Orthop Surg* 2000;8:253-265.

A-6: A collegiate golfer sustained a hook of the hamate fracture. After 12 weeks of splinting and therapy, the hand is still symptomatic. What is the most appropriate management to allow return to competitive activity?

1. Continued observation
2. Open reduction and internal fixation of the fracture
3. Excision of the hook of the hamate
4. Carpal tunnel release
5. Guyon canal release

PREFERRED RESPONSE: 3

DISCUSSION: Excision of the fracture fragment typically leads to rapid return to function. Fixation techniques are difficult to perform because of the size of the bone; hardware prominence is common. Nerve deficits are not typically noted in this injury. The motor branch of the ulnar nerve in Guyon canal must be protected during the surgical approach.

REFERENCES: Kulund DN, McCue FC III, Rockwell DA, et al: Tennis injuries: Prevention and treatment: A review. *Am J Sports Med* 1979;7:249-253.

Morgan WJ, Slowman LS: Acute hand and wrist injuries in athletes: Evaluation and management. *J Am Acad Orthop Surg* 2001;9:389-400.

A-7: A 20-year-old man sustained a closed tibial fracture and is treated with a reamed intramedullary nail. What is the most common complication associated with this treatment?

1. Nonunion
2. Malunion
3. Infection
4. Knee pain
5. Compartment syndrome

PREFERRED RESPONSE: 4

DISCUSSION: The most common complication is anterior knee pain (57%). The knee pain is activity related (92%) and exacerbated by kneeling (83%). Although knee pain is the most common complication, most patients rate it as mild to moderate and only 10% are unable to return to previous employment. Some authors report less knee pain with a peritendinous approach when compared to a tendon-splitting approach. In one study, nail removal resolved pain in 27%, improved it in 70%, and made it worse in 3%. The incidence of the other complications was: infection 0% to 3%, nonunion 0% to 6%, and malunion 2% to 13%. Compartment syndrome is rare after nailing.

REFERENCES: Court-Brown CM: Reamed intramedullary tibial nailing: An overview and analysis of 1106 cases. *J Orthop Trauma* 2004;18:96-101.

McQueen MM, Gaston P, Court-Brown CM: Acute compartment syndrome: Who is at risk? *J Bone Joint Surg Br* 2000;82:200-203.

Keating JF, Orfaly R, O'Brien PJ: Knee pain after tibial nailing. *J Orthop Trauma* 1997;11:10-13.

A-8: What is the most likely complication following treatment of the humeral shaft fracture shown in Figure 2?

1. Nonunion
2. Shoulder pain
3. Infection
4. Elbow injury
5. Radial nerve injury

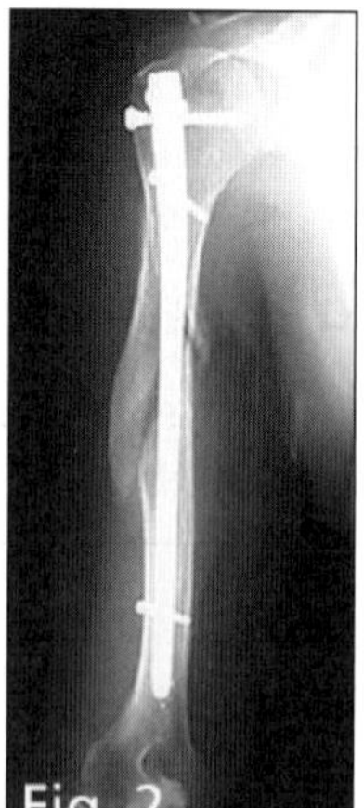
Fig. 2

PREFERRED RESPONSE: 2

DISCUSSION: The humerus was treated with an intramedullary nail. Findings from two prospective randomized studies of intramedullary nailing or compression plating of acute humeral fractures have shown approximately a 30% incidence of shoulder pain with antegrade humeral nailing. This is the most common complication in both of these series. Nonunions are present in approximately 5% to 10% of humeral fractures treated with an intramedullary nail. Infection has an incidence of approximately 1%. Elbow injury is unlikely unless the nail is excessively long. Rarely, injury to the radial nerve is possible if it is trapped in the intramedullary canal.

(continued on next page)

(A-8: *continued*)

REFERENCES: Chapman JR, Henley MB, Agel J, et al: Randomized prospective study of humeral shaft fracture fixation: Intramedullary nails versus plates. *J Orthop Trauma* 2000;14:162-166.

McCormack RG, Brien D, Buckley RE, et al: Fixation of fractures of the shaft of the humerus by dynamic compression plate or intramedullary nail: A prospective, randomised trial. *J Bone Joint Surg Br* 2000;82:336-339.

A-9: A 16-year-old girl sustained the injury shown in Figure 3A. CT scans are shown in Figures 3B through 3D. The results of treatment of this injury have been shown to correlate most with which of the following factors?

1. Surgical approach
2. Location of the transverse fracture
3. Timing of surgery
4. Accuracy of reduction
5. Use of skeletal traction

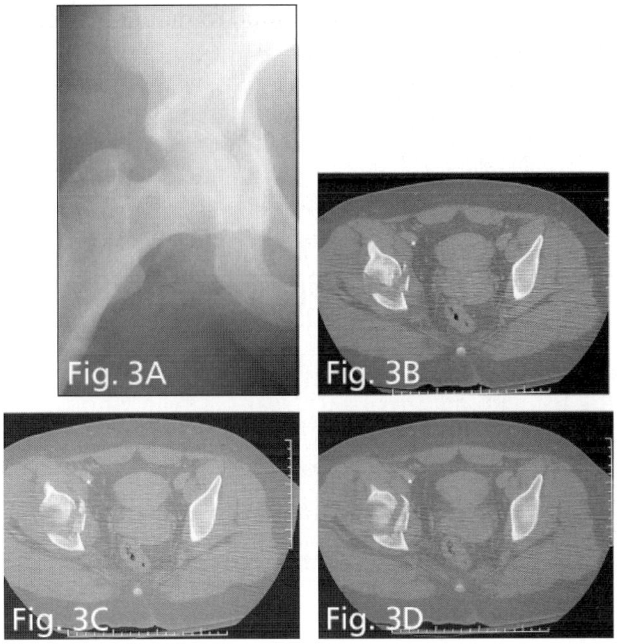

PREFERRED RESPONSE: 4

DISCUSSION: The patient has a very low T-type acetabular fracture; however, the head is not congruent under the dome so surgical reduction is necessary. The anterior and posterior columns are displaced and will move independently of each other. The extended iliofemoral is the only approach allowing for visualization and reduction of each column. A combined anterior and posterior approach may also be used. The timing of surgery should be within the first 3 weeks of injury to optimize chances of obtaining an accurate reduction because this is an important factor in determining outcome.

REFERENCES: Letournel E, Judet R, eds: *Fractures of the Acetabulum*, ed 2. Berlin, Germany, Springer-Verlag, 1991.

Matta JM: Fractures of the acetabulum: Accuracy of reduction and clinical results in patients managed operatively within three weeks after the injury. *J Bone Joint Surg Am* 1996;78:1632-1645.

A-10: An active 49-year-old woman who sustained a diaphyseal fracture of the clavicle 8 months ago now reports persistent shoulder pain with daily activities. An AP radiograph is shown in Figure 4. Management should consist of

1. external electrical stimulation.
2. external ultrasound stimulation.
3. implanted electrical stimulation.
4. closed reduction and percutaneous fixation.
5. open reduction and internal fixation with bone graft.

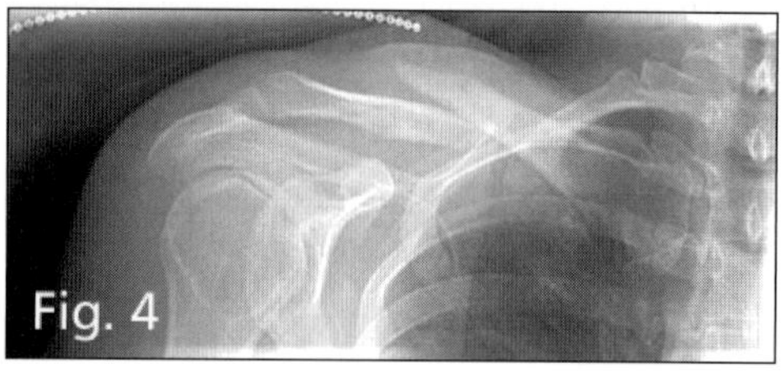
Fig. 4

PREFERRED RESPONSE: 5

DISCUSSION: The radiograph reveals an atrophic nonunion of the diaphysis of the clavicle. Electrical or ultrasound stimulation may be an option in diaphyseal nonunions that have shown some healing response with callus formation, but these techniques are not successful in an atrophic nonunion. The preferred technique for achieving union is open reduction and internal fixation with bone graft. Percutaneous fixation has no role in treatment of nonunions of the clavicle.

REFERENCES: Boyer MI, Axelrod TS: Atrophic nonunion of the clavicle: Treatment by compression plating, lag-screw fixation and bone graft. *J Bone Joint Surg Br* 1997;79:301-303.

Simpson NS, Jupiter JB: Clavicular nonunion and malunion: Evaluation and surgical management. *J Am Acad Orthop Surg* 1996;4:1-8.

A-11: Examination of a 25-year-old man who was injured in a motor vehicle accident reveals a fracture-dislocation of C5-6 with a Frankel B spinal cord injury. He also has a closed right femoral shaft fracture and a grade II open ipsilateral midshaft tibial fracture. Assessment of his vital signs reveals a pulse rate of 45/min, blood pressure of 80/45 mm Hg, and respirations of 25/min. A general surgeon has assessed the abdomen, and peritoneal lavage results are negative. His clinical presentation is most consistent with what type of shock?

1. Neurogenic
2. Hemorrhagic
3. Spinal
4. Septic
5. Hypovolemic

PREFERRED RESPONSE: 1

DISCUSSION: Assessment of the acutely injured patient follows the Advanced Trauma Life Support protocol. Cervical cord injury is often associated with a disruption in sympathetic outflow. Absent sympathetic input to the lower extremities leads to vasodilatation, decreased venous return to the heart, and subsequent hypotension. With hypotension, the physiologic response of tachycardia is not possible because of the unopposed vagal tone. This results in bradycardia. Patient positioning, fluid support, pressor agents, and atropine are used to treat neurogenic shock.

REFERENCE: Sutton DC, Siveri CP, Cotler JM: Initial evaluation and management of the spinal injured patient, in Cotler JM, Simpson JM, An HS, et al, eds: *Surgery of Spinal Trauma*. Philadelphia, PA, Lippincott Williams & Wilkins, 2000, pp 113-126.

A-12: A 32-year-old woman sustained an injury to her left upper extremity in a motor vehicle accident. Examination reveals a 2-cm wound in the midportion of the dorsal surface of the upper arm and deformities at the elbow and forearm; there are no other injuries. Her vital signs are stable, and she has a base deficit of -1 and a lactate level of less than 2. Radiographs are shown in Figures 5A and 5B. In addition to urgent débridement of the humeral shaft fracture, management should include

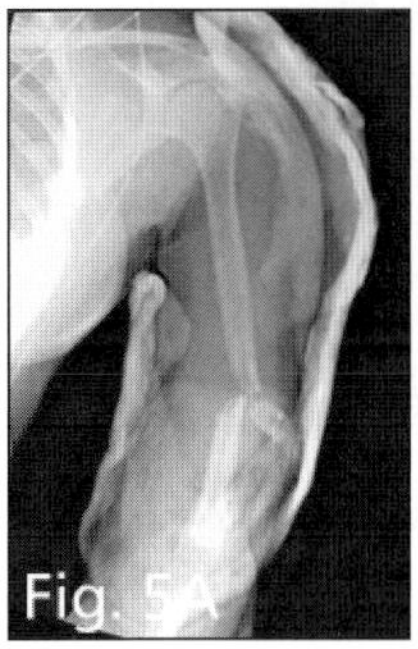

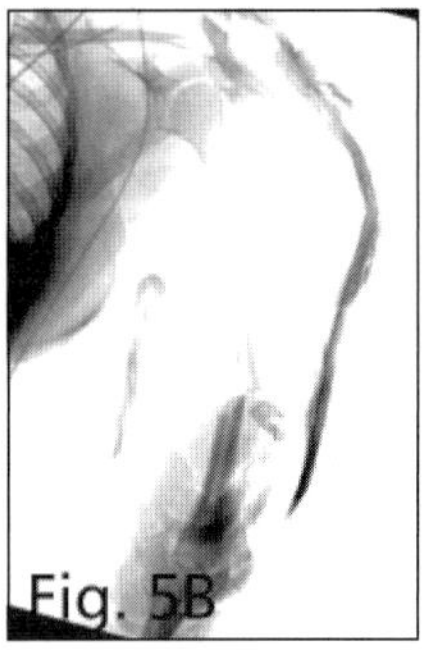

1. closed management of the medial condyle and humeral shaft fractures and open reduction and internal fixation of the both-bones forearm fracture.
2. closed management of the humeral shaft fracture and open reduction and internal fixation of the medial condyle and the both-bones forearm fractures.
3. open reduction and internal fixation of the humeral shaft, medial condyle, and the both-bones forearm fractures.
4. open reduction and internal fixation of the medial condyle and both-bones forearm fractures, and external fixation of the humeral shaft fracture.
5. delayed stabilization of all fractures after the open wound has healed.

PREFERRED RESPONSE: 3

DISCUSSION: With a severe injury to the upper extremity, the best opportunity for achieving a good functional result for a floating elbow is immediate débridement of the open fracture, followed by internal fixation of the fractures. The ability to do this depends on the patient's physiologic status. In this patient, the procedure is acceptable because she has normal vital signs and no chest or abdominal injuries, and normal physiologic parameters (base excess and lactate) show adequate peripheral perfusion. The surgical approaches will be determined by the associated injury patterns and open wounds. In this patient, the humerus was débrided and stabilized through a posterior approach as was the medial condyle fracture. The ulna was fixed through an extension of the posterior incision and the radius through a separate dorsal approach.

REFERENCES: Solomon HB, Zadnik M, Eglseder WA: A review of outcomes in 18 patients with floating elbow. *J Orthop Trauma* 2003;17:563-570.

Pape HC, Hildebrand F, Pertschy S, et al: Changes in the management of femoral shaft fractures in polytrauma patients: From early total care to damage control orthopedic surgery. *J Trauma* 2002;53:452-461.

A-13: A patient sustained the injuries shown in the radiographs and clinical photograph seen in Figures 6A through 6C. The neurovascular examination is normal. The first step in emergent management of the extremity injuries should consist of

1. application of a femoral traction pin.
2. intramedullary nailing of the femur and tibia.
3. surgical irrigation and débridement.
4. external fixation of the femoral fracture.
5. reduction of the femoral head.

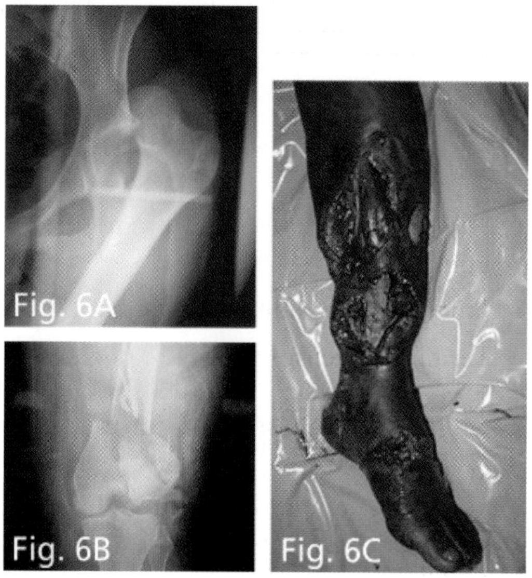

PREFERRED RESPONSE: 5

DISCUSSION: The figures show an open tibial fracture, a femoral shaft fracture, and femoral head dislocation. The most urgent treatment is reduction of the femoral head, as timing to reduction has been correlated with preventing osteonecrosis. After reduction of the femoral head, the next priority is wound management, followed by stabilization of the femoral and tibial fractures with either splinting, traction, or external fixation.

REFERENCES: Sahin V, Karakas ES, Aksu S, et al: Traumatic dislocation and fracture-dislocation of the hip: A long-term follow-up study. *J Trauma* 2003;54:520-529.

Moed BR, WillsonCarr SE, Watson JT: Results of operative treatment of fractures of the posterior wall of the acetabulum. *J Bone Joint Surg Am* 2002;84:752-758.

A-14: A 25-year-old patient sustains the injury shown in Figures 7A through 7C after falling off a curb. Initial management should consist of

1. weight bearing as tolerated in a hard-soled shoe.
2. weight bearing as tolerated in an ankle lacer.
3. weight bearing as tolerated in a short leg cast.
4. no weight bearing in a hard-soled shoe.
5. no weight bearing in a short leg cast.

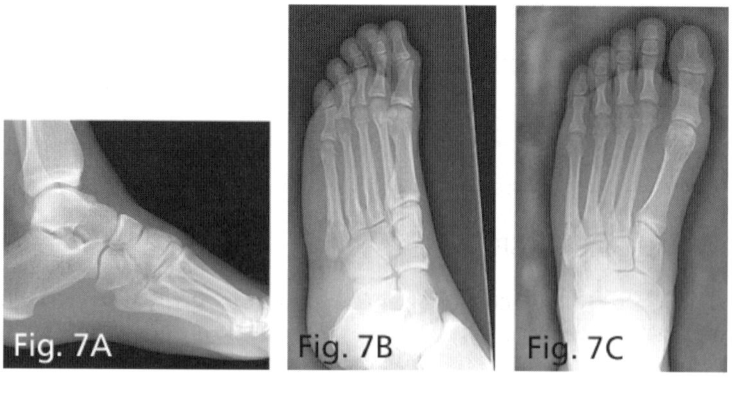

PREFERRED RESPONSE: 5

DISCUSSION: The radiographs reveal a fracture entering the 4-5 intermetatarsal articulation, consistent with a zone 2 injury. This classically is also referred to as a Jones fracture. The history and radiographic findings indicate this is an acute fracture, which guides management. A zone 1 fracture enters the fifth tarsometatarsal joint, and a zone 3 fracture is a proximal diaphyseal fracture distal to the 4-5 articulation. Initial management is usually nonsurgical and consists of no weight bearing in a short leg cast. This method has been shown to result in a better healing rate compared to weight bearing as tolerated.

(continued on next page)

(A-14: *continued*)

REFERENCES: Rosenberg GA, Sterra JJ: Treatment strategies for acute fractures and nonunions of the proximal fifth metatarsal. *J Am Acad Orthop Surg* 2000;8:332-338.

Lawrence SJ, Botte MJ: Jones' fracture and related fractures of the proximal fifth metatarsal. *Foot Ankle* 1993;14:358-365.

A-15: What structure is most often injured in a volar proximal interphalangeal joint dislocation?

1. Sagittal bands
2. Central slip
3. Lumbrical
4. Juncturae tendinum
5. Terminal extensor tendon

PREFERRED RESPONSE: 2

DISCUSSION: Closed ruptures of the central slip of the extensor tendon may occur with volar proximal interphalangeal joint dislocation, forced flexion of the proximal interphalangeal joint, or blunt trauma to the dorsum of the proximal interphalangeal joint. The other structures are not typically injured in proximal interphalangeal joint dislocations. Treatment typically requires static splinting of the proximal interphalangeal joint. In the more common dorsal proximal interphalangeal joint dislocation, the volar plate is injured, and early range of motion may be started after reduction.

REFERENCES: Doyle JR: Extensor tendons: Acute injuries, in Green DP, Hotchkiss RN, eds: *Operative Hand Surgery*, ed 3. New York, NY, Churchill Livingstone, 1993, p 1925.

Newport ML: Extensor tendon injuries in the hand. *J Am Acad Orthop Surg* 1997;5:59-66.

A-16: What patient factor is predictive of better outcomes for surgical management of a displaced calcaneal fracture compared to nonsurgical management?

1. Young man injured at the work site
2. Young woman injured during recreational activities
3. Heavy smoker
4. Patient older than 50 years
5. Patient with bilateral fractures

PREFERRED RESPONSE: 2

DISCUSSION: A recent randomized trial of surgical versus nonsurgical management of calcaneal fractures showed that patients who were on workers' compensation did poorly with surgical care. These patients had less favorable outcomes regardless of their initial management. Factors such as age, smoking, and vasculopathies compromise skin healing, leading to greater surgical risks. The best results were obtained in patients who are younger than age 40 years, have unilateral injuries, and are injured during noncompensable activities. Women tend to do better with surgery than men.

REFERENCES: Howard JL, Buckley R, McCormack R, et al: Complications following management of displaced intra-articular calcaneal fractures: A prospective randomized trial comparing open reduction internal fixation with nonoperative management. *J Orthop Trauma* 2003;17:241-249.

Buckley R, Tough S, McCormack R, et al: Operative compared with nonoperative treatment of displaced intra-articular calcaneal fractures: A prospective, randomized, controlled multicenter trial. *J Bone Joint Surg Am* 2002;84:1733-1744.

A-17: Figures 8A and 8B show the initial radiographs of an 18-year-old man who fell while snowboarding. Figures 8C and 8D show the radiographs obtained following closed reduction. Examination reveals that the elbow is stable with range of motion. Management should now consist of

1. immediate return to unrestricted activity.
2. a posterior long arm splint for 7 to 10 days, followed by elbow range-of-motion exercises.
3. a long arm cast for 4 weeks.
4. immediate surgical repair of the collateral ligaments.
5. immediate surgical repair of the collateral ligaments and placement of a hinged external fixator.

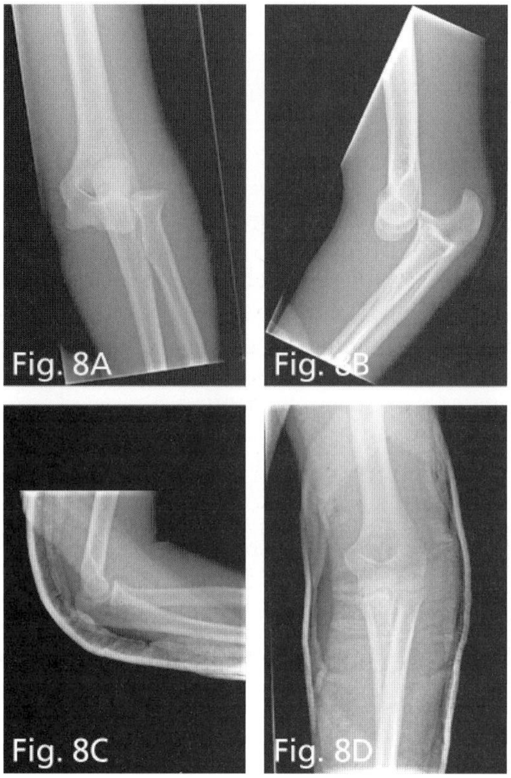

PREFERRED RESPONSE: 2

DISCUSSION: The initial radiographs reveal a simple elbow dislocation without associated fractures. After successful closed reduction, the range of stability should be assessed. If the elbow is stable, nonsurgical management should consist of a short period of immobilization followed by range-of-motion exercises. Immobilization for more than 3 weeks results in significant elbow stiffness. Surgical repair is indicated for dislocations that are irreducible, have associated fractures, or where stability cannot be maintained with closed treatment.

REFERENCES: Cohen MS, Hastings H II: Acute elbow dislocations: Evaluation and management. *J Am Acad Orthop Surg* 1998;6:15-23.

O'Driscoll SW: Elbow dislocations, in Morrey BF, ed: *The Elbow and Its Disorders*, ed 3. Philadelphia, PA, WB Saunders, 2000, pp 409-420.

A-18: Which of the following is an advantage of unreamed nailing of the tibia compared to reamed nailing?

1. Less surgical time
2. Lower risk of nonunion
3. Lower rate of malunion
4. Faster time to union
5. Less secondary procedures to achieve union

PREFERRED RESPONSE: 1

DISCUSSION: The debate between reamed versus unreamed intramedullary nailing of the tibia continues. Although unreamed nailing was proposed for open fractures to minimize infection, its simplicity made it appealing for closed fractures. However, most studies to date show that the only advantage of unreamed nailing is less surgical time. All studies show higher nonunion rates with increased hardware failure and increased time to union for unreamed nailing. Even in open fractures graded up to Gustilo grade IIIA, the reamed tibial nail performs better.

REFERENCES: Larsen LB, Madsen JE, Hoiness PR, et al: Should insertion of intramedullary nails for tibial fractures be with or without reaming? A prospective, randomized study with 3.8 years' follow-up. *J Orthop Trauma* 2004;18: 144-149.

Blachut PA, O'Brien PJ, Meek RN, et al: Interlocking intramedullary nailing with or without reaming for the treatment of closed fractures of the tibial shaft: A prospective randomized study. *J Bone Joint Surg Am* 1997;79:640-646.

A-19: An otherwise healthy 35-year-old woman reports dorsal wrist pain and has trouble extending her thumb after sustaining a minimally displaced fracture of the distal radius 3 months ago. What is the most appropriate next step in management?

1. Neurophysiologic test to evaluate the posterior interosseous nerve
2. Transfer of the extensor indicis proprius to the extensor pollicis longus tendon
3. Interphalangeal joint arthrodesis of the thumb
4. Extension splinting of the thumb
5. Fine-cut CT of the distal radius to evaluate Lister tubercle

PREFERRED RESPONSE: 2

DISCUSSION: Extensor pollicis longus tendon rupture can occur after a fracture of the distal radius, even a minimally displaced one. Poor vascularity of the tendon within the third dorsal compartment is the suspected etiology, not the displaced fracture fragments. Tendon transfer will suitably restore active extension of the thumb interphalangeal joint.

REFERENCES: Christophe K: Rupture of the extensor pollicis longus tendon following Colles fracture. *J Bone Joint Surg Am* 1953;35:1003-1005.

Hove LM: Delayed rupture of the thumb extensor tendon: A 5-year study of 18 consecutive cases. *Acta Orthop Scand* 1994;65:199-203.

A-20: Figure 9A is a radiograph from a 34-year-old woman who sustained a basicervical fracture of the femoral neck. The fracture was treated with a compression screw and side plate. Seven months postoperatively, she continues to have significant hip pain and cannot bear full weight on her hip. A recent radiograph is shown in Figure 9B. Management should now consist of

1. continued non-weight-bearing and a bone stimulator.
2. removal of the hardware, bone grafting of the femoral neck, and refixation.
3. removal of the hardware and hemiarthroplasty.
4. removal of the hardware and total hip arthroplasty.
5. removal of the hardware and a valgus osteotomy.

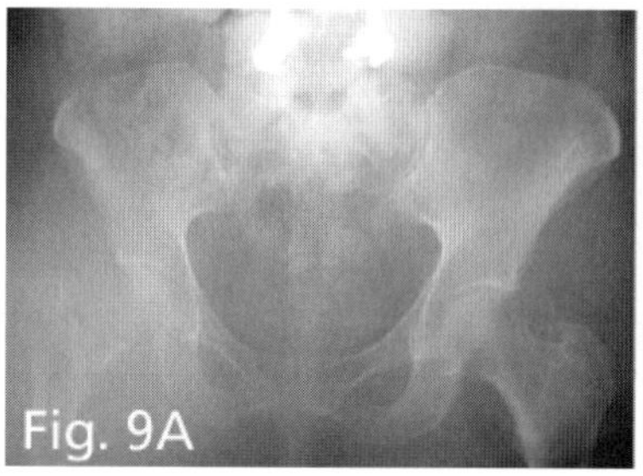
Fig. 9A

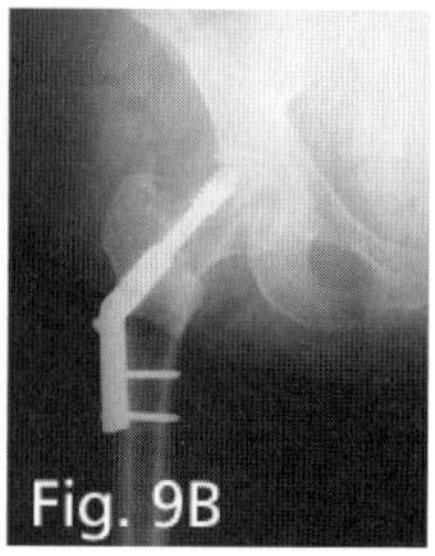
Fig. 9B

PREFERRED RESPONSE: 5

DISCUSSION: The patient sustained a high-angle femoral neck fracture. The follow-up clinical findings and radiograph show that she now has a nonunion with failed internal fixation. The joint appears preserved. In a healthy, young patient, arthroplasty of the femoral head, although possible, is not ideal. Excellent healing and function can be obtained in 70% to 80% of patients with femoral neck nonunion with a valgus intertrochanteric osteotomy.

REFERENCES: Marti RK, Schuller HM, Raaymakers EL: Intertrochanteric osteotomy for non-union of the femoral neck. *J Bone Joint Surg Br* 1989;71:782-787.

Ballmer FT, Ballmer PM, Baumgaertel F, et al: Pauwels osteotomy for nonunions of the femoral neck. *Orthop Clin North Am* 1990;21:759-767.

A-21: An 18-year-old man was in a motor vehicle accident and sustained a closed head injury, right displaced scapular body and glenoid fractures, a right proximal humeral fracture, fractures of ribs one through three, facial fractures, and bilateral pubic rami fractures with minimal displacement. He has a systolic blood pressure of 80/40 mm Hg despite fluid resuscitation. A radiograph is shown in Figure 10. Spiral CT does not identify any thoracic or abdominal injuries. What is the most appropriate next step in management?

1. Pelvic angiography
2. Intracranial pressure monitoring
3. Pelvic external fixation
4. Evaluation of peripheral pulses
5. Urgent open stabilization of the clavicular and humeral fractures

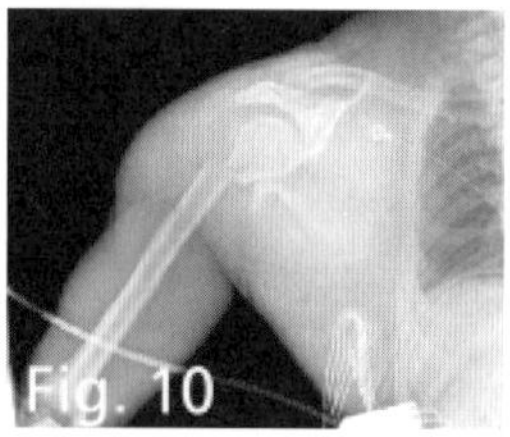
Fig. 10

PREFERRED RESPONSE: 4

DISCUSSION: The patient has sustained high-energy upper extremity and chest injuries. He continues to remain hemodynamically unstable with no obvious thoracic or abdominal injury responsible for bleeding. The pelvic fracture is unlikely to be causing significant bleeding. A scapulothoracic dissociation and possible disruption of one of the great vessels of the upper extremity should be considered. Evaluation of peripheral pulses or blood pressure indices bilaterally in the upper extremities is a simple way to evaluate the need for further work-up. If there is any discrepancy or further concern, angiography of the involved extremity is necessary.

(continued on next page)

(A-21: *continued*)

REFERENCES: Althausen PL, Lee MA, Finkemeier CG: Scapulothoracic dissociation: Diagnosis and treatment. *Clin Orthop* 2003;416:237-244.

Witz M, Korzets Z, Lehmann J: Traumatic scapulothoracic dissociation. *J Cardiovasc Surg* 2000;41:927-929.

A-22: What is the major difference in outcome following open reduction and internal fixation (ORIF) of the tibial plafond at 2 to 5 days versus 10 to 20 days?

1. Improved ankle range of motion
2. Increased risk of wound complications
3. Decreased ankle pain
4. Decreased risk of nerve injuries
5. Decreased risk of development of traumatic arthritis

PREFERRED RESPONSE: 2

DISCUSSION: Long-term outcomes following tibial plafond fractures treated with ORIF are satisfactory in most patients despite a high incidence of posttraumatic osteoarthritis. If ORIF is delayed until 10 to 20 days following injury, the major difference in outcomes is fewer complications associated with wound healing. Ankle strength, pain, range of motion, and the development of arthritis are equal regardless of the time until fixation.

REFERENCES: Sirkin M, Sanders R, DePasquale T, et al: A staged protocol for soft tissue management in the treatment of complex pilon fractures. *J Orthop Trauma* 1999;13:78-84.

Pollak AN, McCarthy ML, Bess RS, et al: Outcomes after treatment of high-energy tibial plafond fractures. *J Bone Joint Surg Am* 2003;85:1893-1900.

A-23: Figure 11 shows the radiograph of a 45-year-old woman who has a painful nonunion. Treatment should consist of

1. revision internal fixation with a longer side plate and bone grafting.
2. open reduction and internal fixation with a 95° fixed angle device and bone grafting.
3. hardware removal and retrograde intramedullary nailing.
4. placement of an implantable bone stimulator.
5. proximal femoral resection and total hip arthroplasty.

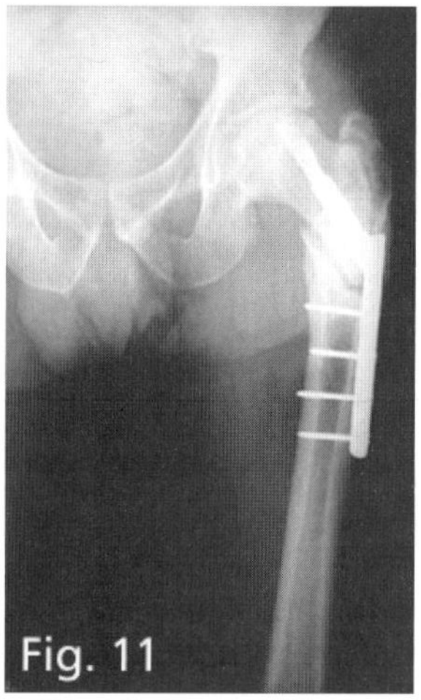
Fig. 11

PREFERRED RESPONSE: 2

DISCUSSION: The radiograph reveals a reverse obliquely subtrochanteric/intertrochanteric fracture. Open reduction and internal fixation should be accomplished with a 95° fixed-angle device. An intramedullary nail with screw fixation into the head is another possible technique. Either method should correct the varus deformity. Exchange of a high-angled screw and plate device to a longer side plate and bone grafting does not afford any improvement in mechanical stability. Hardware removal and retrograde intramedullary nailing is not indicated for this level of proximal femoral injury. Placement of an implantable bone stimulator may change local biologic factors but would not enhance mechanical stability. The patient's femoral head is intact without signs of collapse; therefore, hardware removal, proximal femoral resection, and total hip arthroplasty are not warranted.

REFERENCES: Haidukewych GJ, Israel TA, Berry DJ: Reverse obliquity fractures of the intertrochanteric region of the femur. *J Bone Joint Surg Am* 2001;83:643-650.

Koval KJ, Zuckerman JD: Intertrochanteric fractures, in *Rockwood & Green's Fractures in Adults*, ed 5. Philadelphia, PA, Lippincott Williams and Wilkins, 2001, pp 1635-1681.

A-24: What is the treatment of choice for the injury shown in Figures 12A through 12C?

1. Closed reduction and a short arm cast
2. Splinting in a functional position and early motion
3. Closed or open reduction and internal fixation with Kirschner wires
4. Open reduction and internal fixation with minifragment screws
5. Primary arthrodeses of the carpometacarpal joints

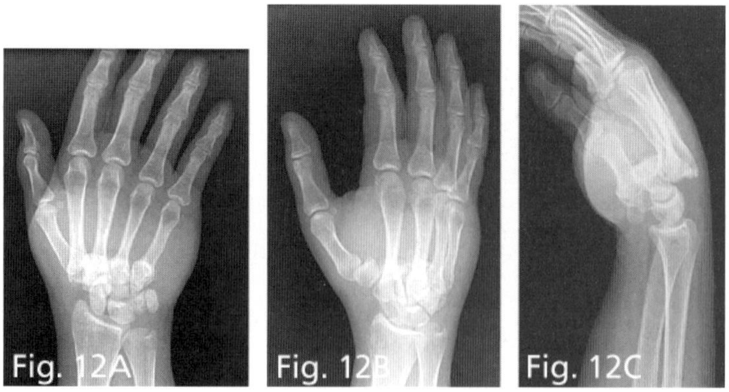
Fig. 12A Fig. 12B Fig. 12C

PREFERRED RESPONSE: 3

DISCUSSION: The radiographs show multiple carpometacarpal dislocations. Reduction is often obtainable but difficult to maintain. Internal fixation is required to maintain the reduction, preferably with Kirschner wires. Closed reduction and percutaneous pinning is preferred by some surgeons. Others recommend open reduction to remove irreconstructable osteochondral fragments from the individual joints and to ensure correct reduction of the carpometacarpal joints. Kirschner wires are removed at 6 to 8 weeks.

(continued on next page)

(A-24: *continued*)

REFERENCES: Prokuski LJ, Eglseder WA Jr: Concurrent dorsal dislocations and fracture-dislocations of the index, long, ring, and small (second to fifth) carpometacarpal joints. *J Orthop Trauma* 2001;15:549-554.

Lawlis JF III, Gunther SF: Carpometacarpal dislocations: Long-term follow-up. *J Bone Joint Surg Am* 1991;73:52-59.

A-25: A 55-year-old woman fell and sustained an elbow dislocation with a coronoid fracture and a radial head fracture. The elbow is reduced and splinted. What is the most common early complication?

1. Brachial artery intimal tear
2. Recurrent dislocation
3. Forearm compartment syndrome
4. Posterior interosseous nerve injury
5. Ulnar nerve palsy

PREFERRED RESPONSE: 2

DISCUSSION: The patient has a dislocation of the elbow with displaced coronoid process and radial head fractures. The elbow is extremely unstable after this injury, and recurrent dislocation in a splint is the most common early complication. Skeletal stabilization of the fractures is required to restore stability of the joint. Characteristics of the fractures will determine the techniques required to restore stability.

REFERENCES: Ring D, Jupiter JB, Zilberfarb J: Posterior dislocation of the elbow with fractures of the radial head and coronoid. *J Bone Joint Surg Am* 2002;84:547-551.

Ring D, Jupiter JB: Fracture-dislocation of the elbow. *J Bone Joint Surg Am* 1998;80:566-580.

A-26: A 25-year-old man sustained the closed injury shown in Figures 13A and 13B. Examination reveals that this is an isolated injury, and the patient is hemodynamically stable. Treatment should consist of

1. multiple flexible intramedullary nails.
2. unreamed intramedullary nailing with static interlocking.
3. unreamed intramedullary nailing with dynamic interlocking.
4. reamed intramedullary nailing with static interlocking.
5. reamed intramedullary nailing with dynamic interlocking.

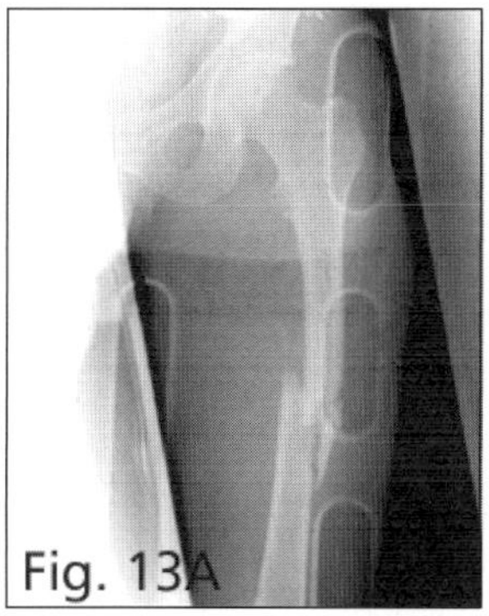
Fig. 13A

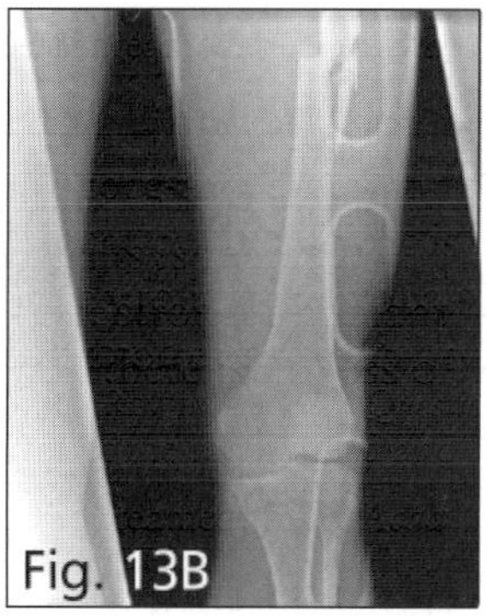
Fig. 13B

PREFERRED RESPONSE: 4

DISCUSSION: The treatment of choice for closed diaphyseal femoral fractures in adults is reamed intramedullary nailing with static interlocking. Reaming allows placement of a larger, stronger implant and offers better healing rates than unreamed nailing. Static interlocking ensures that there is no loss of reduction because of underappreciated fracture lines or comminution.

REFERENCES: Brumback RJ, Virkus WW: Intramedullary nailing of the femur: Reamed versus nonreamed. *J Am Acad Orthop Surg* 2000;8:83-90.

Brumback RJ, Ellison TS, Poka A, et al: Intramedullary nailing of femoral shaft fractures: Part III. Long-term effects of static interlocking fixation. *J Bone Joint Surg Am* 1992;74:106-112.

A-27: Figure 14 shows the radiograph of an elderly man who fell on his right arm. What is the most important determinate of a good outcome following this injury?

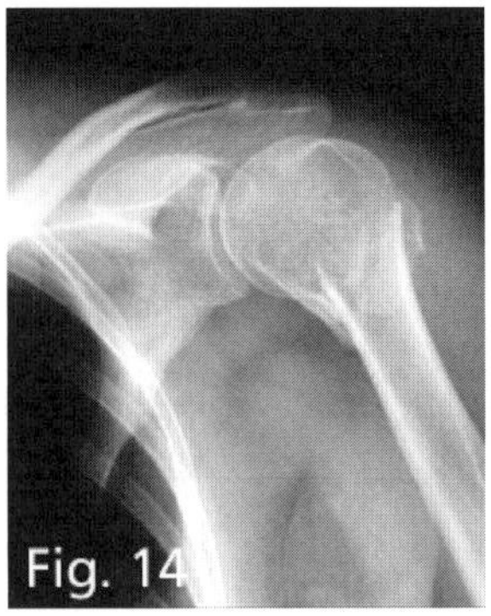
Fig. 14

1. Early open reduction and internal fixation
2. Initiation of physical therapy and passive motion within 2 weeks of the injury
3. Fracture involvement of the greater tuberosity
4. Immobilization with a sling and swathe for 4 weeks
5. Age younger than 70 years

PREFERRED RESPONSE: 2

DISCUSSION: Minimally displaced fractures of the proximal humerus have a good outcome if physical therapy is initiated within 2 weeks of the injury. Results are not affected by age, open reduction and internal fixation, or involvement of the greater tuberosity. Immobilization for longer than 3 weeks will often result in stiffness.

REFERENCES: Koval KJ, Gallagher MA, Marsicano JG, et al: Functional outcome after minimally displaced fractures of the proximal part of the humerus. *J Bone Joint Surg Am* 1997;79:203-207.

Hodgson SA, Mawson SJ, Stanley D: Rehabilitation after two-part fractures of the neck of the humerus. *J Bone Joint Surg Br* 2003;85:419-422.

A-28: A 40-year-old man was involved in a motor vehicle accident and sustained the pelvic injury seen in Figures 15A and 15B. Definitive management of the injury should consist of reduction by

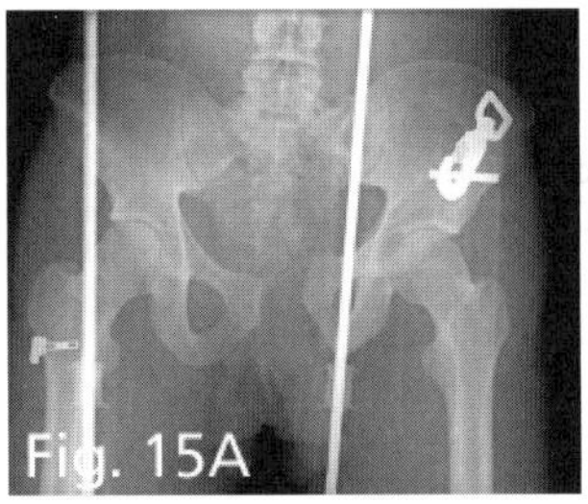
Fig. 15A

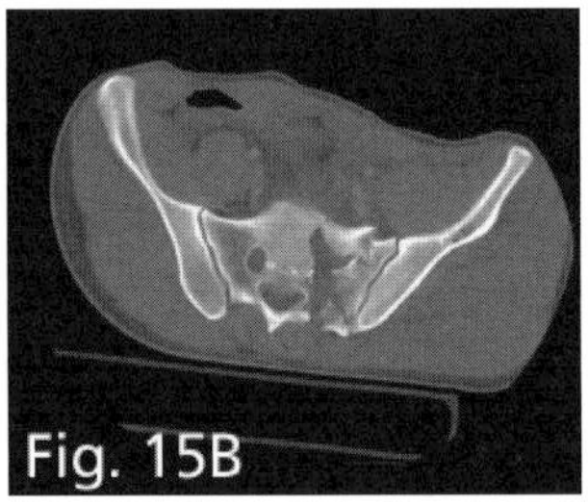
Fig. 15B

1. skeletal traction, and bed rest.
2. anterior external fixation.
3. internal fixation of the symphysis pubis.
4. internal fixation of the symphysis pubis with supplemental external fixation.
5. internal fixation of the symphysis pubis and sacral fracture.

PREFERRED RESPONSE: 5

DISCUSSION: The radiograph reveals disruption of the symphysis pubis and a displaced left sacral fracture. A posterior injury with displacement of greater than 1 cm is unstable, and a sacral fracture is particularly unstable. Surgical stabilization is required for these unstable anterior and posterior injuries. External fixation provides little stability to an unstable posterior pelvic injury. Reduction and internal fixation of the symphysis pubis and sacral fracture will provide the most stable pelvis with the least resultant deformity and allow patient mobilization.

REFERENCES: Tile M: Management of pelvic ring injuries, in Tile M, Helfet DL, Kellam JF, eds: *Fractures of the Pelvis and Acetabulum*, ed 3. Philadelphia, PA, Lippincott Williams & Wilkins, 2003, pp 168-202.

Kabak S, Halici M, Tuncel M, et al: Functional outcome of open reduction and internal fixation for completely unstable pelvic ring fractures (type C): A report of 40 cases. *J Orthop Trauma* 2003;17:555-562.

A-29: A 35-year-old patient sustained a bimalleolar ankle fracture. What is the most reliable method of predicting a tear of the interosseous membrane?

1. Level of the fibular fracture
2. Lauge-Hansen fracture class
3. Intraoperative stress testing
4. Widening of the medial clear space
5. Talar dislocation

PREFERRED RESPONSE: 3

DISCUSSION: The Weber and Lauge-Hansen fracture classifications suggest that the interosseous membrane (IOM) is torn with certain fracture patterns. In a recent study that evaluated ankle fractures with MRI, Nielson and associates identified 30 patients with IOM tears. Ten of the tears did not correspond with the level of the fibular fracture. The authors concluded that stability of the syndesmosis should not be based on the level of the fibular fracture alone but should also include an intraoperative stress test. Transsyndesmotic fixation should be considered for those fractures where the intraoperative stress test demonstrates instability. A widened medial clear space may occur with a deltoid injury and distal fibular fracture in the absence of a significant tear of the interosseous membrane.

REFERENCE: Nielson JH, Sallis JG, Potter HG, et al: Correlation of interosseous membrane tears to the level of the fibular fracture. *J Orthop Trauma* 2004;18:68-74.

A-30: A distal radius fracture in an elderly man is strongly predictive for what subsequent injury?

1. Another distal radius fracture
2. Insufficiency fracture of the spine
3. Insufficiency fracture of the pelvis
4. Hip fracture
5. Proximal humerus fracture

PREFERRED RESPONSE: 4

DISCUSSION: Fractures of the distal radius increase the relative risk of a subsequent hip fracture significantly more in men than in women. A previous spinal fracture has an equally important effect on the risk of a subsequent hip fracture in both sexes.

REFERENCE: Haentjens P, Autier P, Collins J, et al: Colles fracture, spine fracture, and subsequent risk of hip fracture in men and women: A meta-analysis. *J Bone Joint Surg Am* 2003;85:1936-1943.

A-31: What measure of physiologic status best evaluates whether an injured patient is fully resuscitated and best predicts that perioperative complications will be minimized following definitive stabilization of long bone fractures?

1. Urine output greater than 100 mL/h
2. Cardiac output greater than 2
3. Serum lactate level less than 2.5 mmol/L
4. Systolic blood pressure greater than 100 mm Hg
5. Hemoglobin level greater than 10 g/dL

PREFERRED RESPONSE: 3

DISCUSSION: Serum lactate levels can be used to evaluate the effectiveness of the resuscitation of patients who have multiple injuries. Even after resuscitation, patients may have occult hypoperfusion as defined by a serum lactate level greater than 2.5 mmol/L. The studies referenced indicate that these patients are at increased risk of perioperative complications such as organ failure or adult respiratory distress syndrome if definitive surgical fixation of the orthopaedic injuries is pursued prior to correction of the occult hypoperfusion. The other markers may be an indication of current physiology but have not been correlated with perioperative risks.

REFERENCES: Blow O, Magliore L, Claridge JA, et al: The golden hour and silver day: Detection and correction of occult hypoperfusion within 24 hours improves outcomes from major trauma. *J Trauma* 1999;47:964-977.

Crowl A, Young JS, Kahler DM, et al: Occult hypoperfusion is associated with increased morbidity in patients undergoing early femur fracture fixation. *J Trauma* 2000;48:260-267.

Shulman AM: Prediction of patients who will develop prolonged occult hypoperfusion following blunt trauma. *J Trauma* 2004;57:725-800.

A-32: In the treatment of ankle fractures, the superficial peroneal nerve is most commonly injured by

1. a posterior-lateral approach.
2. a lateral approach.
3. a medial approach.
4. an anterior-medial approach.
5. rigid cast immobilization.

PREFERRED RESPONSE: 2

DISCUSSION: In the treatment of ankle fractures, the superficial peroneal nerve is most commonly injured by the use of a direct lateral approach to the ankle. The superficial peroneal nerve and its branches exit the fascial hiatus approximately 9 cm to 10 cm proximal to the tip of the distal fibula with a range of 4 cm to 13 cm, and their course is typically anterior to the midlateral plane of the fibula. However, small branches may course across the surgical plane directly laterally. A posterior-lateral approach diminishes the risk of injury to the superficial peroneal nerve and its branches; however, by moving farther posterior, the sural nerve and its branches may be at increased risk. Cast immobilization may injure the cutaneous nerves about the ankle; however, the risks are greater with surgical intervention. A medial or anterior-medial approach to the ankle will not injure the superficial peroneal nerve at the ankle level.

(continued on next page)

(A-32: *continued*)

REFERENCES: Redfern DJ, Sauve PS, Sakellariou A: Investigation of incidence of superficial peroneal nerve injury following ankle fracture. *Foot Ankle Int* 2003;24:771-774.

Miller SD: Ankle fractures, in Myerson MS, ed: *Foot and Ankle Disorders*. Philadelphia, PA, WB Saunders, 2000, pp 1341-1366.

A-33: A 54-year-old man sustained a small superficial abrasion over the left acromioclavicular joint after falling from his bicycle. Examination reveals no other physical findings. Radiographs show a displaced fracture of the lateral end of the clavicle distal to a line drawn vertically to the coracoid process. Management should consist of

1. open reduction and plate fixation.
2. a figure-of-8 bandage for 4 to 6 weeks.
3. a sling for comfort, followed by physical therapy when pain free.
4. excision of the outer end of the clavicle.
5. a tension band and Kirschner wires.

PREFERRED RESPONSE: 3

DISCUSSION: Displaced clavicular fractures lateral to the coracoid process (Neer type II and III) are best managed nonsurgically with sling immobilization and physical therapy, starting with pendulum exercises and progressing to active-assisted exercises when comfortable. Supervised therapy should be performed for 3 months or until full painless motion is achieved. In a study by Robinson and Cairns, this form of treatment provided patients with an 86% chance of avoiding a secondary reconstructive procedure.

REFERENCES: Robinson CM, Cairns DA: Primary nonoperative treatment of displaced lateral fractures of the clavicle. *J Bone Joint Surg Am* 2004;86:778-782.

Deafenbaugh MK, Dugdale TW, Staeheli JW, et al: Nonoperative treatment of Neer type II distal clavicle fractures: A prospective study. *Contemp Orthop* 1990;20:405-413.

A-34: A 47-year-old man sustained a degloving injury over the pretibial surface and anterior ankle region in a motor vehicle accident. After débridement and irrigation, there is inadequate tissue for closure of the exposed anterior tibial tendon and tibia. Prior to definitive soft-tissue coverage, management should consist of

1. immediate split-thickness skin grafting.
2. immediate xenograft application.
3. a vacuum-assisted closure device.
4. dressing changes with sulfasalazine cream.
5. a cross-leg flap.

PREFERRED RESPONSE: 3

DISCUSSION: With soft-tissue loss, local or free flap coverage may be necessary to treat exposed tendon and bone. However, a vacuum-assisted closure device is a good temporizing dressing. It prevents external contamination, reduces edema around the wound, increases oxygen tension in the wound, and promotes the formation of granulation tissue. The use of this negative pressure device has been described in both acute traumatic and in chronic wound scenarios. If sufficient granulation tissue forms, closure may be by split graft, avoiding a more complex coverage procedure. Immediate skin grafting over the exposed anterior tibial tendon and tibia would have a low likelihood of success. Dressing changes with sulfasalazine may be beneficial in a burn wound to assist with removal of skin slough; however, in a granulating wound, the material may be toxic to early epithelialization. Xenograft is a foreign body and should not be applied to an acute contaminated open wound. Historically, a cross-leg flap was a treatment alternative for lower extremity soft-tissue loss; however, its current applications are extremely limited.

REFERENCES: Webb LX: New techniques in wound management: Vacuum assisted wound closure. *J Am Acad Orthop Surg* 2002;10:303-311.

Clare MP, Fitzgibbons TC, McMullen ST, et al: Experience with the vacuum assisted closure negative pressure technique in the treatment of non-healing diabetic and dysvascular wounds. *Foot Ankle Int* 2002;23:
896-901.

A-35: The humeral nonunion shown in Figure 16 is most likely to unite when using what method of treatment?

1. Intramedullary nail
2. Pulsed electromagnetic fields
3. Compression plate
4. Intramedullary nail and bone graft
5. Compression plate and bone graft

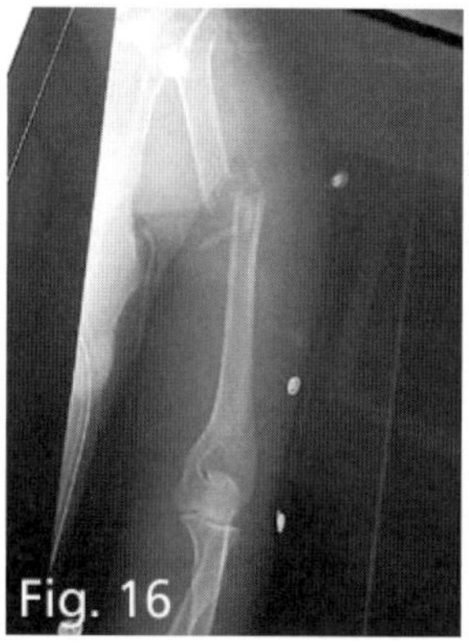

PREFERRED RESPONSE: 5

DISCUSSION: The radiograph shows an atrophic nonunion of the humeral shaft. The management of humeral nonunions has been studied with compression plates and bone graft, as well as intramedullary nailing and bone graft. Compression plating with bone graft results in the highest rate of union. Compression plating by itself is not adequate, given the bone loss and lack of callus in this nonunion. Pulsed electromagnetic fields is a viable option for hypertrophic nonunions where there is inherent

(continued on next page)

(A-35: *continued*)

stability. Intramedullary nailing does not provide as much compression and stability as that achieved with compression plating.

REFERENCES: Pugh DM, McKee MD: Advances in the management of humeral nonunion. *J Am Acad Orthop Surg* 2003;11:48-59.

McKee MD, Miranda MA, Riemer BL, et al: Management of humeral nonunion after the failure of locking intramedullary nails. *J Orthop Trauma* 1996;10:492-499.

A-36: An adult with a distal humeral fracture underwent open reduction and internal fixation. What is the most common postoperative complication?

1. Loss of elbow range of motion
2. Nonunion
3. Malunion
4. Infection
5. Ulnar nerve dysfunction

PREFERRED RESPONSE: 1

DISCUSSION: Most patients lose elbow range of motion after open reduction and internal fixation of a distal humeral fracture. Ulnar nerve dysfunction, nonunion, and infection all occur less commonly.

REFERENCES: Webb LX: Distal humerus fractures in adults. *J Am Acad Orthop Surg* 1996;4:336-344.

McKee MD, Wilson TL, Winston L, et al: Functional outcome following surgical treatment of intra-articular distal humeral fractures through a posterior approach. *J Bone Joint Surg Am* 2000;82:1701-1707.

A-37: The radiographs and CT scan seen in Figures 17A through 17D reveal what type of acetabular fracture pattern?

1. Transverse
2. Transverse with posterior wall
3. Both column
4. Posterior wall anterior hemitransverse
5. T-type

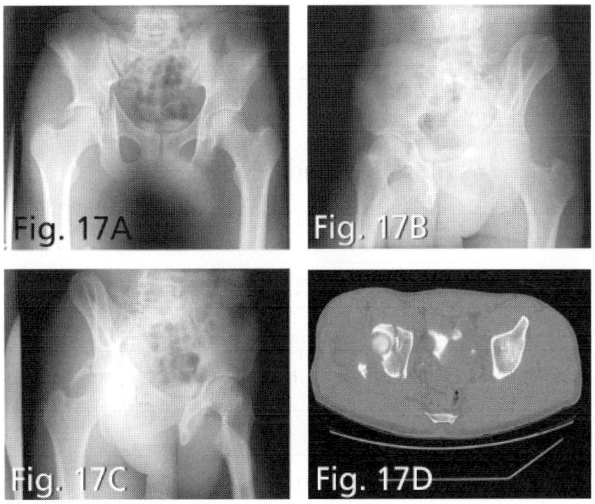

Fig. 17A Fig. 17B Fig. 17C Fig. 17D

PREFERRED RESPONSE: 2

DISCUSSION: The AP, obturator oblique, and iliac oblique views of the pelvis reveal a fracture that disrupts the iliopectineal and ilioischial lines, indicating a fracture that involves both anterior and posterior columns. However, it does not have the other features of anterior or posterior column fracture patterns. A displaced posterior wall fracture is

(continued on next page)

(A-37: *continued*)

also present, best seen on the obturator oblique view. The anterior to posterior directed fracture line on the CT scan indicates a transverse fracture; therefore, the patient has a transverse with posterior wall fracture pattern. A T-type fracture would be similar but would have a break into the obturator ring.

REFERENCES: Tile M: Describing the injury: Classification of acetabular fractures, in Tile M, Helfet DL, Kellam JF, eds: *Fractures of the Pelvis and Acetabulum*, ed 3. Philadelphia, PA, Lippincott Williams & Wilkins, 2003, pp 427-475.

Brandser E, Marsh JL: Acetabular fractures: Easier classification with a systematic approach. *Am J Roentgenol* 1998;171: 1217-1228.

A-38: A 26-year-old man sustained an isolated injury to his left hip joint in a motor vehicle accident. Closed reduction was performed, and the postreduction radiograph is shown in Figure 18. Management should now consist of

1. emergent open reduction and fixation of the fracture.
2. skeletal traction and expedient open reduction and fixation of the fracture.
3. skeletal traction for 6 weeks, followed by physical therapy.
4. crutches and no weight bearing for 6 weeks.
5. bed rest for 1 week and follow-up radiographs to determine if the fragment has moved.

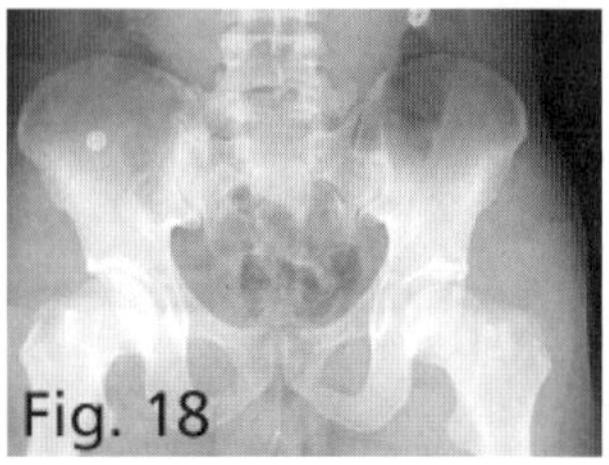

Fig. 18

PREFERRED RESPONSE: 2

DISCUSSION: The patient has a posterior fracture-dislocation of the hip and following reduction, an incarcerated fragment of bone resulted in an incongruent reduction. Whereas expedient removal of the fragment is required to limit articular cartilage damage, this situation is not an emergency and the procedure may be performed when the appropriate surgical team is available and the patient's condition stabilized. Skeletal traction through either the femur or tibia may relieve some pressure on the joint and prevent articular damage. Nonsurgical care for incarcerated fragments is contraindicated.

REFERENCES: Tile M, Olson SA: Decision making: Non operative and operative indications for acetabular fractures, in Tile M, Helfet DL, Kellam JF, eds: *Fractures of the Pelvis and Acetabulum*. Philadelphia, PA, Lippincott Williams and Wilkins, 2003, pp 496-532.

Letournel E, Judet R: *Fractures of the Acetabulum*, ed 2. Berlin, Germany, Springer-Verlag, 1993, pp 337-339, p 507.

A-39: A 35-year-old man is brought to the emergency department following a motorcycle accident. He is breathing spontaneously and has a systolic blood pressure of 80 mm Hg, a pulse rate of 120/min, and a temperature of 98.6° F (37° C). Examination suggests an unstable pelvic fracture; AP radiographs confirm an open book injury with vertical displacement on the left side. Ultrasound evaluation of the abdomen is negative. Despite administration of 4 L of normal saline solution, he still has a systolic pressure of 90 mm Hg and a pulse rate of 110. Urine output has been about 20 mL since arrival 35 minutes ago. What is the best next course of action?

1. Continued resuscitation with fluids and blood
2. Ongoing resuscitation and pelvic angiography
3. Application of an external fixator in the emergency department
4. A pelvic binder and continued resuscitation
5. A pelvic binder, skeletal traction, and continued resuscitation

PREFERRED RESPONSE: 5

DISCUSSION: The patient is at risk for pelvic vascular injury and major hemorrhage. This type of complication of pelvic trauma is highest in motorcyclists. Once it is recognized that the pelvic ring has opened, it is important to close that ring to tamponade any venous bleeding with a pelvic binder and to add a skeletal traction pin to the limb on the involved side. This will correct any translational displacement. The noninvasive pelvic binders or sheets are easy to apply and are very effective. They do not compromise future care and allow the surgeons access to the abdomen. External fixation or pelvic resuscitation clamps require a certain amount of skill to apply and are not always available. If the pelvic stabilization does not improve the hemodynamic parameters in 10 to 15 minutes, angiography is necessary.

REFERENCE: Mayo K, Kellam JK: Pelvic ring disruptions, in Browner BD, ed: *Skeletal Trauma*, ed 3. Philadelphia, PA, WB Saunders, 2003, pp 1052-1108.

A-40: A healthy 25-year-old man sustains a grade IIIB open tibial fracture. Following appropriate débridement, irrigation, and stabilization with an external fixator, the soft-tissue injury is shown in Figure 19. What is the most appropriate definitive soft-tissue coverage procedure?

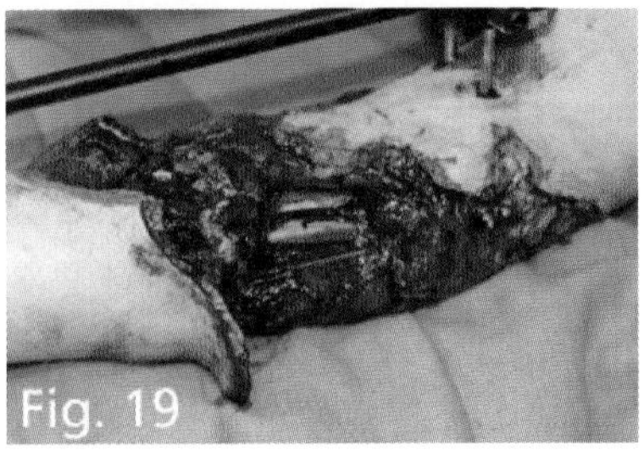
Fig. 19

1. Split-thickness skin graft
2. Full-thickness skin graft
3. Soleus rotation flap
4. Medial gastrocnemius rotation flap
5. Free latissimus dorsi flap with microvascular anastomosis

PREFERRED RESPONSE: 5

DISCUSSION: This is a very large, near-circumferential defect with posterior as well as anterior skin and muscle injury. Bone is exposed. The posterior muscles cannot be rotated because they are part of the zone of injury. The bone and other poorly vascularized areas of this wound would not accept a skin graft. The best chance for limb salvage will be to obtain soft-tissue coverage with a free tissue transfer using the latissimus dorsi.

REFERENCES: Mathes SJ, Nahai F: Vascular anatomy of muscle: Classification and applications, in Mathes SJ, Nahai F, eds: *Clinical Application for Muscle and Musculocutaneous Flaps*. St Louis, MO, CV Mosby, 1982, p 20.

Bos GD, Buehler MJ: Lower-extremity local flaps. *J Am Acad Orthop Surg* 1994;2:342-351.

A-41: A 25-year-old woman undergoes surgical treatment of a displaced proximal humeral fracture via a deltopectoral approach. At the first postoperative visit, she reports a tingling numbness along the anterolateral aspect of the forearm. What structure is most likely injured?

1. Medial cord of the brachial plexus
2. Radial nerve
3. Median nerve
4. Axillary nerve
5. Musculocutaneous nerve

PREFERRED RESPONSE: 5

DISCUSSION: Sensation along the anterolateral aspect of the forearm is supplied by the lateral antebrachial cutaneous nerve, the terminal branch of the musculocutaneous nerve. The musculocutaneous nerve can be injured by proximal humeral fractures or dislocations, and is also at risk during surgical exposure if excessive retraction is placed on the conjoint tendon. The musculocutaneous nerve enters the conjoint tendon 1 cm to 5 cm distal to the coracoid process.

REFERENCES: McIlveen SJ, Duralde XA, D'Alessandro DF, et al: Isolated nerve injuries about the shoulder. *Clin Orthop* 1994;306:54-63.

Warner JP: Frozen shoulder: Diagnosis and management. *J Am Acad Orthop Surg* 1997;5:130-140.

A-42: A 32-year-old man sustained a fracture of his upper arm in a motor vehicle accident. Radiographs are shown in Figure 20. Because of other associated injuries, surgical stabilization is chosen. What technique will result in the fewest complications and the best outcome?

1. Retrograde locked intramedullary nail
2. Antegrade reamed locked intramedullary nail
3. Flexible nails
4. Open reduction and plate fixation
5. External fixation

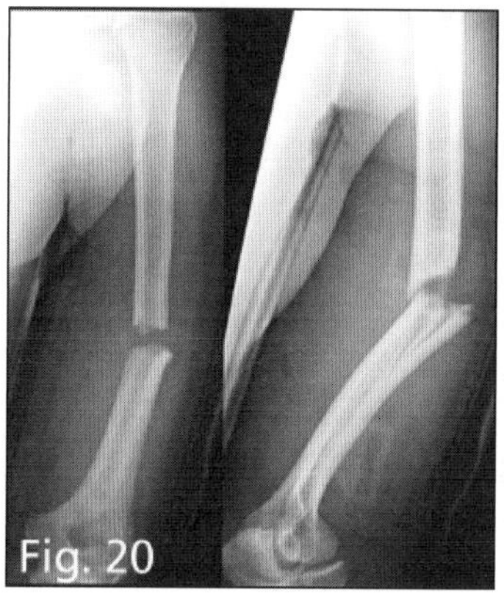
Fig. 20

PREFERRED RESPONSE: 4

DISCUSSION: Most humeral fractures will heal with nonsurgical functional brace management. When the initial pain has subsided in a coaptation splint, the patient is converted to a functional brace and allowed to use the arm for activities. The fracture should heal within 6 to 12 weeks with acceptable results. Surgery is indicated if there is vascular injury, open injury, floating elbow, chest injury, bilateral humeral fractures, or if a reduction cannot be obtained or maintained. The surgical treatment of choice is either antegrade reamed locked intramedullary nailing or plate osteosynthesis. Plate osteosynthesis appears to offer better results with respect to union, function, and risk of complications.

REFERENCES: Schemitsch EH, Bhandari M: Fractures of the humeral shaft, in Browner BD: *Skeletal Trauma*, ed 3. Philadelphia, PA, WB Saunders, 2003, pp 1481-1511.

Chapman JR, Henley MB, Agel J: Randomized prospective study of humeral shaft fracture fixation: Intramedullary nails versus plates. *J Orthop Trauma* 2000;14:162-166.

A-43: During a posterior approach to the glenoid with retraction as shown in Figure 21, care should be taken during superior retraction to avoid injury to which of the following structures?

1. Axillary artery
2. Axillary nerve
3. Branch of the circumflex scapular artery
4. Profunda brachii artery
5. Suprascapular nerve and artery

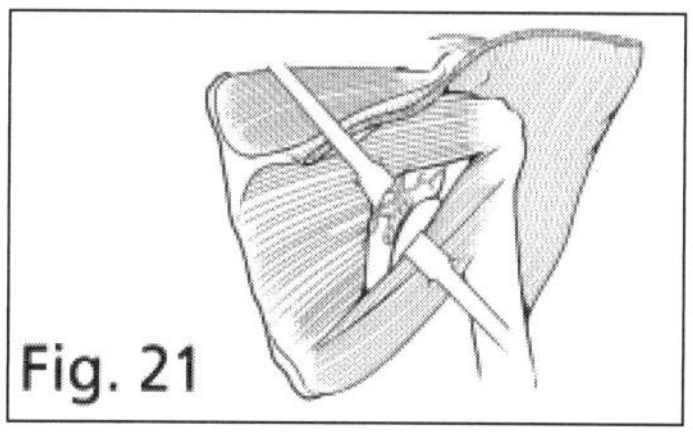
Fig. 21

PREFERRED RESPONSE: 5

DISCUSSION: During a posterior approach to the shoulder for either a scapular fracture, glenoid fracture, or posterior shoulder pathology, the interval between the teres minor and infraspinatus is split. Excessive superior retraction on the infraspinatus, or excessive dissection superomedially under the infraspinatus muscle and tendon can cause injury to the suprascapular nerve and/or artery. During dissection in this interval, the axillary artery and axillary nerve are well protected. A branch of the circumflex scapular artery ascends between the teres minor and infraspinatus muscle, but it is at risk during dissection on the scapula in the midportion of the interval and not during superior retraction. The profunda brachii artery is not present in this interval.

(continued on next page)

(A-43: *continued*)

REFERENCES: Jerosch JJ, Greig M, Peuker ET, et al: The posterior subdeltoid approach: A modified access to the posterior glenohumeral joint. *J Shoulder Elbow Surg* 2001;10:265-268.

Judet R: Surgical treatment of scapular fractures. *Acta Orthop Belg* 1964;30:673-678.

Kavanagh BF, Bradway JK, Cofield RH: Open reduction and internal fixation of displaced intra-articular fractures of the glenoid fossa. *J Bone Joint Surg Am* 1993;75:479-484.

A-44: A 42-year-old woman sustained a closed, displaced talar neck fracture in a motor vehicle accident. Which of the following is an avoidable complication of surgical treatment?

1. Posttraumatic arthritis of the subtalar joint
2. Posttraumatic arthritis of the ankle joint
3. Malunion of the talus
4. Osteonecrosis of the talus
5. Complex regional pain syndrome

PREFERRED RESPONSE: 3

DISCUSSION: Malunion of the talus is a devastating complication that leads to malpositioning of the foot and subsequent arthrosis of the subtalar joint complex. This is considered an avoidable complication in that accurate surgical reduction will minimize its development. Posttraumatic arthritis of the subtalar joint, osteonecrosis of the talus, posttraumatic arthritis of the ankle joint, and complex regional pain syndrome all may develop as a result of the initial traumatic event and may not be avoidable despite anatomic reduction.

REFERENCES: *Rockwood and Green's Fractures in Adults*, ed 5. Philadelphia, PA, Lippincott, Williams and Wilkins, 2001, pp 2091-2132.

Daniels TR, Smith JW, Ross TI: Varus malalignment of the talar neck: Its affects on the position of the foot and on subtalar motion. *J Bone Joint Surg Am* 1996;78:1559-1567.

A-45: Figures 22A and 22B show the radiographs of a 48-year-old woman who smokes cigarettes and sustained a segmental femoral shaft fracture in a motor vehicle accident 9 months ago. Initial management consisted of stabilization with a reamed statically locked intramedullary nail. She now reports lower leg pain that increases with activity. In addition to advising the patient to quit smoking, management should include

1. ultrasonic stimulation for 3 months.
2. removal of the nail and plate fixation.
3. continued observation.
4. removal of the distal locking screws to dynamize the nail.
5. exchange reamed nailing with bone graft.

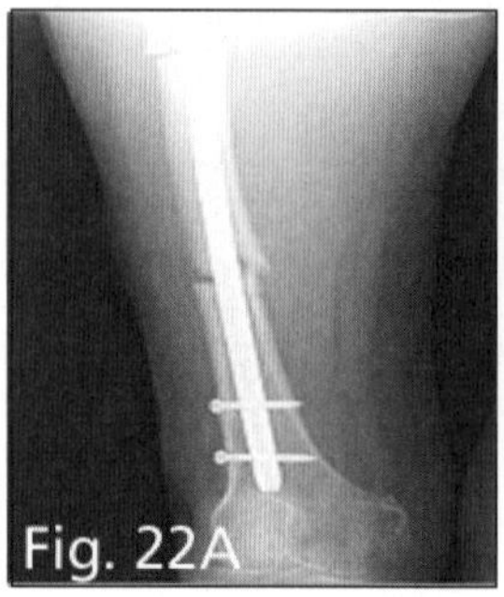
Fig. 22A

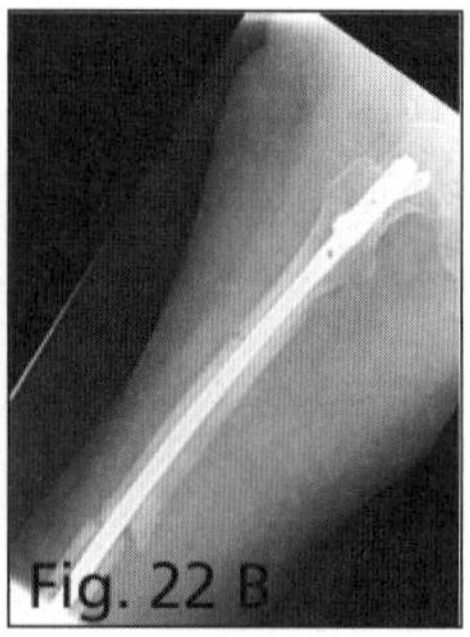
Fig. 22 B

(continued on next page)

(A-45: *continued*)

PREFERRED RESPONSE: 5

DISCUSSION: The patient has an oligotrophic nonunion of the distal femoral fracture. Although the proximal fracture appears incompletely united, it was stable at exchange nailing. The treatment of choice is exchange reamed nailing to at least 2 mm above the nail in place. Bone grafting is debatable. Recent studies have shown a 70% to 75% success rate with exchange nailing only, so in nonhypertrophic nonunions, bone grafting can be considered. Nonsurgical management consisting of observation or external stimulation runs the risk of implant failure. Plate fixation is acceptable but is considered a second choice because of the need to consider stabilization of the proximal fracture until union is achieved. Also, plate fixation definitely requires bone grafting.

REFERENCES: Webb LX, Winquist RA, Hansen ST: Intramedullary nailing and reaming for delayed union or nonunion of the femoral shaft: A report of 105 consecutive cases. *Clin Orthop* 1986;212:133-141.

Weresh MJ, Hakanson R, Stover MD, et al: Failure of exchange reamed intramedullary nailing for ununited femoral shaft fractures. *J Orthop Trauma* 2000;14:335-338.

Hak DG, Lee SS, Goulet JA: Success of exchange reamed intramedullary nailing for femoral shaft nonunion or delayed union. *J Orthop Trauma* 2000;14:178-182.

A-46: A 34-year-old man sustained a tibial fracture in a motorcycle accident. What perioperative variable is associated with the greatest relative risk for reoperation to achieve bone union?

1. Sex
2. Delay in initial surgical treatment
3. Use of NSAIDs
4. Smoking
5. Cortical contact of ≤ 50%

PREFERRED RESPONSE: 5

DISCUSSION: In a recent analysis of 200 patients with tibial fractures, Bhandari and associates attempted to identify variables that were predictive of reoperation. The variables in the study were type of injury (fracture pattern), degree of open injury, mechanism of injury, cortical bone contact, postoperative complications, polytrauma, anti-inflammatory drug use, nail insertion technique (reamed versus nonreamed), smoking history, alcohol use, diabetes mellitus, peripheral vascular disease, age, disability status preinjury, sex, surgeon, time to surgery, steroid use, phenytoin use, antibiotic use, anticoagulant use, and type of fixation used. Three variables were statistically significant predictors of reoperation to achieve bone union in the first postinjury year: transverse fracture pattern, open fracture, and cortical contact of 50% or less. Using these three variables, four reoperation risk groups were identified based on the number of these three variables present: 0, 1, 2, or 3. The risk for reoperation was 0%, 18%, 47%, and 94%, respectively. The authors concluded that these statistics can provide prognostic information to patients and help identify those high-risk patients where early intervention to achieve union is indicated. In addition, the data highlight the significance of achieving cortical contact at the time of initial fixation.

REFERENCE: Bhandari M, Tornetta P III, Sprague S, et al: Predictors of reoperation following operative management of fractures of the tibial shaft. *J Orthop Trauma* 2003;17:353-361.

A-47: A 17-year-old boy sustained a 5-mm laceration on the lateral aspect of the hindfoot while working on a farm. Examination in the emergency department revealed no fractures. Twenty-four hours later, he returns to the emergency department with increasing foot pain. A thin, brown drainage is seen emanating from the wound. He has a temperature of 102.0° F (38.9° C), a pulse rate of 120, and a blood pressure of 80/40 mm Hg. Examination of the foot reveals diffuse swelling, ecchymosis, tenderness, and crepitus with palpation. Current radiographs are shown in Figures 23A and 23B. Management should now consist of

1. intravenous antibiotics.
2. hyperbaric oxygen therapy and intravenous antibiotics.
3. surgical débridement, primary wound closure, and intravenous antibiotics.
4. surgical débridement, closure of the wound over drains, and intravenous antibiotics.
5. surgical débridement, leaving the wound open, and intravenous antibiotics.

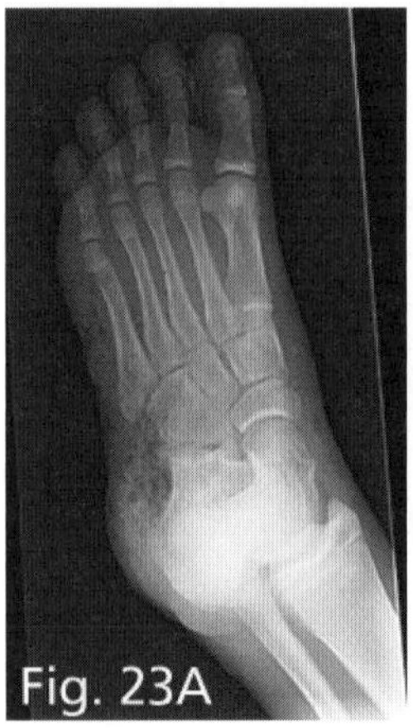
Fig. 23A

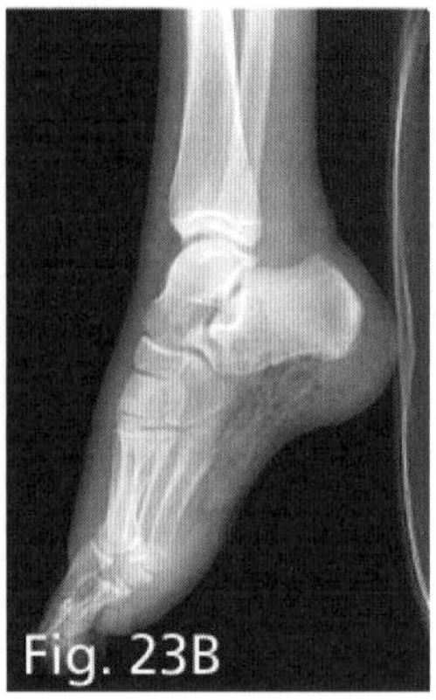
Fig. 23B

PREFERRED RESPONSE: 5

DISCUSSION: The mechanism and environment in which the injury occurred, the clinical picture, and the radiographic findings of gas in the tissues suggest an anaerobic gram-positive bacterial infection. This can be a life- and limb-threatening infection. Treatment should consist of wide débridement of all devitalized tissue, and intravenous antibiotics should be started. Wounds should be left open to allow bacterial effluent and increase oxygen tension in the wound. Hyperbaric oxygen may be used as an adjuvant but is no substitute for débridement.

REFERENCES: Pellegrini VD, Reid JS, Evarts CM: Complications, in Rockwood CA, Green DP, Bucholz RW, et al, eds: *Rockwood and Green's Fractures in Adults*, ed 4. Philadelphia, PA, Lippincott-Raven, 1996, vol 1, pp 458-463.

Ayers DC, Murray DC: Complications of the treatment of fractures and dislocations: General considerations, in Epps CH Jr, ed: *Complications in Orthopedic Surgery*, ed 4. Philadelphia, PA, JB Lippincott, 1994, pp 3-48.

A-48: A healthy, active, independent 74-year-old woman fell and sustained the elbow injury shown in Figures 24A and 24B. Management should consist of

1. a sling and early elbow range-of-motion exercises.
2. a long arm cast for 6 weeks.
3. open reduction and internal fixation.
4. total elbow arthroplasty.
5. elbow arthrodesis.

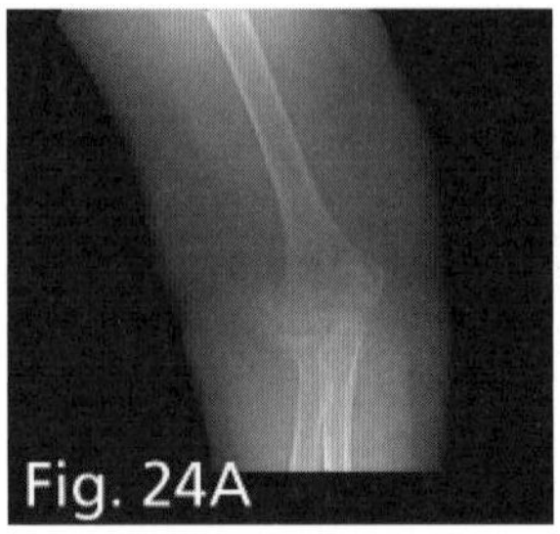
Fig. 24A

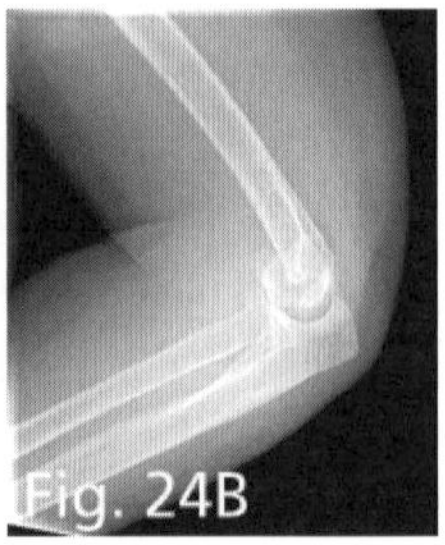
Fig. 24B

PREFERRED RESPONSE: 4

DISCUSSION: Open reduction and internal fixation of distal humeral fractures in elderly patients often fails. These fractures characteristically have a very small distal segment and poor bone quality, resulting in failure of fixation and nonunion. Nonunion is often painful and functionally debilitating. Total elbow arthroplasty provides good results when used for distal humeral fractures in elderly patients with

(continued on next page)

(A-48: *continued*)

osteopenic bone and fracture patterns thought to be irreconstructable. Long arm casting may result in union, but the resulting stiffness is unacceptable for an active patient. Elbow arthrodesis has few indications. A sling and range-of-motion exercises will often result in a painful and debilitating nonunion at the fracture site.

REFERENCES: Frankle MA, Herscovici D Jr, DiPasquale TG, et al: A comparison of open reduction and internal fixation and primary total elbow arthroplasty in the treatment of intra-articular distal humerus fractures in women older than 65. *J Orthop Trauma* 2003;17:473-480.

Cobb TK, Morrey BF: Total elbow arthroplasty as primary treatment for distal humerus fractures in elderly patients. *J Bone Joint Surg Am* 1997;79:826-832.

Obremskey WT, Bhandari M, Dirschl DR, et al: Internal fixation versus arthroplasty of comminuted fractures of the distal humerus. *J Orthop Trauma* 2003;17:463-465.

A-49: A 25-year-old man is brought to the emergency department following a motor vehicle accident. Extrication time was 2 hours, and in the field he had a systolic blood pressure by palpation of 90 mm Hg. Intravenous therapy was started, and on arrival to the emergency department his systolic blood pressure is 90 mm Hg with a pulse rate of 130. Examination reveals a flail chest and a femoral diaphyseal fracture. Ultrasound of the abdomen is positive. The trauma surgeons take him to the operating room for an exploratory laparotomy. At the conclusion of the procedure, systolic pressure of 100 mm Hg with a pulse rate of 110. Oxygen saturation is 90% on 100% oxygen, and the patient's temperature is 95.0° F (35° C). What is the recommended treatment of the femoral fracture at this time?

1. Reamed intramedullary nail
2. Unreamed intramedullary nail
3. Percutaneous plate fixation
4. Skeletal traction
5. External fixation

PREFERRED RESPONSE: 5

DISCUSSION: This is a borderline trauma patient for whom serious consideration for damage control orthopaedic surgery is required. His prolonged hypotension, abdominal injury, and chest injury put him at higher risk for serious postinjury complications. Further surgery, such as definitive fracture fixation, adds metabolic load and injury to his system. It is prudent to consider femoral fracture stabilization with an external fixator until he is physiologically recovered as evidenced by a normal base excess and/or lactate acid levels, as well as all other parameters of resuscitation. A borderline patient has been described as polytrauma with an Injury Severity Score (ISS) > 20 and thoracic trauma (Abbreviated Injury Scale [AIS] > 2); polytrauma and abdominal/pelvic trauma (Moore > 3) and hemodynamic shock (initial blood pressure < 90 mm Hg); ISS > 40; bilateral lung contusions on radiographs; initial mean pulmonary arterial pressure > 24 mm Hg; pulmonary artery pressure increase during intramedullary nailing > 6 mm Hg. Factors that worsen the situation following surgery include multiple long bones and truncal injury (AIS > 2), estimated surgery time of more than 6 hours, arterial injury and hemodynamic instability, and exaggerated inflammatory response (eg, interleukin-6 > 800 pg/mL). It is incumbent on the orthopaedic surgeon who is a member of the trauma team to make sure that he or she is aware of these factors and guides the team to the best patient care.

(continued on next page)

(A-49: *continued*)

REFERENCES: Pape HC, Hildebrand F, Pertschy S, et al: Changes in the management of femoral shaft fractures in polytrauma patients: From early total care to damage control orthopaedic surgery. *J Trauma* 2002;53:452-461.

Bosse M, Kellam JF: Orthopaedic decision making in the multiple trauma patient, in Browner BD, ed: *Skeletal Trauma*, ed 3. Philadelphia, PA, WB Saunders, 2003, pp 133-146.

A-50: A 26-year-old man was thrown from a car and sustained the injury seen in Figures 25A and 25B. Nonsurgical management of this injury is recommended. Which of the following factors increases the risk of nonunion?

1. Male sex
2. Diaphyseal location
3. Comminuted displaced fracture
4. Young age
5. Associated injuries

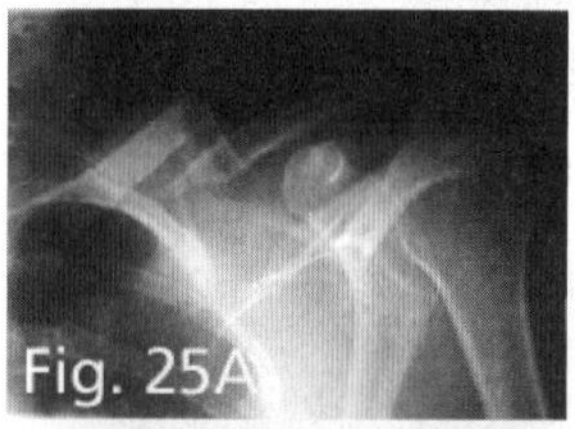

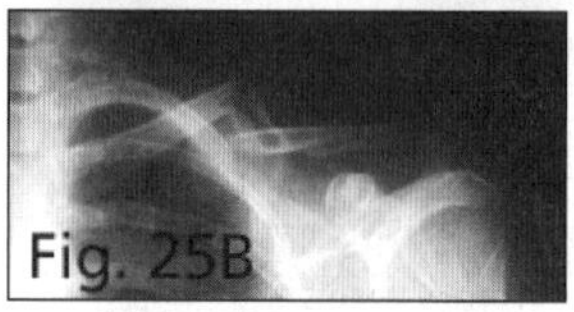

PREFERRED RESPONSE: 3

DISCUSSION: The patient has a displaced comminuted clavicle middle one-third fracture from a high-energy mechanism. Recent literature on high-energy clavicular fractures suggests a higher rate of nonunion than previously reported. A nonunion rate of 30% has been reported by Hill and associates when the fracture fragments are displaced more than 1.5 cm. In addition, several patients had neurologic symptoms related to the injury. Robinson and associates reported an increased risk of nonunion in women, elderly patients, comminuted fractures, and injuries with a lack of cortical contact.

REFERENCES: Hill JM, McGuire MH, Crosby LA: Closed treatment of displaced middle-third fractures of the clavicle gives poor results. *J Bone Joint Surg Br* 1997;79:537-539.

Wick M, Muller EJ, Kollig E: Midshaft fractures of the clavicle with a shortening of more than 2 cm predispose to nonunion. *Arch Orthop Trauma Surg* 2001;121:207-211.

Robinson CM, Court-Brown CM, McQueen MM, et al: Estimating the risk of nonunion following nonoperative treatment of a clavicular fracture. *J Bone Joint Surg Am* 2004;86:1359-1365.

Orthopaedic Oncology/ Systemic Disease

Q-1: The arrow in Figure 1 points toward a finding consistent with which of the following?

1. Metastatic disease
2. Hemangioma
3. Flexion-compression fracture
4. Infection
5. Diastematomyelia

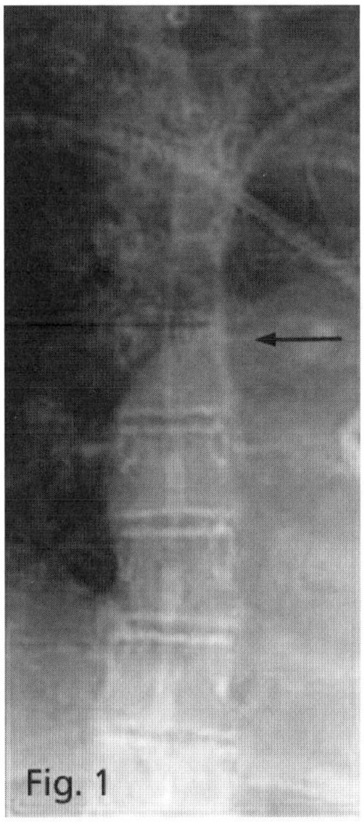

Fig. 1

Q-2: A 62-year-old woman reports diffuse aches and pains of the hip and pelvis. She denies any significant trauma but does have a history of chronic anemia. Figure 2A shows a radiograph of the pelvis, and Figures 2B and 2C show T2-weighted MRI scans. What is the most likely diagnosis?

1. Chondrosarcoma
2. Diffuse fibrous dysplasia
3. Multiple myeloma
4. Osteoporosis
5. Bone infarcts

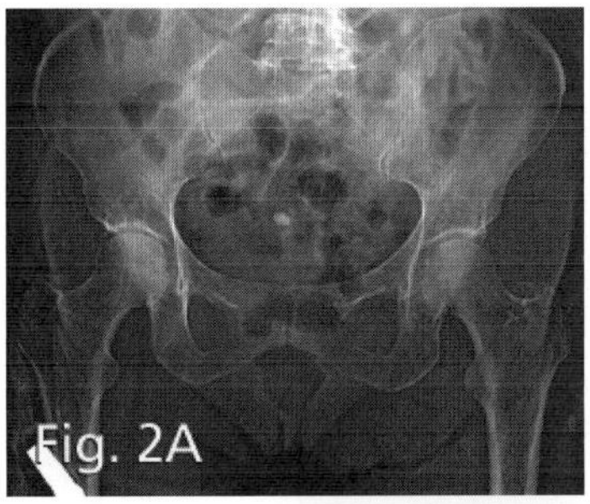

Fig. 2A

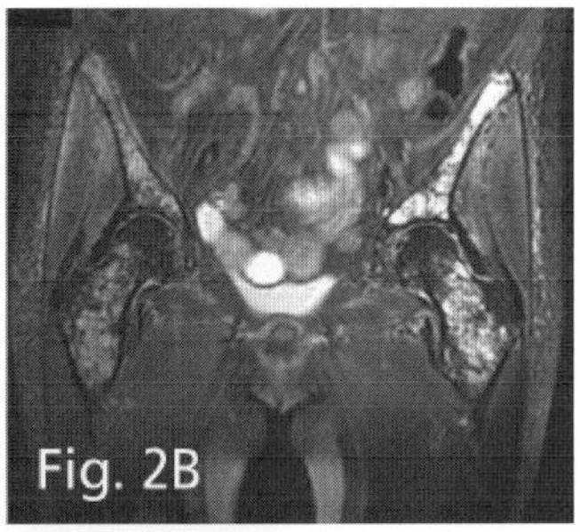

Fig. 2B

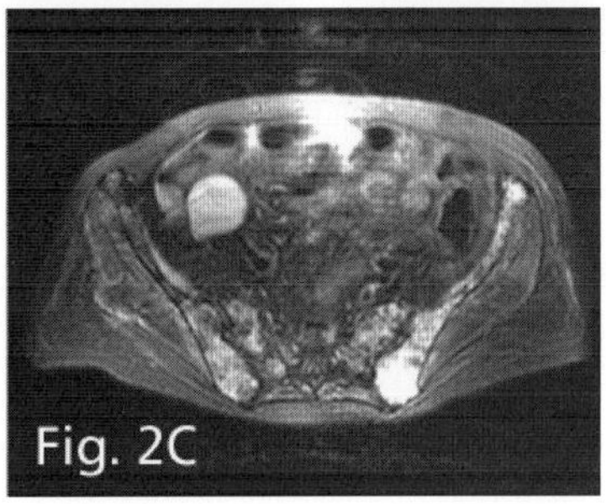

Fig. 2C

Q-3: A 23-year-old woman reports right knee pain and fullness. The pain is worse with activity but is also present at rest. Radiographs are shown in Figures 3A and 3B. What is the most likely diagnosis?

1. Osteosarcoma
2. Chondroblastoma
3. Stress fracture
4. Posttraumatic changes
5. Chondrosarcoma

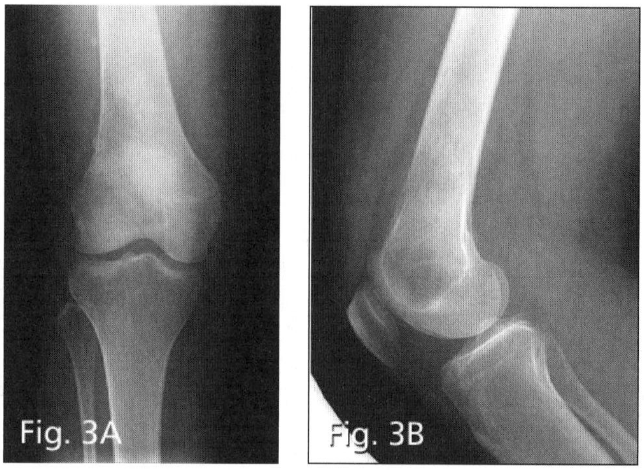

Fig. 3A Fig. 3B

Q-4: Figures 4A through 4C show the coronal T1-weighted, T2-weighted fat-saturated, and T1-weighted fat-saturated gadolinium MRI scans of the proximal thigh of a 52-year-old woman who reports a mass in the medial thigh and groin area. She notes that the fullness of the mass has increased over the course of many months. Based on these findings, what is the most likely diagnosis?

1. Malignant fibrous histiocytoma
2. Liposarcoma
3. Synovial cell sarcoma
4. Leiomyosarcoma
5. Clear cell sarcoma

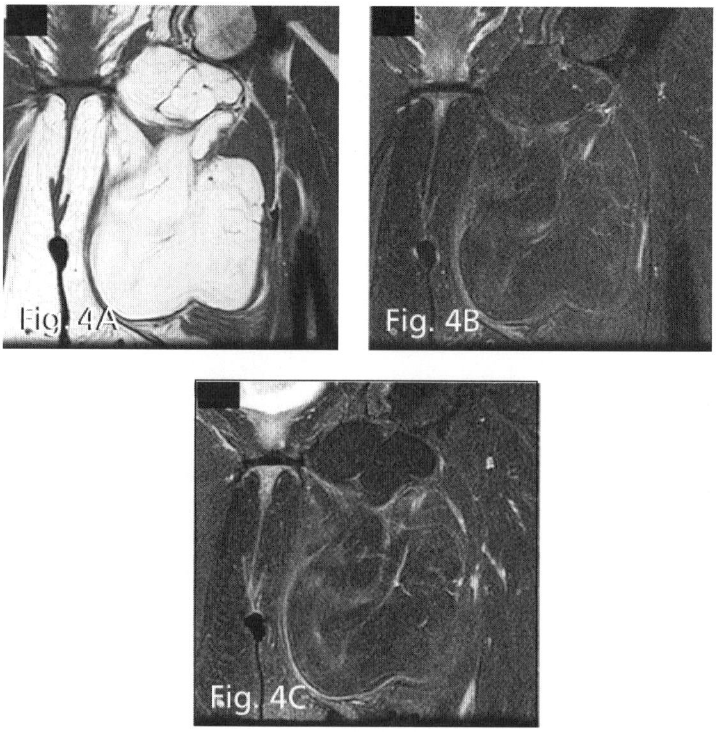

Fig. 4A Fig. 4B Fig. 4C

Q-5: Figures 5A and 5B show the radiographs of a left proximal femoral lesion noted serendipitously following minor trauma to the left hip. The patient has no thigh pain and is fully active without limitation. What is the most likely diagnosis of this bony lesion?

1. Chondroblastoma
2. Enchondroma
3. Giant cell tumor
4. Fibrous dysplasia
5. Osteoblastoma

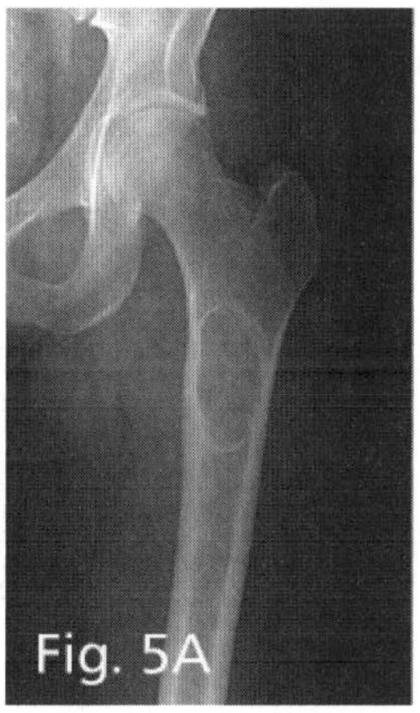
Fig. 5A

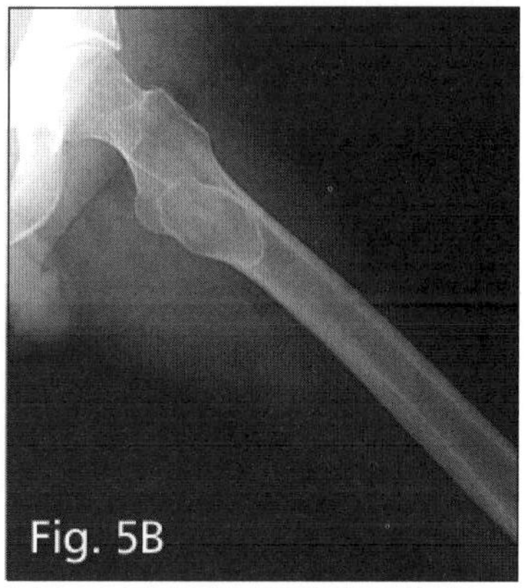
Fig. 5B

Q-6: A 13-year-old girl has had increasing left hip pain for the past 4 months. A radiograph, bone scan, MRI scan, and photomicrograph are shown in Figures 6A through 6D. Which of the following immunohistochemistry results would confirm the most likely diagnosis?

1. Cytokeratin positive
2. PAS negative
3. Reticulin positive
4. MIC-2 positive
5. Vimentin negative

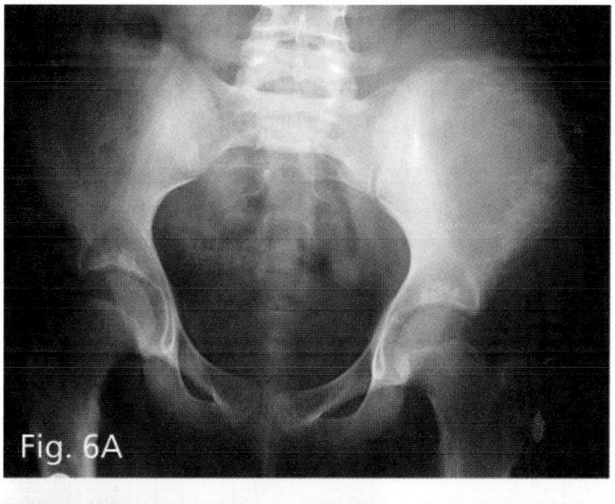
Fig. 6A

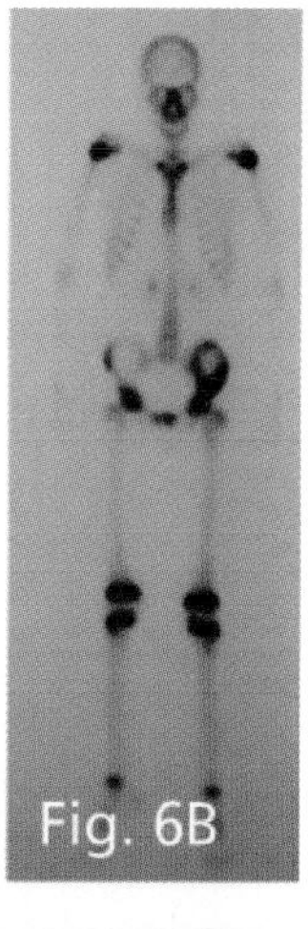
Fig. 6B

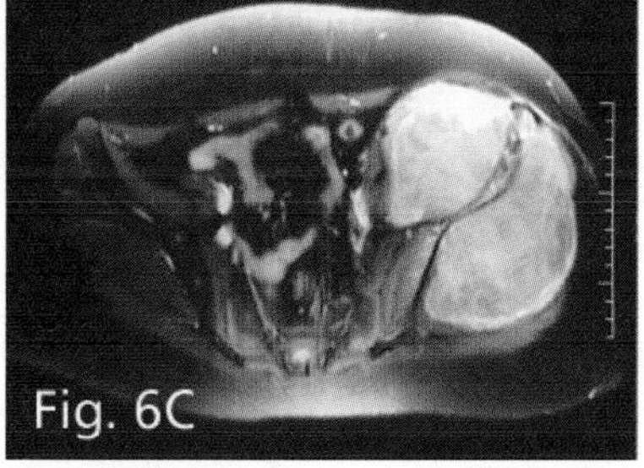
Fig. 6C

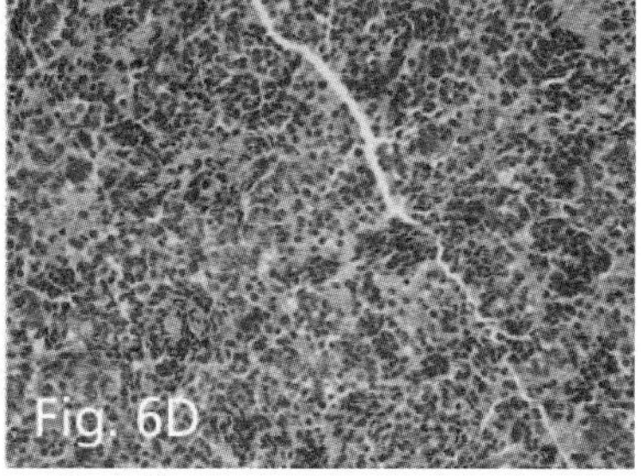
Fig. 6D

Q-7: Which of the following is the preferred treatment for symptomatic localized pigmented villonodular synovitis (PVNS) of the knee?

1. Observation
2. External beam radiation therapy
3. Intra-articular radiation therapy
4. Resection of nodule only
5. Open complete synovectomy

Q-8: A healthy 52-year-old woman is seeking professional advice about management of osteoporosis. She has no risk factors for osteoporosis. What is the best recommendation for bone health for this patient?

1. Bone mineral density testing performed semiannually
2. No treatment
3. A healthy diet high in calcium
4. 1,000 to 1,500 mg calcium supplement plus 400 to 800 IU vitamin D per day
5. Estrogen therapy

Q-9: A 37-year-old man pulled his hamstring playing softball 3 weeks ago. The patient had not noted any mass prior to his injury. MRI scans of the posterior thigh are shown in Figures 7A and 7B. Figure 7C shows the biopsy specimen from a needle biopsy. What is the most likely diagnosis?

1. Intramuscular hematoma
2. Lipoma
3. Myositis ossificans
4. Malignant fibrous histiocytoma
5. Liposarcoma

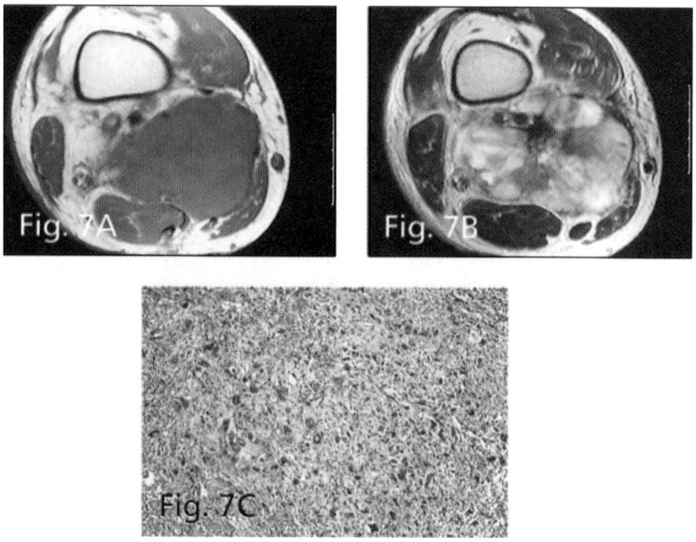
Fig. 7A
Fig. 7B
Fig. 7C

Q-10: A 16-year-old boy has had left knee pain and swelling after sustaining a minor twisting injury while playing basketball 2 weeks ago. Figures 8A through 8E show the radiograph, MRI scans, and biopsy specimens. What is the most likely diagnosis?

1. Osteomyelitis
2. Tuberculosis
3. Osteosarcoma
4. Ewing sarcoma
5. Malignant fibrous histiocytoma (MFH)

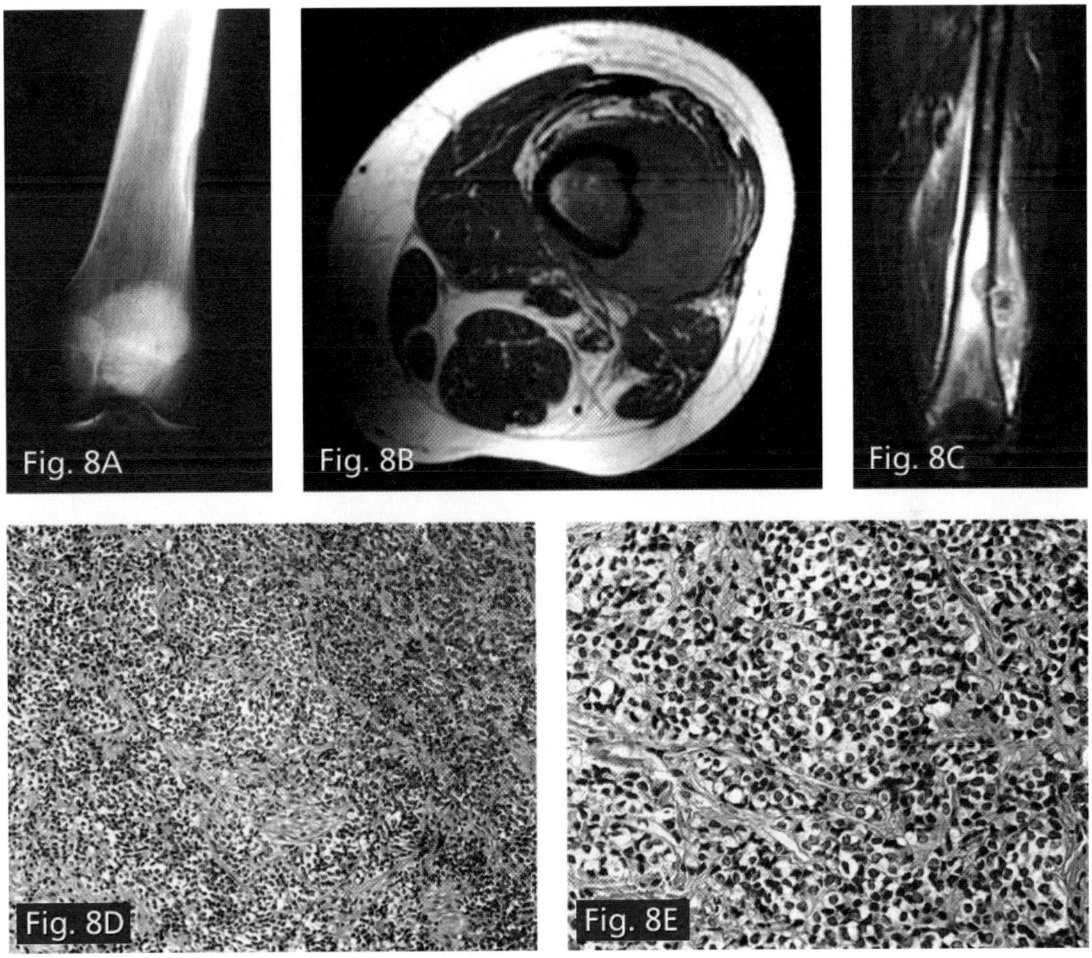

Q-11: A 13-year-old boy has a painless "knot" over his left hip. History reveals that he injured his left hip playing soccer 4 months ago. A radiograph and MRI scan obtained at the time of injury are shown in Figures 9A and 9B. He is very active and is currently asymptomatic. A current radiograph is shown in Figure 9C. What is the next most appropriate step in management?

1. Observation
2. Anti-inflammatory medication
3. Referral to a rheumatologist
4. Biopsy
5. Resection of the lesion

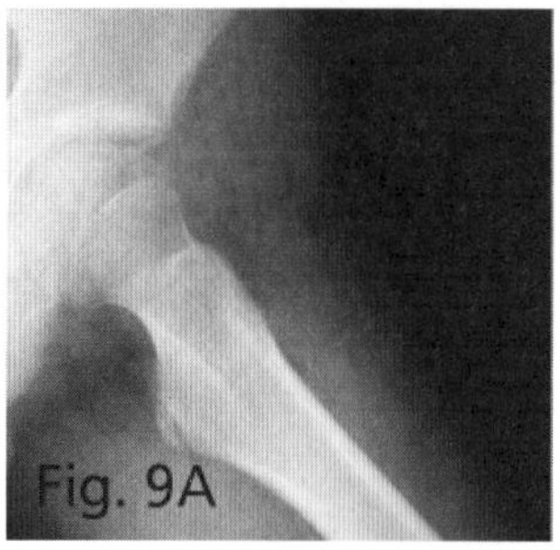
Fig. 9A

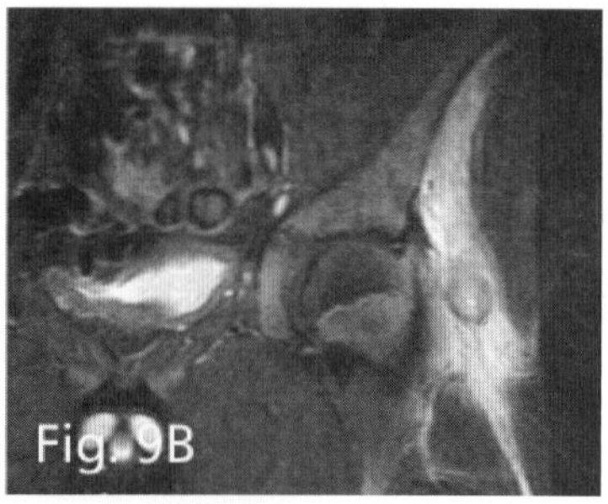
Fig. 9B

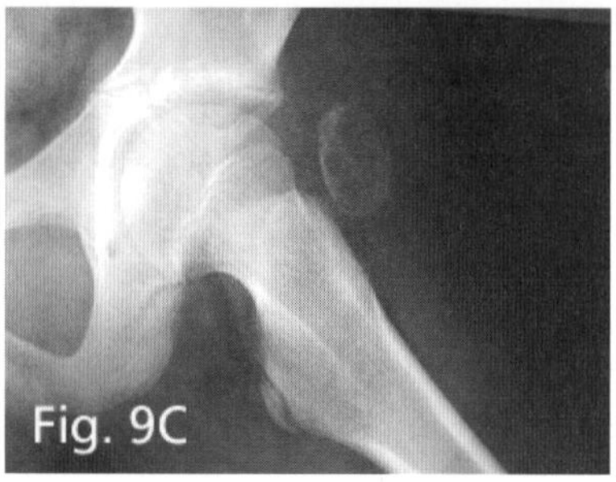
Fig. 9C

Q-12: Figure 10A shows the clinical photograph of an 83-year-old woman who has an enlarging left forearm mass. MRI scans are shown in Figures 10B and 10C. What is the next most appropriate step in management?

1. Radiation therapy
2. Needle biopsy
3. Marginal resection
4. Chemotherapy
5. Amputation

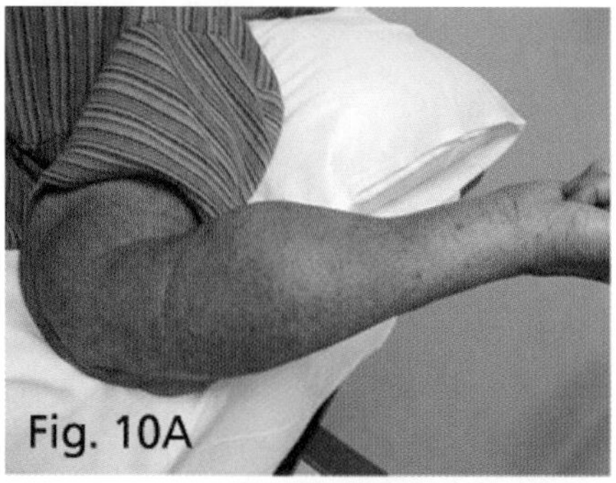
Fig. 10A

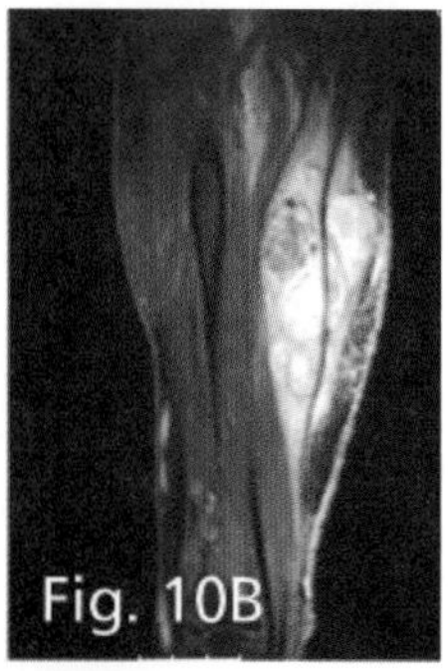
Fig. 10B

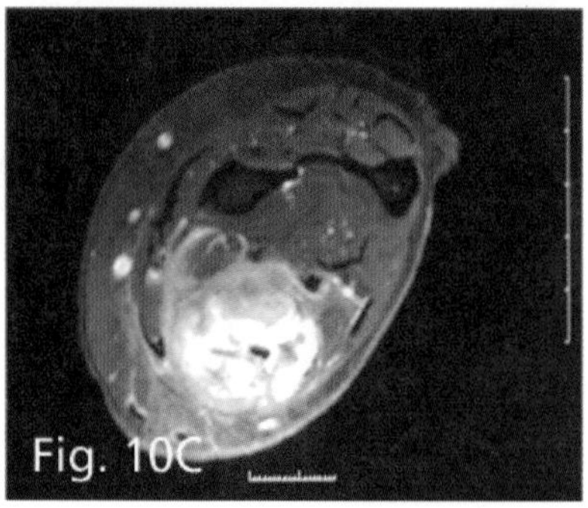
Fig. 10C

Q-13: A 20-year-old man has a large soft-tissue mass behind his knee. MRI scans are shown in Figures 11A through 11C. Figure 11D shows a clinical photograph of his chest. The patient's condition is most likely a result of a defect in what gene?

1. *NF1*
2. *EWS*
3. *EXT1*
4. *P53*
5. *Rb*

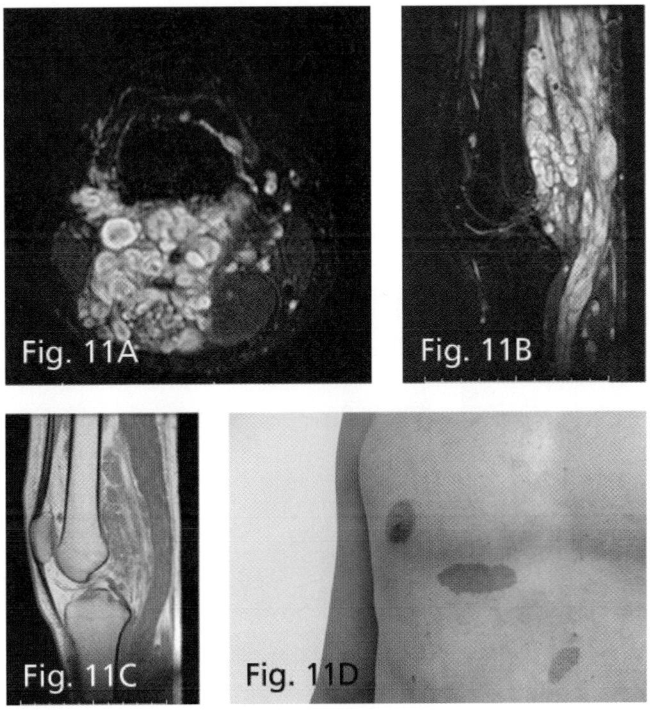

Q-14: A 35-year-old man reports the development of a painful 2-cm nodule on his dorsal wrist over the past 3 years. A surgeon excised the lesion with a presumptive diagnosis of a ganglion cyst. Histology sections from the excision are shown in Figures 12A and 12B. What is the most likely diagnosis?

1. Ganglion cyst
2. Clear cell sarcoma
3. Epithelioid sarcoma
4. Epidermal inclusion cyst
5. Synovial sarcoma

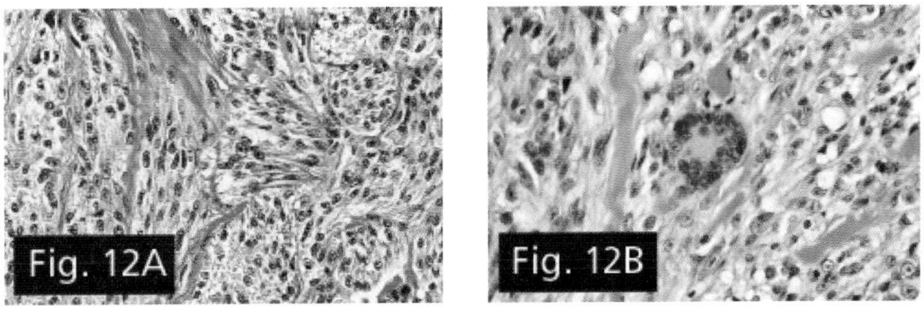

Orthopaedic Oncology/Systemic Disease: Questions

Q-15: Figures 13A through 13E show the radiograph, MRI scans, and histology sections of a 17-year-old boy. What is the most likely diagnosis?

1. Giant cell tumor
2. Chondroblastoma
3. Clear cell chondrosarcoma
4. Osteosarcoma
5. Tuberculous septic arthritis

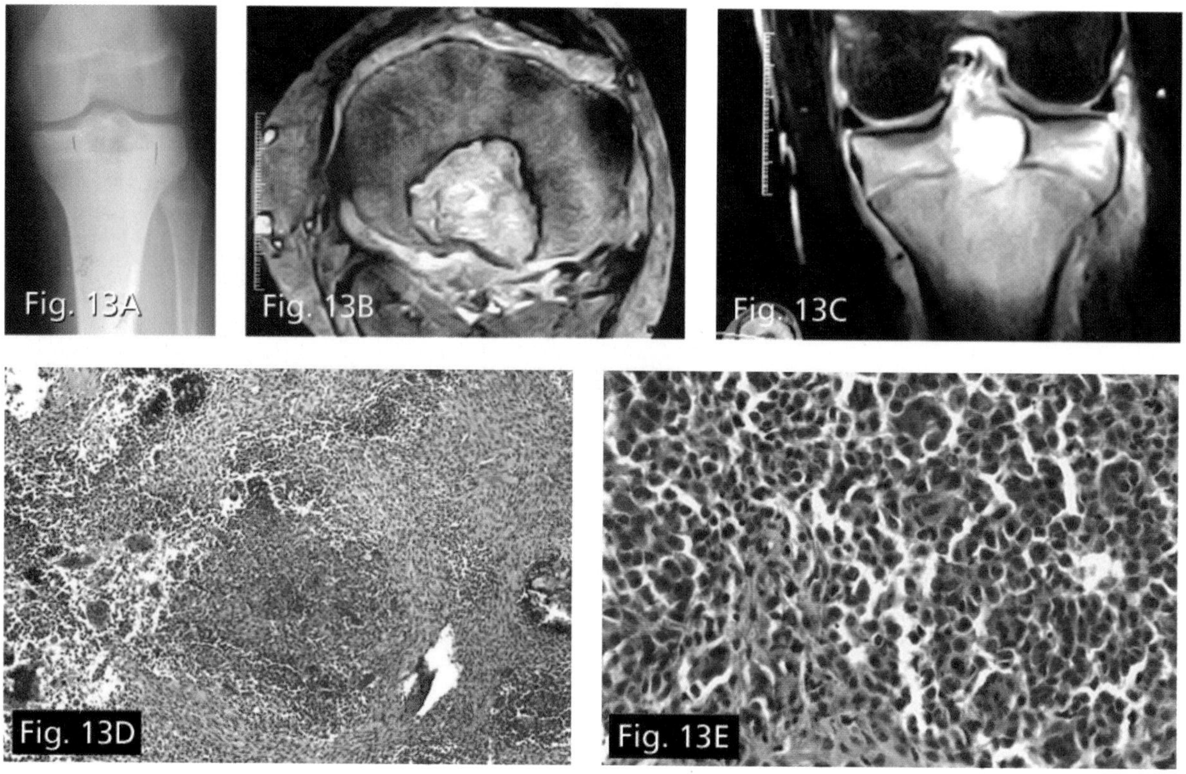

Fig. 13A Fig. 13B Fig. 13C Fig. 13D Fig. 13E

Q-16: An 18-year-old boy reports increasing pain with weight bearing on his right leg and at night. Examination reveals swelling around the right midcalf. Radiographs and an MRI scan are shown in Figures 14A through 14C, and a histology section is shown in Figure 14D. What is the preferred treatment?

1. Chemotherapy and surgical resection
2. Débridement and intravenous antibiotics
3. Chemotherapy alone
4. Radiation therapy alone
5. Surgical resection alone

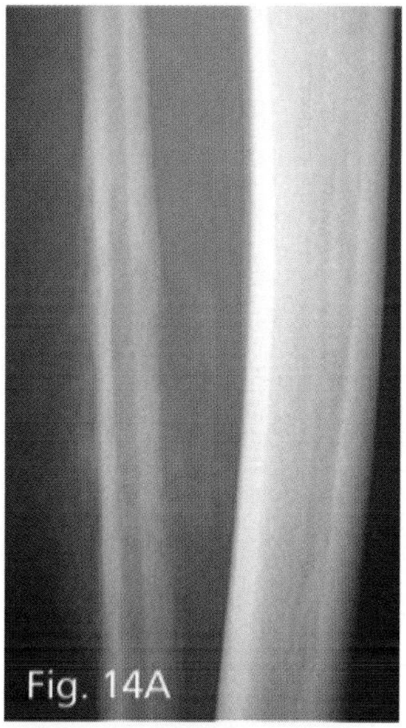
Fig. 14A

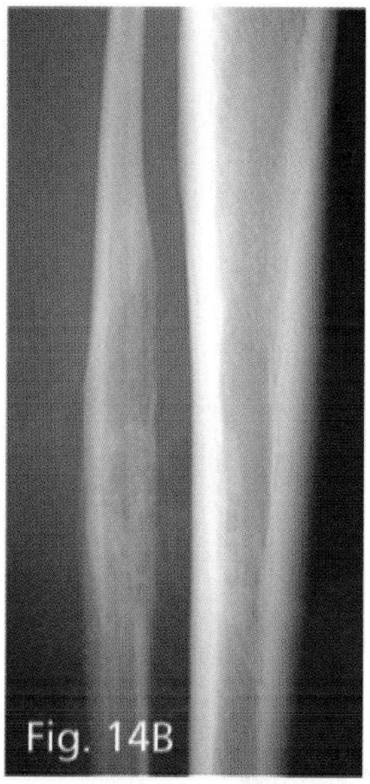
Fig. 14B

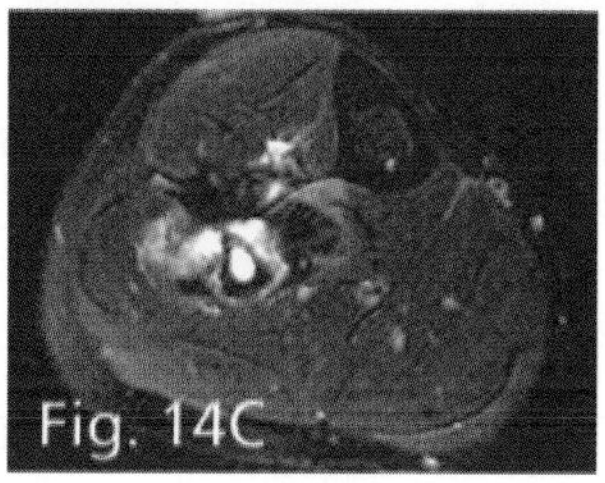
Fig. 14C

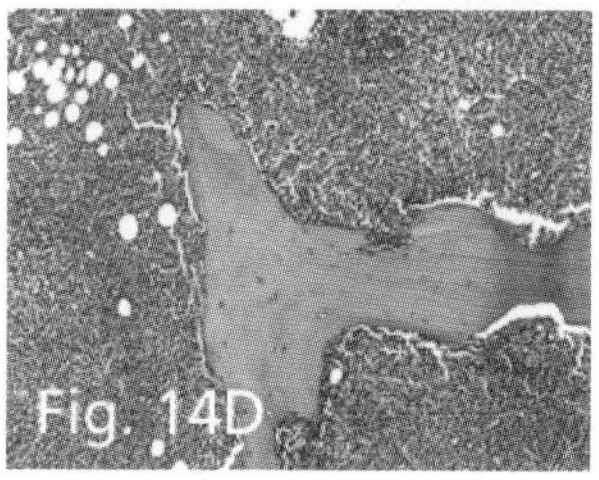
Fig. 14D

Q-17: A 54-year-old woman reports worsening pain in her buttock, especially when sitting for long periods of time. She has occasional pain and paresthesias radiating down her posterior leg. She has no significant medical history. MRI scans are shown in Figures 15A and 15B and a histology section is shown in Figure 15C. What is the most likely diagnosis?

1. Myxoid liposarcoma
2. Myxoma
3. Malignant fibrous histiocytoma
4. Fibromatosis
5. Neurofibroma

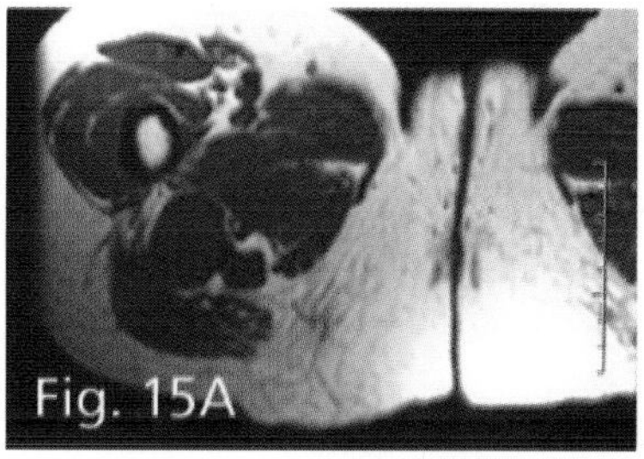
Fig. 15A

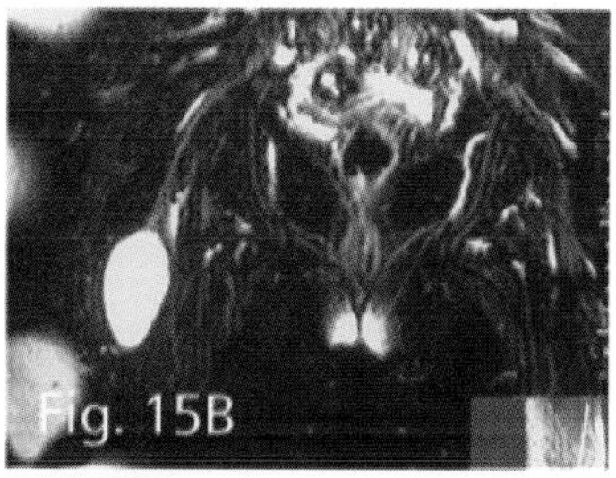
Fig. 15B

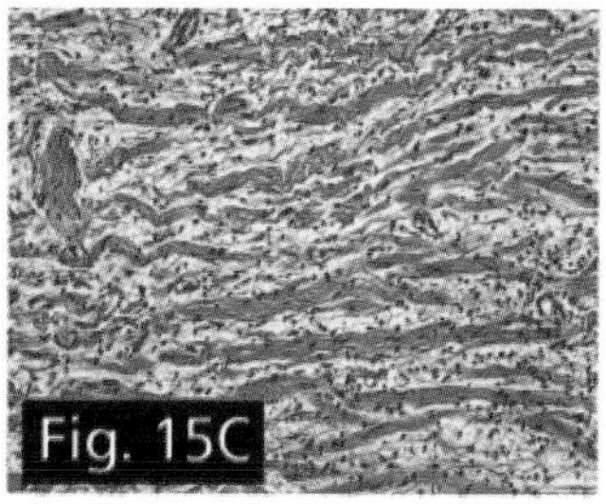
Fig. 15C

Q-18: It has been shown that bisphosphonate-based supportive therapy (pamidronate or zoledronate) reduces skeletal events (onset or progression of osteolytic lesions) both in patients with multiple myeloma and in cancer patients with bone metastasis. The use of bisphosphonate therapy has been associated with

1. increased medical complications of treatment.
2. osteonecrosis of the jaw.
3. improved long-term survival rates.
4. anorexia.
5. decreased quality-of-life measures.

Q-19: A 12-year-old girl has had pain in her right knee for 1 month that started as activity-related and progressed to night pain. Radiographs are shown in Figures 16A and 16B, and a histology section is shown in Figure 16C. What is the recommended treatment?

1. Resection of the distal femur and postoperative chemotherapy
2. Preoperative chemotherapy followed by radiation therapy, then resection of the distal femur
3. Preoperative chemotherapy followed by surgical resection of the lesion and postoperative chemotherapy
4. Preoperative chemotherapy followed by radiation therapy, resection of the distal femur, then postoperative chemotherapy
5. Resection of the distal femur followed by radiation therapy

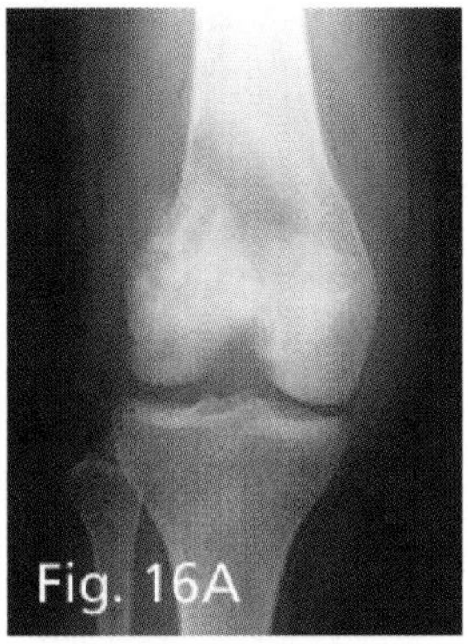
Fig. 16A

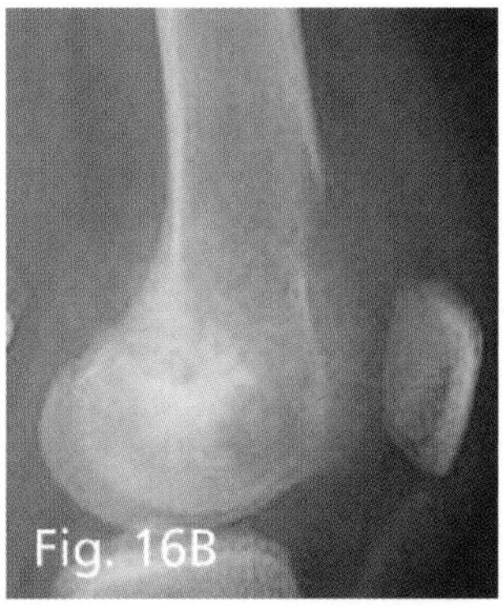
Fig. 16B

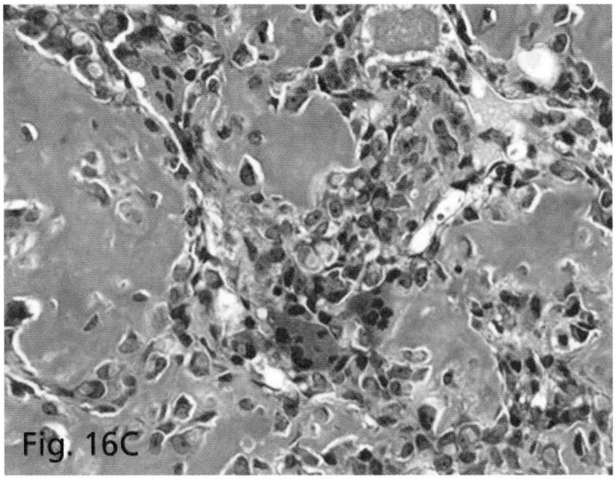
Fig. 16C

Q-20: Figure 17A shows the clinical photograph of a 31-year-old man who has a slowly growing nodule on his right middle finger. It is minimally tender, and there is no erythema on examination. A histology section is shown in Figure 17B. What is the most likely diagnosis?

1. Clear cell sarcoma
2. Clear cell carcinoma
3. Epidermal inclusion cyst
4. Nora tumor (BPOP)
5. Epithelioid sarcoma

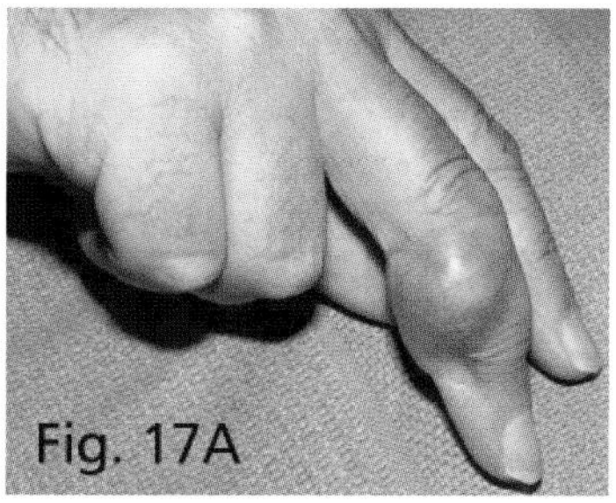
Fig. 17A

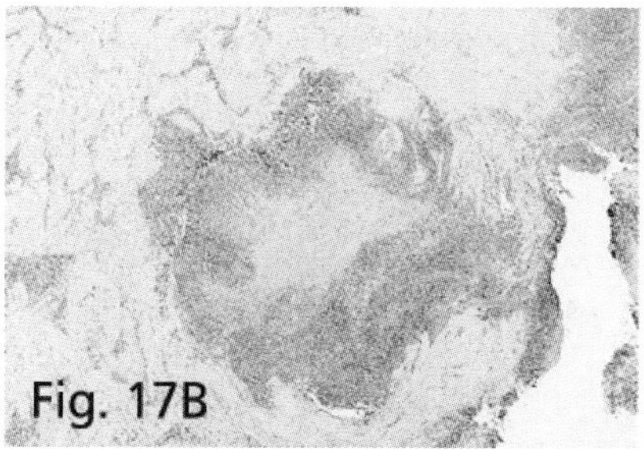
Fig. 17B

Q-21: A 17-year-old girl who initially presented during childhood with multiple skeletal lesions, café-au-lait spots, and precocious puberty now has bone pain. A recent bone scan reveals multiple areas of increased scintigraphic uptake, including bilateral proximal femurs. A radiograph is shown in Figure 18. In addition to activity modification, what is the best next line of treatment for decreasing her pain?

1. Bisphosphonates
2. Calcitonin
3. Parathyroid hormone
4. Vitamin D and calcium
5. Methotrexate

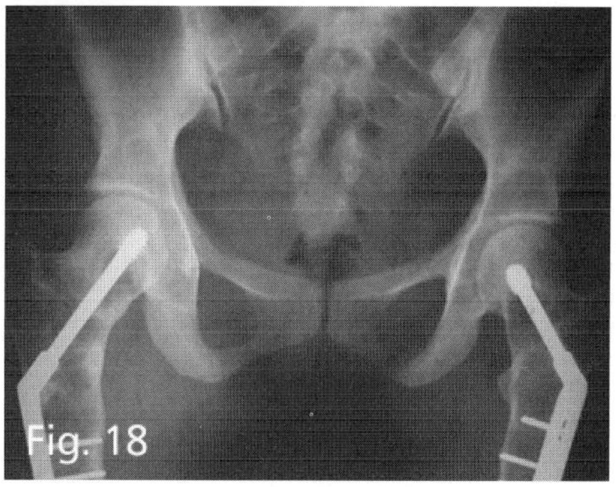
Fig. 18

Q-22: What are the four most common soft-tissue sarcomas to spread via the lymph node system?

1. Rhabdomyosarcoma, malignant fibrous histiocytoma, epithelioid sarcoma, clear cell sarcoma
2. Malignant fibrous histiocytoma, synovial sarcoma, clear cell sarcoma, epithelioid sarcoma
3. Liposarcoma, rhabdomyosarcoma, synovial sarcoma, clear cell sarcoma
4. Rhabdomyosarcoma, clear cell sarcoma, epithelioid sarcoma, synovial sarcoma
5. Liposarcoma, clear cell sarcoma, rhabdomyosarcoma, epithelioid sarcoma

Orthopaedic Oncology/Systemic Disease: Questions

Q-23: Figures 19A and 19B show the AP and lateral radiographs of a 62-year-old man who has had hip pain for the past 3 weeks. Figure 19C shows a CT scan of the abdomen and pelvis. A needle biopsy was performed and the histology is shown in Figure 19D. Preoperative management should include which of the following?

1. Lymphoscintigraphy
2. Colonoscopy
3. Bronchoscopy
4. Embolization of the femoral lesion
5. Bone marrow aspiration

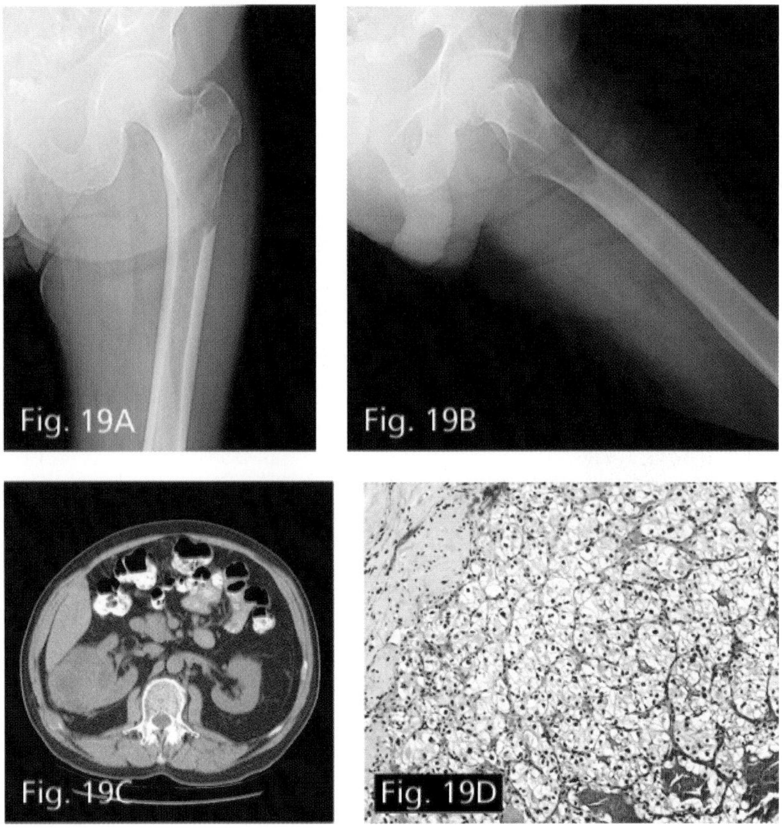
Fig. 19A Fig. 19B Fig. 19C Fig. 19D

Q-24: A 58-year-old woman has a fracture through a metacarpal lesion after a motor vehicle accident. She denies any preinjury symptoms and the fracture heals uneventfully. Based on the radiograph and MRI scans shown in Figures 20A through 20C obtained following fracture healing, follow-up management should consist of

1. curettage.
2. radiation therapy.
3. observation.
4. bisphosphonates.
5. ray resection.

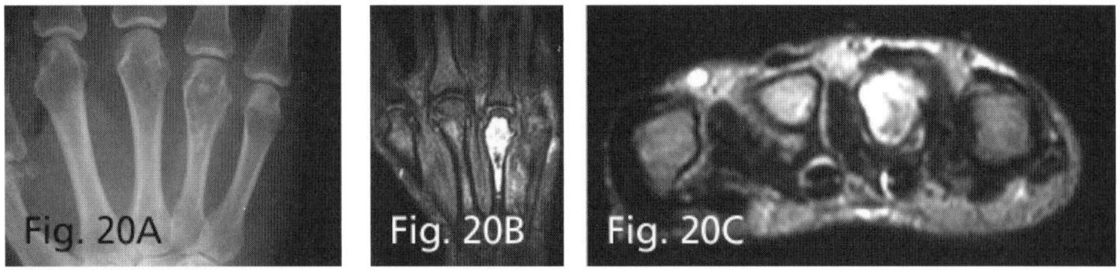
Fig. 20A Fig. 20B Fig. 20C

Q-25: A 13-year-old boy has knee pain after sustaining a mild twisting injury while playing basketball 4 weeks ago. Radiographs and MRI scans are shown in Figures 21A through 21D, and histology sections are shown in Figures 21E and 21F. Treatment should consist of

1. neoadjuvant chemotherapy followed by surgical resection and reconstruction.
2. chemotherapy followed by radiation therapy.
3. Intravenous antibiotics for 4 weeks, followed by oral antibiotics for 4 weeks.
4. surgical resection and reconstruction followed by chemotherapy.
5. radiation therapy alone.

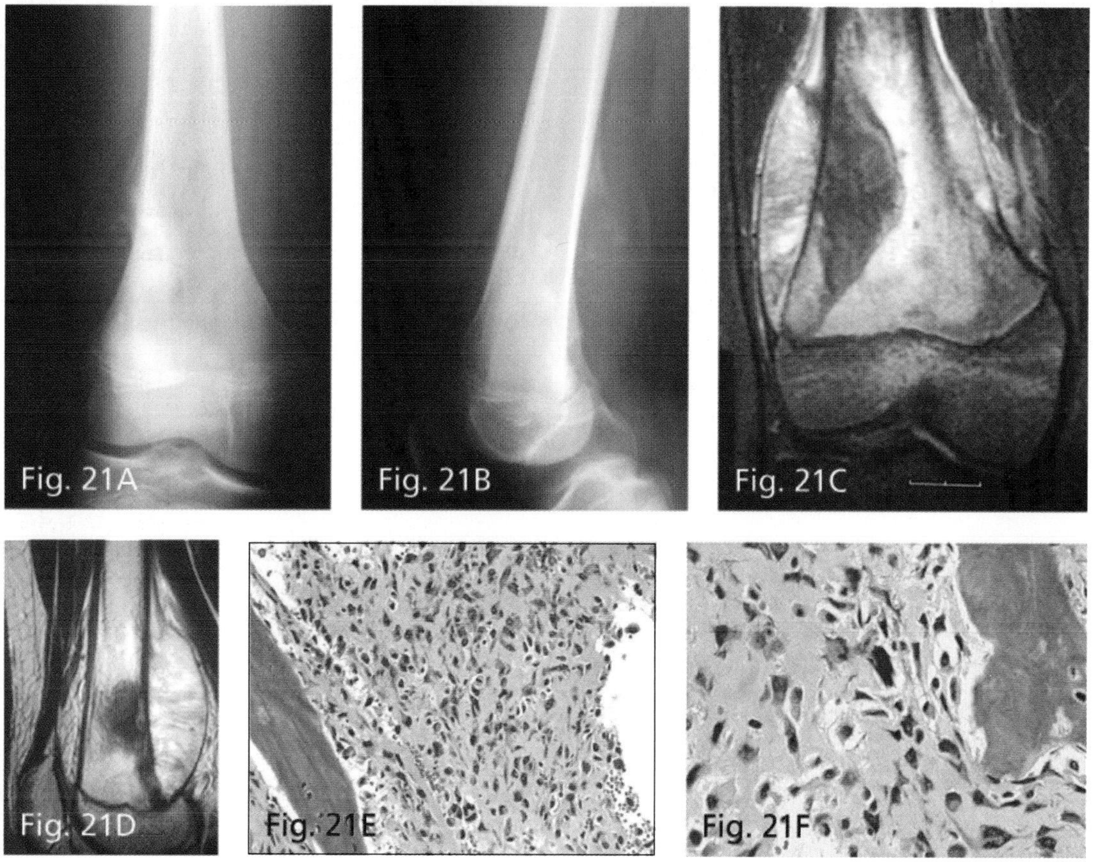
Fig. 21A Fig. 21B Fig. 21C Fig. 21D Fig. 21E Fig. 21F

Q-26: A 64-year-old man has had increasing pain in the left hip for the past 6 months. A radiograph and MRI scan are shown in Figures 22A and 22B. Biopsy specimens are shown in Figures 22C and 22D. What is the recommended treatment?

1. Chemotherapy and internal hemipelvectomy
2. Chemotherapy and hindquarter amputation
3. Radiation therapy and internal hemipelvectomy
4. Radiation therapy and hindquarter amputation
5. Hindquarter amputation or internal hemipelvectomy

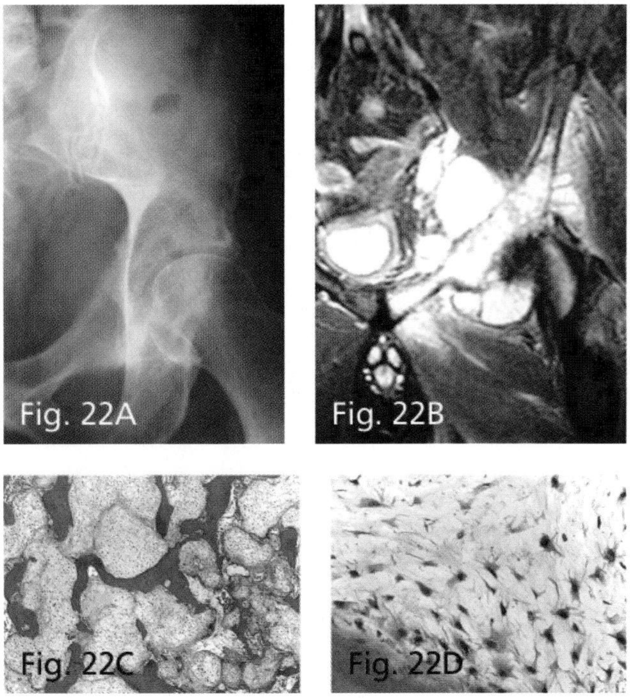

Fig. 22A Fig. 22B Fig. 22C Fig. 22D

Q-27: The scoring system for impending pathologic fractures devised by Mirels involves assessment of which of the following factors?

1. Lesion location, amount of pain, lesion type, lesion size (lucent/blastic)
2. Patient's functional status, lesion location, amount of pain, lesion size
3. Lesion type (lucent/blastic), patient's functional status, lesion location, amount of pain
4. Lesion size, lesion type (lucent/blastic), lesion location, patient's functional status
5. Amount of pain, patient's functional status, lesion type (lucent/blastic), lesion size

Q-28: Figures 23A and 23B show the radiograph and MRI scan of a 22-year-old man with knee pain. What is the most likely diagnosis?

1. Osteochondroma
2. Osteoblastoma
3. Osteosarcoma
4. Chondrosarcoma
5. Malignant fibrous histiocytoma of bone

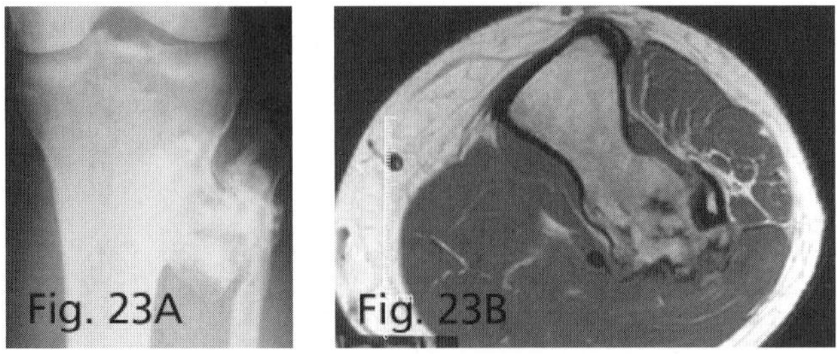

Fig. 23A Fig. 23B

Q-29: Which of the following malignant tumors most commonly contains soft-tissue calcifications seen on radiographs or CT?

1. Hemangioma
2. Ewing sarcoma
3. Clear cell sarcoma
4. Malignant fibrous histiocytoma
5. Synovial sarcoma

Q-30: Which of the following is most associated with local recurrence of the lesion seen in the radiograph and MRI scan shown in Figures 24A and 24B?

1. Effectiveness of chemotherapy
2. Effect of local adjuvant
3. Open physes
4. Presence of giant cells
5. Effectiveness of embolization

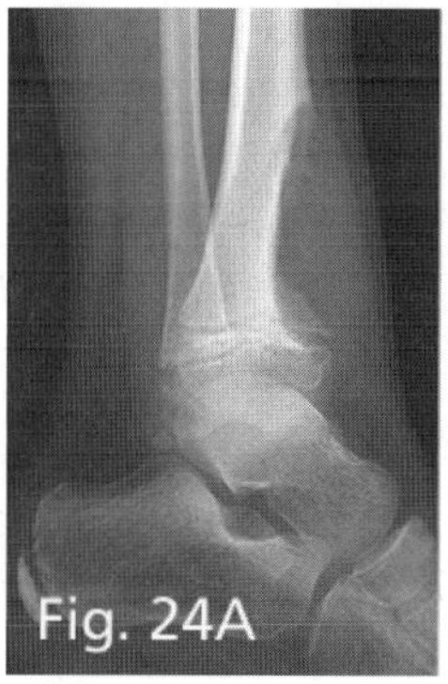

Fig. 24A

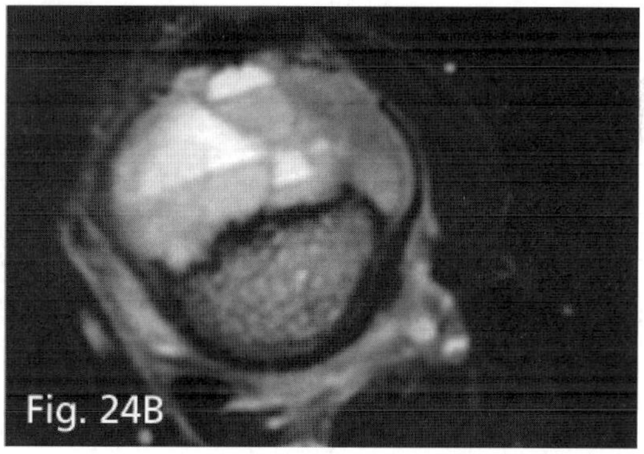

Fig. 24B

Q-31: A 33-year-old woman reports a mass on the right hand that has been enlarging for 1 year. An intraoperative photograph is shown in Figure 25A, and a histology section is shown in Figure 25B. What is the most likely diagnosis?

1. Ganglion cyst
2. Abscess
3. Hematoma
4. Giant cell tumor of tendon sheath
5. Synovial sarcoma

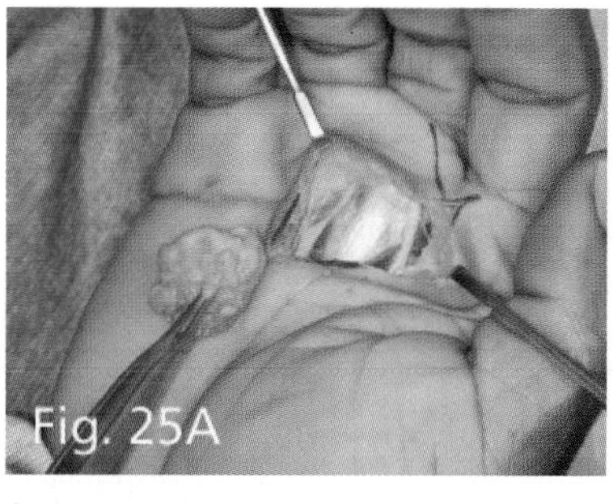

Fig. 25A

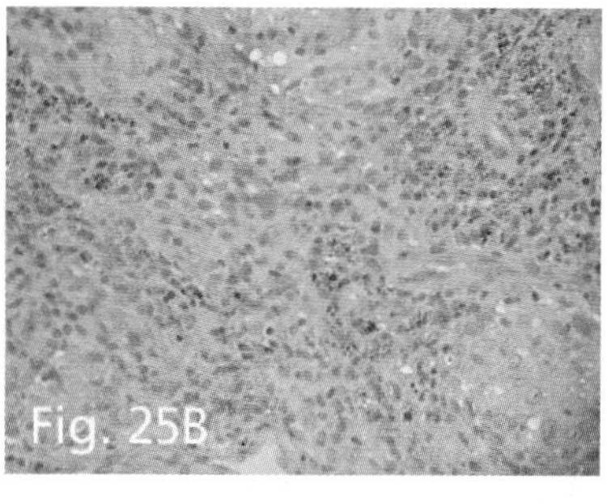

Fig. 25B

Q-32: A 15-year-old girl has had a painful mass on the medial aspect of her left thigh for the past 5 years. The pain is present only when she is performing athletic activities and is completely relieved with rest. A radiograph and MRI scan are shown in Figures 26A and 26B. The patient and her parents would like to have the mass removed. What further diagnostic studies are required prior to considering surgical resection?

1. Bone scan
2. CT
3. Needle biopsy
4. Incisional biopsy
5. No further tests are needed

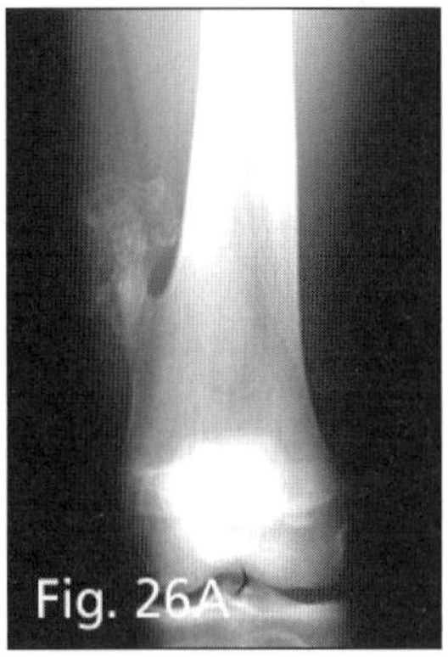
Fig. 26A

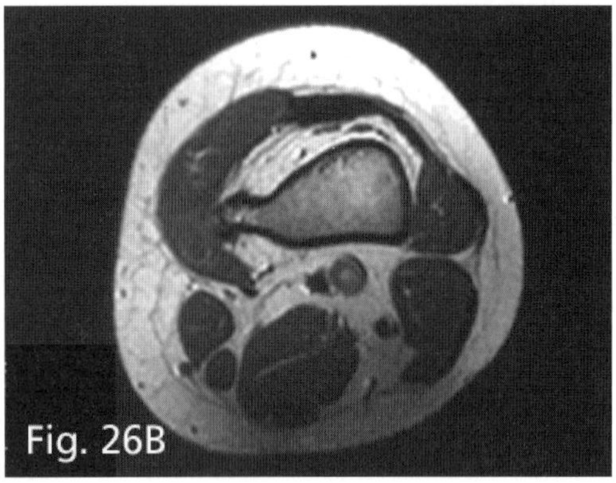
Fig. 26B

Q-33: A 22-year-old man has mild hip pain bilaterally and multiple skeletal lesions. Based on the pelvic radiograph shown in Figure 27, what is the inheritance pattern for his disorder?

1. X-linked
2. Autosomal recessive
3. Autosomal dominant
4. Mitochondral inheritance
5. Germline mutation

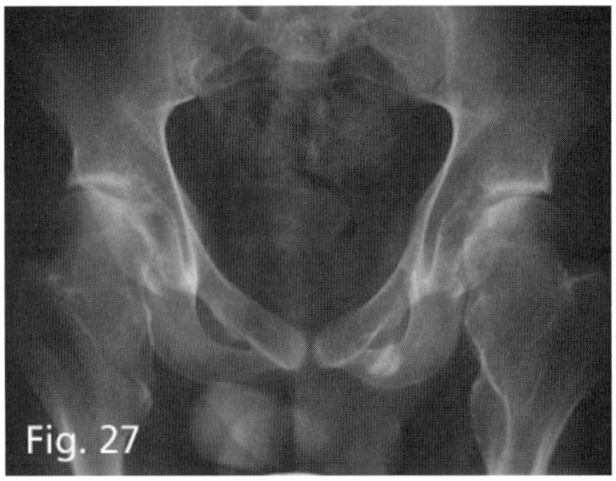
Fig. 27

Q-34: An 80-year-old woman notes a painless mass posterior to her left knee. MRI scans are shown in Figures 28A and 28B. What is the best course of action?

1. Observation
2. Medical management
3. Needle biopsy
4. Incisional biopsy
5. Resection

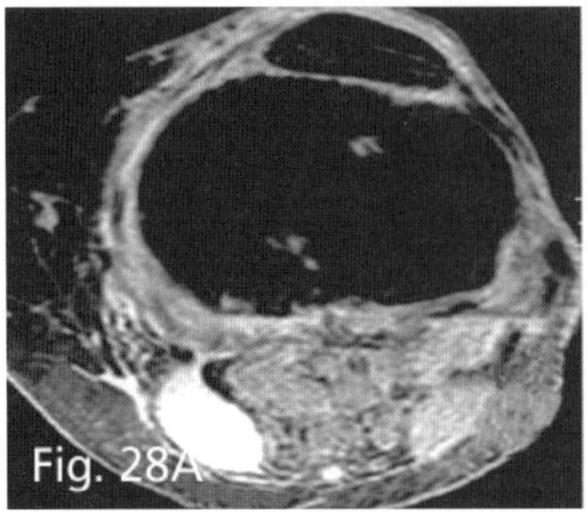
Fig. 28A

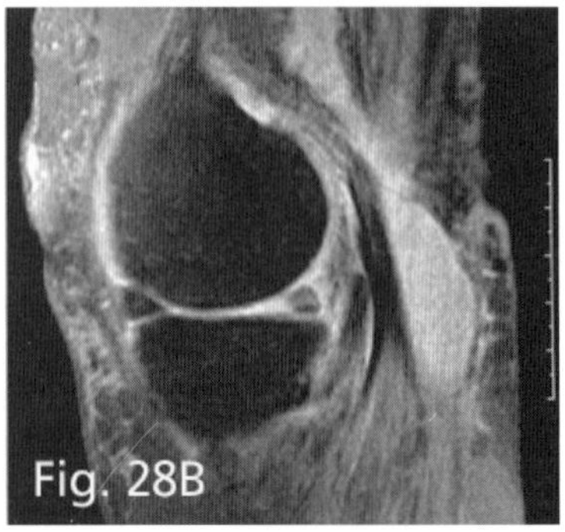
Fig. 28B

Orthopaedic Oncology/Systemic Disease: Questions

Q-35: What is the most common malignancy involving the hand?

1. Epithelioid sarcoma
2. Synovial sarcoma
3. Metastatic lung carcinoma
4. Chondrosarcoma
5. Squamous cell carcinoma

Q-36: A 35-year-old man has had progressive right knee pain for the past 2 months. An AP radiograph, bone scan, MRI scan, and photomicrograph are shown in Figures 29A through 29D. What is the most appropriate treatment of this lesion?

1. Observation
2. Extended curettage with adjuvant treatment
3. Wide resection
4. Radiation therapy
5. Multimodal treatment including chemotherapy and surgery

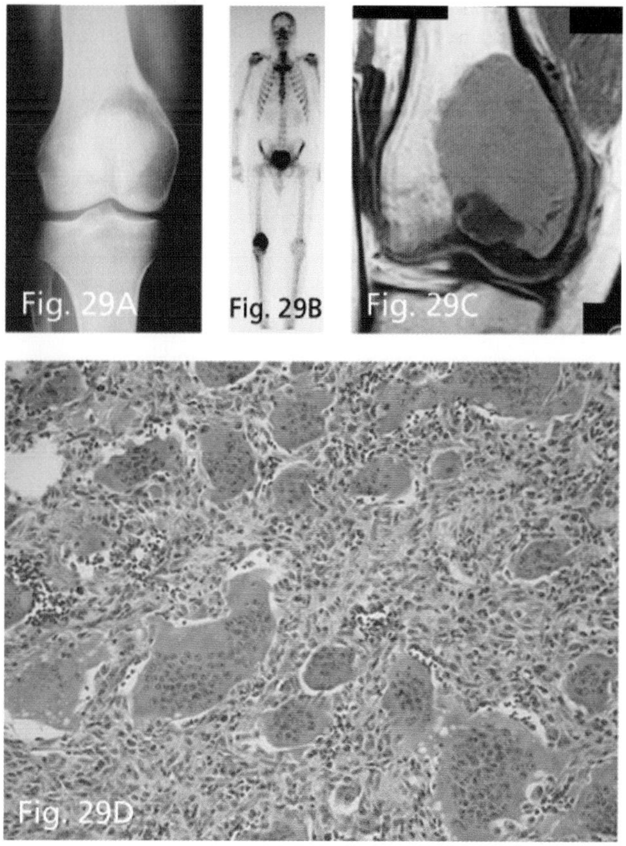

Q-37: What is the most common bone tumor in the hand?

1. Periosteal chondroma
2. Subungual exostosis
3. Chondrosarcoma
4. Osteoid osteoma
5. Enchondroma

Q-38: A 75-year-old woman has had severe shoulder pain for the past month. Her medical history includes hypertension and a total nephrectomy for renal cell carcinoma 7 years ago. Radiographs and sagittal MRI scans are shown in Figures 30A through 30D. A bone scan reveals this to be an isolated lesion. Biopsy findings are consistent with metastatic renal cell carcinoma. What is the most appropriate treatment for this patient?

1. Prophylactic stabilization with an intramedullary rod
2. Radiation therapy alone
3. Embolization alone
4. Wide resection and prosthetic reconstruction
5. Prophylactic stabilization with a locking plate and polymethyl methacrylate cement

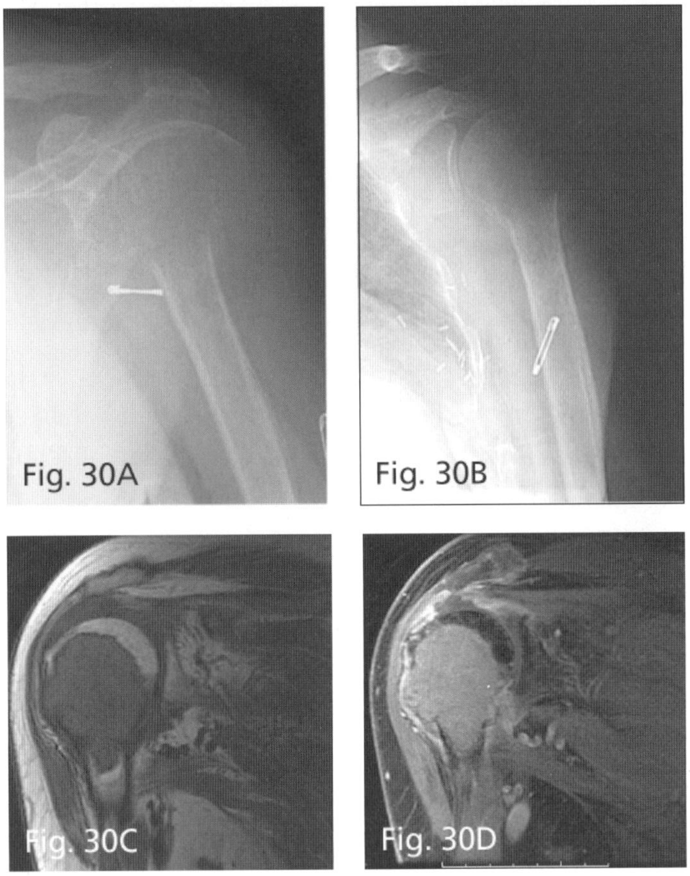

Fig. 30A Fig. 30B Fig. 30C Fig. 30D

Q-39: A patient undergoes a simple excision of a 3-cm superficial mass in the thigh at another institution. The final pathology reveals a leiomyosarcoma, without reference to the margins. What is the recommendation for definitive treatment?

1. Repeat wide excision of the tumor bed
2. Observation
3. Radiation therapy to the tumor bed only
4. Chemotherapy
5. Radiation therapy and chemotherapy

Q-40: A 14-year-old girl reports a 3-week history of anterior thigh pain and a palpable mass after sustaining a soccer-related injury. Examination reveals a tender, firm mass in the midportion of the rectus femoris. MRI scans are shown in Figures 31A through 31C. What is the most appropriate management?

1. Incision and drainage of the abscess
2. NSAIDs, physical therapy, and a repeat MRI scan in 6 to 8 weeks
3. Open biopsy
4. Hematoma evacuation and musculotendinous repair
5. Primary wide resection followed by radiation therapy

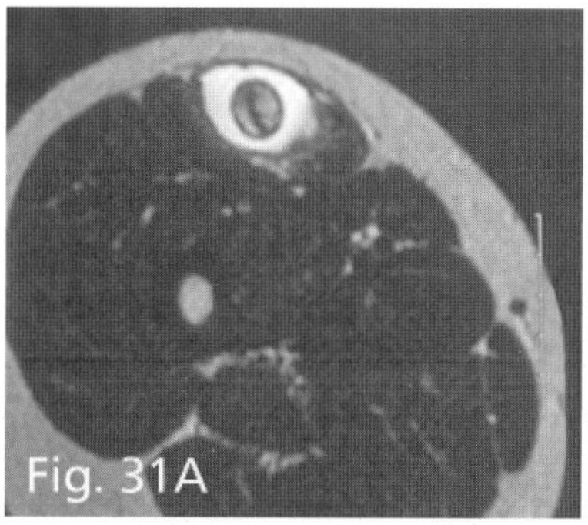
Fig. 31A

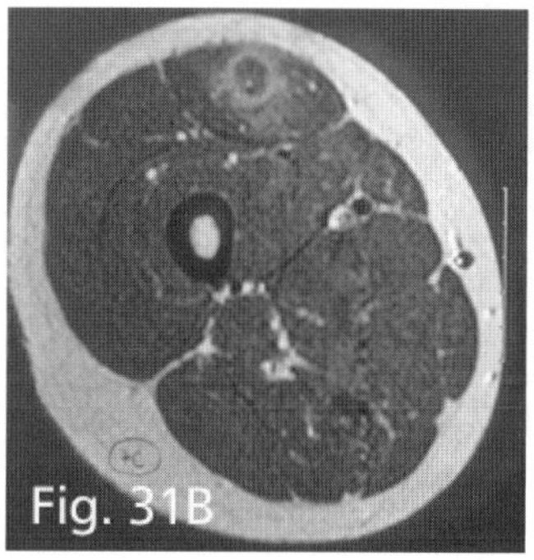
Fig. 31B

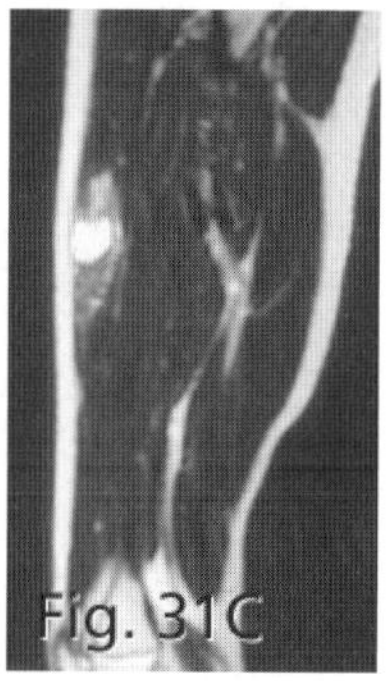
Fig. 31C

Q-41: A 7-year-old girl has had a painful forearm for the past 2 months. Examination reveals fullness on the volar aspect of the forearm. Radiographs and an MRI scan are shown in Figures 32A through 32C. Histology sections are shown in Figures 32D and 32E. What is the most likely diagnosis?

1. Synovial sarcoma
2. Liposarcoma
3. Rhabdomyosarcoma
4. Hemangioma
5. Wilms tumor

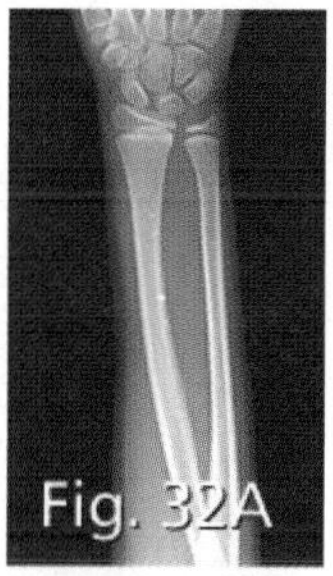
Fig. 32A

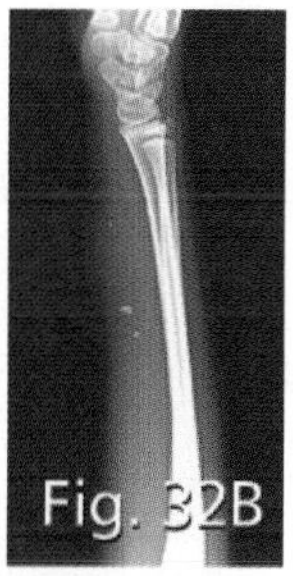
Fig. 32B

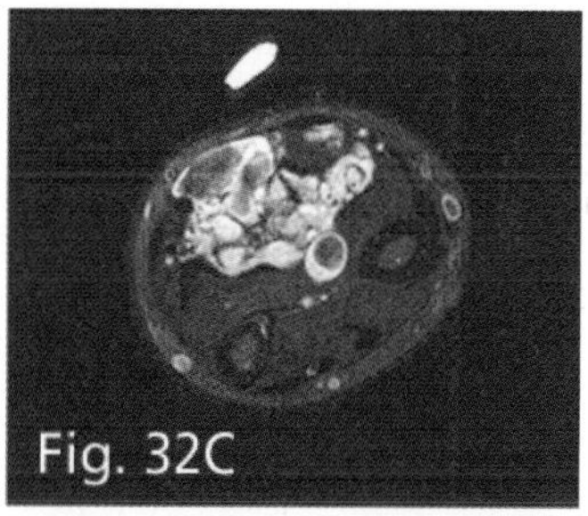
Fig. 32C

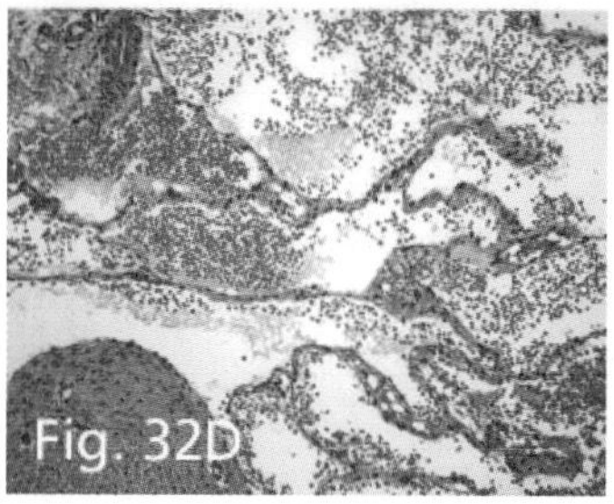
Fig. 32D

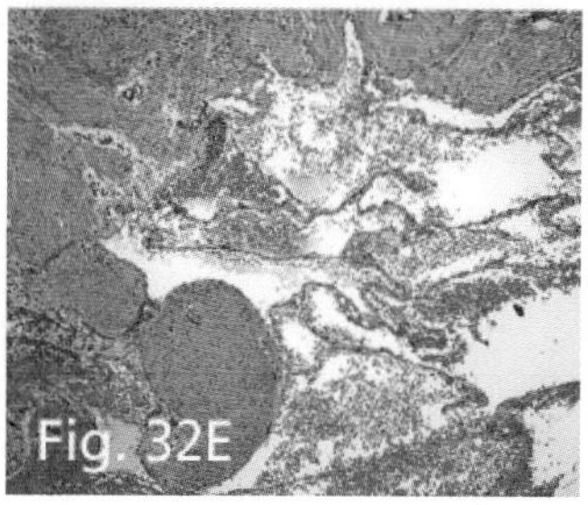
Fig. 32E

Q-42: Which of the following is an important factor in performing a proper biopsy?

1. Staying carefully in the proper intermuscular planes
2. Placing multiple drains
3. Dissecting and protecting critical neurovascular structures
4. Using longitudinal incisions in the extremity
5. Avoiding the use of a tourniquet

Q-43: A 16-year-old girl has had painless swelling in her posterior left arm for the past 4 months. A radiograph, MRI scans, and histology from an incisional biopsy specimen are shown in Figures 33A through 33D. What is the cytogenetic translocation most commonly associated with this tumor?

1. (X;18) (p11;q11)
2. (11;22) (q24;q12)
3. (12;22) (q13;q12)
4. (2;13) (q35;q14)
5. (12;16) (q13;p11)

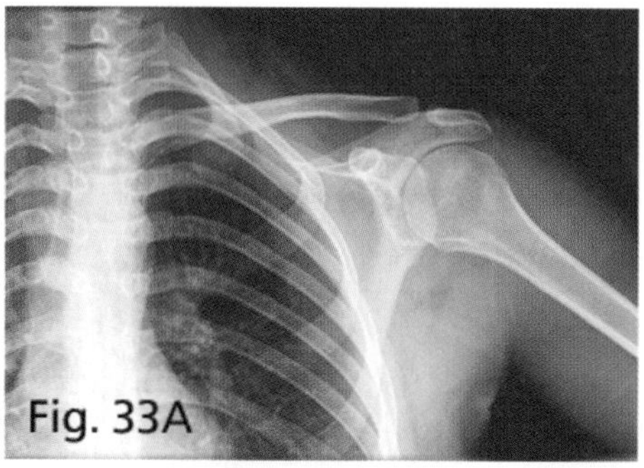
Fig. 33A

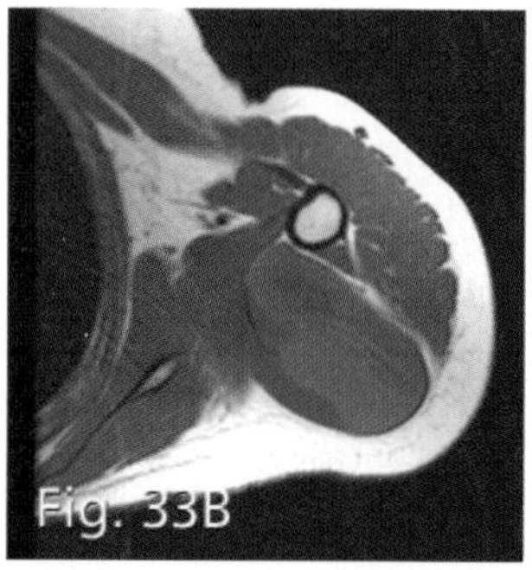
Fig. 33B

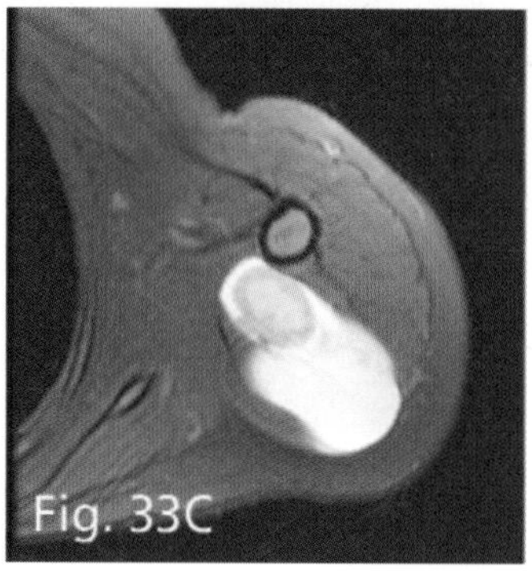
Fig. 33C

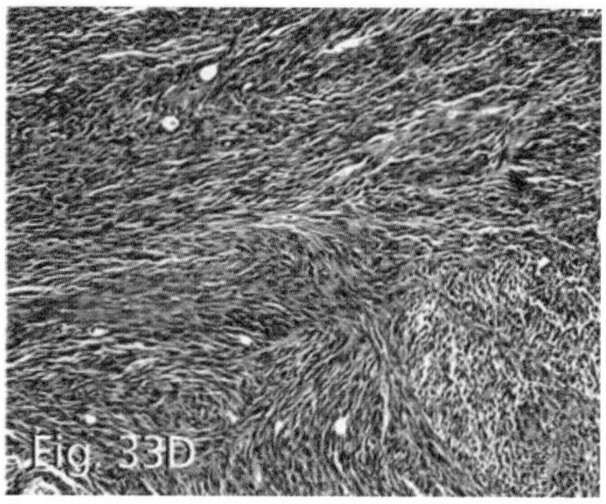
Fig. 33D

Q-44: A 43-year-old woman is referred after excisional biopsy of a cutaneous soft-tissue mass from her left shoulder. Based on the histology from biopsy specimens shown in Figures 34A and 34B, what is the best course of action?

1. Marginal resection
2. Observation
3. Wide tumor bed resection
4. Radiation therapy
5. Chemotherapy

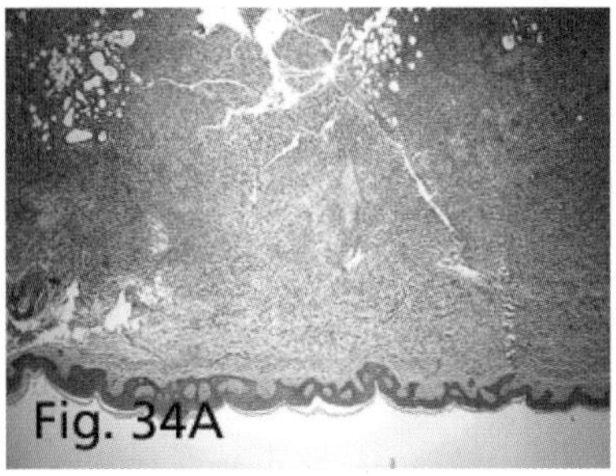
Fig. 34A

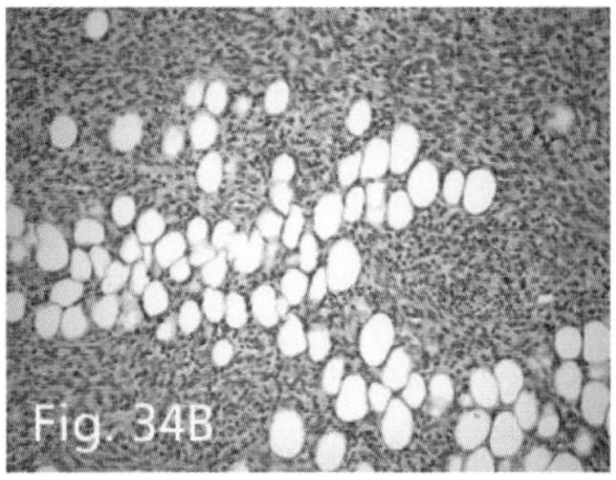
Fig. 34B

Q-45: A 33-year-old man reports an enlarging, painful soft-tissue mass in his right forearm. A radiograph and MRI scans are shown in Figures 35A through 35C. Treatment should consist of

1. core biopsy.
2. wide resection.
3. radiation therapy.
4. marginal resection.
5. incisional biopsy.

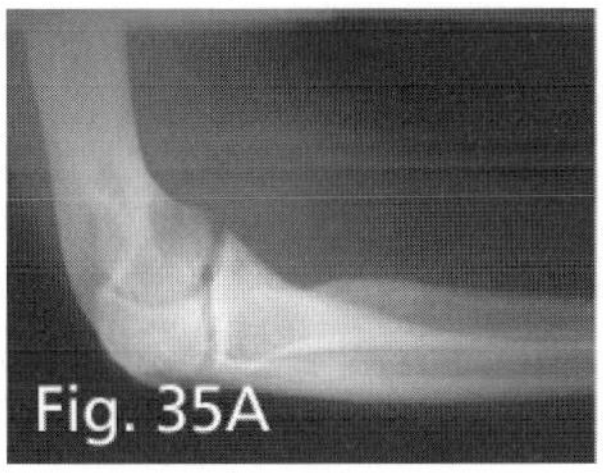
Fig. 35A

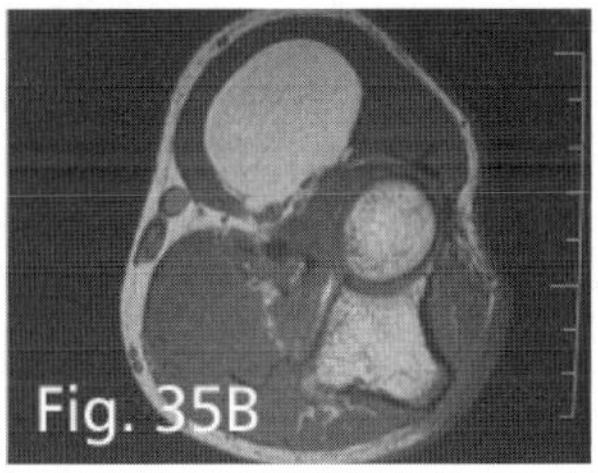
Fig. 35B

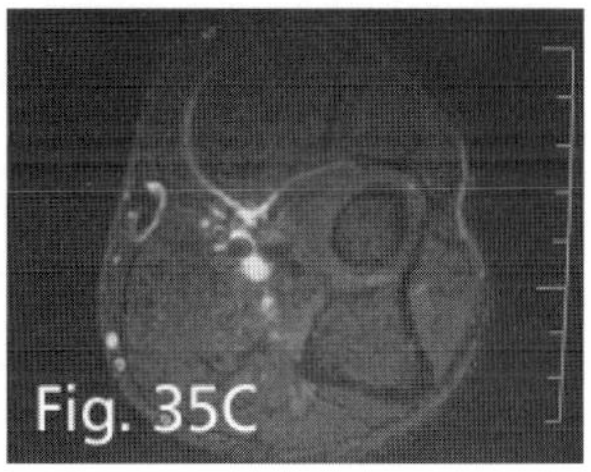
Fig. 35C

Q-46: What is the most common location for localized pigmented villonodular synovitis (PVNS) to occur?

1. Ankle
2. Anterior knee
3. Posterior knee
4. Hip
5. Elbow

Q-47: An 11-year-old boy sustained an injury to his arm in gym class. He denies prior pain in the arm. Radiographs are shown in Figures 36A and 36B. What is the next most appropriate step in the management of this lesion?

1. Open biopsy followed by curettage and bone grafting
2. MRI, whole-body bone scan, CT of the chest, followed by incisional biopsy
3. Allow the fracture to heal with nonsurgical management and serial radiographs
4. Open biopsy followed by wide resection and reconstruction with osteoarticular allograft
5. Open biopsy followed by wide resection and endoprosthetic replacement

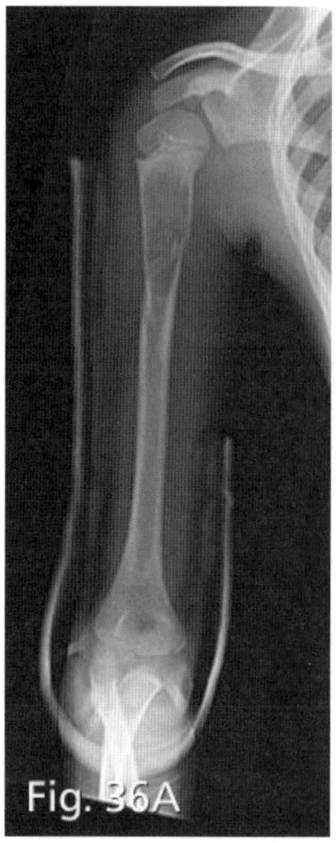
Fig. 36A

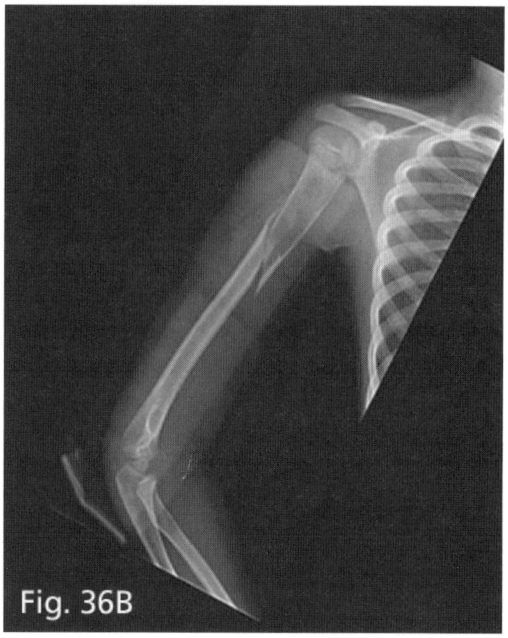
Fig. 36B

Q-48: An 83-year-old woman reports pain in her left middle finger after a minor injury. Laboratory studies show a white blood cell count of 7,000/mm^3, an erythrocyte sedimentation rate of 3 mm/hour, a uric acid level of 10.4 mg/dL, and a normal serum protein electrophoresis level. Radiographs are shown in Figures 37A and 37B. Histology from a core biopsy specimen is shown is Figure 37C. In addition to treatment of the finger fracture, treatment should include

1. colchicine and indomethacin
2. radiation therapy to the left hand.
3. systemic chemotherapy.
4. intravenous antibiotics.
5. through-the-wrist amputation.

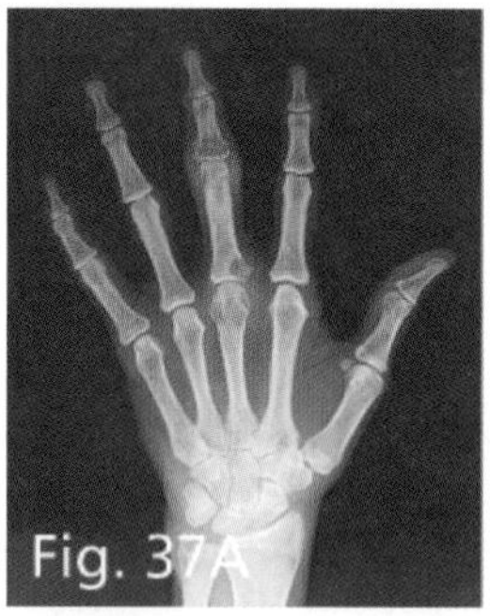
Fig. 37A

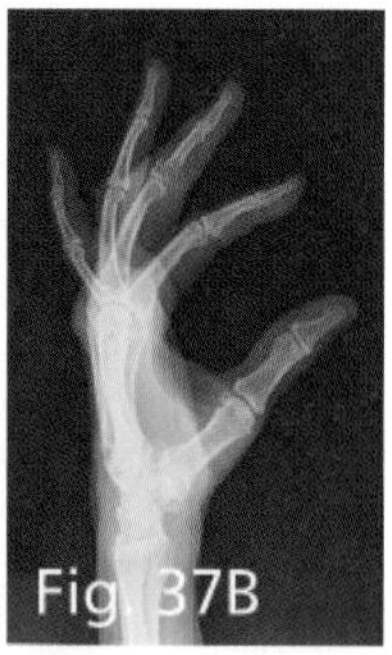
Fig. 37B

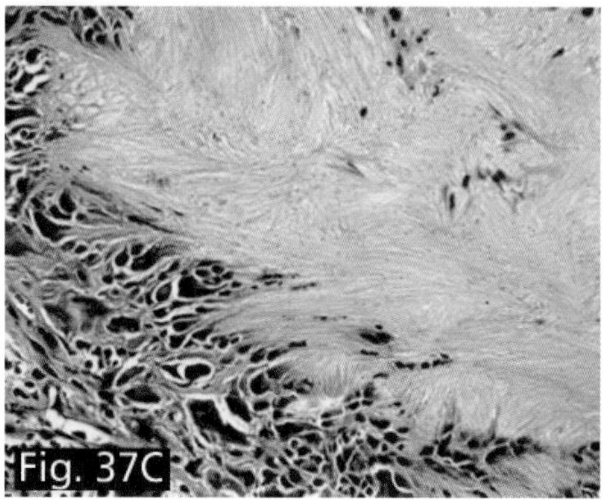
Fig. 37C

Q-49: A 29-year-old woman reports shoulder pain after sustaining a minor fall 6 weeks ago. She has a history of celiac sprue. Radiographs of the forearm and shoulder are shown in Figures 38A and 38B. Which of the following serum abnormalities would be expected?

1. Elevated calcium level
2. Elevated parathyroid hormone level
3. Elevated 1,25 dihydroxyvitamin D
4. Elevated phosphate level
5. Low alkaline phosphatase level

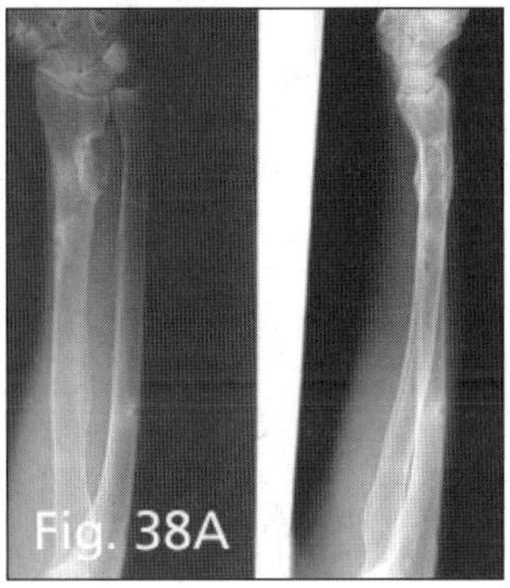
Fig. 38A

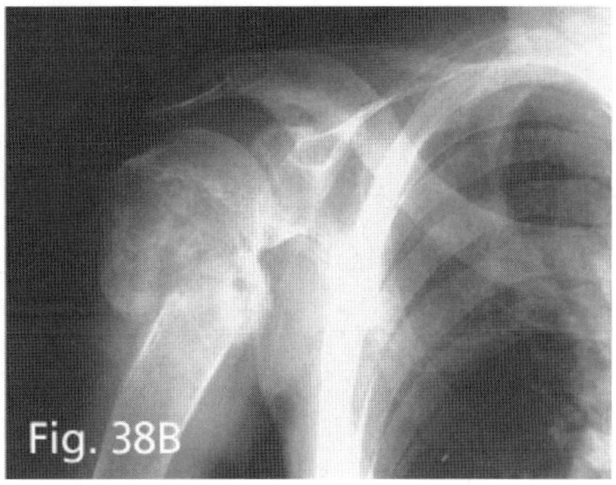
Fig. 38B

A-1: The arrow in Figure 1 points toward a finding consistent with which of the following?

1. Metastatic disease
2. Hemangioma
3. Flexion-compression fracture
4. Infection
5. Diastematomyelia

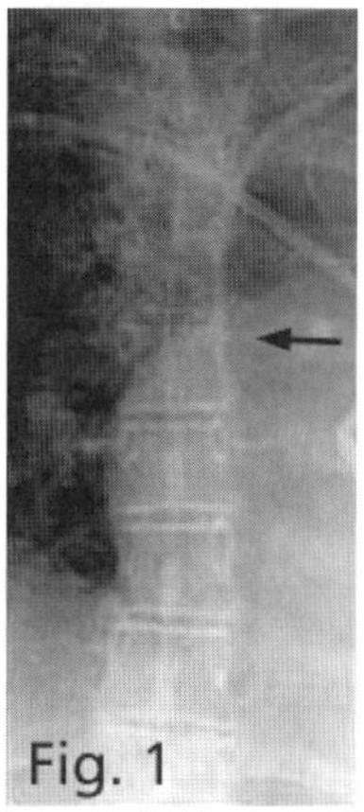
Fig. 1

PREFERRED RESPONSE: 1

DISCUSSION: The finding of a unilateral absent pedicle is often referred to as a winking owl sign and is a manifestation of pedicle destruction from metastatic disease. As the vertebral body is destroyed from the neoplastic process, it extends into the pedicle and destroys the cortical rim that normally creates the oval ring of the pedicle on an AP image.

REFERENCES: McLain R, Weinstein J, eds: Rothman-Simeone: *The Spine*, ed 4. Philadelphia, PA, WB Saunders, 1999, p 1173.

Cohen DB: Tumors of the spine, in Koval KJ, ed: *Orthopaedic Knowledge Update*, ed 7. Rosemont, IL, American Academy of Orthopaedic Surgeons, 2002, p 674.

A-2: A 62-year-old woman reports diffuse aches and pains of the hip and pelvis. She denies any significant trauma but does have a history of chronic anemia. Figure 2A shows a radiograph of the pelvis, and Figures 2B and 2c show T2-weighted MRI scans. What is the most likely diagnosis?

1. Chondrosarcoma
2. Diffuse fibrous dysplasia
3. Multiple myeloma
4. Osteoporosis
5. Bone infarcts

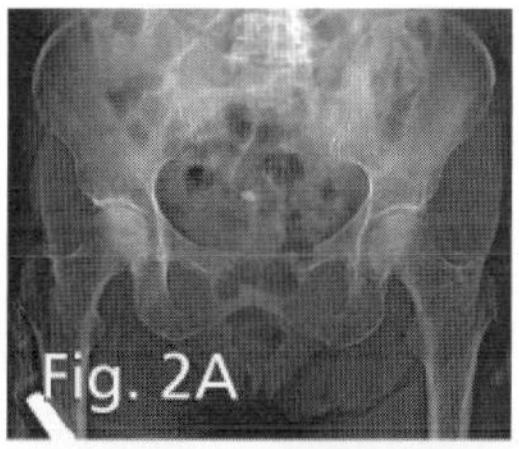
Fig. 2A

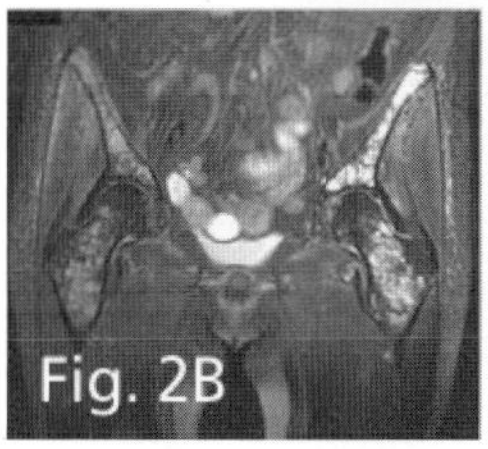
Fig. 2B

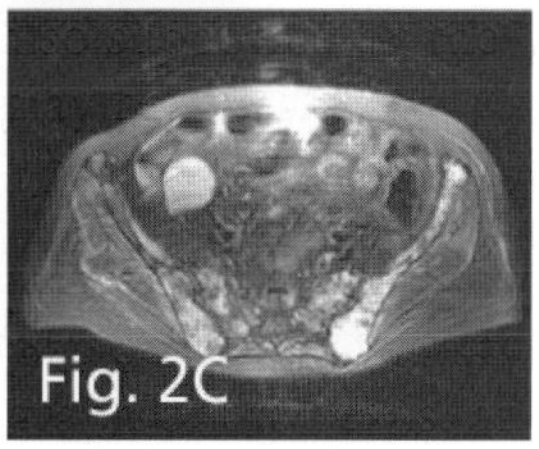
Fig. 2C

PREFERRED RESPONSE: 3

DISCUSSION: The radiograph reveals diffuse osteopenia and areas in the proximal femora that are moth-eaten in appearance. The extent of the marrow-replacing process is evident on the MRI scans, which reveal signal abnormality throughout the entire pelvis and both proximal femora. This represents a marrow-packing process, of which multiple myeloma is the best choice. This diagnosis is also supported by the anemia noted in the patient's history. Metastatic carcinoma and lymphoma also may have a similar presentation.

REFERENCE: Resnick D, ed: *Diagnosis of Bone and Joint Disorders*. Philadelphia, PA, WB Saunders, 2002, pp 2189-2216.

A-3: A 23-year-old woman reports right knee pain and fullness. The pain is worse with activity but is also present at rest. Radiographs are shown in Figures 3A and 3B. What is the most likely diagnosis?

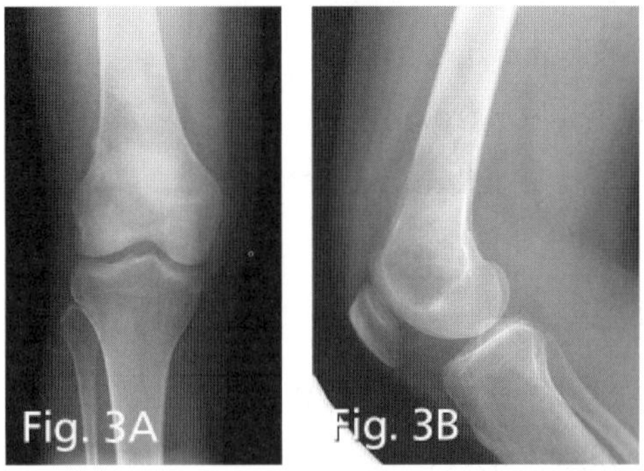
Fig. 3A Fig. 3B

1. Osteosarcoma
2. Chondroblastoma
3. Stress fracture
4. Posttraumatic changes
5. Chondrosarcoma

PREFERRED RESPONSE: 1

DISCUSSION: The radiographs reveal a predominantly lytic, destructive lesion of the distal femur, although there is a hint of some blastic change as well. The lesion has violated the cortex, and there is mineralization outside the cortex laterally. The lateral radiograph suggests a soft-tissue density. These aggressive changes on radiographs in this age group are strongly suggestive of osteosarcoma.

REFERENCES: Sanders TG, Parsons TW: Radiographic imaging of musculoskeletal neoplasia. *Cancer Control* 2001;8:221-231.

Gebhardt MC, Hornicek FJ: Osteosarcoma, in Menendez LR, ed: *Orthopaedic Knowledge Update: Musculoskeletal Tumors*. Rosemont, IL, American Academy of Orthopaedic Surgeons, 2002, pp 175-186.

A-4: Figures 4A through 4C show the coronal T1-weighted, T2-weighted fat-saturated, and T1-weighted fat-saturated gadolinium MRI scans of the proximal thigh of a 52-year-old woman who reports a mass in the medial thigh and groin area. She notes that the fullness of the mass has increased over the course of many months. Based on these findings, what is the most likely diagnosis?

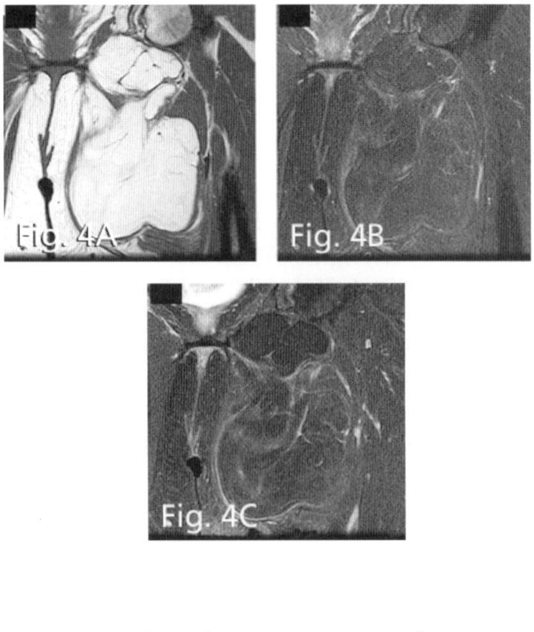
Fig. 4A Fig. 4B Fig. 4C

1. Malignant fibrous histiocytoma
2. Liposarcoma
3. Synovial cell sarcoma
4. Leiomyosarcoma
5. Clear cell sarcoma

PREFERRED RESPONSE: 2

DISCUSSION: The images show a complex, lobular lesion of the thigh that has signal characteristics that follow fat. The size of the lesion, the areas of stranding within the mass, along with mild uptake on the gadolinium sequences and the mild edema within the lesion on the T2-weighted image make liposarcoma the most likely diagnosis and simple intramuscular lipoma far less likely. All other diagnoses listed would not follow fat characteristics shown on the MRI sequences.

REFERENCE: Sanders TG, Parsons TW: Radiographic imaging of musculoskeletal neoplasia. *Cancer Control* 2001;8:221-231.

A-5: Figures 5A and 5B show the radiographs of a left proximal femoral lesion noted serendipitously following minor trauma to the left hip. The patient has no thigh pain and is fully active without limitation. What is the most likely diagnosis of this bony lesion?

1. Chondroblastoma
2. Enchondroma
3. Giant cell tumor
4. Fibrous dysplasia
5. Osteoblastoma

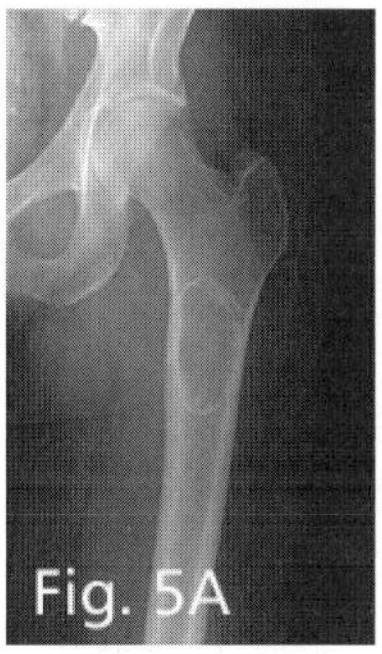
Fig. 5A

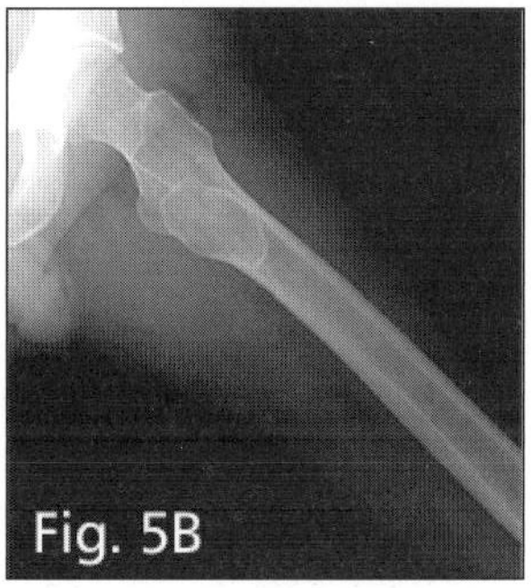
Fig. 5B

PREFERRED RESPONSE: 4

DISCUSSION: The radiographs reveal a geographic lesion of the proximal femur with the classic ground glass appearance noted in fibrous dysplasia. This intramedullary lesion is modestly expansile, demonstrates some minimal cortical thinning, and has no aggressive features. Chondroblastoma, giant cell tumor, and osteoblastoma are more lytic in appearance, and the location is not typical for giant cell tumor or chondroblastoma. Although enchondroma may be considered, the uniform ground glass appearance, lack of punctate mineralization, and distinct margination of the lesion make that diagnosis less likely.

REFERENCE: Parsons TW: Benign bone tumors, in Fitzgerald R Jr, Kaufer H, Malkani A, eds: *Orthopaedics*. Philadelphia, PA, Mosby International, 2002, pp 1027-1035.

A-6: A 13-year-old girl has had increasing left hip pain for the past 4 months. A radiograph, bone scan, MRI scan, and photomicrograph are shown in Figures 6A through 6D. Which of the following immunohistochemistry results would confirm the most likely diagnosis?

1. Cytokeratin positive
2. PAS negative
3. Reticulin positive
4. MIC-2 positive
5. Vimentin negative

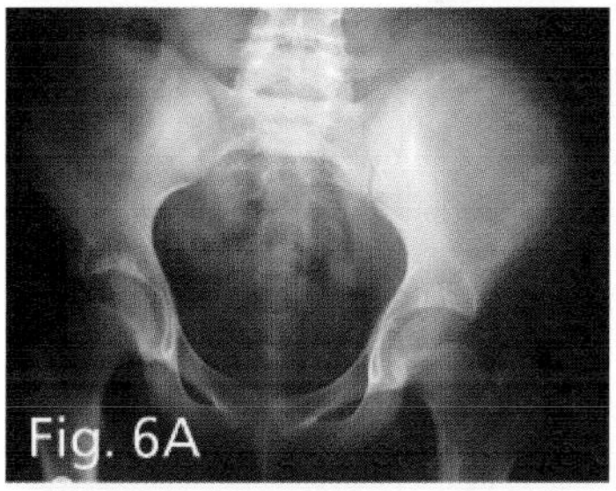
Fig. 6A

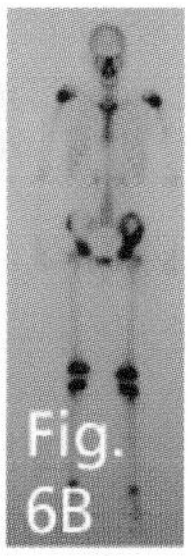
Fig. 6B

PREFERRED RESPONSE: 4

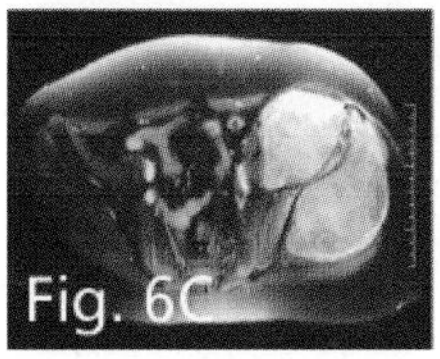
Fig. 6C

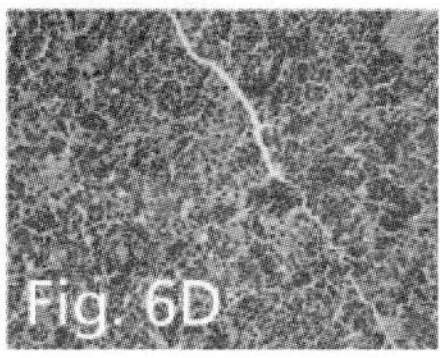
Fig. 6D

DISCUSSION: The imaging studies show a permeative lesion of the left hemipelvis with a large soft-tissue mass. The photomicrograph demonstrates a small blue cell tumor with pseudorosettes. The most likely diagnosis is primitive neuroectodermal tumor (Ewing sarcoma family of tumors). MIC-2 is a highly sensitive and specific marker for this family of tumors. Cytokeratin is an epithelial marker. Vimentin is a mesenchymal marker. Thus, Ewing sarcomas are cytokeratin negative and vimentin positive. Before discovery of the MIC-2 antigen, PAS and reticulin stains were commonly used to help differentiate Ewing sarcoma from lymphoma. In contrast to lymphoma, Ewing sarcomas are typically PAS positive and reticulin negative.

REFERENCES: Halliday BE, Slagel DD, Elsheikh TE, et al: Diagnostic utility of MIC-2 immunocytochemical staining in the differential diagnosis of small blue cell tumors. *Diagn Cytopathol* 1998;19:410-416.

(continued on next page)

Orthopaedic Oncology/Systemic Disease: Answers

(A-6: *continued*)

Llombart-Bosch A, Navarro S: Immunohistochemical detection of EWS and FLI-1 proteins is Ewing sarcoma and primitive neuroectodermal tumors: Comparative analysis with CD99 (MIC-2) expression. *Appl Immunohistochem Mol Morphol* 2001;9:255-260.

A-7: Which of the following is the preferred treatment for symptomatic localized pigmented villonodular synovitis (PVNS) of the knee?

1. Observation
2. External beam radiation therapy
3. Intra-articular radiation therapy
4. Resection of nodule only
5. Open complete synovectomy

PREFERRED RESPONSE: 4

DISCUSSION: Localized PVNS is a variant of the disease process where the synovial proliferation occurs in one area and usually presents as a discrete mass. It has been effectively treated with complete excision. This may be performed arthroscopically or with arthrotomy. Complete synovectomy and radiation therapy are unnecessary to eradicate the localized form of PVNS.

REFERENCES: Tyler WK, Vidal AF, Williams RJ, et al: Pigmented villonodular synovitis. *J Am Acad Orthop Surg* 2006;14:376-385.

Kim SJ, Shin SJ, Choi NH, et al: Arthroscopic treatment for localized pigmented villonodular synovitis of the knee. *Clin Orthop Relat Res* 2000;379:224-230.

A-8: A healthy 52-year-old woman is seeking professional advice about management of osteoporosis. She has no risk factors for osteoporosis. What is the best recommendation for bone health for this patient?

1. Bone mineral density testing performed semiannually
2. No treatment
3. A healthy diet high in calcium
4. 1,000 to 1,500 mg calcium supplement plus 400 to 800 IU vitamin D per day
5. Estrogen therapy

PREFERRED RESPONSE: 4

DISCUSSION: Women older than 50 years should receive daily supplementation with calcium and vitamin D to help preserve bone density. Bone mineral density testing is recommended for women age 65 years or older and postmenopausal women with at least one risk factor for osteoporotic fractures: prior fragility fracture, low estrogen levels, premature menopause, long-term secondary amenorrhea, glucocorticoid therapy, maternal history of hip fracture, or low body mass index. Hormone therapy is not approved for the treatment of osteoporosis.

REFERENCES: Gass M, Dawson-Hughes B: Preventing osteoporosis-related fractures: An overview. *Am J Med* 2006;119:S3-S11.

Lin JT, Lane JM: Osteoporosis: A review. *Clin Orthop Relat Res* 2004;425:126-134.

A-9: A 37-year-old man pulled his hamstring playing softball 3 weeks ago. The patient had not noted any mass prior to his injury. MRI scans of the posterior thigh are shown in Figures 7A and 7B. Figure 7C shows the biopsy specimen from a needle biopsy. What is the most likely diagnosis?

1. Intramuscular hematoma
2. Lipoma
3. Myositis ossificans
4. Malignant fibrous histiocytoma
5. Liposarcoma

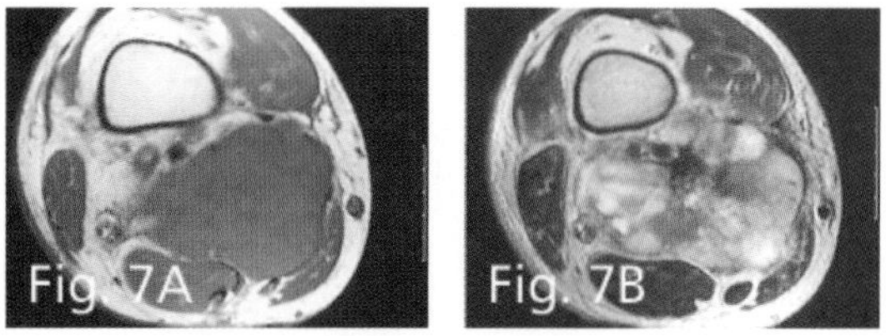

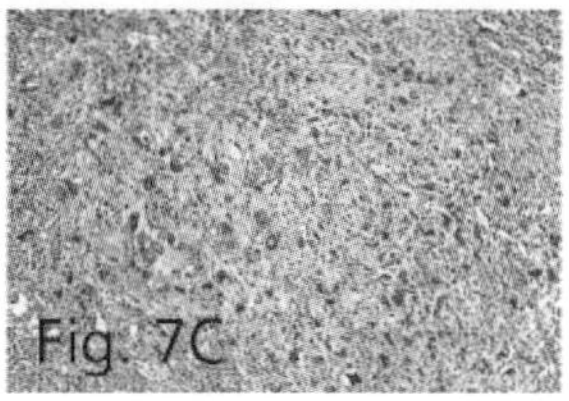

PREFERRED RESPONSE: 4

DISCUSSION: Malignant fibrous histiocytoma (MFH) is the most common soft-tissue sarcoma. MFH typically presents as a large mass, deep to the fascia with heterogeneous signal on MRI. The MRI scans show a heterogeneous lesion in the posterior thigh. There is significant high signal uptake on the T2-weighted image. The histology shows malignant histiocytic cells with marked atypia and pleomorphism. Histology of a hematoma would show only old hemorrhage and some granulation tissue. Lipoma and liposarcoma are both seen as a fat-containing lesion on histology. No significant fat tissue is seen in this histologic specimen. Histology of myositis ossificans would show bone formation.

REFERENCES: Springfield DS, Bolander ME, Friedlaender GE, Lane N: Molecular and cellular biology of inflammation and neoplasia, in Simon SR, ed: *Orthopaedic Basic Science*. Rosemont, IL, American Academy of Orthopaedic Surgeons, 1994, pp 219-276.

Campanacci M: *Bone and Soft Tissue Tumors*, ed 2. New York, NY, Springer-Verlag, 1999, pp 965-981.

A-10: A 16-year-old boy has had left knee pain and swelling after sustaining a minor twisting injury while playing basketball 2 weeks ago. Figures 8A through 8E show the radiograph, MRI scans, and biopsy specimens. What is the most likely diagnosis?

1. Osteomyelitis
2. Tuberculosis
3. Osteosarcoma
4. Ewing's sarcoma
5. Malignant fibrous histiocytoma (MFH)

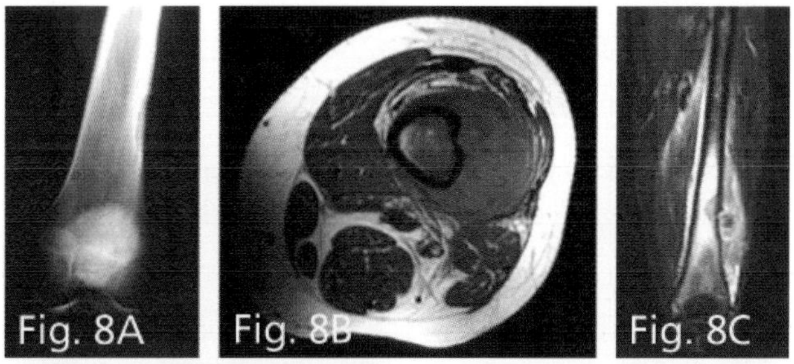

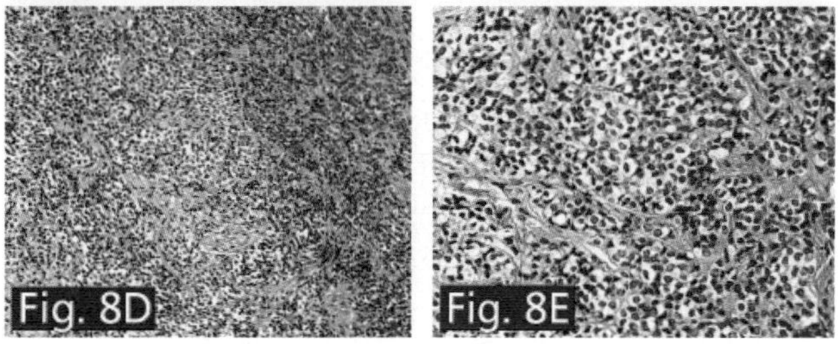

PREFERRED RESPONSE: 4

DISCUSSION: The imaging studies and histology are most consistent with Ewing sarcoma. Tuberculosis can show small round blue cells on histology (lymphocytes associated with chronic infection) but would more typically involve the knee joint and periarticular bone. Osteosarcoma and MFH do not have small round blue cells histologically.

REFERENCES: Sissons HA, Murray RO, Kemp HBS: *Orthopaedic Diagnosis*. Berlin, Springer-Verlag, 1984, pp 254-256.

Wafa H, Grimer RJ: Surgical options and outcomes in bone sarcoma. *Expert Rev Anticancer Ther* 2006;6:239-248.

Orthopaedic Oncology/Systemic Disease: Answers

A-11: A 13-year-old boy has a painless "knot" over his left hip. History reveals that he injured his left hip playing soccer 4 months ago. A radiograph and MRI scan obtained at the time of injury are shown in Figures 9A and 9B. He is very active and is currently asymptomatic. A current radiograph is shown in Figure 9C. What is the next most appropriate step in management?

1. Observation
2. Anti-inflammatory medication
3. Referral to a rheumatologist
4. Biopsy
5. Resection of the lesion

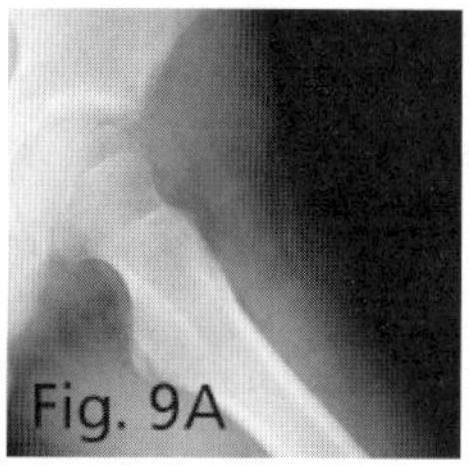
Fig. 9A

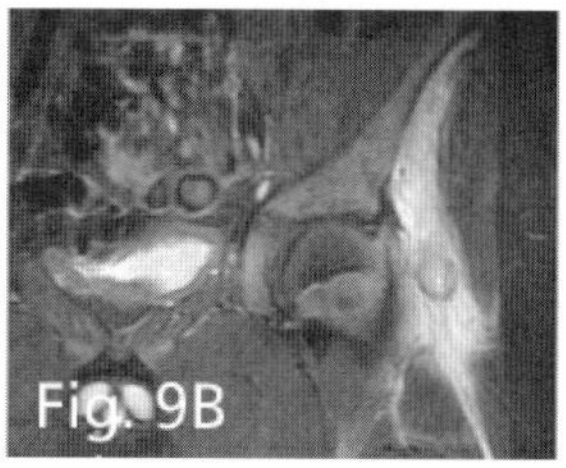
Fig. 9B

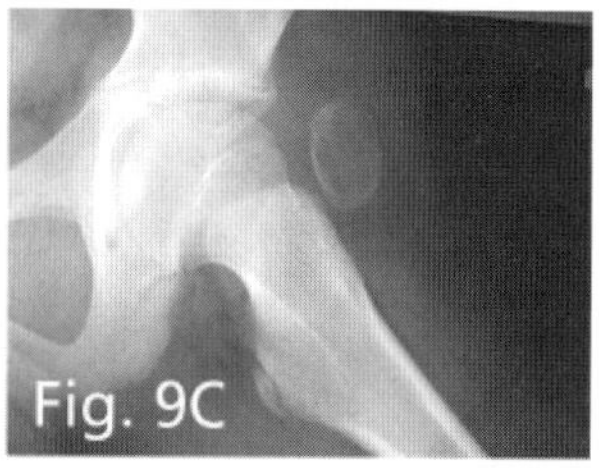
Fig. 9C

PREFERRED RESPONSE: 1

DISCUSSION: The diagnosis is myositis ossificans resulting from an injury. The initial radiograph reveals a small amount of mineralization in the soft tissues overlying the left hip. The MRI scan shows signal abnormality of the entire gluteus minimus muscle with a mineralized mass in the center. The current radiograph shows a lesion within the abductor musculature with mature ossification peripherally. The imaging studies are diagnostic and the patient is asymptomatic; therefore, the management of choice is observation with no further evaluation or treatment indicated.

REFERENCES: Miller AE, Davis BA, Beckley OA: Bilateral and recurrent myositis ossificans in an athlete: A case report and review of treatment options. *Arch Phys Med Rehabil* 2006;87:286-290.

West RV, Fu FH: Soft-tissue physiology and repair, in Vaccaro AR, ed: *Orthopaedic Knowledge Update*, ed 8. Rosemont, IL, American Academy of Orthopaedic Surgeons, 2005, pp 15-27.

A-12: Figure 10A shows the clinical photograph of an 83-year-old woman who has an enlarging left forearm mass. MRI scans are shown in Figures 10B and 10C. What is the next most appropriate step in management?

1. Radiation therapy
2. Needle biopsy
3. Marginal resection
4. Chemotherapy
5. Amputation

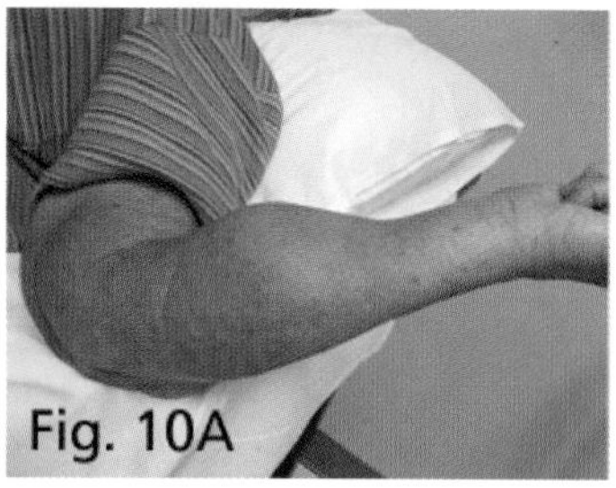
Fig. 10A

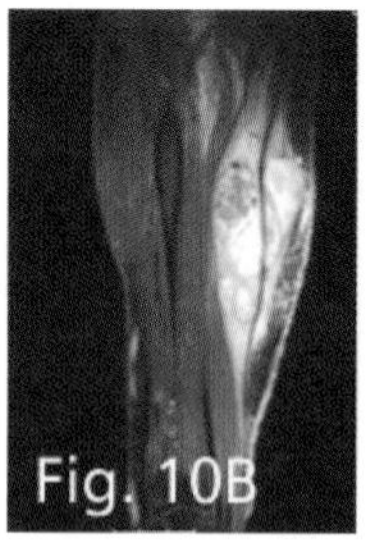
Fig. 10B

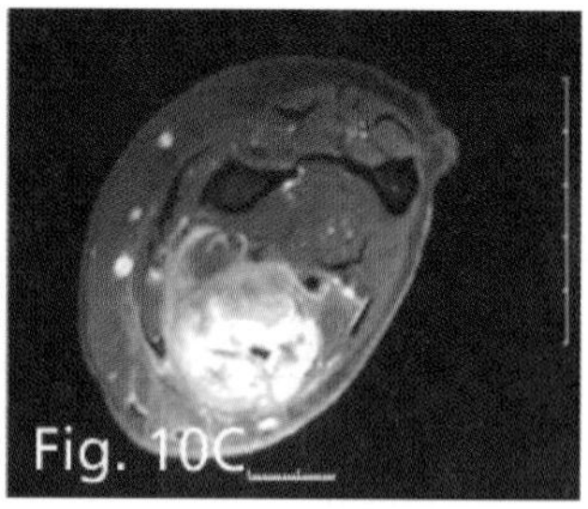
Fig. 10C

PREFERRED RESPONSE: 2

DISCUSSION: Any large (greater than 5 cm), deep, heterogeneous mass in the extremities should be considered a sarcoma until proven otherwise. Sarcomas are rare, and without a high index of suspicion, the lesions may be misdiagnosed or there may be a delay in diagnosis. Needle biopsies can obtain sufficient tissue for diagnosis and are associated with less morbidity than open biopsy. Marginal resections or excisional biopsies should be reserved for a few select benign lesions and locations.

REFERENCES: Damron TA, Beauchamp CP, Rougraff BT, et al: Soft-tissue lumps and bumps. *Instr Course Lect* 2004;53:625-637.

Sim FH, Frassica FJ, Frassica DA: Soft-tissue tumors: Diagnosis, evaluation, and management. *J Am Acad Orthop Surg* 1994;2:202-211.

A-13: A 20-year-old man has a large soft-tissue mass behind his knee. MRI scans are shown in Figures 11A through 11C. Figure 11D shows a clinical photograph of his chest. The patient's condition is most likely a result of a defect in what gene?

1. *NF1*
2. *EWS*
3. *EXT1*
4. *P53*
5. *Rb*

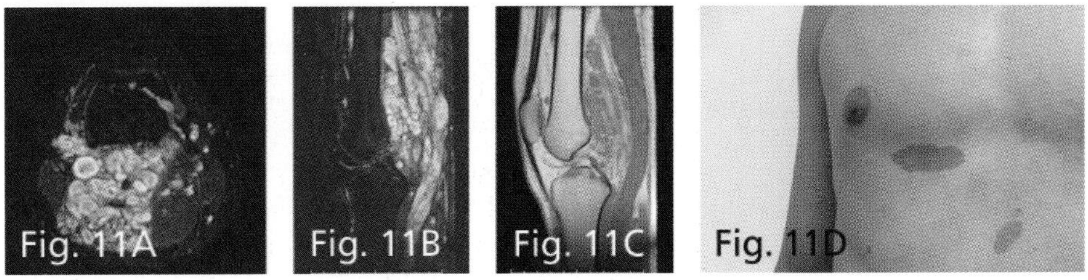

PREFERRED RESPONSE: 1

DISCUSSION: The patient has a plexiform neurofibroma and multiple café-au-lait spots, all characteristic of von Recklinghausen neurofibromatosis. This disease has been linked to a defect of the gene *NF1* on chromosome 17. *EWS* is one of the genes associated with the 11;22 translocation found in Ewing sarcoma and several other sarcomas. *EXT1* is the most common gene affecting patients with multiple hereditary exostosis. *P53* and *Rb* are tumor suppressor genes whose inactivation has been associated with tumors in conditions such as Li-Fraumeni syndrome and retinoblastoma, respectively.

REFERENCES: Theos A, Korf BR, American College of Physicians, et al: Pathophysiology of neurofibromatosis Type 1. *Ann Intern Med* 2006;144:842-849.

Lin PP: Cellular and molecular biology of musculoskeletal tumors, in Menendez LR: *Orthopaedic Knowledge Update: Musculoskeletal Tumors*. Rosemont, IL, American Academy of Orthopaedic Surgeons, 2002, pp 11-20.

A-14: A 35-year-old man reports the development of a painful 2-cm nodule on his dorsal wrist over the past 3 years. A surgeon excised the lesion with a presumptive diagnosis of a ganglion cyst. Histology sections from the excision are shown in Figures 12A and 12B. What is the most likely diagnosis?

1. Ganglion cyst
2. Clear cell sarcoma
3. Epithelioid sarcoma
4. Epidermal inclusion cyst
5. Synovial sarcoma

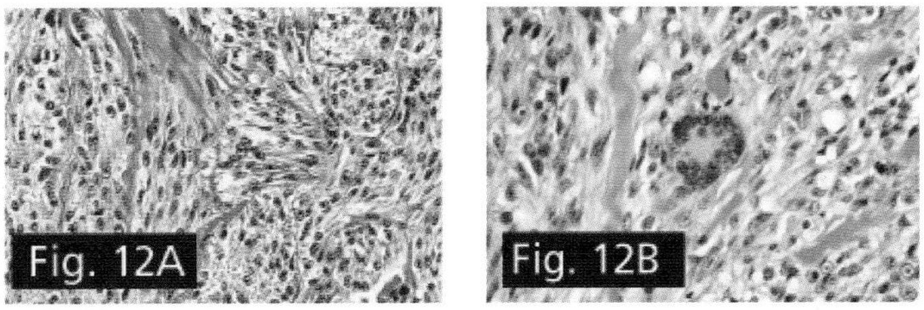

PREFERRED RESPONSE: 2

DISCUSSION: The histologic appearance of the soft-tissue lesion reveals compact nests of cells with a clear cytoplasm surrounded by a delicate border of fibrocollagenous tissue. There can be scattered multinucleated giant cells. This is consistent with a clear cell sarcoma, also called malignant melanoma of soft parts. This tumor is usually positive for S-100 and HMB45 (a melanoma-associated antigen). These tumors are frequently found around the foot and ankle. Similar to epithelioid sarcoma, it is usually intimately bound to tendons or tendon sheaths. Often the tumors are present for many years. The classic histologic appearance of this lesion differentiates it from the other choices.

REFERENCES: Enzinger FM, Weiss SW: *Soft Tissue Tumors*, ed 3. St Louis, MO, Mosby, 1995, p 913.

Lucas DR, Nascimento AG, Sim FH: Clear cell sarcoma of soft tissues: Mayo Clinic experience with 35 cases. *Am J Surg Pathol* 1992;16:1197-1204.

Orthopaedic Oncology/Systemic Disease: Answers

A-15: Figures 13A through 13E show the radiograph, MRI scans, and histology section of a 17-year-old boy. What is the most likely diagnosis?

1. Giant cell tumor
2. Chondroblastoma
3. Clear cell chondrosarcoma
4. Osteosarcoma
5. Tuberculous septic arthritis

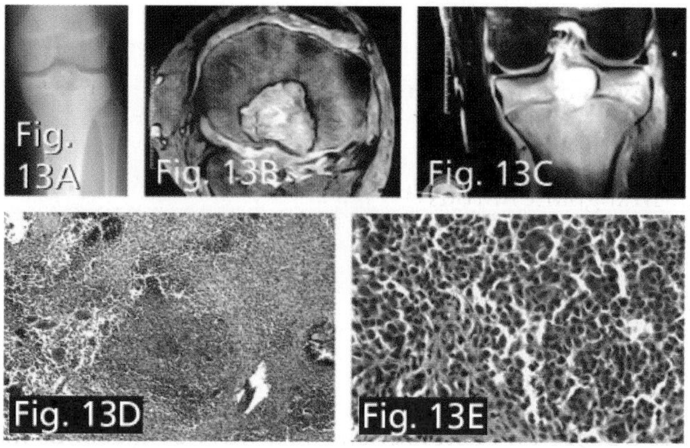

Fig. 13A Fig. 13B Fig. 13C Fig. 13D Fig. 13E

PREFERRED RESPONSE: 2

DISCUSSION: The images show an epiphyseal lesion. The MRI scans show extensive bone edema surrounding the lesion, consistent with chondroblastoma. Histology shows polygonal chondroblasts in a cobblestone-like pattern and areas of calcification consistent with chondroblastoma. Although some giant cells are seen, the age of the patient and the polygonal chondroblasts differentiate this lesion from giant cell tumor. Clear cell chondrosarcoma is an epiphyseal lesion that occurs in an older population, and the cells have clear cytoplasm. This lesion is not producing bone on imaging or histologic specimen, eliminating osteosarcoma. Tuberculous septic arthritis can be an epiphyseal lesion, but granulomas would be seen on histology.

REFERENCES: Gitelis S, Soorapanth C: Benign chondroid tumors, in Menendez LR, ed: *Orthopaedic Knowledge Update: Musculoskeletal Tumors*. Rosemont, IL, American Academy of Orthopaedic Surgeons, 2002, pp 103-111.

Campanacci M: *Bone and Soft Tissue Tumors*, ed 2. New York, NY, Springer-Verlag, 1999, pp 247-263.

A-16: An 18-year-old boy reports increasing pain with weight bearing on his right leg and at night. Examination reveals swelling around the right midcalf. Radiographs and an MRI scan are shown in Figures 14A through 14C, and a histology section is shown in Figure 14D. What is the preferred treatment?

1. Chemotherapy and surgical resection
2. Débridement and intravenous antibiotics
3. Chemotherapy alone
4. Radiation therapy alone
5. Surgical resection alone

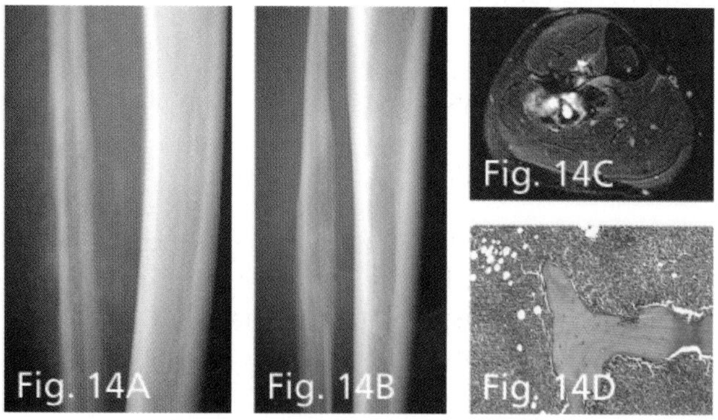

Fig. 14A Fig. 14B Fig. 14C Fig. 14D

PREFERRED RESPONSE: 1

DISCUSSION: The findings are consistent with Ewing sarcoma. The radiographs reveal a lytic lesion in the diaphysis of the right fibula. There is elevation of the periosteum and evidence of a surrounding soft-tissue mass. Histology shows diffuse small round blue cells surrounding the lamellar bone. It is the second most common malignant bone tumor in children. The most common treatment regimen consists of chemotherapy followed by surgical resection and/or radiation therapy. Surgical resection is used when the lesion can be removed with wide margins and causes less morbidity than radiation therapy.

REFERENCES: McCarthy EF, Frassica FJ: *Pathology of Bone and Joint Disorders With Clinical and Radiographic Correlation*. Philadelphia, PA, WB Saunders, 1998, p 258.

Gibbs CP Jr, Weber K, Scarborough MT: Malignant bone tumors. *Instr Course Lect* 2002;51:413-428.

Orthopaedic Oncology/Systemic Disease: Answers

A-17: A 54-year-old woman reports worsening pain in her buttock, especially when sitting for long periods of time. She has occasional pain and paresthesias radiating down her posterior leg. She has no significant medical history. MRI scans are shown in Figures 15A and 15B and a histology section is shown in Figure 15C. What is the most likely diagnosis?

1. Myxoid liposarcoma
2. Myxoma
3. Malignant fibrous histiocytoma
4. Fibromatosis
5. Neurofibroma

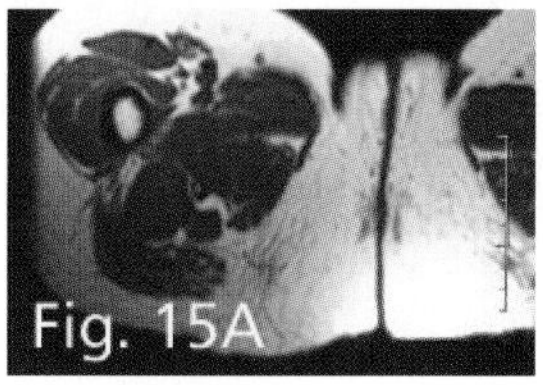
Fig. 15A

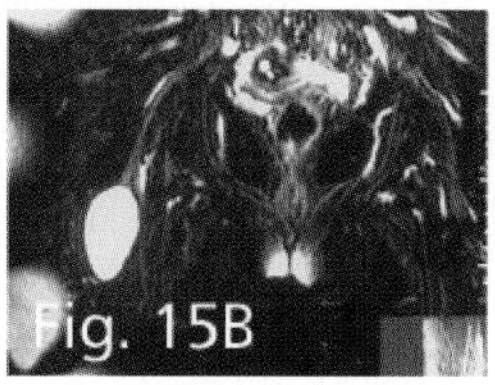
Fig. 15B

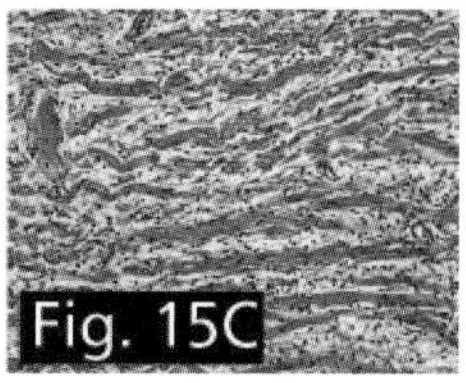
Fig. 15C

PREFERRED RESPONSE: 5

DISCUSSION: Histology shows a wavy collagenous matrix with elongated cells; this is most consistent with neurofibroma. The patient has a mass in the region of the sciatic nerve. Imaging characteristics, homogeneous and very low signal on T1-weighted and very high signal on the T2-weighted sequences, are consistent with a myxoid-type lesion. These include myxoma, myxoid sarcomas, and nerve sheath tumors.

REFERENCES: Campanacci M: *Bone and Soft Tissue Tumors*, ed 2. New York, NY, Springer-Verlag, 1999, pp 1135-1136.

Randall RL: Surgical management of benign soft-tissue tumors, in Menendez LR: *Orthopaedic Knowledge Update: Musculoskeletal Tumors*. Rosemont, IL, American Academy of Orthopaedic Surgeons, 2002, p 251.

A-18: It has been shown that bisphosphonate-based supportive therapy (pamidronate or zoledronate) reduces skeletal events (onset or progression of osteolytic lesions) both in patients with multiple myeloma and in cancer patients with bone metastasis. The use of bisphosphonate therapy has been associated with

1. increased medical complications of treatment.
2. osteonecrosis of the jaw.
3. improved long-term survival rates.
4. anorexia.
5. decreased quality-of-life measures.

PREFERRED RESPONSE: 2

DISCUSSION: The use of bisphosphonates has been recently associated with the development of osteonecrosis of the jaw. Length of exposure seems to be the most important risk factor for this complication. The type of bisphosphonate may play a role and previous dental procedures may be a precipitating factor. Bisphosphonates (such as alendronate) are a class of therapeutic agents originally designed to treat loss of bone density. The primary mechanism of action of these drugs is inhibition of osteoclastic activity, and it has been shown that these drugs are useful in diseases with propensities toward osseous metastases. In particular, they are effective in diseases in which there is clear upregulation of osteoclastic or osteolytic activity, such as breast cancer and multiple myeloma, and have developed into a mainstay of treatment for individuals with these diseases. Although shown to reduce skeletal events, there has been no improvement in patient survival.

REFERENCES: Bamias A, Kastritis E, Bamia C, et al: Osteonecrosis of the jaw in cancer after treatment with bisphosphonates: Incidence and risk factors. *J Clin Oncol* 2005;23:8580-8587.

Thakkar SG, Isada C, Smith J, et al: Jaw complications associated with bisphosphonate use in patients with plasma cell dyscrasias. *Med Oncol* 2006;23:51-56. Van Poznak C: The phenomenon of osteonecrosis of the jaw in patients with metastatic breast cancer. *Cancer Invest* 2006;24:110-112.

A-19: A 12-year-old girl has had pain in her right knee for 1 month that started as activity-related and progressed to night pain. Radiographs are shown in Figures 16A and 16B, and a histology section is shown in Figure 16C. What is the recommended treatment?

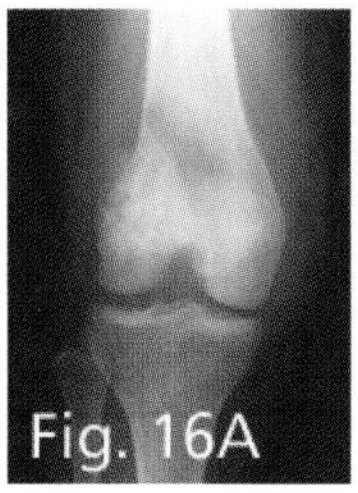
Fig. 16A

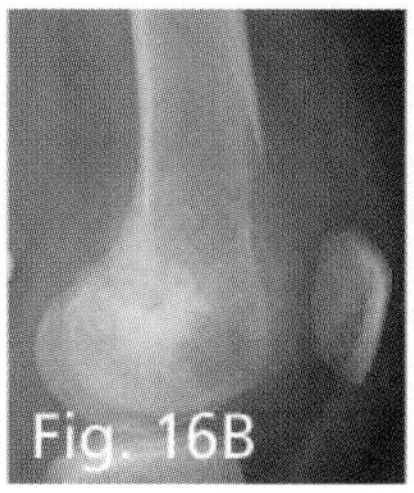
Fig. 16B

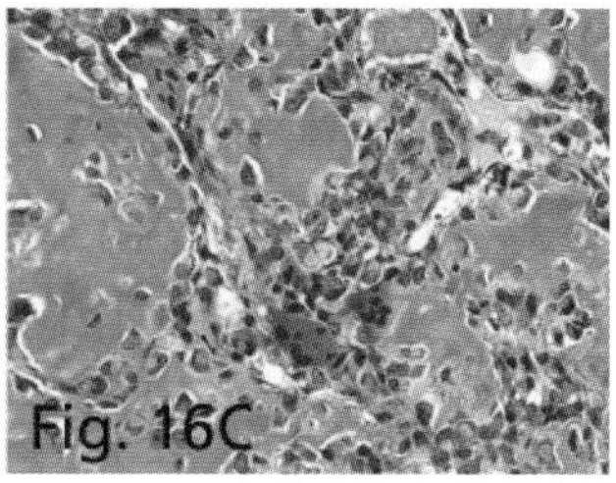
Fig. 16C

1. Resection of the distal femur and postoperative chemotherapy
2. Preoperative chemotherapy followed by radiation therapy, then resection of the distal femur
3. Preoperative chemotherapy followed by surgical resection of the lesion and postoperative chemotherapy
4. Preoperative chemotherapy followed by radiation therapy, resection of the distal femur, then postoperative chemotherapy
5. Resection of the distal femur followed by radiation therapy

PREFERRED RESPONSE: 3

DISCUSSION: This is a classic appearance for an osteosarcoma. The radiographs reveal a mixed osteolytic and osteoblastic lesion in a skeletally immature patient in the distal right femoral metaphysis. The pain pattern with progressive symptoms leading to the presence of night pain is also typical for this condition. Histology reveals pleomorphic cells and the presence of osteoid. The current standard of care in the treatment of osteosarcoma is neoadjuvant chemotherapy followed by surgical resection or amputation followed by additional postoperative chemotherapy. Osteosarcoma is not radiosensitive.

REFERENCES: Wold LE, Adler CP, Sim FH, et al: *Atlas of Orthopedic Pathology*, ed 2. Philadelphia, PA, WB Saunders, 2003, p 179.

McCarthy EF, Frassica FJ: *Pathology of Bone and Joint Disorders with Clinical and Radiographic Correlation*. Philadelphia, PA, WB Saunders, 1998, p 205.

A-20: Figure 17A shows the clinical photograph of a 31-year-old man who has a slowly growing nodule on his right middle finger. It is minimally tender, and there is no erythema on examination. A histology section is shown in Figure 17B. What is the most likely diagnosis?

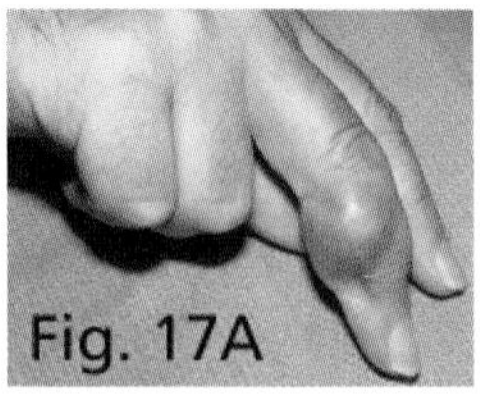
Fig. 17A

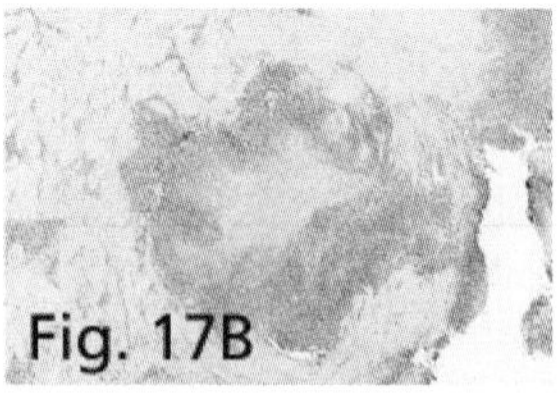
Fig. 17B

1. Clear cell sarcoma
2. Clear cell carcinoma
3. Epidermal inclusion cyst
4. Nora's tumor (BPOP)
5. Epithelioid sarcoma

PREFERRED RESPONSE: 5

DISCUSSION: Epithelioid sarcoma is the most common soft-tissue sarcoma in the hand and most commonly occurs in young adults. The tumors can be superficial and may become ulcerated. Deeper lesions are often attached to tendons, tendon sheaths, or fascial structures. These are usually minimally symptomatic. The biopsy specimen reveals the typical appearance of a nodular pattern with central necrosis. They can mimic a necrotizing granulomatous process. Usually there are chronic inflammatory cells along the margin of the tumor nodules. This biopsy specimen does not have the clear cells necessary for

(continued on next page)

(A-20: *continued*)

a clear cell carcinoma or sarcoma. Nora tumor is a bizarre parosteal osteochondromatous proliferation (BPOP) first described in 1983 by the pathologist, Nora. The lesion is defined as a reactive heterotopic ossification and is mostly found in the hands or feet of adults in the third decade of life.

REFERENCES: Enzinger FM, Weiss SW: *Soft Tissue Tumors*, ed 3. St. Louis, MO, Mosby, 1995, p 1074.

Halling AC, Wollan PC, Pritchard DJ, et al: Epithelioid sarcoma: A clinicopathologic review of 55 cases. *Mayo Clin Proc* 1996;71:636-642.

A-21: A 17-year-old girl who initially presented during childhood with multiple skeletal lesions, café-au-lait spots, and precocious puberty now has bone pain. A recent bone scan reveals multiple areas of increased scintigraphic uptake, including bilateral proximal femurs. A radiograph is shown in Figure 18. In addition to activity modification, what is the best next line of treatment for decreasing her pain?

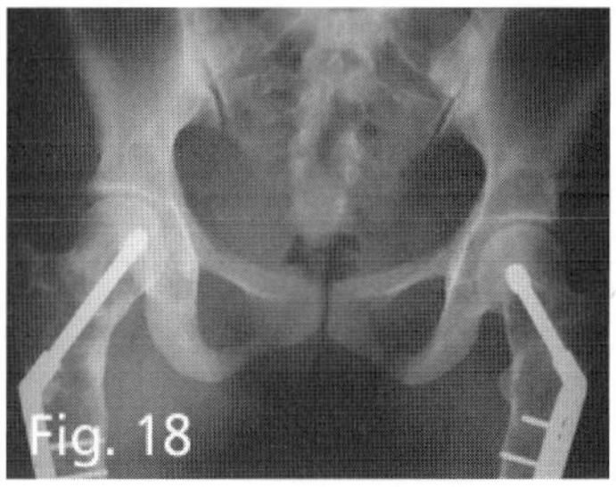

1. Bisphosphonates
2. Calcitonin
3. Parathyroid hormone
4. Vitamin D and calcium
5. Methotrexate

PREFERRED RESPONSE: 1

DISCUSSION: McCune-Albright syndrome is the combination of polyostotic fibrous dysplasia, café-au-lait lesions, and endocrine dysfunction. The most common endocrine presentation is precocious development of secondary sexual characteristics. Compared with bone lesions in patients without polyostotic disease, the skeletal lesions in patients with the syndrome tend to be larger, more persistent, and associated with more complications. Bisphosphonate therapy has been shown in several studies to decrease the pain associated with the skeletal lesions of fibrous dysplasia.

REFERENCES: DiCaprio MR, Enneking WF: Fibrous dysplasia: Pathophysiology, evaluation and treatment. *J Bone Joint Surg Am* 2005;87:1848-1864.

Zacharin M, O'Sullivan M: Intravenous pamidronate treatment of polyostotic fibrous dysplasia associated with McCune Albright syndrome. *J Pediatr* 2000;137:403-409.

A-22: What are the four most common soft-tissue sarcomas to spread via the lymph node system?

1. Rhabdomyosarcoma, malignant fibrous histiocytoma, epithelioid sarcoma, clear cell sarcoma
2. Malignant fibrous histiocytoma, synovial sarcoma, clear cell sarcoma, epithelioid sarcoma
3. Liposarcoma, rhabdomyosarcoma, synovial sarcoma, clear cell sarcoma
4. Rhabdomyosarcoma, clear cell sarcoma, epithelioid sarcoma, synovial sarcoma
5. Liposarcoma, clear cell sarcoma, rhabdomyosarcoma, epithelioid sarcoma

PREFERRED RESPONSE: 4

DISCUSSION: Soft-tissue sarcomas most frequently metastasize to the lung, but certain histologic types have a predilection for the lymph node system as well. Rhabdomyosarcoma, clear cell sarcoma, epitheli-

(continued on next page)

(A-22: *continued*)

oid sarcoma, and synovial sarcoma are four of the most common types to spread in this fashion. Careful evaluation and/or sentinel lymph node biopsy play a role in disease staging and prognosis.

REFERENCES: Riad S, Griffin AM, Liberman B, et al: Lymph node metastasis in soft-tissue sarcoma in an extremity. *Clin Orthop Relat Res* 2004;426:129-134.

Blazer DG III, Sabel MS, Sondak VK: Is there a role for sentinel lymph node biopsy in the management of sarcoma? *Surg Oncol* 2003;12:201-206.

A-23: Figures 19A and 19B show the AP and lateral radiographs of a 62-year-old man who has had hip pain for the past 3 weeks. Figure 19C shows a CT scan of the abdomen and pelvis. A needle biopsy was performed and the histology is shown in Figure 19D. Preoperative management should include which of the following?

1. Lymphoscintigraphy
2. Colonoscopy
3. Bronchoscopy
4. Embolization of the femoral lesion
5. Bone marrow aspiration

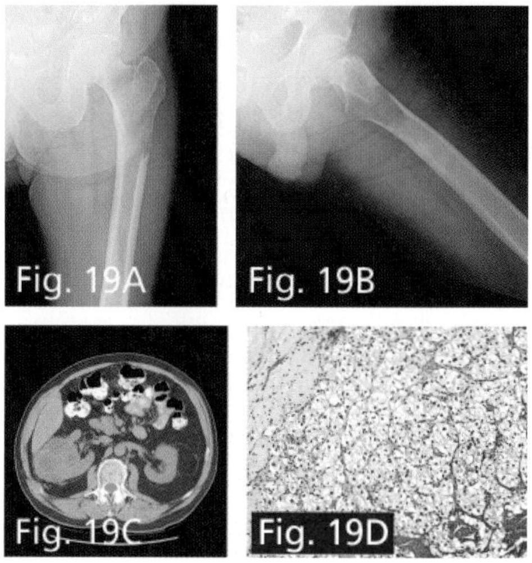
Fig. 19A Fig. 19B Fig. 19C Fig. 19D

PREFERRED RESPONSE: 4

DISCUSSION: The histology shows findings consistent with metastatic renal cell carcinoma. Renal cell carcinoma metastases are extremely vascular. Preoperative embolization helps minimize the amount of blood loss during curettage of these lesions.

REFERENCES: Chatziioannou AN, Johnson ME, Pneumaticos SG, et al: Preoperative embolization of bone metastases from renal cell carcinoma. *Eur Radiol* 2000;10:593-596.

Sun S, Lang EV: Bone metastases from renal cell carcinoma: Preoperative embolization. *J Vasc Interv Radiol* 1998;9:263-269.

A-24: A 58-year-old woman has a fracture through a metacarpal lesion after a motor vehicle accident. She denies any preinjury symptoms and the fracture heals uneventfully. Based on the radiograph and MRI scans shown in Figures 20A through 20C obtained following fracture healing, follow-up management should consist of

1. curettage.
2. radiation therapy.
3. observation.
4. bisphosphonates.
5. ray resection.

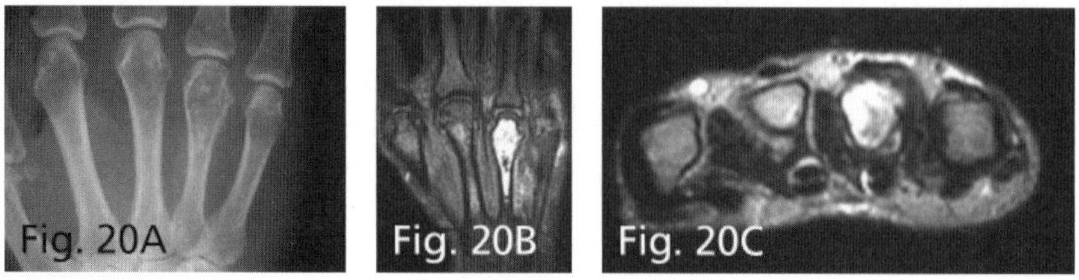
Fig. 20A Fig. 20B Fig. 20C

(continued on next page)

(A-24: *continued*)

PREFERRED RESPONSE: 3

DISCUSSION: Enchondromas are the most common benign skeletal lesions identified in the bones of the hand. Most are incidentally found or initially become clinically evident after a pathologic fracture. If the patient has a fracture, the hand is immobilized until union. If the lesion is large and further pathologic fractures are expected, then an intralesional curettage and grafting procedure may be warranted. In this patient, the lesion has not significantly altered the size, shape, or morphology of the involved metacarpal head and recurrent fracture is unlikely. Observation with follow-up radiographs is considered appropriate management.

REFERENCES: Campanacci M: *Bone and Soft Tissue Tumors*, ed 2. New York, NY, Springer-Verlag, 1999, pp 213-228.

Marco RA, Gitelis S, Brebach GT, et al: Cartilage tumors: Evaluation and treatment. *J Am Acad Orthop Surg* 2000;8:292-304.

A-25: A 13-year-old boy has knee pain after sustaining a mild twisting injury while playing basketball 4 weeks ago. Radiographs and MRI scans are shown in Figures 21A through 21D, and histology sections are shown in Figures 21E and 21F. Treatment should consist of

1. neoadjuvant chemotherapy followed by surgical resection and reconstruction.
2. chemotherapy followed by radiation therapy.
3. intravenous antibiotics for 4 weeks, followed by oral antibiotics for 4 weeks.
4. surgical resection and reconstruction followed by chemotherapy.
5. radiation therapy alone.

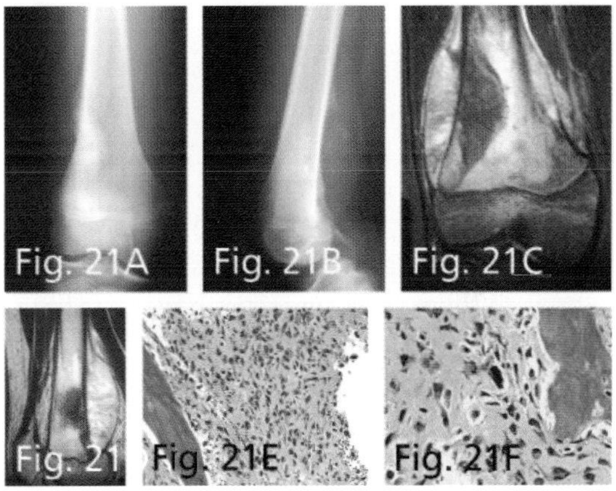

PREFERRED RESPONSE: 1

DISCUSSION: The imaging studies and histology are consistent with high-grade osteosarcoma. The standard treatment for osteosarcoma is neoadjuvant chemotherapy combined with wide surgical resection that can be performed with amputation or limb salvage depending on characteristics unique to each tumor and each patient. In most patients, limb salvage surgery can be performed with reconstruction using allografts and/or megaprostheses. Osteosarcoma is poorly responsive to radiation therapy. Chemotherapy alone, in the absence of appropriate surgery, has not proven effective.

REFERENCES: Simon MA, Springfield DS: *Surgery for Bone and Soft-Tissue Tumors*. Philadelphia, PA, Lippincott-Raven, 1998, pp 265-274.

Gibbs CP, Weber K, Scarborough MT: Malignant bone tumors. *Instr Course Lect* 2002;51:413-428.

A-26: A 64-year-old man has had increasing pain in the left hip for the past 6 months. A radiograph and MRI scan are shown in Figures 22A and 22B. Biopsy specimens are shown in Figures 22C and 22D. What is the recommended treatment?

1. Chemotherapy and internal hemipelvectomy
2. Chemotherapy and hindquarter amputation
3. Radiation therapy and internal hemipelvectomy
4. Radiation therapy and hindquarter amputation
5. Hindquarter amputation or internal hemipelvectomy

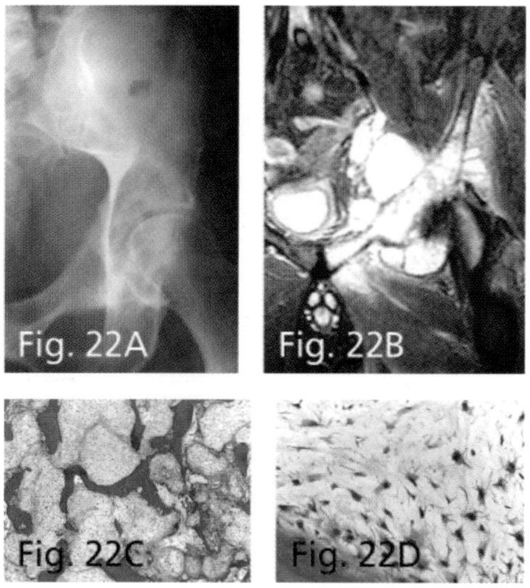

PREFERRED RESPONSE: 5

DISCUSSION: The radiograph shows a lytic lesion in the left periacetabular area consistent with chondrosarcoma. A large soft-tissue mass is present along with extension through the supra-acetabular region and pubic ramus. The histology shows a hypercellular lesion infiltrating through the bony trabeculae with a basophilic cytoplasm. This is classified as a grade 2 chondrosarcoma. The treatment of a pelvic chondrosarcoma is wide resection via either an internal hemipelvectomy or amputation. Chondrosarcoma requires surgical resection for control and does not traditionally respond to chemotherapy or external beam irradiation therapy.

REFERENCES: Pring M, Weber, KL, Unni KK, et al: Chondrosarcoma of the pelvis: A review of sixty-four cases. *J Bone Joint Surg* 2001;83:1630-1642.

Wold LE, Adler CP, Sim FH, et al: *Atlas of Orthopedic Pathology*, ed 2. Philadelphia, PA, WB Saunders, 2003, p 255.

A-27: The scoring system for impending pathologic fractures devised by Mirels involves assessment of which of the following factors?

1. Lesion location, amount of pain, lesion type, lesion size (lucent/blastic)
2. Patient's functional status, lesion location, amount of pain, lesion size
3. Lesion type (lucent/blastic), patient's functional status, lesion location, amount of pain
4. Lesion size, lesion type (lucent/blastic), lesion location, patient's functional status
5. Amount of pain, patient's functional status, lesion type (lucent/blastic), lesion size

PREFERRED RESPONSE: 1

DISCUSSION: The scoring system published by Mirels in 1989 is based on the following characteristics: the location of the lesion, the amount of pain the patient is experiencing, the type of lesion (either lucent, mixed, or blastic), and the lesion size. The tumor is scored from 1 to 3 in each category and a total score is obtained that correlates to fracture risk. Prophylactic fixation is advised for lesions with scores higher than 8, and consideration for stabilization should be strongly considered for scores of 8. The Mirels scoring system can be useful as an adjunct to clinical decision making.

REFERENCES: Mirels H: Metastatic disease in long bones: A proposed scoring system for diagnosing impending pathologic fractures. 1989. *Clin Orthop Relat Res* 2003;415:S4-S13.

Damron TA, Morgan H, Prakash D, et al: Critical evaluation of Mirels' rating system for impending pathologic fractures. *Clin Orthop Relat Res* 2003;415:S201-S207.

A-28: Figures 23A and 23B show the radiograph and MRI scan of a 22-year-old man with knee pain. What is the most likely diagnosis?

1. Osteochondroma
2. Osteoblastoma
3. Osteosarcoma
4. Chondrosarcoma
5. Malignant fibrous histiocytoma of bone

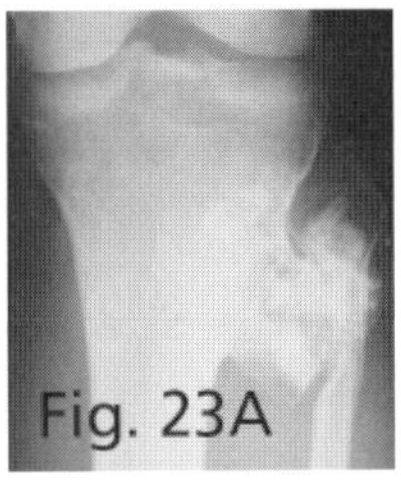
Fig. 23A

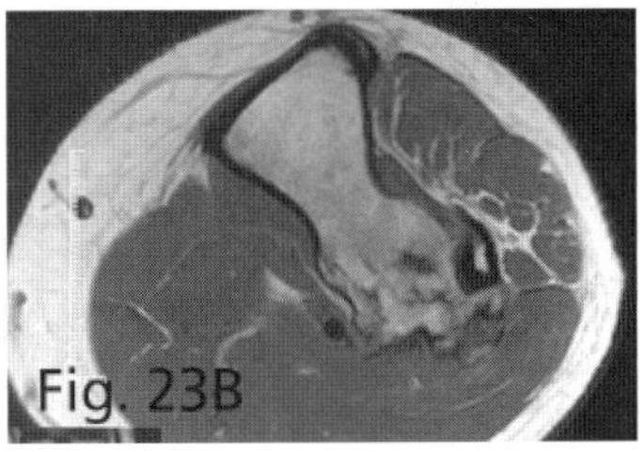
Fig. 23B

PREFERRED RESPONSE: 1

DISCUSSION: The lesion is an osteochondroma. This is demonstrated by a pedunculated bone-forming lesion where the medullary space of the lesion communicates with the medullary space of the host bone. The cortex of the exostosis is in continuity with the cortex of the underlying bone. The MRI scan reveals that there is no significant cartilage cap, alleviating concern for malignant conversion to a chondrosarcoma. Osteoblastoma and osteosarcoma typically have mixed areas of bone formation and bone destruction. Malignant fibrous histiocytoma of bone is usually purely lytic.

REFERENCES: Lackman RD: Musculoskeletal oncology, in Vaccaro AR, ed: *Orthopaedic Knowledge Update*, ed 8. Rosemont, IL, American Academy of Orthopaedic Surgeons, 2005, pp 197-215.

Gitelis S, Soorapanth G: Benign chondroid tumors, in Menendez LR, ed: *Orthopaedic Knowledge Update: Musculoskeletal Tumors*. Rosemont, IL, American Academy of Orthopaedic Surgeons, 2002, pp 103-111.

A-29: Which of the following malignant tumors most commonly contains soft-tissue calcifications seen on radiographs or CT?

1. Hemangioma
2. Ewing sarcoma
3. Clear cell sarcoma
4. Malignant fibrous histiocytoma
5. Synovial sarcoma

PREFERRED RESPONSE: 5

DISCUSSION: Focal calcifications causing small radiopacities are found in 15% to 20% of synovial sarcomas. Their irregular contours differentiate them from the phleboliths found in a benign hemangioma. Ewing sarcoma, clear cell sarcoma, and malignant fibrous histiocytoma do not commonly have calcifications within the lesions.

REFERENCES: Enzinger FM, Weiss SW: *Soft Tissue Tumors*, ed 3. St. Louis, MO, Mosby, 1995, p 761.

Bullough PG: *Atlas of Orthopedic Pathology With Clinical and Radiologic Correlations*, ed 2. New York, NY, Gower, 1992, p 17.23.

A-30: Which of the following is most associated with local recurrence of the lesion seen in the radiograph and MRI scan shown in Figures 24A and 24B?

1. Effectiveness of chemotherapy
2. Effect of local adjuvant
3. Open physes
4. Presence of giant cells
5. Effectiveness of embolization

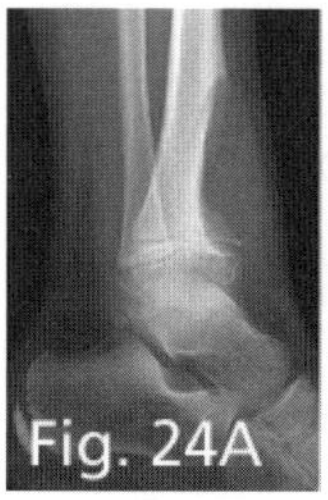
Fig. 24A

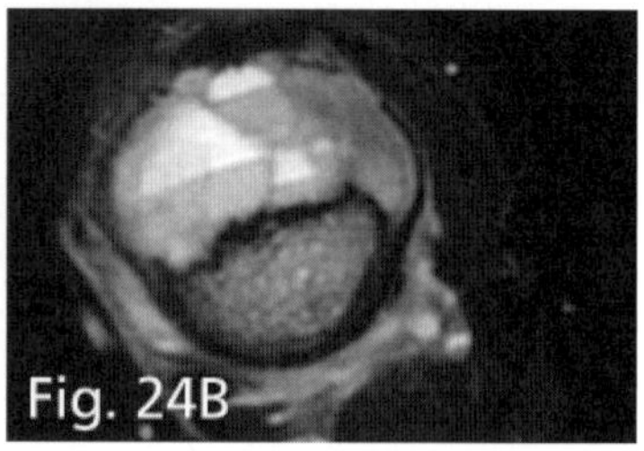
Fig. 24B

PREFERRED RESPONSE: 3

DISCUSSION: The lesion is an aneurysmal bone cyst. These lesions are known to have a local recurrence rate of 5% to 50%. Young age, open physes, stage, and type of surgical removal and resulting margin have all been shown to affect the recurrence rate. Chemotherapy is not used in the treatment of aneurysmal bone cysts.

REFERENCES: Gibbs CP Jr, Hefele MC, Peabody TD, et al: Aneurysmal bone cyst of the extremities: Factors related to local recurrence after curettage with a high-speed burr. *J Bone Joint Surg Am* 1999;81:1671-1678.

Vergel De Dios AM, Bond JR, Shives TC, et al: Aneurysmal bone cyst: A clinicopathologic study of 238 cases. *Cancer* 1992;69:2921-2931.

A-31: A 33-year-old woman reports a mass on the right hand that has been enlarging for 1 year. An intraoperative photograph is shown in Figure 25A, and a histology section is shown in Figure 25B. What is the most likely diagnosis?

1. Ganglion cyst
2. Abscess
3. Hematoma
4. Giant cell tumor of tendon sheath
5. Synovial sarcoma

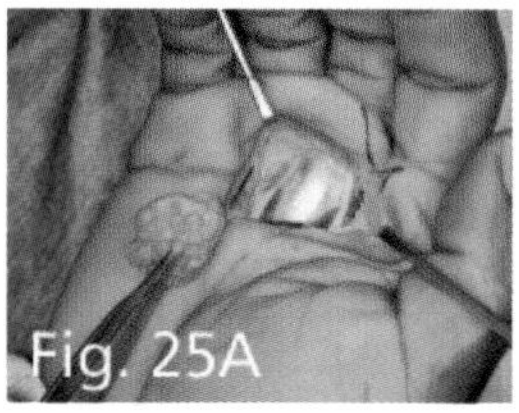
Fig. 25A

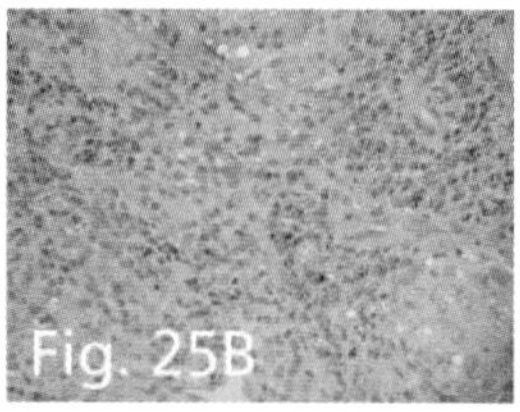
Fig. 25B

PREFERRED RESPONSE: 4

DISCUSSION: Giant cell tumor of the tendon sheath is the most common solid soft-tissue mass in the hand. These tumors are slow growing and may be present for months or years before coming to medical attention. Patients usually report mechanical difficulties because of the size or position of the tumor. The gross appearance is that of a lobulated mass that may be multicolored; typically yellow, brown, red, and gray. Histologically the lesion consists of multinucleated giant cells, polygonal mononuclear cells, and histiocytes that may contain abundant hemosiderin or lipid.

REFERENCES: Walsh EF, Mechrefe A, Akelman E, et al: Giant cell tumor of tendon sheath. *Am J Orthop* 2005;34: 116-121.

Weiss SW, Goldblum JR, eds: *Enzinger and Weiss's Soft Tissue Tumors*, ed 4. St. Louis, MO, Mosby, 2001, pp 1038-1047.

A-32: A 15-year-old girl has had a painful mass on the medial aspect of her left thigh for the past 5 years. The pain is present only when she is performing athletic activities and is completely relieved with rest. A radiograph and MRI scan are shown in Figures 26A and 26B. The patient and her parents would like to have the mass removed. What further diagnostic studies are required prior to considering surgical resection?

1. Bone scan
2. CT
3. Needle biopsy
4. Incisional biopsy
5. No further tests are needed

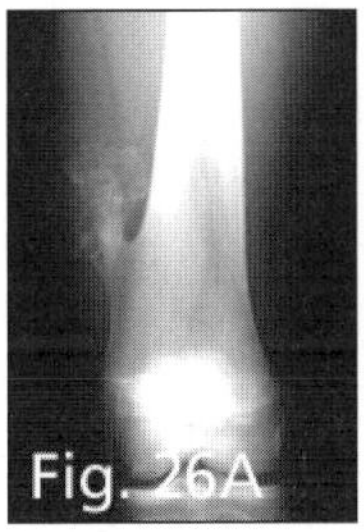

Fig. 26A

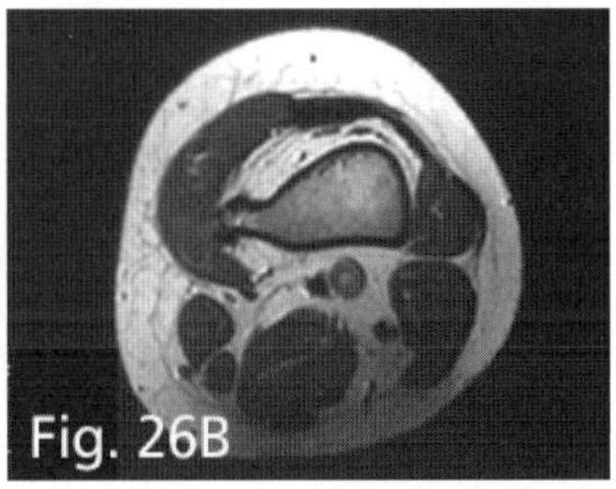

Fig. 26B

PREFERRED RESPONSE: 5

DISCUSSION: The radiograph and MRI scan show a pedunculated lesion arising from the medial aspect of the distal femoral metaphysis. The cortex of the lesion is contiguous with the cortex of the underlying normal bone. Similarly, the medullary canal of the lesion is contiguous with that of the normal bone. These findings are diagnostic of osteochondroma. Rarely a secondary chondrosarcoma can arise in a preexisting osteochondroma. This diagnosis is suggested by identifying a cartilage cap that is greater than 1.5 cm thick in a skeletally mature patient. MRI is the best study to rule out a secondary chondrosarcoma. CT also may be used for this purpose but is not indicated in this patient because an MRI has already been obtained. A bone scan is not useful to identify a secondary chondrosarcoma. Similarly, there is no role for biopsy in this patient. No further tests are needed.

REFERENCES: Menendez LR, ed: *Orthopaedic Knowledge Update: Musculoskeletal Tumors.* Rosemont, IL, American Academy of Orthopaedic Surgeons, 2002, pp 103-111.

Murphey MD, Choi JJ, Kransdorf, MJ, et al: Imaging of osteochondroma: Variants and complications with radiologic-pathologic correlation. *Radiographics* 2000;20:1407-1434.

A-33: A 22-year-old man has mild hip pain bilaterally and multiple skeletal lesions. Based on the pelvic radiograph shown in Figure 27, what is the inheritance pattern for his disorder?

1. X-linked
2. Autosomal recessive
3. Autosomal dominant
4. Mitochondrial inheritance
5. Germline mutation

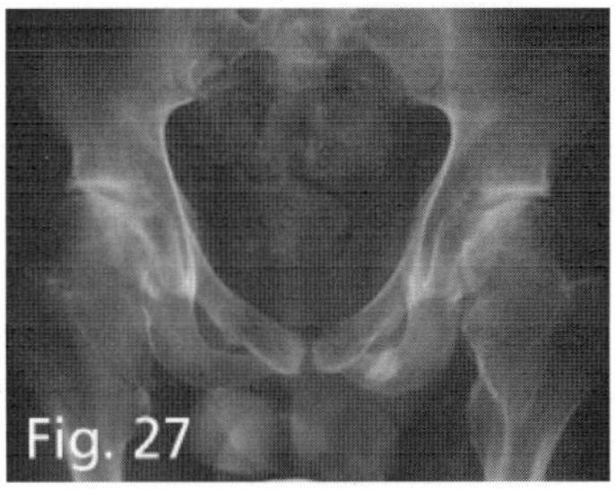

Fig. 27

PREFERRED RESPONSE: 3

DISCUSSION: Multiple hereditary exostoses (MHE) is an autosomal dominant disorder manifested by multiple osteochondromas and characteristic skeletal involvement. *EXT1* on 8q24.1 and *EXT2* on 11p13 are the two genes most strongly associated with MHE. Mutations in these genes affect proper development of endochondral bone, such that in all affected individuals exostoses develop adjacent to the growth plates of long bones, and some exhibit additional bone deformities. Defects in the *EXT* genes result in increased chondrocyte proliferation and delayed hypertrophic differentiation.

(continued on next page)

(A-33: *continued*)

REFERENCES: Stieber JR, Dormans JP: Manifestations of hereditary multiple exostoses. *J Am Acad Orthop Surg* 2005;13:110-120.

Hilton MJ, Gutierrez L, Martinez DA, et al: EXT1 regulates chondrocyte proliferation and differentiation during endochondral bone development. *Bone* 2005;36:379-386.

A-34: An 80-year-old woman notes a painless mass posterior to her left knee. MRI scans are shown in Figures 28A and 28B. What is the best course of action?

1. Observation
2. Medical management
3. Needle biopsy
4. Incisional biopsy
5. Resection

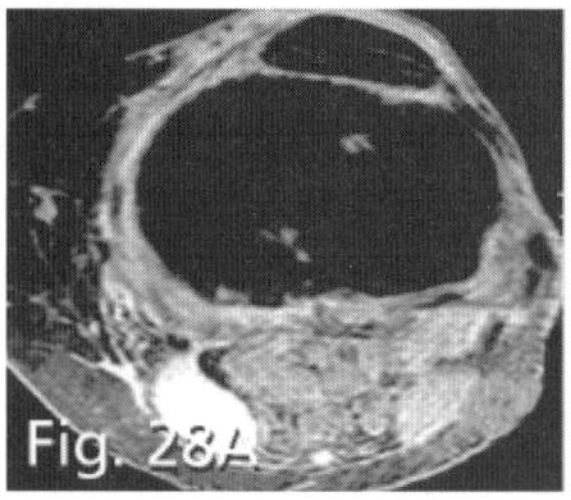
Fig. 28A

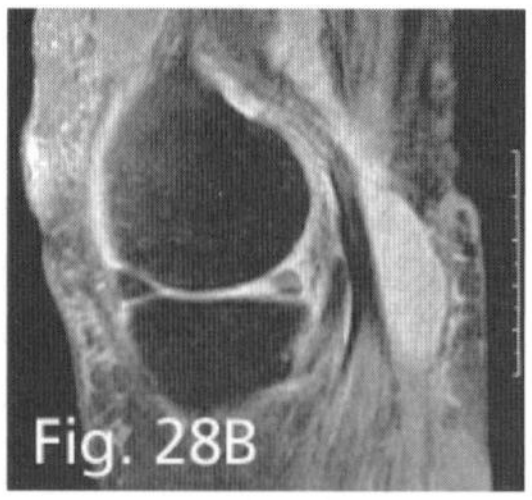
Fig. 28B

PREFERRED RESPONSE: 1

DISCUSSION: The MRI scans show a popliteal cyst (Baker cyst) in its most common location. The cyst emerges from the knee joint between the medial head of the gastrocnemius muscle and the tendon of the semimembranosus muscle. These images are diagnostic; therefore, no further work-up is indicated. Because the patient is asymptomatic, no treatment is necessary.

REFERENCES: Dlabach JA: Nontraumatic soft tissue disorders, in Canale ST, ed: *Campbell's Operative Orthopaedics*, ed 10. Philidelphia, PA, Mosby, 2003, vol 1, pp 885-969.

Fritschy D, Fasel J, Imbert JC, et al: The popliteal cyst. *Knee Surg Sports Traumatol Arthrosc* 2006;14:623-628.

A-35: What is the most common malignancy involving the hand?

1. Epithelioid sarcoma
2. Synovial sarcoma
3. Metastatic lung carcinoma
4. Chondrosarcoma
5. Squamous cell carcinoma

PREFERRED RESPONSE: 5

DISCUSSION: Skin cancers far outnumber primary musculoskeletal malignancies of the hand and the most common of these is squamous cell carcinoma. Metatastic lung carcinoma, although classic for the carcinoma that metastasizes to the hand, does so at an extremely low rate.

REFERENCES: Fink JA, Akelman E: Nonmelanotic malignant skin tumors of the hand. *Hand Clin* 1995;11:255-264.
Fleegler EJ: Skin tumors, in Green DP, Hotchkiss RN, Pederson WC, eds: *Green's Operative Hand Surgery*, ed 4. Philadelphia, PA, Churchill Livingstone, 1999, vol 2, pp 2184-2205.

A-36: A 35-year-old man has had progressive right knee pain for the past 2 months. An AP radiograph, bone scan, MRI scan, and photomicrograph are shown in Figures 29A through 29D. What is the most appropriate treatment of this lesion?

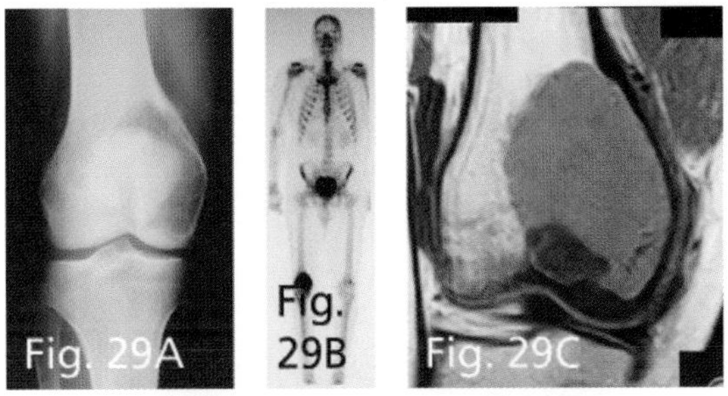

1. Observation
2. Extended curettage with adjuvant treatment
3. Wide resection
4. Radiation therapy
5. Multimodal treatment including chemotherapy and surgery

PREFERRED RESPONSE: 2

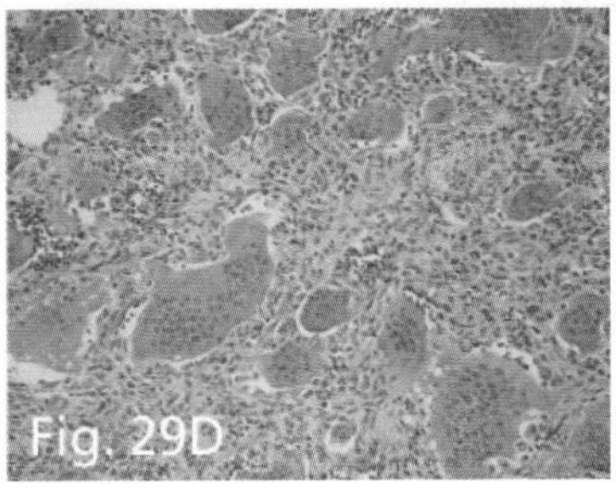

DISCUSSION: This is a classic case of giant cell tumor of bone. The radiograph and the MRI scan reveal a purely lytic lesion in the medial femoral condyle. The lesion is well demarcated without a rim of sclerotic bone. It is eccentrically located and abuts the subchondral bone. The lesion demonstrates increased uptake on a technetium Tc-99m bone scan. These imaging studies are highly suggestive of giant cell tumor arising in its most common location. The photomicrograph confirms the diagnosis of giant cell tumor. Based on these findings, the most widely accepted treatment is extended curettage plus a local adjuvant such as polymethyl methacrylate bone cement, argon beam coagulation, liquid nitrogen, and/or phenol.

REFERENCES: Lackman RD, Hosalkar HS, Ogilvie CM, et al: Intralesional curettage for grades II and III giant cell tumors of bone. *Clin Orthop Relat Res* 2005;438:123-127.

Ward WG Sr, Li G III: Customized treatment algorithm for giant cell tumor of bone: Report of a series. *Clin Orthop Relat Res* 2002;397:259-270.

A-37: What is the most common bone tumor in the hand?

1. Periosteal chondroma
2. Subungual exostosis
3. Chondrosarcoma
4. Osteoid osteoma
5. Enchondroma

PREFERRED RESPONSE: 5

DISCUSSION: The most common bone tumor in the hand is an enchondroma. Forty-two percent of these lesions occur in the small tubular bones. They frequently present with a fracture in these locations. Fractures are usually treated nonsurgically. Indications for surgery include patients with symptomatic lesions or those who are considered high risk for recurrent fracture. The histologic appearance of an enchondroma in the hand is more cellular than enchondromas found in the long bones.

REFERENCES: Gitelis S, Sooropanth C: Benign chondroid tumors, in Menendez LR, ed: *Orthopaedic Knowledge Update: Musculoskeletal Tumors*. Rosemont, IL, American Academy of Orthopaedic Surgeons, 2002, p 103.

Kuur E, Hansen SL, Lindequist S: Treatment of solitary enchondromas in fingers. *J Hand Surg Br* 1989;14:109-112.

A-38: A 75-year-old woman has had severe shoulder pain for the past month. Her medical history includes hypertension and a total nephrectomy for renal cell carcinoma 7 years ago. Radiographs and sagittal MRI scans are shown in Figures 30A through 30D. A bone scan reveals this to be an isolated lesion. Biopsy findings are consistent with metastatic renal cell carcinoma. What is the most appropriate treatment for this patient?

1. Prophylactic stabilization with an intramedullary rod
2. Radiation therapy alone
3. Embolization alone
4. Wide resection and prosthetic reconstruction
5. Prophylactic stabilization with a locking plate and polymethyl methacrylate cement

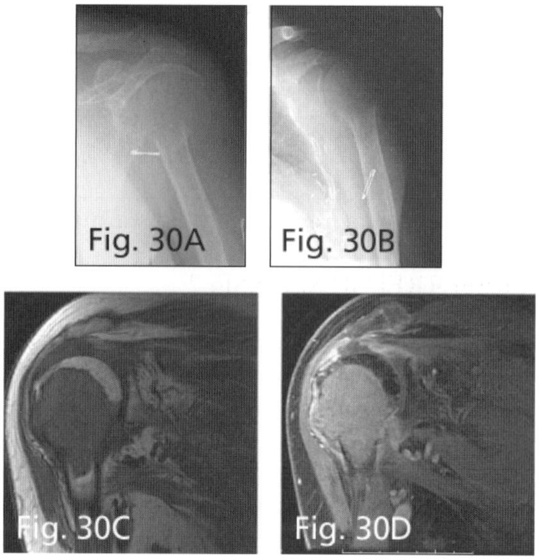

Fig. 30A Fig. 30B Fig. 30C Fig. 30D

PREFERRED RESPONSE: 4

DISCUSSION: Resection and reconstruction of this very proximal lesion provides the best chance to avoid hardware complications that may be associated with stabilization procedures. Wide resection of isolated renal cell carcinoma metastasis, which presents distant to the nephrectomy, may improve long-term survival.

REFERENCES: Fuchs B, Trousdale RT, Rock MG: Solitary bony metastasis from renal cell carcinoma: Significance of surgical treatment. *Clin Orthop Relat Res* 2005;431:187-192.

Jung ST, Ghert MA, Harrelson JM, et al: Treatment of osseous metastases in patients with renal cell carcinoma. *Clin Orthop Relat Res* 2003;409:223-231.

A-39: A patient undergoes a simple excision of a 3-cm superficial mass in the thigh at another institution. The final pathology reveals a leiomyosarcoma, without reference to the margins. What is the recommendation for definitive treatment?

1. Repeat wide excision of the tumor bed
2. Observation
3. Radiation therapy to the tumor bed only
4. Chemotherapy
5. Radiation therapy and chemotherapy

PREFERRED RESPONSE: 1

DISCUSSION: Treatment of patients with unplanned excision of soft-tissue sarcomas is challenging. If the margins are positive or unclear, the patient is best managed with repeat excision of the tumor bed, and radiation therapy if the repeat excision does not yield wide margins. In patients with no detectable tumor on physical examination or imaging after unplanned excision, some studies have shown that up to 35% of patients will have residual disease and a poorer local recurrence rate (22% versus 7%). Therefore, whenever feasible, a reexcision of the tumor bed is recommended.

REFERENCE: Noria S, Davis A, Kandel R, et al: Residual disease following unplanned excision of soft-tissue sarcoma of an extremity. *J Bone Joint Surg Am* 1996;78:650-655.

A-40: A 14-year-old girl reports a 3-week history of anterior thigh pain and a palpable mass after sustaining a soccer-related injury. Examination reveals a tender, firm mass in the midportion of the rectus femoris. MRI scans are shown in Figures 31A through 31C. What is the most appropriate management?

1. Incision and drainage of the abscess
2. NSAIDs, physical therapy, and a repeat MRI scan in 6 to 8 weeks
3. Open biopsy
4. Hematoma evacuation and musculotendinous repair
5. Primary wide resection followed by radiation therapy

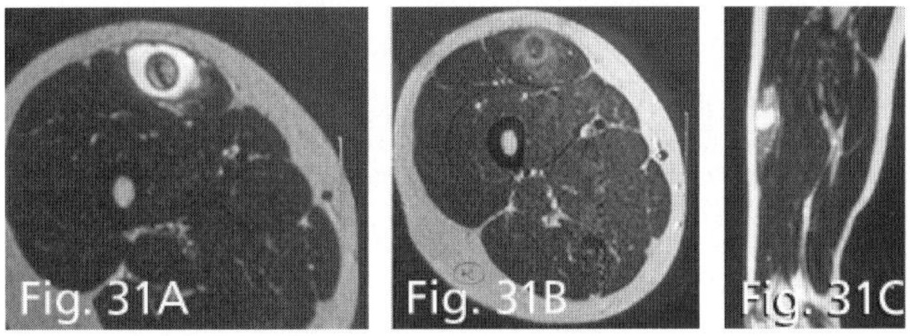
Fig. 31A Fig. 31B Fig. 31C

PREFERRED RESPONSE: 2

DISCUSSION: The history, examination, and MRI findings are consistent with a midsubstance partial rupture of the rectus femoris muscle. This is an injury masquerading as a pseudotumor. The lack of an appreciable mass effect on the T1-weighted MRI scan, the defined fluid signal on the T2-weighted scans, and the lack of significant contrast enhancement after gadolinium are all most consistent with injury rather than a neoplasm. Most of these injuries respond to nonsurgical management; a few will benefit from late débridement and repair if symptoms fail to resolve in 3 to 6 months. The treatment of choice is nonsurgical management with a follow-up MRI scan to verify that the findings are resolving.

REFERENCES: Hughes C IV, Hasselman CT, Best TM, et al: Incomplete, intrasubstance strain injuries of the rectus femoris muscle. *Am J Sports Med* 1995;23:500-506.

Temple HT, Kuklo TR, Sweet DE, et al: Rectus femoris muscle tear appearing as a pseudotumor. *Am J Sports Med* 1998;26:544-548.

A-41: A 7-year-old girl has had a painful forearm for the past 2 months. Examination reveals fullness on the volar aspect of the forearm. Radiographs and an MRI scan are shown in Figures 32A through 32C. Histology sections are shown in Figures 32D and 32E. What is the most likely diagnosis?

1. Synovial sarcoma
2. Liposarcoma
3. Rhabdomyosarcoma
4. Hemangioma
5. Wilms tumor

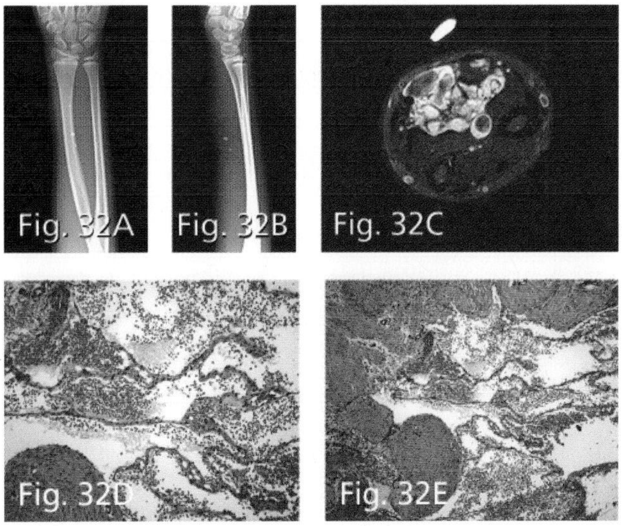
Fig. 32A Fig. 32B Fig. 32C Fig. 32D Fig. 32E

PREFERRED RESPONSE: 4

DISCUSSION: The radiographs reveal phleboliths on the volar side of the forearm consistent with hemangioma. The MRI scan reveals a rather well circumscribed in size, irregular in shape, intramuscular soft-tissue mass in the volar aspect of the distal right forearm within the flexor group musculature. The mass demonstrates heterogeneous mixed signal intensity

(continued on next page)

Orthopaedic Oncology/Systemic Disease: Answers

(A-41: *continued*)

in both T1- and T2-weighted sequences with increased signal intensity on the T1, suggesting fat within the tumor, typical of hemangioma. The postgadolinium-enhanced sequences demonstrate heterogeneous enhancement. The MRI findings are consistent with a soft-tissue hemangioma.

REFERENCES: Garzon M: Hemangiomas: Update on classification, clinical presentation and associate anomalies. *Cutis* 2000;66:325-328.

Kurkcuoglu IC, Eroglu A, Karaoglanoglu N, et al: Soft tissue hemangioma is a common soft tissue neoplasm. *Eur J Radiol* 2004;49:179-181.

A-42: Which of the following is an important factor in performing a proper biopsy?
1. Staying carefully in the proper intermuscular planes
2. Placing multiple drains
3. Dissecting and protecting critical neurovascular structures
4. Using longitudinal incisions in the extremity
5. Avoiding the use of a tourniquet

PREFERRED RESPONSE: 4

DISCUSSION: There are a number of important technical details in performing a biopsy. Incisions should always be longitudinal in the extremity. Good hemostasis is important in avoiding contamination from hematoma. The approach should avoid neurovascular structures, and go through a single muscle belly when possible. Although a frozen section should be obtained to ensure adequate viable tissue has been obtained, definitive diagnosis is not necessary at the time of the frozen section.

REFERENCES: Lackman RD: Musculoskeletal oncology, in Vaccaro AR, ed: *Orthopaedic Knowledge Update*, ed 8. Rosemont, IL, American Academy of Orthopaedic Surgeons, 2005, pp 197-215. Athanasian EA: Biopsy of musculoskeletal tumors, in Menendez LR, ed: *Orthopaedic Knowledge Update: Musculoskeletal Tumors*. Rosemont, IL, American Academy of Orthopaedic Surgeons, 2002, pp 29-34.

A-43: A 16-year-old girl has had painless swelling in her posterior left arm for the past 4 months. A radiograph, MRI scans, and histology from an incisional biopsy specimen are shown in Figures 33A through 33D. What is the cytogenetic translocation most commonly associated with this tumor?

1. (X;18) (p11;q11)
2. (11;22) (q24;q12)
3. (12;22) (q13;q12)
4. (2;13) (q35;q14)
5. (12;16) (q13;p11)

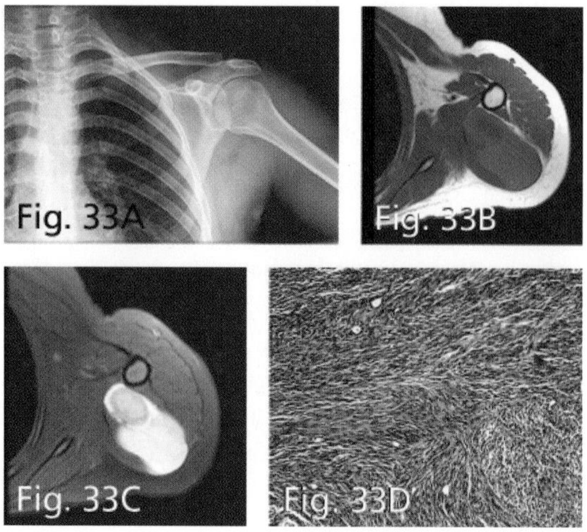
Fig. 33A Fig. 33B Fig. 33C Fig. 33D

PREFERRED RESPONSE: 1

DISCUSSION: This is a case of synovial sarcoma. The radiograph shows some soft-tissue swelling in the upper arm. The MRI scans show a lesion that has increased signal on T2-weighted images and low signal on T1-

(continued on next page)

(A-43: *continued*)

weighted images. There is a suggestion of a large cystic component to this lesion. The histology shows a biphasic population of cells, a spindle cell component, and an epithelioid component. Up to 20% of synovial cell sarcomas have areas of cyst formation. The most common cytogenetic translocation with synovial cell sarcoma is X;18. The 11;22 translocation is most commonly associated with Ewing's sarcomas; the 12;22 translocation is most commonly associated with clear cell sarcomas; the 2;13 translocation is most commonly associated with alveolar rhabdomyosarcomas, and the 12;16 translocation is most commonly associated with myxoid liposarcomas.

REFERENCES: Kawai A, Woodruff J, Healey JH, et al: SYT-SSX gene fusion as a determinant of morphology and prognosis in synovial sarcoma. *N Engl J Med* 1998;338:153-160.

Sandberg AA: Cytogenetics and molecular genetics of bone and soft tissue tumors. *Am J Med Genet* 2002;115:189-193.

A-44: A 43-year-old woman is referred after excisional biopsy of a cutaneous soft-tissue mass from her left shoulder. Based on the histology from biopsy specimens shown in Figures 34A and 34B, what is the best course of action?

1. Marginal resection
2. Observation
3. Wide tumor bed resection
4. Radiation therapy
5. Chemotherapy

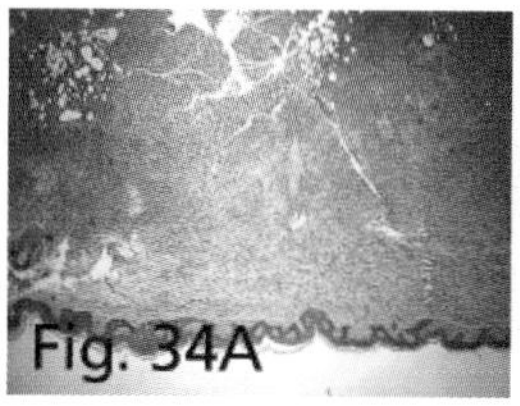
Fig. 34A

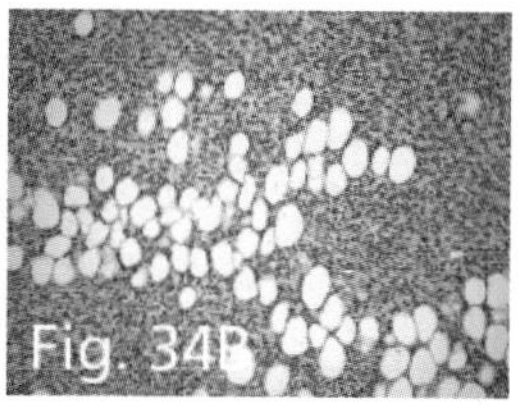
Fig. 34B

PREFERRED RESPONSE: 3

DISCUSSION: Dermatofibrosarcoma protuberans (DFSP) is a rare superficial sarcoma that is frequently misdiagnosed at presentation. It is frequently excised prior to suspecting that the lesion is a sarcoma and if not appropriately treated with tumor bed resection to obtain wide margins, these lesions have a high incidence of local recurrence. It is recommended that the wide excision include the deep fascia and a 2.5- to 3-cm cuff of normal-appearing skin. Distant disease spread is rare and usually occurs in the face of a multiply recurrent lesion. Despite the apparent gross circumscription of these lesions, the tumor diffusely infiltrates the dermis and subcutaneous tissues. A characteristic histologic finding can be seen in the deep margins of the tumor where it intricately interdigitates with normal fat.

REFERENCES: Lindner NJ, Scarborough MT, Powell GJ, et al: Revision surgery in dermatofibrosarcoma protuberans of the trunk and extremities. *Eur J Surg Oncol* 1999;25:392-397.

Weiss SW, Goldblum JR, Enzinger FM: *Enzinger and Weiss's Soft Tissue Tumors*, ed 4. Philadelphia, PA, Elsevier, 2001, pp 491-505.

A-45: A 33-year-old man reports an enlarging painful soft-tissue mass in his right forearm. A radiograph and MRI scans are shown in Figures 35A through 35C. Treatment should consist of

1. core biopsy.
2. wide resection.
3. radiation therapy.
4. marginal resection.
5. incisional biopsy.

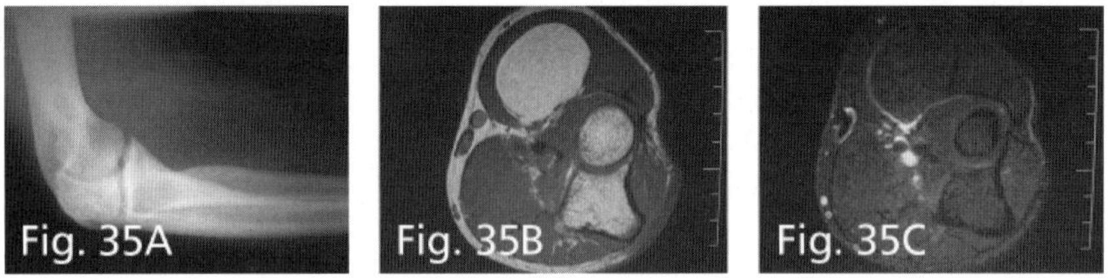
Fig. 35A Fig. 35B Fig. 35C

PREFERRED RESPONSE: 4

DISCUSSION: An intramuscular lipoma is a benign soft-tissue lesion that can grow and has a small risk of progressing to a liposarcoma. Radiographs usually show a globular radiolucent mass adjacent to higher density muscle tissue shadows. When the patient has symptoms and reports an increase in size of the mass, the treatment of choice after appropriate radiographic analysis is complete excision of the mass with marginal resection. Sampling error is a problem with fatty lesions and core or incisional biopsies are frequently unnecessary, especially if an MRI scan of the lesion shows signal intensity that matches subcutaneous fat on all sequences.

REFERENCES: Damron TA: What to do with deep lipomatous tumors. *Instr Course Lect* 2004;53:651-655.

Gaskin CM, Helms CA: Lipomas, lipoma variants, and well-differentiated liposarcomas (atypical lipomas): Results of MRI evaluations of 126 consecutive fatty masses. *Am J Roentgenol* 2004;182:733-739.

Rozental TD, Khoury LD, Donthineni-Rao R, et al: Atypical lipomatous masses of the extremities: Outcome of surgical treatment. *Clin Orthop Relat Res* 2002;398:203-211.

A-46: What is the most common location for localized pigmented villonodular synovitis (PVNS) to occur?

1. Ankle
2. Anterior knee
3. Posterior knee
4. Hip
5. Elbow

PREFERRED RESPONSE: 2

DISCUSSION: Localized PVNS is a form of the disease in which synovial proliferation is restricted to one area of a joint and causes the formation of a small mass-like lesion. The true incidence of this is unknown but is probably less common than the diffuse form of the disease. PVNS presents as a usually painful discrete mass. The anterior compartment of the knee is the most common location.

REFERENCES: Tyler WK, Vidal AF, Williams RJ, et al: Pigmented villonodular synovitis. *J Am Acad Orthop Surg* 2006;14:376-385.

Kim SJ, Shin SJ, Choi NH, et al: Arthroscopic treatment for localized pigmented villonodular synovitis of the knee. *Clin Orthop Relat Res* 2000;379:224-230.

A-47: An 11-year-old boy sustained an injury to his arm in gym class. He denies prior pain in the arm. Radiographs are shown in Figures 36A and 36B. What is the next most appropriate step in the management of this lesion?

1. Open biopsy followed by curettage and bone grafting
2. MRI, whole-body bone scan, CT of the chest, followed by incisional biopsy
3. Allow the fracture to heal with nonsurgical management and serial radiographs
4. Open biopsy followed by wide resection and reconstruction with osteoarticular allograft
5. Open biopsy followed by wide resection and endoprosthetic replacement

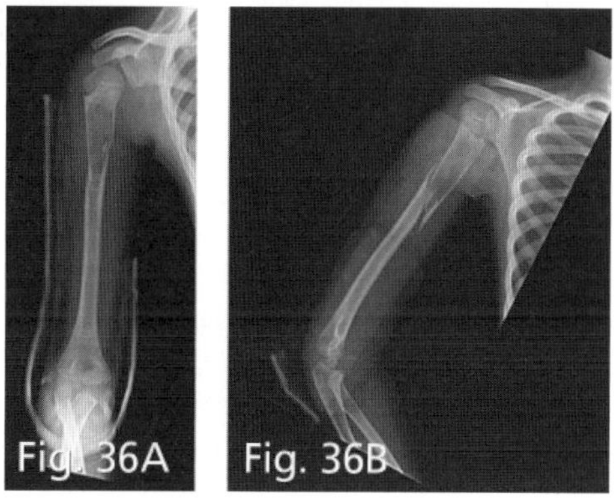
Fig. 36A Fig. 36B

PREFERRED RESPONSE: 3

DISCUSSION: This radiolucent lesion with a "fallen leaf sign" is typical for a unicameral bone cyst (UBC). The most appropriate treatment is to allow the fracture to heal with clinical and radiographic observation. Curettage and bone grafting is not the best initial management for UBC. Wide resection is not indicated for UBC. The proximal humerus is the most common site for UBC. Although staging studies consisting of MRI, bone scan, and CT of the chest are appropriate for lesions suspected of being malignant, the classic appearance of this UBC is such that this work-up is not necessary initially. Following fracture healing, aspiration and injection of the cyst may be indicated.

REFERENCES: Dormans JP, Pill SG: Fractures through bone cysts: Unicameral bone cysts, aneurysmal bone cysts, fibrous cortical defects, and nonossifying fibromas. *Instr Course Lect* 2002;51:457-467.

Deyoe L, Woodbury DF: Unicameral bone cyst with fracture. *Orthopedics* 1985;8:529-531.

A-48: An 83-year-old woman reports pain in her left middle finger after a minor injury. Laboratory studies show a white blood cell count of 7,000/mm^3, an erythrocyte sedimentation rate of 3 mm/hour, a uric acid level of 10.4 mg/dL, and a normal serum protein electrophoresis level. Radiographs are shown in Figures 37A and 37B. Histology from a core biopsy specimen is shown is Figure 37C. In addition to treatment of the finger fracture, treatment should include

1. colchicine and indomethacin
2. radiation therapy to the left hand.
3. systemic chemotherapy.
4. intravenous antibiotics.
5. through-the-wrist amputation.

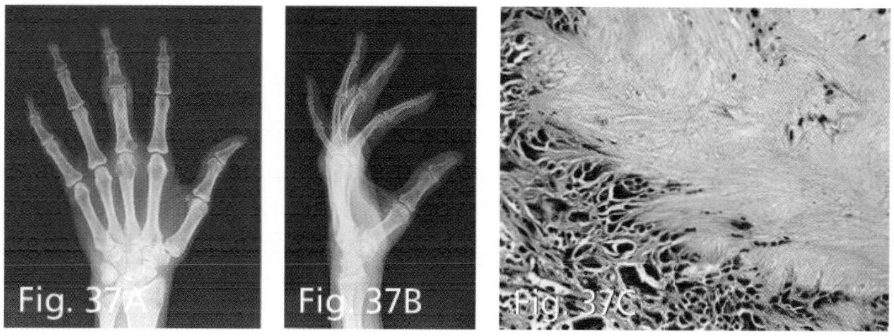
Fig. 37A Fig. 37B Fig. 37C

PREFERRED RESPONSE: 1

DISCUSSION: This clinical picture is most consistent with periarticular erosions from gout. The patient has multiple periarticular lytic lesions in the hand. The laboratory studies show an elevated serum uric acid level, and histology demonstrates acute and chronic inflammation with prominent clefts. Therefore, the preferred treatment is systemic control of her gout. Radiation therapy, chemotherapy, and/or amputation should be considered for a malignancy; however, the histology does not demonstrate any evidence

(continued on next page)

(A-48: *continued*)

of pleomorphism, high nuclear-to-cytoplasmic ratio, nuclear atypia, or mitotic activity. Antibiotics for an infectious process is a consideration, but the minimal elevation in the white blood cell count and erythrocyte sedimentation rate does not support an infectious process.

REFERENCES: Wise CM: Crystal-associated arthritis in the elderly. *Clin Geriatr Med* 2005;21:491-511.
Mudgal CS: Management of tophaceous gout of the distal interphalangeal joint. *J Hand Surg Br* 2006;31:101-103.

A-49: A 29-year-old woman reports shoulder pain after sustaining a minor fall 6 weeks ago. She has a history of celiac sprue. Radiographs of the forearm and shoulder are shown in Figures 38A and 38B. Which of the following serum abnormalities would be expected?

1. Elevated calcium level
2. Elevated parathyroid hormone level
3. Elevated 1,25 dihydroxyvitamin D
4. Elevated phosphate level
5. Low alkaline phosphatase level

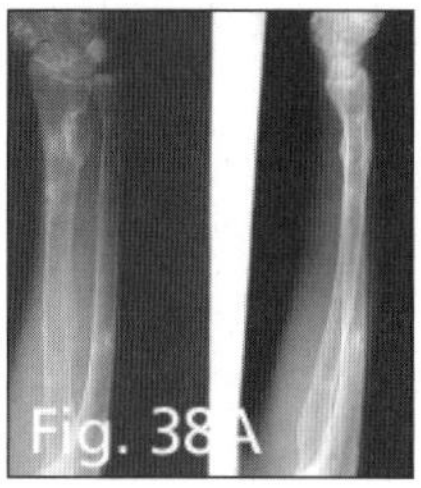
Fig. 38A

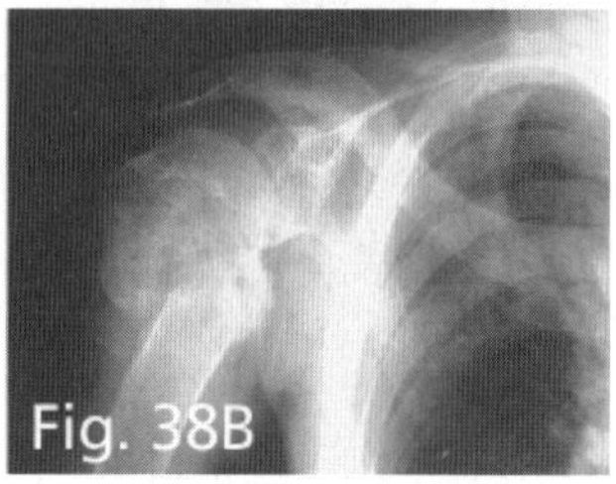
Fig. 38B

PREFERRED RESPONSE: 2

DISCUSSION: Celiac sprue results in rapid gastrointestinal transit and fatty stools that impair the absorption of calcium and vitamin D and result in nutritional-deficiency osteomalacia with secondary hyperparathyroidism. The radiographs show marked osteopenia with brown tumors. A pathologic fracture is seen in the proximal humerus through a large brown tumor. Serum findings include low or normal calcium, low phosphate, elevated alkaline phosphatase, low 1,25 dihydroxyvitamin D, and increased parathyroid hormone levels. Secondary hyperparathyroidism is associated with a variety of conditions including malabsorption syndromes.

REFERENCES: Potts JT: Parathyroid hormone: Past and present. *J Endocrinol* 2005;187:311-325.

Corazza GR, Di Stefano M, Maurino E, et al: Bones in coeliac disease: Diagnosis and treatment. *Best Pract Res Clin Gastroenterol* 2005;19:453-465.

Mankin HJ, Mankin CJ: Metabolic bone disease: An update. *Instr Course Lect* 2003;52:769-784.

Pediatric Orthopaedics

Q-1: A 9-year-old child sustains a proximal tibial physeal fracture with a hyperextension mechanism. What structure is at most risk for serious injury?

1. Tibial nerve
2. Popliteal artery
3. Common peroneal nerve
4. Posterior cruciate ligament
5. Popliteus muscle

Q-2: In a juvenile Tillaux ankle fracture, what ligament causes the displacement of the fracture fragment?

1. Anterior tibiofibular
2. Posterior tibiofibular
3. Deltoid
4. Calcaneofibular
5. Talonavicular

Q-3: A 4-month-old infant is unable to flex her elbow as a result of an obstetric brachial plexus palsy. This most likely illustrates a predominant injury to what structure?

1. C4
2. Upper trunk
3. Posterior cord
4. Lateral cord
5. Musculocutaneous nerve

Q-4: A 13-year-old boy injured his knee playing basketball and is now unable to bear weight. Examination reveals tenderness and swelling at the proximal anterior tibia, with a normal neurologic examination. AP and lateral radiographs are shown in Figures 1A and 1B. Management should consist of

1. MRI.
2. a long leg cast.
3. fasciotomy of the anterior compartment.
4. open reduction and internal fixation.
5. patellar advancement.

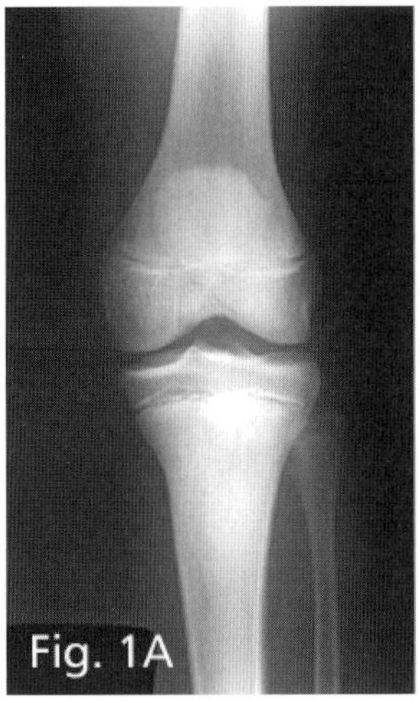
Fig. 1A

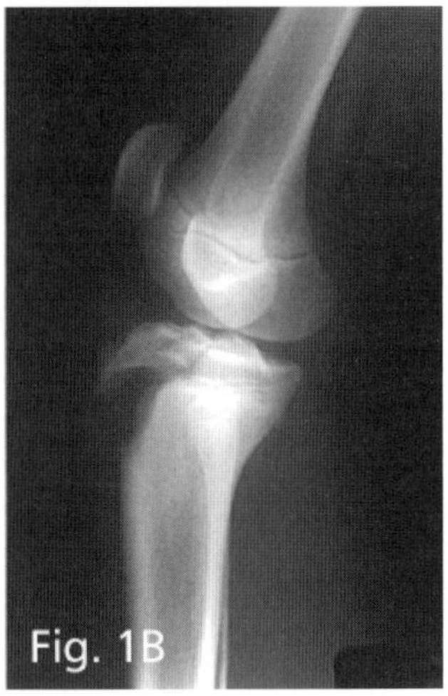
Fig. 1B

Q-5: A 6-year-old child sustained a closed nondisplaced proximal tibial metaphyseal fracture 1 year ago. She was treated with a long leg cast with a varus mold, and the fracture healed uneventfully. She now has a 15° valgus deformity. What is the next step in management?

1. Proximal tibial/fibular osteotomy with acute correction and pin fixation
2. Proximal tibial/fibular osteotomy with gradual correction and external fixation
3. MRI of the proximal tibial physis
4. Medial proximal tibial hemiepiphysiodesis
5. Continued observation

Q-6: A 6-year-old girl is referred for the elbow injury seen in Figure 2. What is the most appropriate treatment?

1. Immobilization in a long arm cast for 3 weeks
2. Immobilization in a long arm cast for 8 weeks
3. Open reduction and immobilization in a long-arm cast for 3 weeks
4. Open reduction and internal fixation with smooth pins
5. Open reduction and internal fixation with a screw

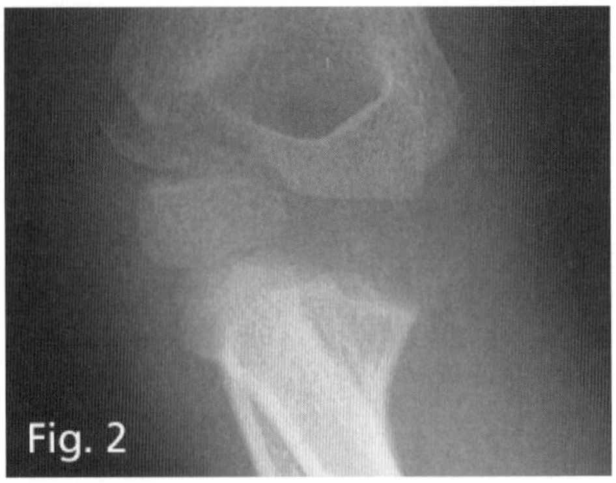
Fig. 2

Q-7: Where is the underlying defect in a rhizomelic dwarf with the findings shown in Figure 3?

1. Type I collagen
2. Type II collagen
3. Collagen oligomeric protein (COMP)
4. Sulfate transport
5. Fibroblast growth factor receptor 3

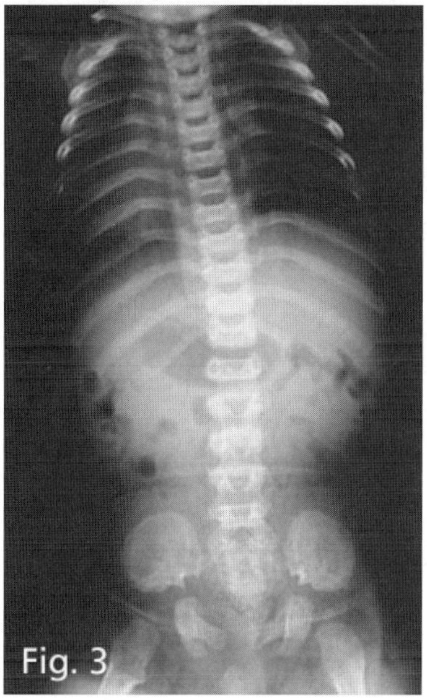

Fig. 3

Q-8: Which of the following findings is most prognostic for the ability of a young child with cerebral palsy to walk?

1. Ability to sit independently by age 2 years
2. Ability to creep by age 2 years
3. Ability to roll by age 2 years
4. Pattern of cerebral palsy (quadriplegia, diplegia, hemiplegia)
5. Type of motor dysfunction (spastic, ataxic, dyskinetic, hypotonic)

Q-9: A 2-year-old girl has had a 2-day history of fever and refuses to move her left shoulder following varicella. Laboratory studies show an erythrocyte sedimentation rate of 75 mm/hour and a peripheral WBC count of 18,000/mm^3. What is the most common organism in this scenario?

1. *Kingella kingae*
2. Group A beta-hemolytic streptococcus
3. Group B streptococcus
4. *Staphylococcus epidermidis*
5. *Staphylococcus aureus*

Q-10: Which of the following is considered the best method to measure limb-length discrepancy in a patient with a knee flexion contracture?

1. Obtain a standard scanogram
2. Obtain a lateral CT scanogram
3. Measure the distance from the anterior superior iliac spine to the medial malleolus
4. Measure the distance from the umbilicus to the medial malleolus
5. Stand the patient on blocks to measure the difference in the heights of the iliac wings

Q-11: A 5-year-old boy sustained an elbow injury. Examination in the emergency department reveals that he is unable to flex the interphalangeal joint of his thumb and the distal interphalangeal joint of his index finger. The radial pulse is palpable at the wrist, and sensation is normal throughout the hand. Radiographs are shown in Figures 4A and 4B. In addition to reduction and pinning of the fracture, initial treatment should include

1. repair of the posterior interosseous nerve.
2. repair of the median nerve at the elbow.
3. neurolysis of the anterior interosseous nerve.
4. observation of the nerve palsy.
5. immediate electromyography and nerve conduction velocity studies.

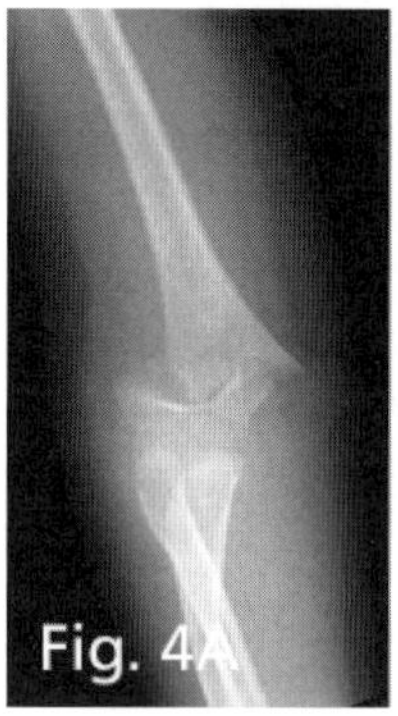

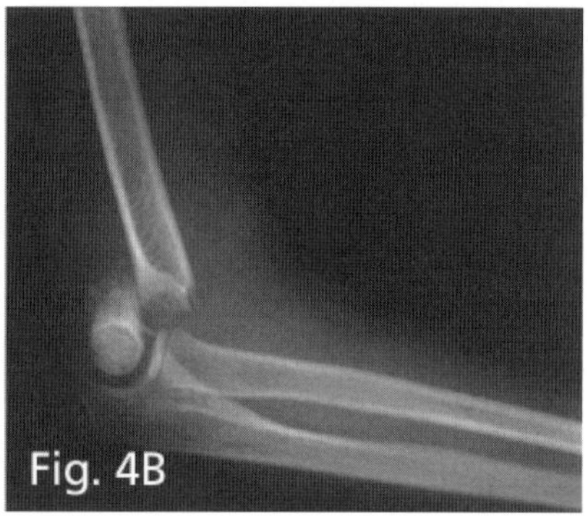

Q-12: An 11-year-old boy who plays basketball reports that he felt a painful pop in the left knee when he stumbled while running. He is unable to bear weight on the extremity and cannot actively extend the knee against gravity. Examination reveals a large knee effusion. A lateral radiograph is shown in Figure 5. Management should consist of

1. physical therapy for quadriceps strengthening exercises.
2. a long leg cast with the knee fully extended.
3. excision of the fragment.
4. suture reattachment of the patellar tendon to the tibial tuberosity.
5. open reduction and tension band fixation.

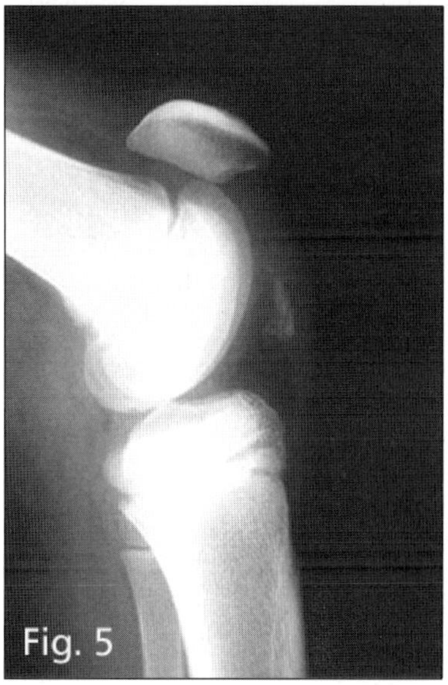

Fig. 5

Q-13: Figures 6A and 6B show the clinical photograph and radiograph of a 4-month-old infant who has a left foot deformity. Examination reveals that the foot deformity is an isolated entity, and the infant has no known neuromuscular conditions or genetic syndromes. Which of the following studies will best confirm the diagnosis?

1. MRI of the foot
2. Static ultrasound examination of the foot in dorsiflexion
3. Lateral radiograph of the foot in maximum plantar flexion
4. Lateral radiograph of the foot in maximum dorsiflexion
5. CT of the foot

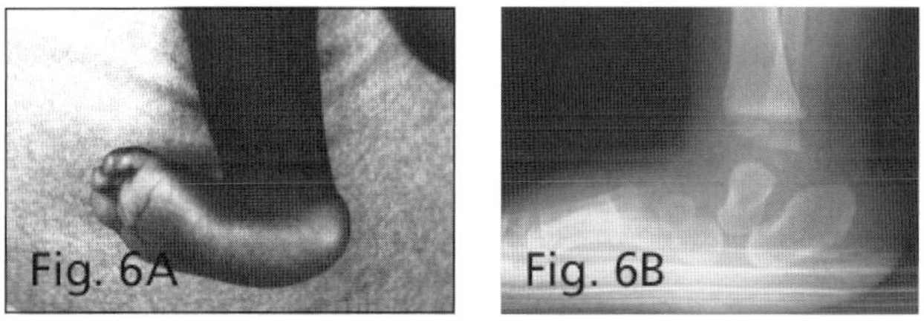

Fig. 6A Fig. 6B

Q-14: An 8-year-old girl was treated for a Salter-Harris type I fracture of the right distal femur 2 years ago. Examination reveals symmetric knee flexion, extension, and frontal alignment compared to the contralateral knee. She has 1 cm of shortening of the right femur. History reveals that she has always been in the 50th percentile for height, and her skeletal age matches her chronologic age. Radiographs are shown in Figure 7. What is the expected consequence at maturity?

1. 6-cm limb-length discrepancy with the right femur longer
2. 6-cm limb-length discrepancy with the left femur longer
3. 12° varus deformity
4. 18° valgus deformity
5. 20° recurvatum deformity

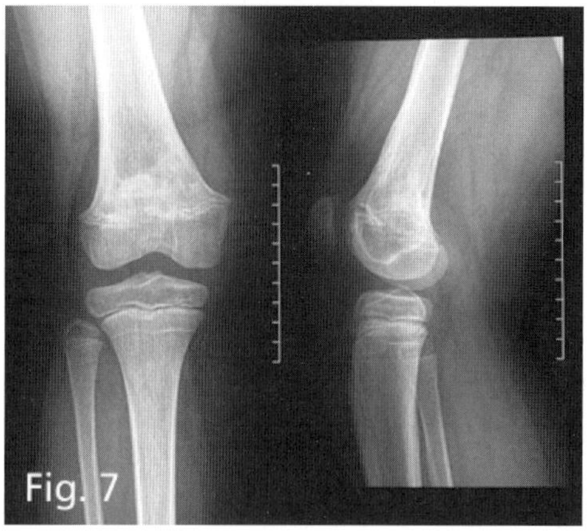

Fig. 7

Q-15: Examination of an obese 3-year-old girl reveals 30° of unilateral genu varum. A radiograph of the involved leg with the patella forward is shown in Figure 8. Management should consist of

1. continued observation until skeletal maturity.
2. fitting for a valgus-producing hinged knee-ankle-foot orthosis.
3. lateral proximal tibial hemiepiphysiodesis.
4. proximal tibiofibular osteotomy and acute correction.
5. proximal tibiofibular epiphysiodesis and osteotomy with lengthening.

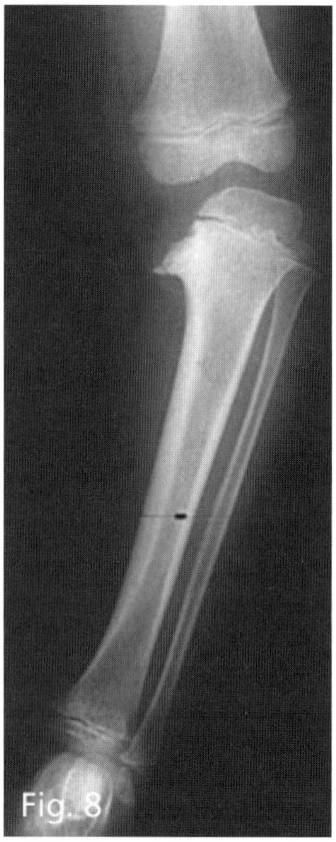

Fig. 8

Q-16: What is the most important consideration in the preoperative evaluation of a child with polyarticular or systemic juvenile rheumatoid arthritis (JRA)?

1. Cervical spine assessment
2. Temporomandibular joint (TMJ)/jaw assessment
3. Dental assessment
4. Stress dosing with corticosteroids
5. Ophthalmology examination

Q-17: Figure 9 shows the radiograph of a 2-year-old child with marked genu varum and tibial bowing. Based on these findings, what is the best initial course of action?

1. Obtain serum phosphorous, calcium, and alkaline phosphatase levels.
2. Obtain a scanogram to assess for limb-length discrepancy.
3. Perform bilateral valgus osteotomies to correct the deformities.
4. Measure the child for a varus prevention orthosis.
5. Educate the family about physiologic genu varum and conduct a follow-up examination in 6 months.

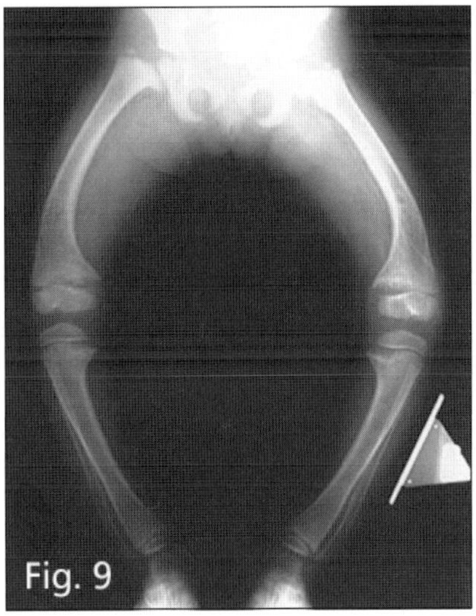

Fig. 9

Q-18: Figure 10 shows the radiograph of a 15-year-old boy with cerebral palsy who has pain at the first metatarsophalangeal joints. He is a community ambulator. Management consisting of accommodative shoes has failed to provide relief. What is the treatment of choice?

1. Custom-molded night orthotics
2. Double osteotomy of the first metatarsals
3. Crescentic osteotomy of the first metatarsals
4. Distal realignment (modified McBride)
5. First metatarsophalangeal joint arthrodeses

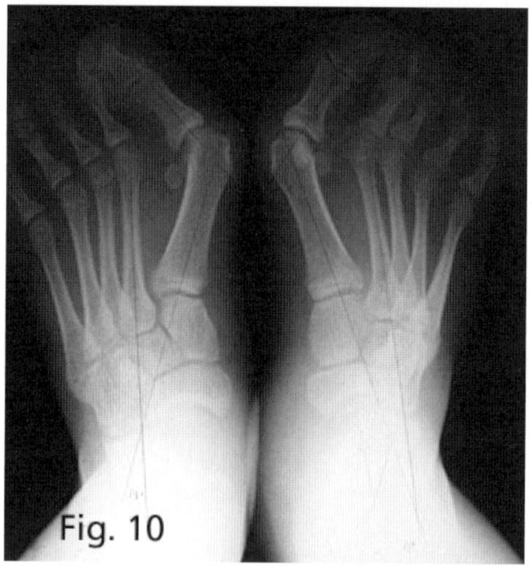
Fig. 10

Q-19: A 2-year-old child is being evaluated for limb-length and girth discrepancy. As a newborn, the patient was large for gestational age and had hypoglycemia. Current examination shows enlargement of the entire right side of the body, including the right lower extremity and foot. The skin shows no abnormal markings, and the neurologic examination is normal. The spine appears normal. Radiographs confirm a 2-cm discrepancy in the lengths of the lower extremities. Additional imaging studies should include

1. bone age of the left wrist.
2. MRI of the spine.
3. MRI of the brain.
4. renal and abdominal ultrasonography.
5. hip ultrasonography.

Q-20: A 12½-year-old boy reports intermittent knee pain and limping that interferes with his ability to participate in sports. He actively participates in football, basketball, and baseball. He denies any history of injury. Examination shows full range of motion without effusion. Radiographs reveal an osteochondritis dissecans (OCD) lesion on the lateral aspect of the medial femoral condyle. MRI scans are shown in Figures 11A and 11B. Initial treatment should consist of

1. immobilization.
2. arthroscopic evaluation of fragment stability.
3. transarticular drilling of the lesion with a 0.045 Kirschner wire.
4. arthroscopic excision of the fragment and microfracture of underlying cancellous bone.
5. excision of the fragment and mosaicplasty.

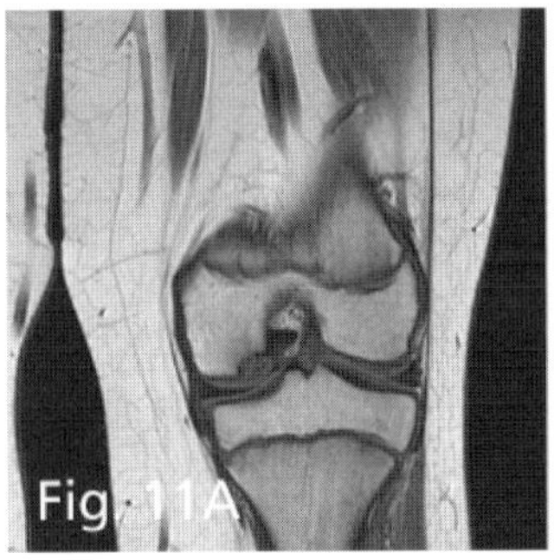

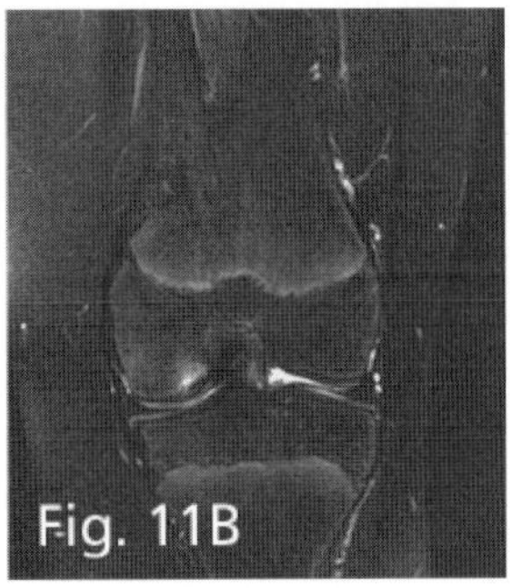

Q-21: A 14-year-old boy undergoes application of a circular frame with tibial and fibular osteotomy for gradual limb lengthening. He initiates lengthening 7 days after surgery. During the first week of lengthening, he reports that turning of the distraction device is becoming increasingly difficult. On the ninth day of lengthening, he is seen in the emergency department after feeling a pop in his leg and noting the acute onset of severe pain. What complication has most likely occurred?

1. Joint subluxation and acute ligament rupture
2. Incomplete corticotomy at the time of surgery with spontaneous completion and acute distraction
3. Premature consolidation of the osteotomy with breakage of bone transfixation wire
4. Fracture through the bone regenerate
5. Fracture of the tibia through a unicortical half-pin track

Q-22: A 10-year-old girl who is Risser stage 0 has back deformity associated with neurofibromatosis type 1 (NF1). She has no back pain. Examination shows multiple café-au-lait nevi with normal lower extremity neurologic function and reflexes. Standing radiographs of the spine show a short 50° right thoracic scoliosis with a kyphotic deformity of 55° (apex T8). A 10° progression in scoliosis has occurred during the past year. There is no cervical deformity. MRI shows mild dural ectasia, primarily in the upper lumbar region. Management should consist of

1. observation with repeat radiographs in 6 months.
2. a thoracolumbosacral orthosis (TLSO).
3. in situ posterior spinal fusion without instrumentation, followed by full-time TLSO bracing.
4. anterior spinal convex hemiepiphysiodesis.
5. combined anterior and posterior spinal arthrodesis with instrumentation.

Q-23: In obstetric brachial plexus palsy, which of the following signs is associated with the poorest prognosis for recovery in a 2-month-old infant?

1. Persistent inability to bring the hand to the mouth with the elbow stabilized at the side
2. Persistent inability to actively abduct the arm past 90°
3. Persistent inability to externally rotate the shoulder past 20°
4. Persistent unilateral ptosis, myosis, and anhydrosis
5. History of clavicle fracture at birth

Q-24: A 6-year-old boy with acute hematogenous osteomyelitis of the distal femur is being treated with intravenous antibiotics. The most expeditious method to determine the early success or failure of treatment is by serial evaluations of which of the following studies?

1. Complete blood count with differential
2. MRI
3. CT
4. Radiographs
5. C-reactive protein (CRP)

Q-25: A 6-year-old girl has a painless spinal deformity. Examination reveals 2+ and equal knee jerks and ankle jerks, negative clonus, and a negative Babinski sign. The straight leg raising test is negative. Abdominal reflexes are asymmetrical. PA and lateral radiographs are shown in Figures 12A and 12B. What is the most appropriate next step in management?

1. MRI of the spinal axis
2. Physical therapy
3. A brace for scoliosis
4. Observation, with reevaluation in 6 to 12 months
5. Posterior spinal fusion from T6 to T12

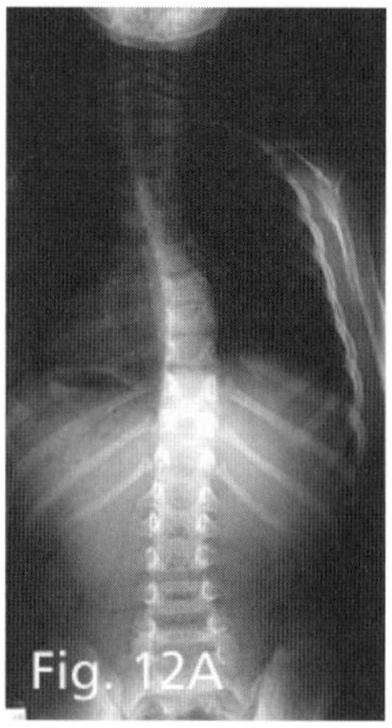
Fig. 12A

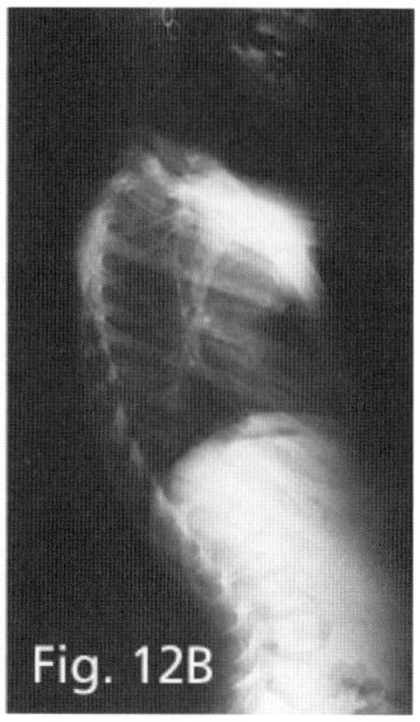
Fig. 12B

Q-26: Figure 13 shows the radiograph of a 7-year-old boy who sustained a pathologic fracture of the left humerus 1 day ago. Initial management should consist of

1. a sling and swathe.
2. needle biopsy of the lesion.
3. a corticosteroid injection of the lesion.
4. curettage and bone packing of the lesion.
5. insertion of an intramedullary rod.

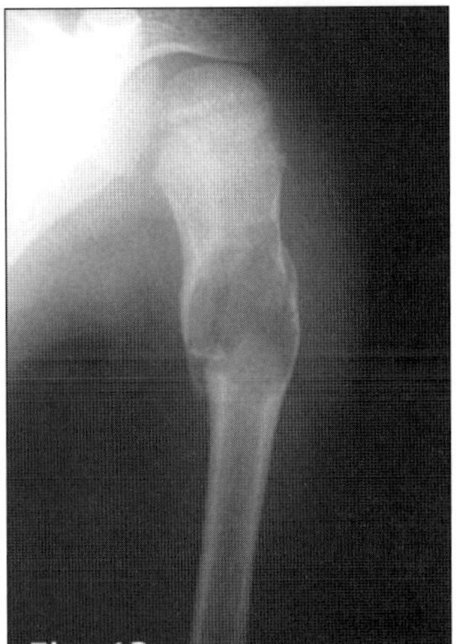

Fig. 13

Q-27: A newborn with myelomeningocele has no movement below the waist and has bilateral hips that dislocate with provocative flexion and adduction. What is the best treatment option for the hip instability?

1. A Pavlik harness with the hips in 90° of flexion and 60° of abduction
2. A spica cast with the hips in 100° of flexion and 70° of abduction
3. Observation with range-of-motion exercises to minimize contractures
4. Open reduction through an anterior hip approach
5. Open reduction through a medial hip approach

Q-28: A 14-year-old boy reports a 4-month history of increasing backache with difficulty walking long distances. His parents state that he walks with his knees slightly flexed and is unable to bend forward and get his hands to his knees. He denies numbness, tingling, and weakness in his legs and denies loss of bladder and bowel control. A lateral radiograph of the lumbosacral spine is shown in Figure 14. What is the best surgical management for this condition?

1. Vertebrectomy of L5
2. Posterior spinal fusion with or without instrumentation from L4 to S1
3. Posterior spinal fusion without instrumentation from L5 to S1
4. Anterior spinal fusion from L4 to L5
5. Direct repair of the spondylolysis defect

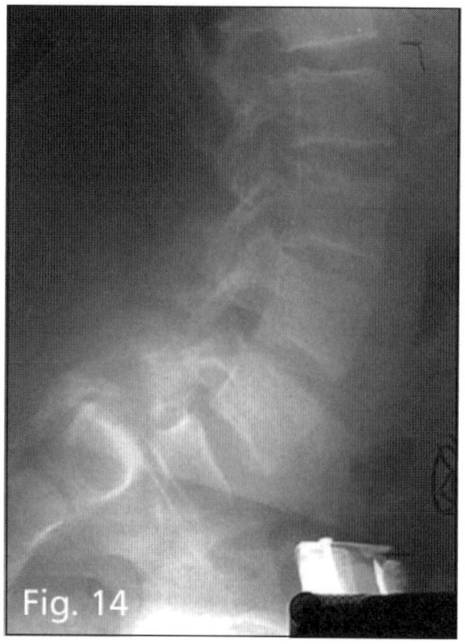

Fig. 14

Q-29: A 12-year-old boy reports limping and chronic knee pain that is now inhibiting his ability to participate in sports. Clinical examination and radiographs of the knee are normal. Additional evaluation should include

1. mechanical alignment radiographs.
2. stress radiographs of the knee.
3. comparison radiographs of both knees.
4. erythrocyte sedimentation rate and C-reactive protein level.
5. examination of the hip.

Q-30: Split posterior tibial tendon transfer is used in the treatment of children with cerebral palsy. Which of the following patients is considered the most appropriate candidate for this procedure?

1. A 6-year-old child with athetosis and a flexible equinovarus deformity of the foot
2. A 6-year-old child with spastic hemiplegia and a rigid equinovarus deformity of the foot
3. A 6-year-old child with spastic hemiplegia and a flexible equinovarus deformity of the foot
4. A 10-year-old child with spastic quadriplegia and rigid valgus deformities of the feet
5. A 15-year-old child with spastic diplegia and rigid equinovalgus deformities of the feet

Q-31: Late surgical treatment of posttraumatic cubitus varus (gunstock deformity) is usually necessitated by the patient reporting problems related to

1. tardy ulnar nerve palsy.
2. posterior glenohumeral subluxation.
3. posterolateral rotatory subluxation of the elbow.
4. poor appearance.
5. snapping medial triceps.

Q-32: What is the incidence and significance of anterior cruciate ligament laxity following tibial eminence fractures in skeletally immature individuals?

1. Common and frequently symptomatic
2. Common and infrequently symptomatic
3. Common but generally resolves spontaneously
4. Rare but when present, usually symptomatic
5. Rare and if present, infrequently symptomatic

Q-33: A full-term newborn has webbing at the knees, rigid clubfeet, a Buddha-like posture of the lower extremities, and no voluntary or involuntary muscle action at and below the knees. Radiographs of the spine and pelvis reveal an absence of the lumbar spine and sacrum. What maternal condition is associated with this diagnosis?

1. Alcoholism
2. Drug abuse
3. Down syndrome
4. Diabetes mellitus
5. Idiopathic scoliosis

Q-34: Figure 15 shows the sitting AP and lateral spinal radiographs of a nonambulatory 12½-year-old boy with Duchenne muscular dystrophy who is being evaluated for scoliosis. The lumbar curve from T12 to L5 measures 36°, and the thoracic curve from T3 to T12 measures 24° on the AP radiograph. He has 5° of pelvic obliquity. His forced vital capacity is 45% of predicted for height and weight. What is the most appropriate treatment for the spinal deformity?

1. Posterior spinal fusion from T2 to L5 with segmental instrumentation
2. Anterior spinal fusion from L1 to L4, followed by posterior spinal fusion from T2 to the sacrum with segmental instrumentation including iliac fixation
3. Custom-molded spinal orthosis worn 23 hours per day until skeletal maturity
4. A spinal orthosis until age 14 years, followed by posterior spinal fusion with segmental instrumentation
5. Adapted wheelchair seating with a custom-molded back support to correct scoliosis and kyphosis

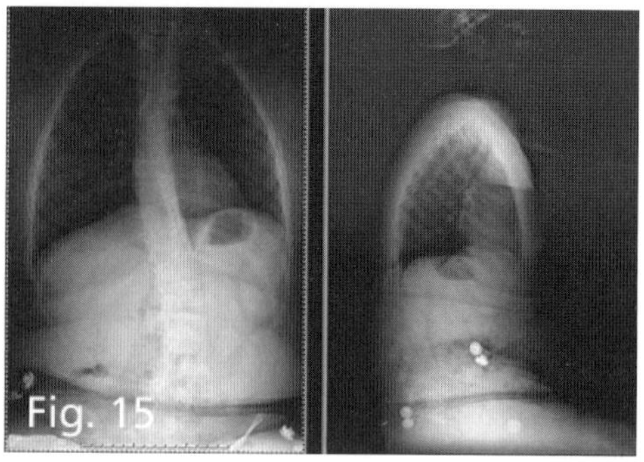
Fig. 15

Q-35: A 3-year-old child has refused to walk for the past 2 days. Examination in the emergency department reveals a temperature of 102.2° F (39° C) and limited range of motion of the left hip. An AP pelvic radiograph is normal. Laboratory studies show a white blood cell (WBC) count of 9,000/mm^3, an erythrocyte sedimentation rate (ESR) of 65 mm/hour, and a C-reactive protein level of 10.5 mg/L (normal < 0.4). What is the next most appropriate step in management?

1. Technetium Tc 99m bone scan
2. Intravenous antibiotics
3. Oral antibiotics
4. CT of the hips
5. Aspiration of the left hip

Q-36: A 12-year-old girl who has a history of frequent tripping and falling also has bilateral symmetric hand weakness, high arched feet, absent patellar and Achilles tendon reflexes, and excessive wear on the lateral border of her shoes. She reports that she has multiple paternal family members with similar deformities. She most likely has a defect of what protein?

1. Peripheral myelin protein-22
2. Dystrophin
3. Type I collagen
4. Alpha-L-iduronidase
5. Cartilage oligomeric matrix protein

Q-37: What acetabular procedure for developmental dysplasia of the hip does not require a concentric reduction of the femoral head in the acetabulum?

1. Salter innominate osteotomy
2. Pemberton innominate osteotomy
3. Dega innominate osteotomy
4. Triple innominate osteotomy
5. Staheli shelf procedure

Q-38: A 5-year-old boy has had pain in the right foot for the past month. Examination reveals tenderness and mild swelling in the region of the tarsal navicular. Radiographs are shown in Figure 16. Management should consist of

1. biopsy of the tarsal navicular.
2. curettage and bone grafting of the tarsal navicular.
3. Complete blood count, C-reactive protein level, erythrocyte sedimentation rate, blood cultures, and intravenous antibiotics.
4. symptomatic treatment with restriction of weight bearing or application of short leg cast.
5. medial column lengthening of the foot through the tarsal navicular.

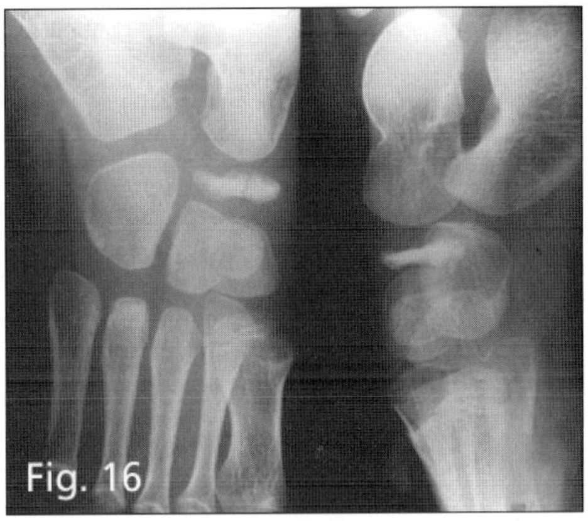
Fig. 16

Q-39: A 9-year-old child sustained a fracture-dislocation of C5 and C6 with a complete spinal cord injury. What is the likelihood that scoliosis will develop during the remaining years of his growth?

1. 10%
2. 20%
3. 50%
4. 70%
5. 100%

Q-40: The husband of a 22-year-old woman has hypophosphatemic rickets. The woman has no orthopaedic abnormalities, but she is concerned about her chances of having a child with the same disease. What should they be told regarding this disorder?

1. Their sons will have a 50% chance of having this X-linked dominant disorder.
2. All of their daughters will be carriers or will have this disorder.
3. They should be advised to not have any children because the risk of having boys with the disorder and girls who will be carriers is too hard for any parent.
4. As long as the woman does not carry the trait, the children will not be affected because the husband has the disease and this is an X-linked dominant disorder.
5. Their sons or daughters may be born with this disorder, but males are more severely affected.

Q-41: A 9-year-old boy sustained a traumatic brain injury and right lower extremity trauma in an accident involving a motor vehicle and a pedestrian. Initial evaluation in the emergency department reveals an obtunded patient who is breathing spontaneously and withdraws appropriately to painful stimuli. After initial resuscitation and stabilization, a CT scan reveals a right parietal intracranial hemorrhage. Radiographs of the swollen right thigh are shown in Figures 17A and 17B. Management of the fractured femur should ultimately consist of

1. immediate hip spica casting.
2. closed reduction and percutaneous pin fixation supplemented by a hip spica cast.
3. placement in 90-90 traction after insertion of a distal femoral traction pin.
4. insertion of a reamed antegrade intramedullary nail starting at the piriformis fossa, stopping the nail short of the distal femoral growth plate.
5. closed reduction and stabilization using retrograde flexible intramedullary nails.

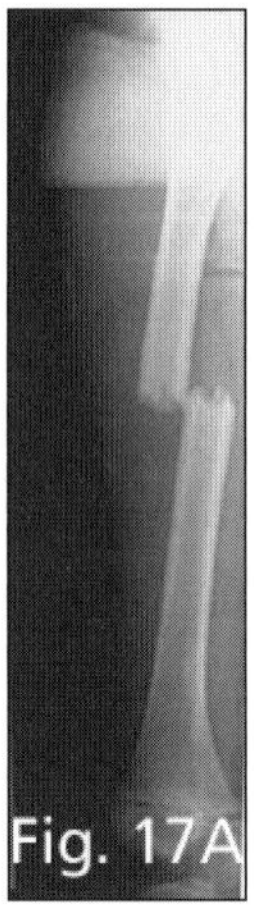
Fig. 17A

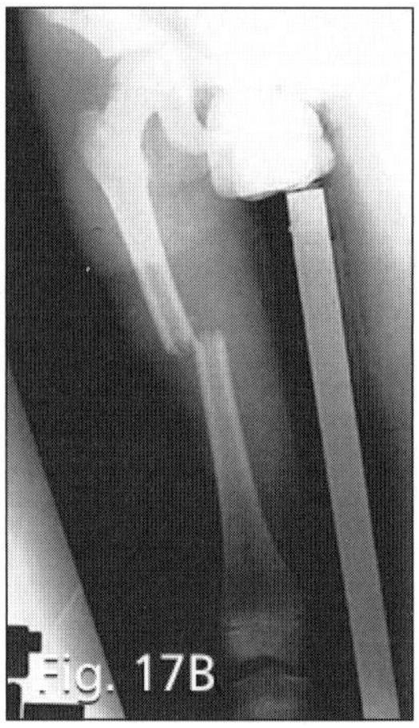
Fig. 17B

Q-42: Figure 18 shows the oblique radiograph of an 11-year-old boy who has a mild left flatfoot deformity. Examination reveals that subtalar motion is limited and painful. Despite casting for 6 weeks, the patient reports foot pain that limits participation in sport activities. A CT scan shows no subtalar joint abnormalities. Management should now include

1. manipulation of the foot under general anesthesia.
2. peroneal lengthening.
3. coalition resection with interposition of fat or muscle.
4. distal calcaneal lengthening osteotomy.
5. triple arthrodesis.

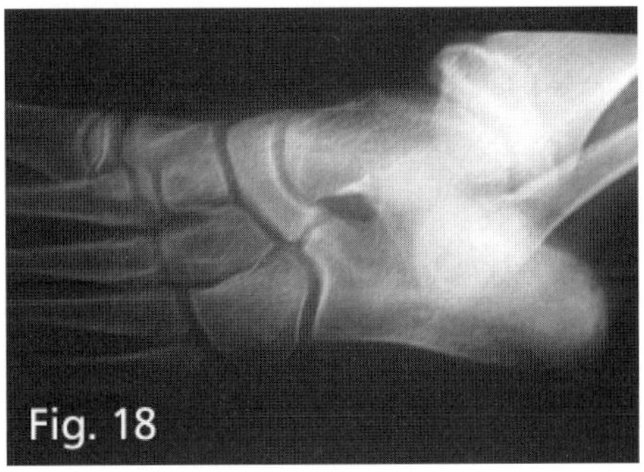
Fig. 18

Q-43: A nonambulatory verbal 6-year-old child with spastic quadriplegic cerebral palsy has progressive bilateral hip subluxation of more than 50%. There is no pain with range of motion, but abduction is limited to 20° maximum. An AP radiograph is seen in Figure 19. Management should consist of

1. percutaneous bilateral adductor tenotomy.
2. oral baclofen.
3. phenol injection into the obturator nerve.
4. open adductor tenotomy with neurectomy of the anterior branch of the obturator nerve.
5. open adductor tenotomy with release of the iliopsoas and bilateral proximal femoral varus derotation osteotomy.

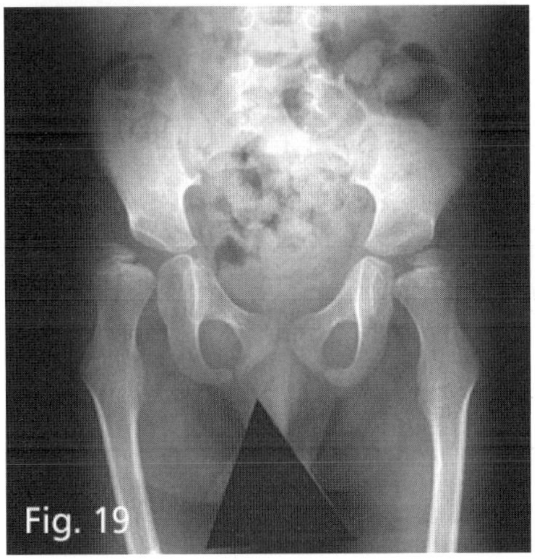
Fig. 19

Q-44: Figures 20A through 20C show the clinical photograph and radiographs of a 15-year-old boy who stubbed his toe 1 day ago while walking barefoot in the yard. Management should consist of

1. buddy taping of the great toe to the second toe for 3 weeks and use of a hard-soled shoe.
2. buddy taping of the great toe to the second toe for 3 weeks and application of a short leg cast.
3. buddy taping of the great toe to the second toe for 3 weeks, use of a hard-soled shoe, and a short course of antibiotics.
4. nail removal in the emergency department, buddy taping of the great toe to the second toe for 3 weeks, and use of a hard-soled shoe.
5. irrigation and open reduction, with or without fixation, and a short course of antibiotics.

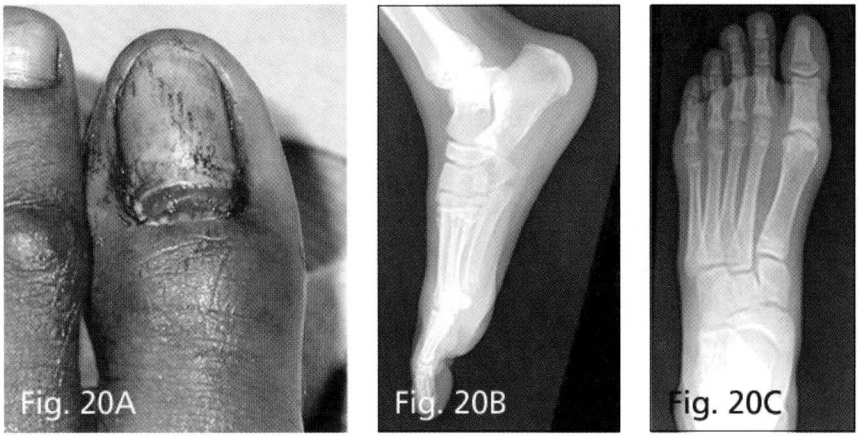

Fig. 20A Fig. 20B Fig. 20C

Q-45: A newborn girl is referred for evaluation of suspected hip instability. What information from her history would place her in the highest risk category?

1. History of maternal diabetes mellitus
2. Frank breech presentation
3. Female sex
4. Concomitant metatarsus adductus
5. Twin gestation

Q-46: Figures 21A and 21B show the current radiographs of an 8-year-old girl who has had pain in the left thigh for the past 3 months. Hypothyroidism was recently diagnosed in this patient and she started treatment 1 week ago. Examination reveals a mild abductor deficiency limp on the left side. She lacks 30° internal rotation on the left hip compared with the right hip. Management should consist of

1. abductor muscle strengthening.
2. a left 1-½ hip spica cast.
3. closed reduction and pinning of the left hip.
4. symptomatic treatment with crutch walking and NSAIDs.
5. in situ pinning of both hips.

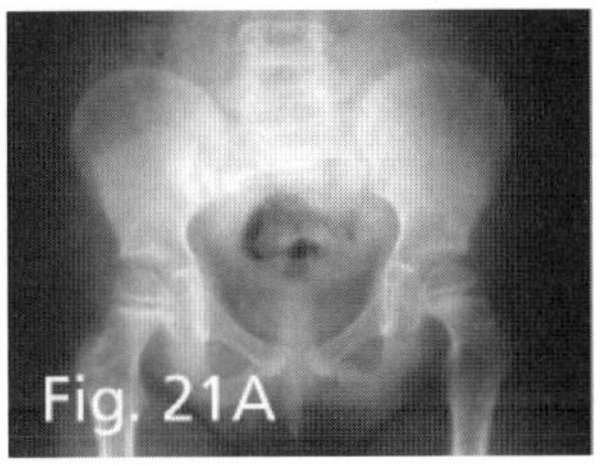

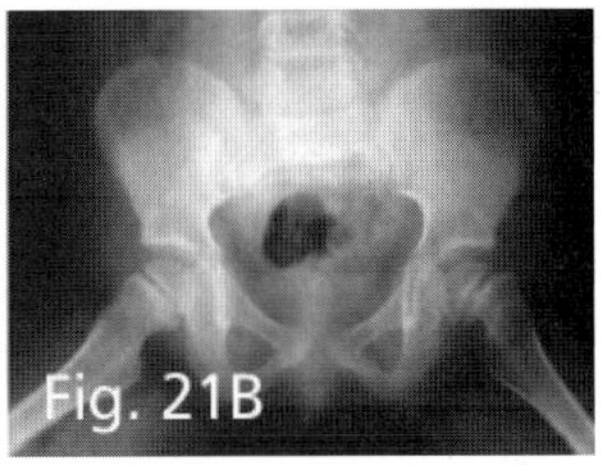

Q-47: A 3-year-old boy had been treated with serial casting for a right congenital idiopathic clubfoot deformity. The parents are concerned because the child now walks on the lateral border of the right foot. Examination shows that the foot passively achieves a plantigrade position with neutral heel valgus and ankle dorsiflexion to 15°. The forefoot inverts during active ankle dorsiflexion. Mild residual metatarsus adductus is present. Management should now consist of

1. additional serial casting.
2. a floor-reaction ankle-foot orthosis.
3. closing wedge cuboid osteotomy.
4. lateral transfer of the anterior tibialis tendon.
5. posterior tibial tendon transfer through the interosseous membrane to the third metatarsal.

Q-48: A 12-month-old boy has right congenital fibular intercalary hemimelia with a normal contralateral limb. A radiograph of the lower extremities shows a limb-length discrepancy of 2 cm. All of the shortening is in the right tibia. Assuming that no treatment is rendered prior to skeletal maturity, the limb-length discrepancy will most likely

1. remain 2 cm at maturity.
2. decrease slowly until the limb lengths equalize.
3. increase at a constant rate of 2 cm per year.
4. increase markedly because of complete failure of tibial growth.
5. increase slowly, with the right lower extremity remaining in proportion to the left lower extremity.

Q-49: What zone of the physis is widened in rickets?

1. Reserve
2. Proliferative
3. Hypertrophic
4. Maturation
5. Primary spongiosa

Q-50: A 7-year-old boy has had low back pain for the past 3 weeks. Radiographs reveal apparent disk space narrowing at L4-5. The patient is afebrile. Laboratory studies show a white blood cell count of 9,000/mm^3 and a C-reactive protein level of 10 mg/L. A lumbar MRI scan confirms the loss of disk height at L4-5 and reveals a small perivertebral abscess at that level. To achieve the most rapid improvement and to lessen the chances of recurrence, management should consist of

1. oral antibiotics.
2. intravenous antibiotics.
3. surgical drainage of the perivertebral abscess and intravenous antibiotics.
4. bed rest.
5. cast immobilization.

A-1: A 9-year-old child sustains a proximal tibial physeal fracture with a hyperextension mechanism. What structure is at most risk for serious injury?

1. Tibial nerve
2. Popliteal artery
3. Common peroneal nerve
4. Posterior cruciate ligament
5. Popliteus muscle

PREFERRED RESPONSE: 2

DISCUSSION: The most serious injury associated with proximal tibial physeal fracture is vascular trauma. The popliteal artery is tethered by its major branches near the posterior surface of the proximal tibial epiphysis. During tibial physeal displacement, the popliteal artery is susceptible to injury. Injuries to the other structures are less common.

REFERENCE: Beaty JH, Kasser JR: *Rockwood and Wilkins Fractures in Children*. Philadelphia, PA, JB Lippincott, 2006, p 961.

A-2: In a juvenile Tillaux ankle fracture, what ligament causes the displacement of the fracture fragment?

1. Anterior tibiofibular
2. Posterior tibiofibular
3. Deltoid
4. Calcaneofibular
5. Talonavicular

PREFERRED RESPONSE: 1

DISCUSSION: The juvenile Tillaux ankle fracture usually occurs because the lateral half of the distal tibial physis remains open. During an external rotational force, the anterior tibiofibular ligament holds the lateral tibial epiphysis, separating it through at the junction of the middle closed physis and lateral open physis.

REFERENCE: Green NE, Swiontkowski MF: *Skeletal Trauma in Children*, ed 3. Philadelphia, PA, WB Saunders, 2003, p 529.

A-3: A 4-month-old infant is unable to flex her elbow as a result of an obstetric brachial plexus palsy. This most likely illustrates a predominant injury to what structure?

1. C4
2. Upper trunk
3. Posterior cord
4. Lateral cord
5. Musculocutaneous nerve

PREFERRED RESPONSE: 2

DISCUSSION: Erb palsy is the most common form of obstetric plexus palsy resulting in C5, C6, or upper trunk deficits. This causes loss of shoulder abduction and elbow flexion. The biceps muscle and the brachialis muscles are predominantly responsible for flexion of the elbow. Each of these muscles is innervated by individual branches of the musculocutaneous nerve, which are supplied predominantly by axons from the C6 nerve root and the upper trunk of the brachial plexus.

REFERENCES: Netter F: *The Ciba Collection of Medical Illustrations: The Musculoskeletal System, Part 1. Anatomy, Physiology and Metabolic Disorders.* West Caldwell, NJ, Ciba-Geigy Corporation, 1987, vol 8, pp 28-29.

Wolock B, Millesi H: Brachial plexus-applied anatomy and operative exposure, in Gelberman RH, ed: *Operative Nerve Repair and Reconstruction.* Philadelphia, PA, JB Lippincott, 1991, pp 1255-1272.

Zancolli E: Reconstructive surgery in brachial plexus sequelae, in Gupta A, Kay S, Scheker L, eds: *The Growing Hand.* London, United Kingdom, Mosby, 1999, p 807.

A-4: A 13-year-old boy injured his knee playing basketball and is now unable to bear weight. Examination reveals tenderness and swelling at the proximal anterior tibia, with a normal neurologic examination. AP and lateral radiographs are shown in Figures 1A and 1B. Management should consist of

1. MRI.
2. a long leg cast.
3. fasciotomy of the anterior compartment.
4. open reduction and internal fixation.
5. patellar advancement.

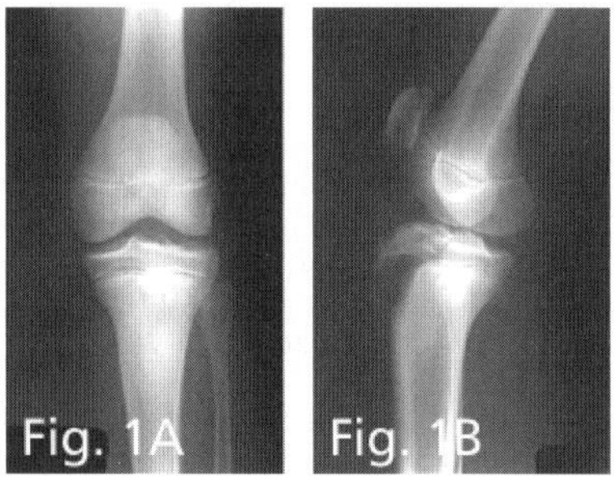

PREFERRED RESPONSE: 4

DISCUSSION: The patient has a displaced intra-articular tibial tuberosity fracture; therefore, the treatment of choice is open reduction and internal fixation. Periosteum is often interposed between the fracture fragments and prevents satisfactory closed reduction. Fortunately, most patients with this injury are close to skeletal maturity and therefore, growth arrest and recurvatum are unusual. Nondisplaced fractures can be treated with a cast, but displaced fractures are best treated with open reduction and internal fixation. Intra-articular fractures can disrupt the joint surface and are sometimes associated with a meniscal tear; therefore, arthroscopy may be needed at the time of open reduction and internal fixation.

REFERENCES: McKoy BE, Stanitski CL: Acute tibial tubercle avulsion fractures. *Orthop Clin North Am* 2003;34: 397-403.

Zionts LE: Fractures around the knee in children. *J Am Acad Orthop Surg* 2002;10:345-355.

A-5: A 6-year-old child sustained a closed nondisplaced proximal tibial metaphyseal fracture 1 year ago. She was treated with a long leg cast with a varus mold, and the fracture healed uneventfully. She now has a 15° valgus deformity. What is the next step in management?

1. Proximal tibial/fibular osteotomy with acute correction and pin fixation
2. Proximal tibial/fibular osteotomy with gradual correction and external fixation
3. MRI of the proximal tibial physis
4. Medial proximal tibial hemiepiphysiodesis
5. Continued observation

PREFERRED RESPONSE: 5

DISCUSSION: The tibia has grown into valgus secondary to the proximal fracture. This occurs in about one half of these injuries, and maximal deformity occurs at 18 months postinjury. The deformity gradually improves over several years, with minimal residual deformity. Therefore, treatment at this age is unnecessary because there is a high rate of recurrence and complications regardless of technique. The valgus deformity is not a result of physeal injury or growth arrest. Medial proximal tibial hemiepiphysiodesis is an excellent method of correcting the residual deformity but is best reserved until close to the end of growth.

REFERENCES: Brougham DI, Nicol RO: Valgus deformity after proximal tibial fractures in children. *J Bone Joint Surg Br* 1987;69:482.

McCarthy JJ, Kim DH, Eilert RE: Posttraumatic genu valgum: Operative versus nonoperative treatment. *J Pediatr Orthop* 1998;18:518-521.

Robert M, Khouri N, Carlioz H, et al: Fractures of the proximal tibial metaphysis in children: Review of a series of 25 cases. *J Pediatr Orthop* 1987;7:444-449.

A-6: A 6-year-old girl is referred for the elbow injury seen in Figure 2. What is the most appropriate treatment?

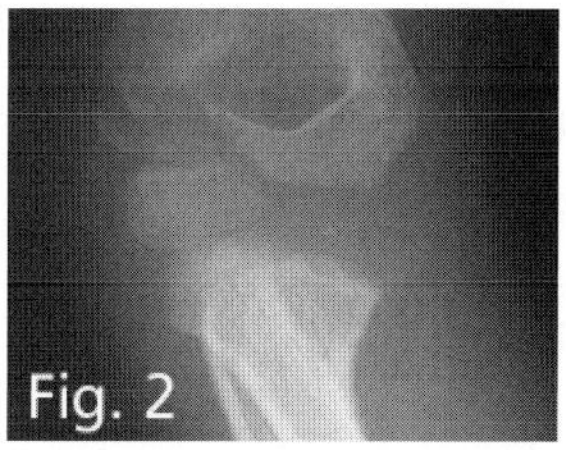
Fig. 2

1. Immobilization in a long arm cast for 3 weeks
2. Immobilization in a long arm cast for 8 weeks
3. Open reduction and immobilization in a long-arm cast for 3 weeks
4. Open reduction and internal fixation with smooth pins
5. Open reduction and internal fixation with a screw

PREFERRED RESPONSE: 4

DISCUSSION: The patient has a displaced lateral condyle fracture; therefore, simple immobilization for 3 to 8 weeks is likely to result in malunion or nonunion. Closed reduction of such injuries is rarely successful. The fracture is unstable, so fixation is required after open reduction. Because the fixation must cross the physis, smooth pins are indicated for the skeletally immature elbow. Open reduction with fixation has been shown to reduce the risk of delayed union and malunion.

(continued on next page)

(A-6: *continued*)

REFERENCES: Beaty JH, Kasser JR: The elbow: Physeal fractures, apophyseal injuries of the distal humerus, avascular necrosis of the trochlea, and T-condylar fractures, in Beaty JH, Kasser JR, eds: *Fractures in Children*, ed 5. Philadelphia, PA, Lippincott Williams & Wilkins, 2001, pp 625-703.

Rutherford A: Fractures of the lateral humeral condyle in children. *J Bone Joint Surg Am* 1985;67:851-856.

Hasler CC, von Laer L: Prevention of growth disturbances after fractures of the lateral humeral condyle in children. *J Pediatr Orthop B* 2001;10:123-130.

A-7: Where is the underlying defect in a rhizomelic dwarf with the findings shown in Figure 3?

1. Type I collagen
2. Type II collagen
3. Collagen oligomeric protein (COMP)
4. Sulfate transport
5. Fibroblast growth factor receptor 3

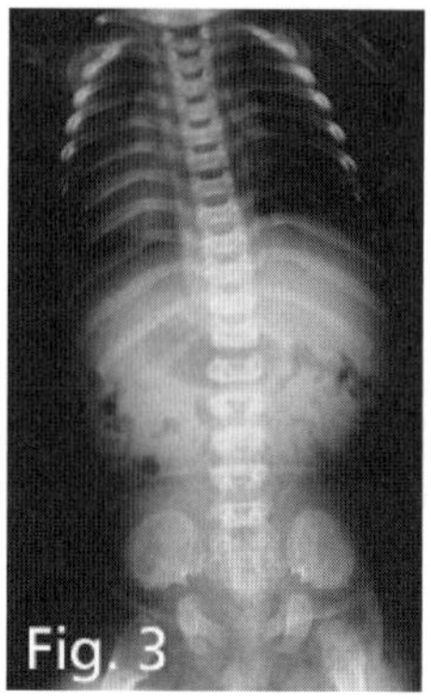

PREFERRED RESPONSE: 5

DISCUSSION: The radiograph shows the typical findings of achondroplasia. The defect is in fibroblast growth factor receptor 3. The pedicles narrow distally in the lumbar spine. The pelvis is low and broad with narrow sciatic notches and ping-pong paddle-shaped iliac wings. This is often called a champagne glass pelvis. Type I collagen abnormalities are typically found in osteogenesis imperfecta, and type II collagen defects are found in spondyloepiphyseal dysplasia and Kneist syndrome. COMP is defective in multiple epiphyseal dysplasia. Sulfate transport defects are seen in diastrophic dysplasia.

REFERENCES: Johnson TR, Steinbach LS: *Essentials of Musculoskeletal Imaging*. Rosemont, IL, American Academy of Orthopaedic Surgeons, 2004, pp 809-812.

Caffey J: Achondroplasia of the pelvis and lumbosacral spine: Some roentgenographic features. *Am J Roentgenol* 1958;80:449.

A-8: Which of the following findings is most prognostic for the ability of a young child with cerebral palsy to walk?

1. Ability to sit independently by age 2 years
2. Ability to creep by age 2 years
3. Ability to roll by age 2 years
4. Pattern of cerebral palsy (quadriplegia, diplegia, hemiplegia)
5. Type of motor dysfunction (spastic, ataxic, dyskinetic, hypotonic)

PREFERRED RESPONSE: 1

DISCUSSION: Several studies have shown that sitting ability by age 2 years is highly prognostic of walking. Molnar and Gordon reported that children not sitting independently by age 2 years had a poor prognosis for walking. Wu and associates reported that children sitting without support by age 2 years had an odds ratio of 26:1 of walking compared with those unable to sit. This was far higher than the odds ratios for cerebral palsy location, motor dysfunction, crawling, creeping, scooting, or rolling.

REFERENCES: Molnar GE, Gordon SU: Cerebral palsy: Predictive value of selected clinical signs for early prognostication of motor function. *Arch Phys Med Rehabil* 1976;57:153-158.

Wu YW, Day SM, Strauss DJ, et al: Prognosis for ambulation in cerebral palsy: A population-based study. *Pediatrics* 2004;114:1264-1271.

A-9: A 2-year-old girl has had a 2-day history of fever and refuses to move her left shoulder following varicella. Laboratory studies show an erythrocyte sedimentation rate of 75 mm/hour and a peripheral WBC count of 18,000/mm^3. What is the most common organism in this scenario?

1. *Kingella kingae*
2. Group A beta-hemolytic streptococcus
3. Group B streptococcus
4. *Staphylococcus epidermidis*
5. *Staphylococcus aureus*

PREFERRED RESPONSE: 2

DISCUSSION: The most common bacterial etiologic agent following varicella is group A beta-hemolytic streptococcus. The other organisms are much less common. Staphylococcus aureus is the most common bone infection organism. *Staphylococcus epidermidis* is increasingly a bone infection organism. Group B streptococcus occurs more commonly in newborns. *Kingella kingae* is a common joint pathogen but is not as common following varicella.

REFERENCES: Schreck P, Schreck P, Bradley J, et al: Musculoskeletal complications of varicella. *J Bone Joint Surg Am* 1996;78:1713-1719.

Mills WJ, Mosca VS, Nizet V: Orthopaedic manifestations of invasive group A streptococcal infections complicating primary varicella. *J Pediatr Orthop* 1996;16:522-528.

A-10: Which of the following is considered the best method to measure limb-length discrepancy in a patient with a knee flexion contracture?

1. Obtain a standard scanogram
2. Obtain a lateral CT scanogram
3. Measure the distance from the anterior superior iliac spine to the medial malleolus
4. Measure the distance from the umbilicus to the medial malleolus
5. Stand the patient on blocks to measure the difference in the heights of the iliac wings

PREFERRED RESPONSE: 2

DISCUSSION: The most effective way to measure a limb-length discrepancy in a patient with a knee flexion contracture is a lateral CT scanogram. All the other methods listed provide inaccurate results with a knee flexion contracture because the measurements are made in the coronal plane.

REFERENCES: Aaron A, Weinstein D, Thickman D, et al: Comparison of orthoroentgenography and computed tomography in the measurement of limb-length discrepancy. *J Bone Joint Surg Am* 1992;74:897-902.

Tachdjian MO: *Clinical Pediatric Orthopaedics: The Art of Diagnosis and Principles of Management.* Stamford, CT, Appleton and Lange, 1997, pp 237-240.

A-11: A 5-year-old boy sustained an elbow injury. Examination in the emergency department reveals that he is unable to flex the interphalangeal joint of his thumb and the distal interphalangeal joint of his index finger. The radial pulse is palpable at the wrist, and sensation is normal throughout the hand. Radiographs are shown in Figures 4A and 4B. In addition to reduction and pinning of the fracture, initial treatment should include

1. repair of the posterior interosseous nerve.
2. repair of the median nerve at the elbow.
3. neurolysis of the anterior interosseous nerve.
4. observation of the nerve palsy.
5. immediate electromyography and nerve conduction velocity studies.

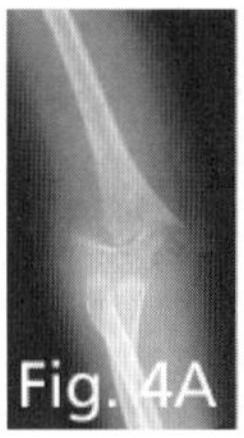
Fig. 4A

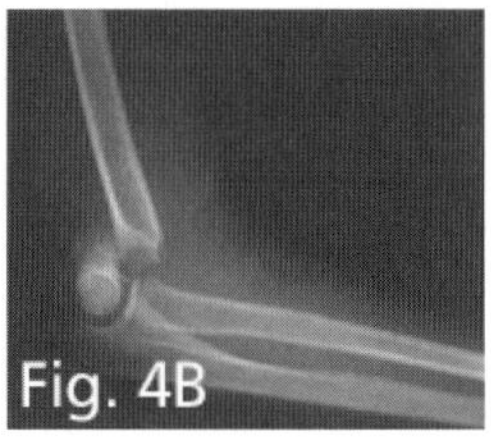
Fig. 4B

PREFERRED RESPONSE: 4

DISCUSSION: The findings are consistent with a neurapraxia of the anterior interosseous branch of the median nerve. This is the most common nerve palsy seen with supracondylar humerus fractures, followed closely by radial nerve palsy. Nearly all cases of neurapraxia following supracondylar humerus fractures resolve spontaneously, and therefore, further diagnostic studies and surgery are not indicated.

REFERENCES: Cramer KE, Green NE, Devito DP: Incidence of anterior interosseous nerve palsy in supracondylar humerus fractures in children. *J Pediatr Orthop* 1993;13:502-505.

Sood MK, Burke FD: Anterior interosseous nerve palsy: A review of 16 cases. *J Hand Surg Br* 1997;22:64-68.

A-12: An 11-year-old boy who plays basketball reports that he felt a painful pop in the left knee when he stumbled while running. He is unable to bear weight on the extremity and cannot actively extend the knee against gravity. Examination reveals a large knee effusion. A lateral radiograph is shown in Figure 5. Management should consist of

1. physical therapy for quadriceps strengthening exercises.
2. a long leg cast with the knee fully extended.
3. excision of the fragment.
4. suture reattachment of the patellar tendon to the tibial tuberosity.
5. open reduction and tension band fixation.

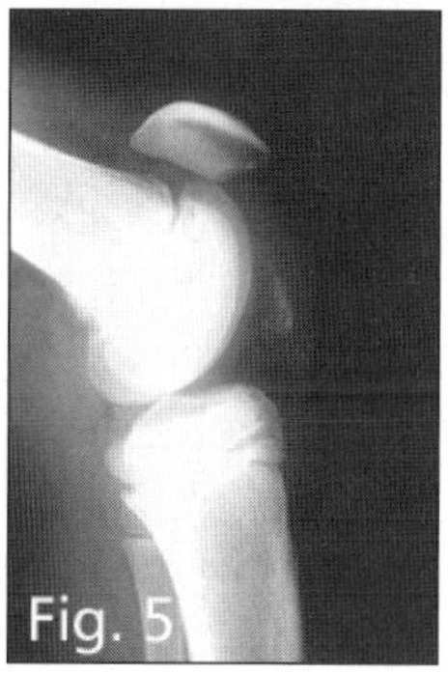

PREFERRED RESPONSE: 5

DISCUSSION: The radiograph shows an avulsion fracture, or sleeve fracture, of the distal pole of the patella. The distal fragment is much larger than it appears on the radiograph because it largely consists of cartilage; therefore, excision of the fragment is contraindicated. The treatment of choice is open reduction and tension band fixation to correct patella alta and restore the extensor mechanism.

REFERENCES: Maguire JK, Canale ST: Fractures of the patella in children and adolescents. *J Pediatr Orthop* 1993;13:567-571.

Grogan DP, Carey TP, Leffers D, et al: Avulsion fractures of the patella. *J Pediatr Orthop* 1990;10:721-730.

A-13: Figures 6A and 6B show the clinical photograph and radiograph of a 4-month-old infant who has a left foot deformity. Examination reveals that the foot deformity is an isolated entity, and the infant has no known neuromuscular conditions or genetic syndromes. Which of the following studies will best confirm the diagnosis?

1. MRI of the foot
2. Static ultrasound examination of the foot in dorsiflexion
3. Lateral radiograph of the foot in maximum plantar flexion
4. Lateral radiograph of the foot in maximum dorsiflexion
5. CT of the foot

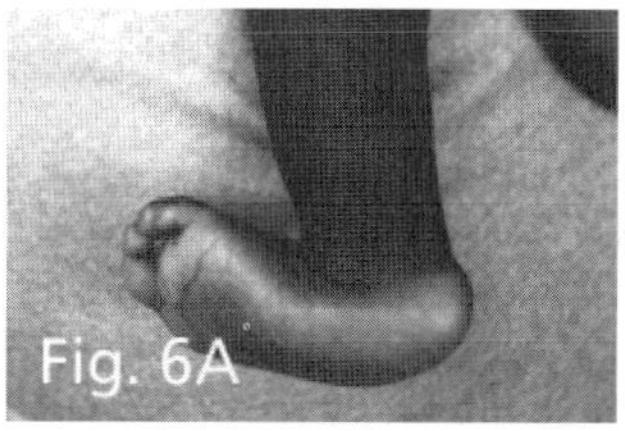

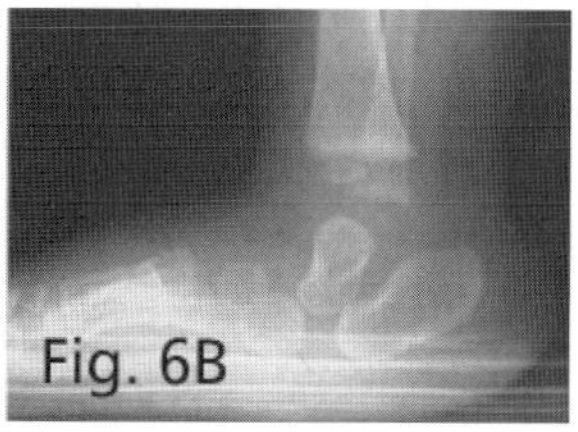

PREFERRED RESPONSE: 3

DISCUSSION: The clinical photograph shows a rocker-bottom deformity, and the lateral radiograph suggests a congenital vertical talus deformity. A lateral radiograph of the foot in maximum plantar flexion is needed to demonstrate the fixed position of the deformity with malalignment of the talar-metatarsal axis. A fixed dislocation of the navicular on the talus differentiates a congenital vertical talus from the oblique talus with talonavicular subluxation.

(continued on next page)

(A-13: *continued*)

REFERENCES: Kumar SJ, Cowell HR, Ramsey PL: Vertical and oblique talus. *Instr Course Lect* 1982;31:235-251.

Kodros SA, Dias LS: Single-stage correction of congenital vertical talus. *J Pediatr Orthop* 1999;19:42-48.

Herring JA: Disorders of the foot, vertical talus, in Herring JA, ed: *Tachdjian's Pediatric Orthopaedics, from the Texas Scottish Rite Hospital for Children*, ed 3. Philadelphia, PA, WB Saunders, 2002, pp 959-967.

A-14: An 8-year-old girl was treated for a Salter-Harris type I fracture of the right distal femur 2 years ago. Examination reveals symmetric knee flexion, extension, and frontal alignment compared to the contralateral knee. She has 1 cm of shortening of the right femur. History reveals that she has always been in the 50th percentile for height, and her skeletal age matches her chronologic age. Radiographs are shown in Figure 7. What is the expected consequence at maturity?

1. 6-cm limb-length discrepancy with the right femur longer
2. 6-cm limb-length discrepancy with the left femur longer
3. 12° varus deformity
4. 18° valgus deformity
5. 20° recurvatum deformity

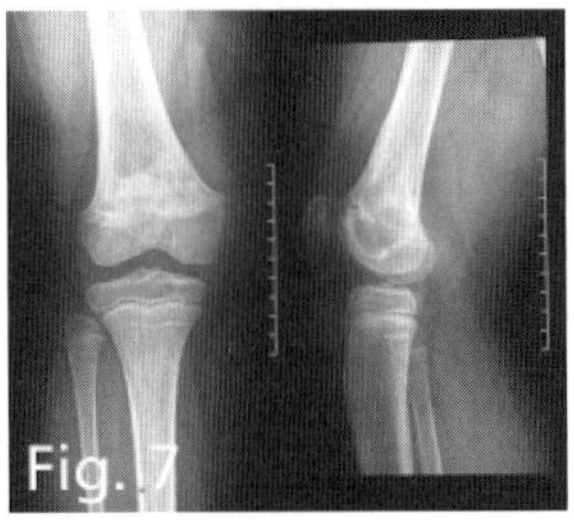

PREFERRED RESPONSE: 2

DISCUSSION: The child has a near-complete central physeal arrest of the distal femur, and worsening limb-length discrepancy will develop. She is growing at the average rate for the population. The distal femoral physis grows at a rate of roughly 9 mm per year. Girls finish their growth at approximately age 14 years. Thus, at maturity the left leg will be 6.4 cm longer than the right. An angular deformity has not developed at this point and her arrest is central; therefore, angular deformity is unlikely to develop in any plane.

REFERENCES: Little DG, Nigo L, Aiona MD: Deficiencies of current methods for the timing of epiphysiodesis. *J Pediatr Orthop* 1996;16:173-179.

Moseley CF: Assessment and prediction in leg-length discrepancy. *Instr Course Lect* 1989;38:325-330.

A-15: Examination of an obese 3-year-old girl reveals 30° of unilateral genu varum. A radiograph of the involved leg with the patella forward is shown in Figure 8. Management should consist of

1. continued observation until skeletal maturity.
2. fitting for a valgus-producing hinged knee-ankle-foot orthosis.
3. lateral proximal tibial hemiepiphysiodesis.
4. proximal tibiofibular osteotomy and acute correction.
5. proximal tibiofibular epiphysiodesis and osteotomy with lengthening.

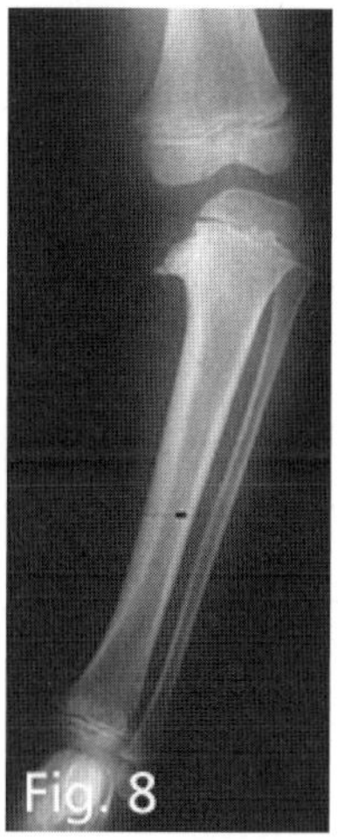

PREFERRED RESPONSE: 4

DISCUSSION: The clinical scenario describes infantile tibia vara (Blount disease). The radiograph shows severe deformity with the characteristic Langenskiöld stage 3 changes of the medial proximal tibial metaphysis that distinguish it from physiologic bowing. The preferred treatment is proximal tibiofibular osteotomy with acute correction into slight valgus to unload the damaged area of the physis. This method provides the best results in patients younger than 4 years. Continued observation would result in progressive deformity. Bracing is most effective in younger children with less severe deformity. Lateral proximal tibial hemiepiphysiodesis relies on growth of the injured medial physis for correction and would result in severe tibial shortening in this young child. Complete epiphysiodesis also produces severe shortening and requires multiple lengthening procedures.

REFERENCES: Johnston CE II: Infantile tibia vara. *Clin Orthop* 1990;255:13-23.

Richards BS, Katz DE, Sims JB: Effectiveness of brace treatment in early infantile Blount's disease. *J Pediatr Orthop* 1998;18:374-380.

A-16: What is the most important consideration in the preoperative evaluation of a child with polyarticular or systemic juvenile rheumatoid arthritis (JRA)?

1. Cervical spine assessment
2. Temporomandibular joint (TMJ)/jaw assessment
3. Dental assessment
4. Stress dosing with corticosteroids
5. Ophthalmology examination

PREFERRED RESPONSE: 1

DISCUSSION: The cervical spine may be involved in a child with polyarticular or systemic JRA; fusion or instability can occur. Radiographic assessment of the cervical spine should include lateral flexion-extension views. The potential exists for spinal cord injury during intubation or positioning in the presence of an unstable cervical spine. Limitations of the TMJ and micrognathia may affect ease of intubation and administration of anesthesia via a mask. If the TMJ and jaw are involved, some patients may have dental findings such as dental caries and even abscesses that can affect surgery. Some children, particularly those with systemic arthritis, may be taking corticosteroids long-term and may need stress dosing with complex surgeries. Although it is important to routinely check for uveitis and iritis in children with JRA, this usually is not needed preoperatively. Uveitis and iritis are less likely in a child with systemic JRA.

(continued on next page)

(A-16: *continued*)

REFERENCES: Cassity JT, Petty RE, eds: *Textbook of Pediatric Rheumatology*, ed 5. Philadelphia, PA, WB Saunders, 2005. Ilowite N: Current treatment of juvenile rheumatoid arthritis. *Pediatrics* 2002;109:109-115.

Ruddy S, Harris ED, Sledge CB, eds: *Kelley's Textbook of Rheumatology*, ed 6. Philadelphia, PA, WB Saunders, 2001.

Hamalainen M: Surgical treatment of juvenile rheumatoid arthritis. *Clin Exp Rheumatol* 1994;12:S107-S112.

A-17: Figure 9 shows the radiograph of a 2-year-old child with marked genu varum and tibial bowing. Based on these findings, what is the best initial course of action?

1. Obtain serum phosphorous, calcium, and alkaline phosphatase levels.
2. Obtain a scanogram to assess for limb-length discrepancy.
3. Perform bilateral valgus osteotomies to correct the deformities.
4. Measure the child for a varus prevention orthosis.
5. Educate the family about physiologic genu varum and conduct a follow-up examination in 6 months.

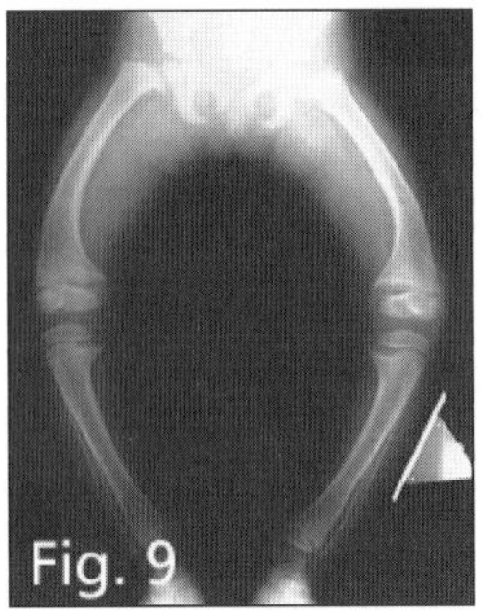
Fig. 9

PREFERRED RESPONSE: 1

DISCUSSION: The radiograph shows multiple wide physes, consistent with a diagnosis of rickets. A low serum phosphorus level and an elevated alkaline phosphatase level are the hallmarks in diagnosing familial hypophosphatemic vitamin D-resistant rickets. Serum calcium level is usually normal or low normal. This disease is inherited as an X-linked dominant trait and usually presents at age 18 to 24 months. The disease results from a poorly defined problem with renal phosphate transport in which normal dietary intake of vitamin D is insufficient to achieve normal bone mineralization. Renal tubular dysfunction is associated with urinary phosphate wasting. Treatment involves oral phosphate supplementation, which can cause hypocalcemia and secondary hyperparathyroidism. To prevent associated problems, high doses of vitamin D are administered. While obtaining a scanogram may be clinically indicated in an associated limb-length discrepancy, and subsequent corrective surgery may be indicated, either of these choices would not be the first course of action. An orthosis may slow the progression of genu varum in this disorder but is less important than establishing the correct diagnosis to begin pharmacologic treatment. This amount of varum and tibial bowing far exceeds the normal limits of physiologic genu varum. Skeletal dysplasias usually are not associated with abnormal laboratory values.

REFERENCES: Herring JA: Metabolic and endocrine bone diseases, in *Tachdjian's Pediatric Orthopaedics*, ed 3. New York, NY, WB Saunders, 2002, pp 1685-1743.

Sillence DO: Disorders of bone density, volume, and mineralization, in Rimoin DL, Conner JM, Pyerite RE, et al, eds: *Principles and Practice of Medical Genetics*, ed 3. New York, NY, Churchill Livingstone, 1995, pp 1996-2002.

A-18: Figure 10 shows the radiograph of a 15-year-old boy with cerebral palsy who has pain at the first metatarsophalangeal joints. He is a community ambulator. Management consisting of accommodative shoes has failed to provide relief. What is the treatment of choice?

1. Custom-molded night orthotics
2. Double osteotomy of the first metatarsals
3. Crescentic osteotomy of the first metatarsals
4. Distal realignment (modified McBride)
5. First metatarsophalangeal joint arthrodeses

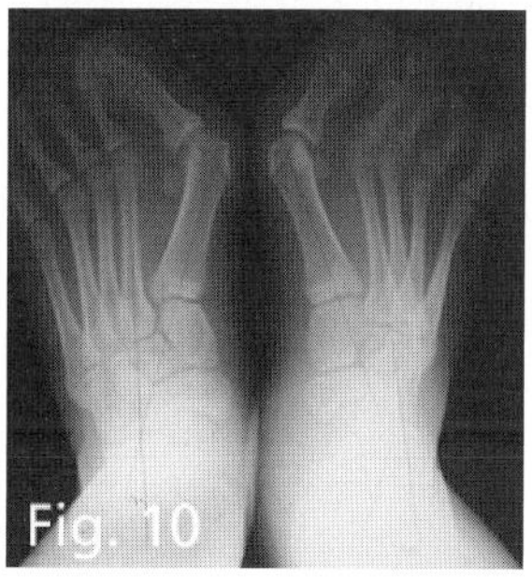

PREFERRED RESPONSE: 5

DISCUSSION: Although other surgeries have provided some success, first metatarsophalangeal joint arthrodesis has the highest overall success rate compared to other surgeries in ambulatory and nonambulatory children with cerebral palsy. The recurrence rate is unacceptably high with the other procedures listed. In contrast, neurologically normal children are amenable to osteotomies and soft-tissue procedures.

REFERENCES: Davids JR, Mason TA, Danko A, et al: Surgical management of hallux valgus deformity in children with cerebral palsy. *J Pediatr Orthop* 2001;21:89-94.

Jenter M, Lipton GE, Miller F: Operative treatment for hallux valgus in children with cerebral palsy. *Foot Ankle Int* 1998;19:830-835.

A-19: A 2-year-old child is being evaluated for limb-length and girth discrepancy. As a newborn, the patient was large for gestational age and had hypoglycemia. Current examination shows enlargement of the entire right side of the body, including the right lower extremity and foot. The skin shows no abnormal markings, and the neurologic examination is normal. The spine appears normal. Radiographs confirm a 2-cm discrepancy in the lengths of the lower extremities. Additional imaging studies should include

1. bone age of the left wrist.
2. MRI of the spine.
3. MRI of the brain.
4. renal and abdominal ultrasonography.
5. hip ultrasonography.

PREFERRED RESPONSE: 4

DISCUSSION: The patient may have Beckwith-Wiedemann syndrome (BWS), which consists of exophthalmos, macroglossia, gigantism, visceromegaly, abdominal wall defects, and neonatal hypoglycemia. Hemihypertrophy develops in approximately 15% of patients with BWS. Patients with hemihypertrophy that is the result of BWS have a 40% chance of developing malignancies such as Wilms tumor or hepatoblastoma; therefore, frequent ultrasound screening is recommended until about age 7 years. The absence of nevi and vascular markings helps to rule out other causes of hemihypertrophy, such as neurofibromatosis, Proteus syndrome, and Klippel-Trenaunay syndrome. Bone age estimations are not accurate at this young age but may become more useful later to help predict the timing of epiphysiodesis procedures.

(continued on next page)

(A-20: *continued*)

REFERENCES: DeBaun MR, Tucker MA: Risk of cancer during the first four years of life in children from The Beckwith-Wiedemann Syndrome Registry. *J Pediatr* 1998;132:398-400.

Ballock RT, Wiesner GL, Myers MT, et al: Hemihypertrophy concepts and controversies. *J Bone Joint Surg Am* 1997;79:1731-1738.

Carpenter CT, Lester EL: Skeletal age determination in young children: Analysis of three regions of the hand/wrist film. *J Pediatr Orthop* 1993;13:76-79.

A-20: A 12½-year-old boy reports intermittent knee pain and limping that interferes with his ability to participate in sports. He actively participates in football, basketball, and baseball. He denies any history of injury. Examination shows full range of motion without effusion. Radiographs reveal an osteochondritis dissecans (OCD) lesion on the lateral aspect of the medial femoral condyle. MRI scans are shown in Figures 11A and 11B. Initial treatment should consist of

1. immobilization.
2. arthroscopic evaluation of fragment stability.
3. transarticular drilling of the lesion with a 0.045 Kirschner wire.
4. arthroscopic excision of the fragment and microfracture of underlying cancellous bone.
5. excision of the fragment and mosaicplasty.

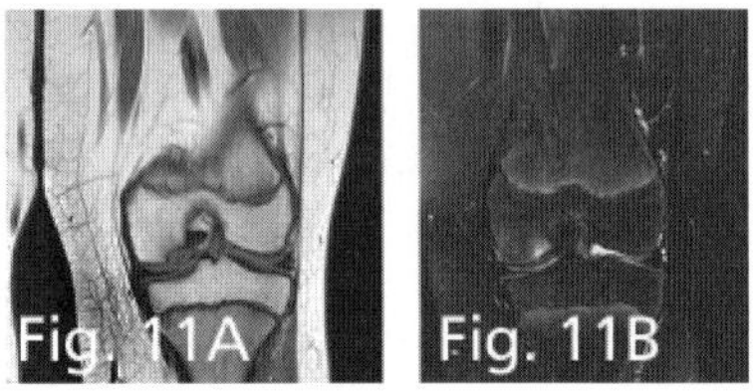
Fig. 11A Fig. 11B

PREFERRED RESPONSE: 1

DISCUSSION: This skeletally immature patient has a small OCD lesion that appears stable, and he has not undergone any treatment. Therefore, a trial of immobilization until pain resolves is the best initial choice. Thereafter, cessation of sport activities for 4 to 6 months may allow healing of the lesion. Surgical treatment of juvenile OCD lesions is reserved for unstable lesions, patients who have not shown radiographic evidence of healing and are still symptomatic after 6 months of nonsurgical management, or patients who are approaching skeletal maturity. Good results with stable in situ lesions that have failed to respond to nonsurgical management have been reported with both transarticular and retroarticular drilling. Results after excision alone are poor at 5-year follow-up, and it is unclear if microfracture will improve the long-term outcome. Mosaicplasty may be the next best option for patients who remain or become symptomatic after excision of the fragment and microfracture.

REFERENCES: Wall E, Von Stein D: Juvenile osteochondritis dissecans. *Orthop Clin North Am* 2003;34:341-353.

Kocher MS, Micheli LJ, Yaniv M, et al: Functional and radiographic outcome of juvenile osteochondritis dissecans of the knee treated with transarticular arthroscopic drilling. *Am J Sports Med* 2001;29:562-566.

A-21: A 14-year-old boy undergoes application of a circular frame with tibial and fibular osteotomy for gradual limb lengthening. He initiates lengthening 7 days after surgery. During the first week of lengthening, he reports that turning of the distraction device is becoming increasingly difficult. On the 9th day of lengthening, he is seen in the emergency department after feeling a pop in his leg and noting the acute onset of severe pain. What complication has most likely occurred?

1. Joint subluxation and acute ligament rupture
2. Incomplete corticotomy at the time of surgery with spontaneous completion and acute distraction
3. Premature consolidation of the osteotomy with breakage of bone transfixation wire
4. Fracture through the bone regenerate
5. Fracture of the tibia through a unicortical half-pin track

PREFERRED RESPONSE: 2

DISCUSSION: Incomplete corticotomy may result from osteotomy with limited soft-tissue stripping and exposure. When the patient begins distraction, tension develops at all wire/half-pin and bone interfaces, leading to increasing difficulty in distraction and limb pain. Sudden spontaneous completion of the osteotomy with continued tension applied by the fixator results in acute distraction of the osteotomy with severe pain. Premature consolidation is unlikely this early following the initial surgery.

REFERENCES: Birch JG, Samchukov ML: Use of the Ilizarov method to correct lower limb deformities in children and adolescents. *J Am Acad Orthop Surg* 2004;12:144-154.

Noonan KJ, Leyes M, Forriol F, et al: Distraction osteogenesis of the lower extremity with use of monolateral external fixation: A study of two hundred and sixty-one femora and tibiae. *J Bone Joint Surg Am* 1998;80:793-806.

A-22: A 10-year-old girl who is Risser stage 0 has back deformity associated with neurofibromatosis type 1 (NF1). She has no back pain. Examination shows multiple café-au-lait nevi with normal lower extremity neurologic function and reflexes. Standing radiographs of the spine show a short 50° right thoracic scoliosis with a kyphotic deformity of 55° (apex T8). A 10° progression in scoliosis has occurred during the past 1 year. There is no cervical deformity. MRI shows mild dural ectasia, primarily in the upper lumbar region. Management should consist of

1. observation with repeat radiographs in 6 months.
2. a thoracolumbosacral orthosis (TLSO).
3. in situ posterior spinal fusion without instrumentation, followed by full-time TLSO bracing.
4. anterior spinal convex hemiepiphysiodesis.
5. combined anterior and posterior spinal arthrodesis with instrumentation.

PREFERRED RESPONSE: 5

DISCUSSION: Scoliotic deformities in patients with NF1 are often dysplastic with short, angular curves. Posterior arthrodesis is made more difficult by the presence of kyphosis and of weak posterior elements caused by dural ectasia. Combined anterior and posterior spinal arthrodesis is generally preferred for progressive dysplastic curves to maximize deformity correction and to decrease the risk of pseudarthrosis. Anterior fusion may also prevent crankshaft phenomenon in young children. Brace treatment is not effective for large, rigid, or dysplastic curves.

(continued on next page)

(A-22: *continued*)

REFERENCES: Kim HW, Weinstein SL: Spine update: The management of scoliosis in neurofibromatosis. *Spine (Phila Pa 1976)* 1997;22:2770-2776.

Funasaki H, Winter RB, Lonstein JB, et al: Pathophysiology of spinal deformities in neurofibromatosis: An analysis of seventy-one patients who had curves associated with dystrophic changes. *J Bone Joint Surg Am* 1994;76:692-700.

A-23: In obstetric brachial plexus palsy, which of the following signs is associated with the poorest prognosis for recovery in a 2-month-old infant?

1. Persistent inability to bring the hand to the mouth with the elbow stabilized at the side
2. Persistent inability to actively abduct the arm past 90°
3. Persistent inability to externally rotate the shoulder past 20°
4. Persistent unilateral ptosis, myosis, and anhydrosis
5. History of clavicle fracture at birth

PREFERRED RESPONSE: 4

DISCUSSION: Persistent Horner sign (ptosis, myosis, and anhydrosis) is a sign of proximal injury, usually avulsion of the roots from the cord, which disrupts the sympathetic chain. Root rupture or avulsion proximal to the myelin sheath has less chance of healing. Two-month-old infants with persistent weakness in the other areas described may still have a good prognosis for recovery. Concurrent clavicle fracture has been shown to have no prognostic value.

REFERENCES: Clarke HM, Curtis CG: An approach to obstetrical brachial plexus injuries. *Hand Clin* 1995;11:563-581.

Narakas AO: Injuries to the brachial plexus, in Bora FW, ed: *The Pediatric Upper Extremity: Diagnosis and Management*. Philadelphia, PA, WB Saunders, 1986, p 247.

A-24: A 6-year-old boy with acute hematogenous osteomyelitis of the distal femur is being treated with intravenous antibiotics. The most expeditious method to determine the early success or failure of treatment is by serial evaluations of which of the following studies?

1. Complete blood count with differential
2. MRI
3. CT
4. Radiographs
5. C-reactive protein (CRP)

PREFERRED RESPONSE: 5

DISCUSSION: Successful antibiotic treatment of osteomyelitis should lead to a rapid decline in CRP level. The CRP level should decline after 48 to 72 hours of appropriate treatment. Imaging studies will take much longer to show resolution of bone infection.

REFERENCES: Unkila-Kallio L, Kallio MJ, Eskola J, et al: Serum C-reactive protein, erythrocyte sedimentation rate, and white blood cell count in acute hematogenous osteomyelitis of children. *Pediatrics* 1994;93:59-62.

Herring JA: *Tachdjian's Pediatric Orthopaedics*, ed 3. Philadelphia, PA, WB Saunders, 2002, vol 3, pp 1841-1860.

A-25: A 6-year-old girl has a painless spinal deformity. Examination reveals 2+ and equal knee jerks and ankle jerks, negative clonus, and a negative Babinski sign. The straight leg raising test is negative. Abdominal reflexes are asymmetrical. PA and lateral radiographs are shown in Figures 12A and 12B. What is the most appropriate next step in management?

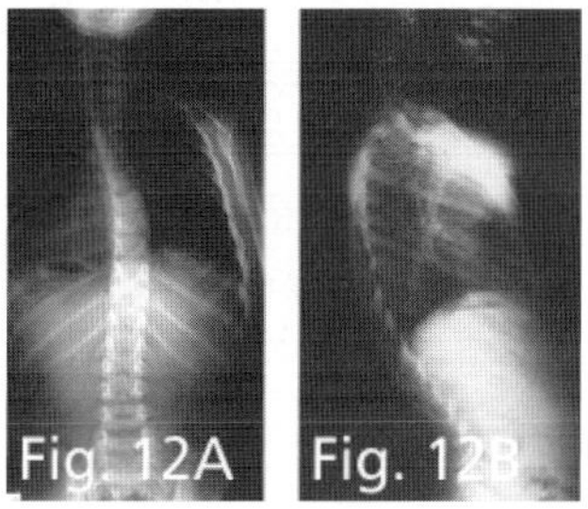

1. MRI of the spinal axis
2. Physical therapy
3. A brace for scoliosis
4. Observation, with reevaluation in 6 to 12 months
5. Posterior spinal fusion from T6 to T12

PREFERRED RESPONSE: 1

DISCUSSION: The patient has an abnormal neurologic examination as shown by the abnormal abdominal reflexes. Furthermore, she has a significant curve and is younger than 10 years. These findings are not consistent with idiopathic scoliosis. MRI will best rule out syringomyelia or an intraspinal tumor. Bracing and surgery are not indicated for this small curvature prior to obtaining an MRI scan.

REFERENCES: Ginsburg GM, Bassett GS: Back pain in children and adolescents: Evaluation and differential diagnosis. *J Am Acad Orthop Surg* 1997;5:67-78.

Schwend RM, Hennrikus W, Hall JE, et al: Childhood scoliosis: Clinical indications for magnetic resonance imaging. *J Bone Joint Surg Am* 1995;77:46-53.

Pediatrics: Answers

A-26: Figure 13 shows the radiograph of a 7-year-old boy who sustained a pathologic fracture of the left humerus 1 day ago. Initial management should consist of

1. a sling and swathe.
2. needle biopsy of the lesion.
3. a corticosteroid injection of the lesion.
4. curettage and bone packing of the lesion.
5. insertion of an intramedullary rod.

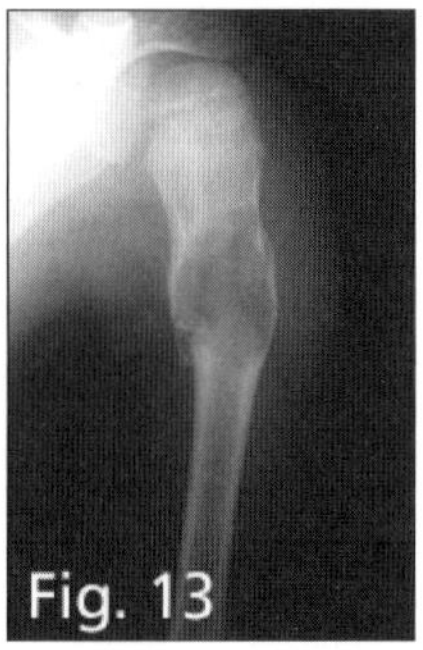

PREFERRED RESPONSE: 1

DISCUSSION: The radiograph shows a pathologic fracture through a unicameral (simple) bone cyst (UBC). This is the most common location and presentation of a UBC. Fewer than 10% of UBCs heal spontaneously following a fracture. Urgent biopsy is not indicated because the lesion appears benign and the histology of fracture callus may be misinterpreted as osteosarcoma. After the fracture heals with the use of a sling and swathe, the UBC may be treated with a minimally invasive procedure such as injection of bone marrow and/or demineralized bone matrix. The chance for success is relatively low in an active cyst located adjacent to the physis. More invasive procedures, such as curettage, Rush rod fixation, or cannulated screw decompression, have been described but are rarely necessary for treatment of upper extremity cysts.

REFERENCES: Rougraff BT, Kling TJ: Treatment of active unicameral bone cysts with percutaneous injection of demineralized bone matrix and autogenous bone marrow. *J Bone Joint Surg Am* 2002;84:921-929.

Robosch A, Saraph V, Linhart WE: Flexible intramedullary nailing for the treatment of unicameral bone cysts in long bones. *J Bone Joint Surg Am* 2000;82:1447-1453.

Wilkins RM: Unicameral bone cysts. *J Am Acad Orthop Surg* 2000;8:217-224.

A-27: A newborn with myelomeningocele has no movement below the waist and has bilateral hips that dislocate with provocative flexion and adduction. What is the best treatment option for the hip instability?

1. A Pavlik harness with the hips in 90° of flexion and 60° of abduction
2. A spica cast with the hips in 100° of flexion and 70° of abduction
3. Observation with range-of-motion exercises to minimize contractures
4. Open reduction through an anterior hip approach
5. Open reduction through a medial hip approach

PREFERRED RESPONSE: 3

DISCUSSION: The status of the hips (located or dislocated) in children with thoracic-level myelomeningocele has no effect on the functional outcome of these patients. Management of unstable hips in this population should be limited to treatment of the contractures that may lead to poor limb positioning in either braces or a wheelchair. The use of the Pavlik harness and/or spica cast is contraindicated because they would promote flexion and abduction contractures. In the past, open reduction either through an anterior or medial approach had been performed with a high incidence of redislocation and other complications, with little functional gain for the child.

(continued on next page)

(A-27: *continued*)

REFERENCES: Gabriel KG: Natural history of hip deformity in spina bifida, in Sarwark JR, Lubicky JP, eds: *Caring for the Child With Spina Bifida*. Rosemont, IL, American Academy of Orthopaedic Surgeons, 2001, pp 89-103.

Schoenecker PL: Surgical management of hip problems in children with myelomeningocele, in Sarwark KR, Lubicky JP, eds: *Caring for the Child With Spina Bifida*. Rosemont, IL, American Academy of Orthopaedic Surgeons, 2001, pp 117-131.

A-28: A 14-year-old boy reports a 4-month history of increasing backache with difficulty walking long distances. His parents state that he walks with his knees slightly flexed and is unable to bend forward and get his hands to his knees. He denies numbness, tingling, and weakness in his legs and denies loss of bladder and bowel control. A lateral radiograph of the lumbosacral spine is shown in Figure 14. What is the best surgical management for this condition?

1. Vertebrectomy of L5
2. Posterior spinal fusion with or without instrumentation from L4 to S1
3. Posterior spinal fusion without instrumentation from L5 to S1
4. Anterior spinal fusion from L4 to L5
5. Direct repair of the spondylolysis defect

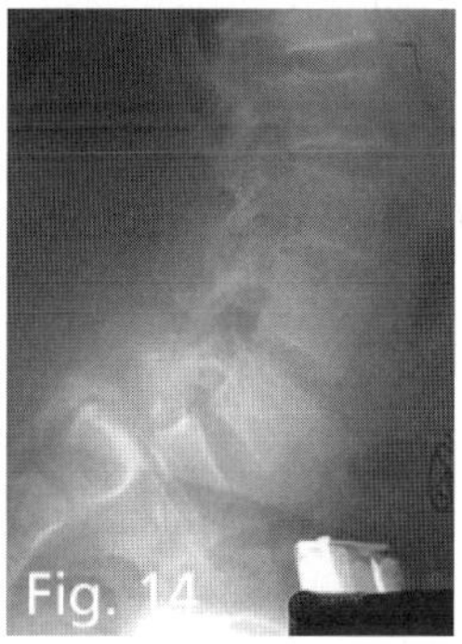
Fig. 14

PREFERRED RESPONSE: 2

DISCUSSION: The patient has a grade 4 spondylolisthesis. Optimal surgical management is posterior spinal fusion from L4 to the sacrum. The use of instrumentation is controversial. Vertebrectomy is typically reserved for spondylo-optosis (grade 5) cases. Spinal fusion from L5 to S1 usually is not successful for a slip that is greater than 50%. Isolated anterior spinal fusion has not been successful, and direct repair of the pars defect is only useful for spondylolysis without spondylolisthesis.

REFERENCES: Lenke LG, Bridwell KH: Evaluation and surgical treatment of high-grade isthmic dysplastic spondylolisthesis. *Instr Course Lect* 2003;52:525-532.

Ginsburg GM, Bassett GS: Back pain in children and adolescents: Evaluation and differential diagnosis. *J Am Acad Orthop Surg* 1997:5:67-78.

Pediatrics: Answers

A-29: A 12-year-old boy reports limping and chronic knee pain that is now inhibiting his ability to participate in sports. Clinical examination and radiographs of the knee are normal. Additional evaluation should include

1. mechanical alignment radiographs.
2. stress radiographs of the knee.
3. comparison radiographs of both knees.
4. erythrocyte sedimentation rate and C-reactive protein level.
5. examination of the hip.

PREFERRED RESPONSE: 5

DISCUSSION: Although all of the answers may be appropriate, radiating pain from hip pathology must be excluded. At this age, a slipped capital femoral epiphysis is likely. Therefore, the hip must be examined.

REFERENCES: Kocher MS, Bishop JA, Weed B, et al: Delay in diagnosis of slipped capital femoral epiphysis. *Pediatrics* 2004;113:322-325.

Matava MJ, Patton CM, Luhmann S, et al: Knee pain as the initial symptom of slipped capital femoral epiphysis: An analysis of initial presentation and treatment. *J Pediatr Orthop* 1999;19:455-460.

A-30: Split posterior tibial tendon transfer is used in the treatment of children with cerebral palsy. Which of the following patients is considered the most appropriate candidate for this procedure?

1. A 6-year-old child with athetosis and a flexible equinovarus deformity of the foot
2. A 6-year-old child with spastic hemiplegia and a rigid equinovarus deformity of the foot
3. A 6-year-old child with spastic hemiplegia and a flexible equinovarus deformity of the foot
4. A 10-year-old child with spastic quadriplegia and rigid valgus deformities of the feet
5. A 15-year-old child with spastic diplegia and rigid equinovalgus deformities of the feet

PREFERRED RESPONSE: 3

DISCUSSION: Split posterior tibial tendon transfers are best performed in patients with spastic cerebral palsy who are between the ages of 4 and 7 years and have flexible equinovarus deformities. Rigid deformities typically require bony reconstruction procedures. Tendon transfers in patients with athetosis are unpredictable.

REFERENCES: Green NE, Griffin PP, Shiavi R: Split posterior tibial-tendon transfer in spastic cerebral palsy. *J Bone Joint Surg Am* 1983;65:748-754.

Herring JA: *Tachdjian's Pediatric Orthopaedics*, ed 3. Philadelphia, PA, WB Saunders, 2002, vol 2, pp 1142-1152.

A-31: Late surgical treatment of posttraumatic cubitus varus (gunstock deformity) is usually necessitated by the patient reporting problems related to

1. tardy ulnar nerve palsy.
2. posterior glenohumeral subluxation.
3. posterolateral rotatory subluxation of the elbow.
4. poor appearance.
5. snapping medial triceps.

PREFERRED RESPONSE: 4

DISCUSSION: Cubitus varus, elbow hyperextension, and internal rotation are all typical components of the gunstock deformity. This deformity results from malunion of a supracondylar fracture of the humerus. All of the problems listed above have been reported as sequelae of a gunstock deformity, although the malunion usually causes no functional limitations. Unacceptable appearance is the most common reason why patients or parents request corrective osteotomy.

REFERENCES: O'Driscoll SW, Spinner RJ, McKee MD, et al: Tardy posterolateral rotatory instability of the elbow due to cubitus varus. *J Bone Joint Surg Am* 2001;83:1358-1369.

Gurkan I, Bayrakci K, Tasbas B, et al: Posterior instability of the shoulder after supracondylar fractures recovered with cubitus varus deformity. *J Pediatr Orthop* 2002;22:198-202.

Spinner RJ, O'Driscoll SW, Davids JR, et al: Cubitus varus associated with dislocation of both the medial portion of the triceps and the ulnar nerve. *J Hand Surg* 1999;24:718-726.

A-32: What is the incidence and significance of anterior cruciate ligament laxity following tibial eminence fractures in skeletally immature individuals?

1. Common and frequently symptomatic
2. Common and infrequently symptomatic
3. Common but generally resolves spontaneously
4. Rare but when present, usually symptomatic
5. Rare and if present, infrequently symptomatic

PREFERRED RESPONSE: 2

DISCUSSION: Measurable anterior cruciate ligament laxity, while frequently seen after tibial eminence fractures, usually does not cause symptoms. It is found even in patients whose fractures have been anatomically reduced and fixed, leading to speculation that it is caused by stretching of the ligament at the time of injury.

REFERENCES: Willis R, Blokker C, Stall TM, et al: Long-term follow-up of anterior eminence fractures. *J Pediatr Orthop* 1993;13:361-364.

Smith JB: Knee instability after fracture of the intercondylar eminence of the tibia. *J Pediatr Orthop* 1984;4:462-464.

A-33: A full-term newborn has webbing at the knees, rigid clubfeet, a Buddha-like posture of the lower extremities, and no voluntary or involuntary muscle action at and below the knees. Radiographs of the spine and pelvis reveal an absence of the lumbar spine and sacrum. What maternal condition is associated with this diagnosis?

1. Alcoholism
2. Drug abuse
3. Down syndrome
4. Diabetes mellitus
5. Idiopathic scoliosis

PREFERRED RESPONSE: 4

DISCUSSION: The history, physical examination, and radiographic findings are consistent with type IV sacral agenesis or caudal regression syndrome. These children are born with no lumbar spine or sacrum. The T12 vertebra is often prominent posteriorly. Popliteal webbing and knee flexion contractures are common with this diagnosis. There is a higher incidence of this diagnosis when the mother has diabetes mellitus. Maternal drug abuse and alcoholism can produce phenotypically unique children but without the findings described here. Maternal idiopathic scoliosis is not associated with caudal regression syndrome.

REFERENCES: Chan BW, Chan KS, Koide T, et al: Maternal diabetes increases the risk of caudal regression caused by retinoic acid. *Diabetes* 2002;51:2811-2816.

Zaw W, Stone DG: Caudal regression syndrome in twin pregnancy with type II diabetes. *J Perinatol* 2002;22:171-174.

A-34: Figure 15 shows the sitting AP and lateral spinal radiographs of a nonambulatory 12½-year-old boy with Duchenne muscular dystrophy who is being evaluated for scoliosis. The lumbar curve from T12 to L5 measures 36°, and the thoracic curve from T3 to T12 measures 24° on the AP radiograph. He has 5° of pelvic obliquity. His forced vital capacity is 45% of predicted for height and weight. What is the most appropriate treatment for the spinal deformity?

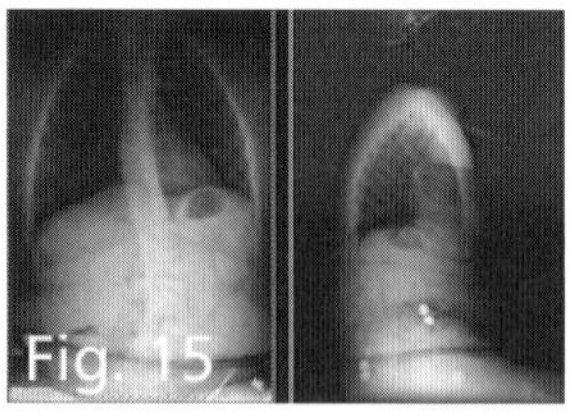

1. Posterior spinal fusion from T2 to L5 with segmental instrumentation
2. Anterior spinal fusion from L1 to L4, followed by posterior spinal fusion from T2 to the sacrum with segmental instrumentation including iliac fixation
3. Custom-molded spinal orthosis worn 23 hours per day until skeletal maturity
4. A spinal orthosis until age 14 years, followed by posterior spinal fusion with segmental instrumentation
5. Adapted wheelchair seating with a custom-molded back support to correct scoliosis and kyphosis

PREFERRED RESPONSE: 1

DISCUSSION: Posterior spinal fusion is the treatment of choice for scoliosis in patients with Duchenne muscular dystrophy after they are no longer able to walk. This treatment improves quality of life and upright wheelchair positioning. Its effect on pulmonary function is less clear, as pulmonary function will

(continued on next page)

(A-34: *continued*)

continue to decline because of the underlying muscle disease. Although bracing and wheelchair modifications may slow the progression of the curve, progression will continue. Surgical intervention at this stage does not have to include the pelvis, which, in general, is indicated in curves of greater than 40°, and when pelvic obliquity is greater than 10°. Fixation to the pelvis should also be considered in lumbar curves where the apex is lower than L1. Surgical treatment usually can be safely performed if the vital capacity is greater than 35%.

REFERENCES: Hahn GV, Mubarak SJ: Muscular dystrophy, in Weinstein SL, ed: *The Pediatric Spine*, ed 2. Philadelphia, PA, Lippincott Williams & Wilkins, 2001, pp 819-832.

Mubarak SJ, Morin WD, Leach J: Spinal fusion in Duchenne muscular dystrophy: Fixation and fusion to the sacropelvis? *J Pediatr Orthop* 1993;13:752-757.

A-35: A 3-year-old child has refused to walk for the past 2 days. Examination in the emergency department reveals a temperature of 102.2° F (39° C) and limited range of motion of the left hip. An AP pelvic radiograph is normal. Laboratory studies show a white blood cell (WBC) count of 9,000/mm^3, an erythrocyte sedimentation rate (ESR) of 65 mm/hour, and a C-reactive protein level of 10.5 mg/L (normal < 0.4). What is the most appropriate next step in management?

1. Technetium Tc 99m bone scan
2. Intravenous antibiotics
3. Oral antibiotics
4. CT of the hips
5. Aspiration of the left hip

PREFERRED RESPONSE: 5

DISCUSSION: Examination reveals an irritable hip, creating a differential diagnosis of transient synovitis versus pyogenic hip arthritis. Kocher and associates described four criteria to help predict the presence of infection: inability to bear weight, fever, ESR of more than 40 mm/hour, and a peripheral WBC count of more than 12,000/mm^3. This patient meets three of the four criteria, with a positive predictive value of 73% to 93% for joint infection. Therefore, aspiration of the hip is warranted, with a high likelihood that emergent hip arthrotomy will be indicated. Ideally, intravenous antibiotics should be administered after culture material has been obtained from needle aspiration of the hip. An urgent bone scan is better indicated as a screening test for sacroiliitis or diskitis. If the arthrocentesis proves negative, CT or MRI of the pelvis may be indicated to rule out a pelvic or psoas abscess.

REFERENCES: Del Beccaro MA, Champoux AN, Bockers T, et al: Septic arthritis versus transient synovitis of the hip: The value of screening laboratory tests. *Ann Emerg Med* 1992;21:1418-1422.

Kocher MS, Mandiga R, Zurakowski D, et al: Validation of a clinical prediction rule for the differentiation between septic arthritis and transient synovitis of the hip in children. *J Bone Joint Surg Am* 2004;86:1629-1635.

Kocher MS, Zurakowski D, Kasser JR: Differentiating between septic arthritis and transient synovitis of the hip in children: An evidence-based clinical prediction algorithm. *J Bone Joint Surg Am* 1999;81:1662-1670.

A-36: A 12-year-old girl who has a history of frequent tripping and falling also has bilateral symmetric hand weakness, high arched feet, absent patellar and Achilles tendon reflexes, and excessive wear on the lateral border of her shoes. She reports that she has multiple paternal family members with similar deformities. She most likely has a defect of what protein?

1. Peripheral myelin protein-22
2. Dystrophin
3. Type I collagen
4. Alpha-L-iduronidase
5. Cartilage oligomeric matrix protein

PREFERRED RESPONSE: 1

DISCUSSION: The girl shows clinical features of hereditary motor sensory neuropathy type 1, Charcot-Marie-Tooth disease. The most common type of this autosomal dominant disease is caused by an underlying defect in the gene coding for peripheral myelin protein-22 on chromosome 17. Many other less common mutations have been identified in this family of neuropathies. Dystrophin is a protein that is abnormal in Duchenne muscular dystrophy, which affects males and is diagnosed earlier. Type I collagen is defective in osteogenesis imperfecta. Alpha-L-iduronidase is defective in mucopolysaccharidosis type I, Hurler syndrome. Defective cartilage oligomeric matrix protein is associated with some forms of multiple epiphyseal dysplasia.

REFERENCES: Patel PI, Roa BB, Welcher AA, et al: The gene for the peripheral myelin protein PMP-22 is a candidate for Charcot-Marie-Tooth disease type 1A. *Nat Genet* 1992;1:159-165.

Harding AE: From the syndrome of Charcot, Marie and Tooth to disorders of peripheral myelin proteins. *Brain* 1995;118:809-818.

A-37: What acetabular procedure for developmental dysplasia of the hip does not require a concentric reduction of the femoral head in the acetabulum?

1. Salter innominate osteotomy
2. Pemberton innominate osteotomy
3. Dega innominate osteotomy
4. Triple innominate osteotomy
5. Staheli shelf procedure

PREFERRED RESPONSE: 5

DISCUSSION: All of the reorientation innominate osteotomies require a concentric reduction of the hip. The Staheli shelf procedure may be performed even with the hip subluxated, but it is a salvage procedure that covers a portion of the femoral head with capsular fibrocartilage rather than hyaline cartilage.

REFERENCES: Staheli LT, Chew DE: Slotted acetabular augmentation in childhood adolescence. *J Pediatr Orthop* 1992;12:569-580.

Herring JA: *Tachdjian's Pediatric Orthopaedics*, ed 3. Philadelphia, PA, WB Saunders, 2002, vol 1, pp 618-650.

A-38: A 5-year-old boy has had pain in the right foot for the past month. Examination reveals tenderness and mild swelling in the region of the tarsal navicular. Radiographs are shown in Figure 16. Management should consist of

1. biopsy of the tarsal navicular.
2. curettage and bone grafting of the tarsal navicular.
3. Complete blood count, C-reactive protein level, erythrocyte sedimentation rate, blood cultures, and IV antibiotics.
4. symptomatic treatment with restriction of weight bearing or application of short leg cast.
5. medial column lengthening of the foot through the tarsal navicular.

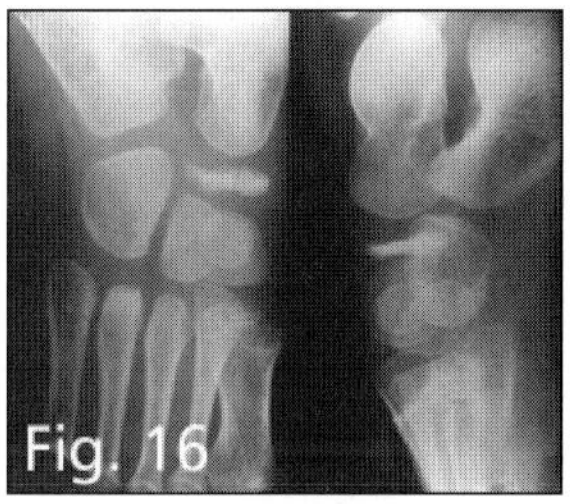

PREFERRED RESPONSE: 4

DISCUSSION: The child has the classic findings of Kohler disease or osteochondrosis of the tarsal navicular. The cause of this condition is not known, but osteonecrosis and mechanical compression have been proposed. Children generally report midfoot pain over the tarsal navicular and limping. Physical findings include tenderness, swelling, and occasionally redness in the region of the tarsal navicular. Radiographs show sclerosis and narrowing of the tarsal navicular. The natural history of the condition is spontaneous resolution and reconstitution of the navicular. Symptomatic treatment with restriction of weight bearing or casting is recommended.

REFERENCES: Karp M: Kohler's disease of the tarsal scaphoid. *J Bone Joint Surg* 1937;19:84-96.

Borges JL, Guille JT, Bowen JR: Kohler's bone disease of the tarsal navicular. *J Pediatr Orthop* 1995;15:596-598.

A-39: A 9-year-old child sustained a fracture-dislocation of C5 and C6 with a complete spinal cord injury. What is the likelihood that scoliosis will develop during the remaining years of his growth?

1. 10%
2. 20%
3. 50%
4. 70%
5. 100%

PREFERRED RESPONSE: 5

DISCUSSION: The incidence of late spinal deformity after complete spinal cord injury in children depends on the level of the spinal cord injury and the age of the patient at the time of injury. If a cervical level injury occurs before age 10 years, paralytic scoliosis will develop in virtually 100% of patients.

REFERENCES: Brown JC, Swank SM, Matta J, et al: Late spinal deformity in quadriplegic children and adolescents. *J Pediatr Orthop* 1984;4:456-461.

Lancourt JE, Dickson JH, Carter RE: Paralytic spinal deformity following traumatic spinal-cord injury in children and adolescents. *J Bone Joint Surg Am* 1981;63:47-53.

Dearolf WW III, Betz RR, Vogel LC, et al: Scoliosis in pediatric spinal cord-injured patients. *J Pediatr Orthop* 1990;10:214-218.

A-40: The husband of a 22-year-old woman has hypophosphatemic rickets. The woman has no orthopaedic abnormalities, but she is concerned about her chances of having a child with the same disease. What should they be told regarding this disorder?

1. Their sons will have a 50% chance of having this X-linked dominant disorder.
2. All of their daughters will be carriers or will have this disorder.
3. They should be advised to not have any children because the risk of having boys with the disorder and girls who will be carriers is too hard for any parent.
4. As long as the woman does not carry the trait, the children will not be affected because the husband has the disease and this is an X-linked dominant disorder.
5. Their sons or daughters may be born with this disorder, but males are more severely affected.

PREFERRED RESPONSE: 2

DISCUSSION: Hypophosphatemia is a rare genetic disease usually inherited as an X-linked dominant trait. The fact that the woman has no skeletal manifestations would indicate that the husband has the X-linked mutation. The disease is more severe in boys than it is in girls. The husband will not transmit the disease to his sons. However, all of their daughters will be affected either with the disease or as carriers. If the woman has the disease or the trait, there is a 50% chance that her sons will inherit the disease and a 50% chance that her daughters will be carriers or have a milder form of the disease. Parents should be advised to have genetic counseling so they can be informed when deciding whether to have children.

REFERENCES: Herring JA: Metabolic and endocrine bone diseases, in *Tachdjian's Pediatric Orthopaedics*, ed 3. New York, NY, WB Saunders, 2002, pp 1685-1743.

Sillence DO: Disorders of bone density, volume, and mineralization, in Rimoin DL, Conner JM, Pyerite RE, et al, eds: *Principles and Practice of Medical Genetics*, ed 4. New York, NY, Churchill Livingstone, 2002.

Staheli LT: *Practice of Pediatric Orthopedics*. Philadelphia, PA, Lippincott Williams & Wilkins, 2001.

A-41: A 9-year-old boy sustained a traumatic brain injury and right lower extremity trauma in an accident involving a motor vehicle and a pedestrian. Initial evaluation in the emergency department reveals an obtunded patient who is breathing spontaneously and withdraws appropriately to painful stimuli. After initial resuscitation and stabilization, a CT scan reveals a right parietal intracranial hemorrhage. Radiographs of the swollen right thigh are shown in Figures 17A and 17B. Management of the fractured femur should ultimately consist of

1. immediate hip spica casting.
2. closed reduction and percutaneous pin fixation supplemented by a hip spica cast.
3. placement in 90-90 traction after insertion of a distal femoral traction pin.
4. insertion of a reamed antegrade intramedullary nail starting at the piriformis fossa, stopping the nail short of the distal femoral growth plate.
5. closed reduction and stabilization using retrograde flexible intramedullary nails.

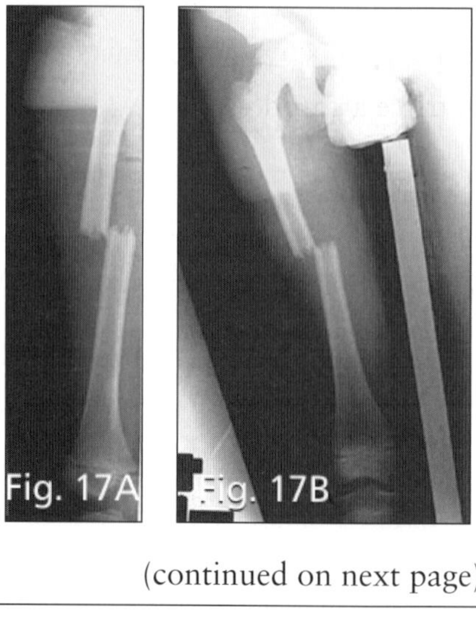
Fig. 17A Fig. 17B

(continued on next page)

(A-41: *continued*)

PREFERRED RESPONSE: 5

DISCUSSION: A child with a traumatic brain injury generally achieves significant neurologic recovery and has a more favorable prognosis than an adult. Early stabilization of fractures facilitates transportation of the child for diagnostic tests and decreases the incidence of shortening and malunion. Surgical treatment of the fracture is indicated when cerebral perfusion pressure has stabilized. Casting or traction is not the most appropriate treatment of a femoral fracture in a child of this age with a brain injury. Fracture reduction is difficult to maintain if the brain injury leads to spasticity, and transportation within the hospital for tests is more difficult. Insertion of a reamed antegrade intramedullary nail inserted at the piriformis fossa is associated with a small risk of osteonecrosis of the femoral head. The transverse femoral fracture in this patient is ideally suited for stabilization with flexible intramedullary nails. Ligier and associates treated 123 femoral shaft fractures in children with flexible intramedullary nails, including 35 patients with head injury. In one patient with hemiplegia and a urinary tract infection, a deep wound infection developed, necessitating nail removal. The remaining patients all healed without major complications. Heinrich and associates treated 78 diaphyseal femoral fractures with flexible intramedullary nails, including 14 with head injury. No major complications were reported and all fractures healed.

REFERENCES: Tolo VT: Management of the multiply injured child, in Rockwood CA, Wilkins KE, Beaty JH, eds: *Fractures in Children*, ed 4. Philadelphia, PA, Lippincott-Raven, 1996, pp 83-95.

Ligier JN, Metaizeau JP, Prevot J, et al: Elastic stable intramedullary nailing of femoral shaft fractures in children. *J Bone Joint Surg Br* 1988;70:74-77.

Heinrich MS, Drvaric DM, Darr K, et al: The operative stabilization of pediatric diaphyseal femur fractures with flexible intramedullary nails: A prospective analysis. *J Pediatric Orthop* 1994;14:501-507.

Canale ST, Tolo VT: Fractures of the femur in children. *Instr Course Lect* 1995;44:255-273.

A-42: Figure 18 shows the oblique radiograph of an 11-year-old boy who has a mild left flatfoot deformity. Examination reveals that subtalar motion is limited and painful. Despite casting for 6 weeks, the patient reports foot pain that limits participation in sport activities. A CT scan shows no subtalar joint abnormalities. Management should now include

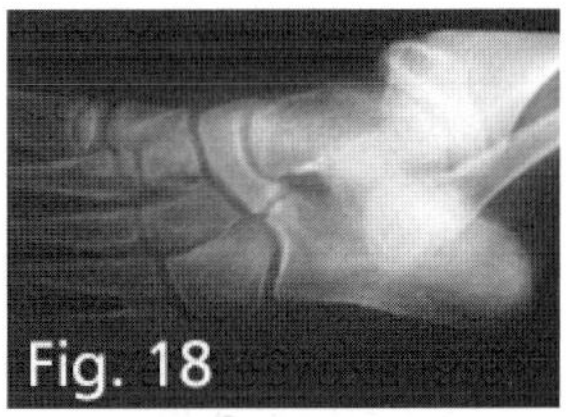

Fig. 18

1. manipulation of the foot under general anesthesia.
2. peroneal lengthening.
3. coalition resection with interposition of fat or muscle.
4. distal calcaneal lengthening osteotomy.
5. triple arthrodesis.

PREFERRED RESPONSE: 3

DISCUSSION: The radiograph shows an incompletely ossified calcaneonavicular coalition. When symptomatic, a trial of cast immobilization is reasonable. If this fails to provide relief, the preferred treatment is resection of the coalition. Before attempting surgery, a CT scan should be obtained to rule out ipsilateral subtalar coalition. Recurrence of the coalition is usually prevented with interposition of autogenous fat graft or with local interposition of the extensor digitorum brevis muscle. Approximately 80% of patients treated in this manner have decreased pain and improved subtalar motion. When the flatfoot deformity is mild, calcaneal lengthening or medial translation osteotomy is unnecessary. Primary triple arthrodesis may be indicated if degenerative changes are present in the subtalar or midfoot joints.

(continued on next page)

(A-42: *continued*)

Peroneal lengthening has been described for treatment of the peroneal spastic flatfoot without demonstrable tarsal coalition.

REFERENCES: Gonzalez P, Kumar SJ: Calcaneonavicular coalition treated by resection and interposition of the extensor digitorum brevis muscle. *J Bone Joint Surg Am* 1990;72:71-77.

Vincent KA: Tarsal coalition and painful flatfoot. *J Am Acad Orthop Surg* 1998;6:274-281.

Luhmann SJ, Rich MM, Schoenecker PL: Painful idiopathic rigid flatfoot in children and adolescents. *Foot Ankle Int* 2000;21:59-66.

A-43: A nonambulatory verbal 6-year-old child with spastic quadriplegic cerebral palsy has progressive bilateral hip subluxation of more than 50%. There is no pain with range of motion, but abduction is limited to 20 degrees maximum. An AP radiograph is seen in Figure 19. Management should consist of

1. percutaneous bilateral adductor tenotomy.
2. oral baclofen.
3. phenol injection into the obturator nerve.
4. open adductor tenotomy with neurectomy of the anterior branch of the obturator nerve.
5. open adductor tenotomy with release of the iliopsoas and bilateral proximal femoral varus derotation osteotomy.

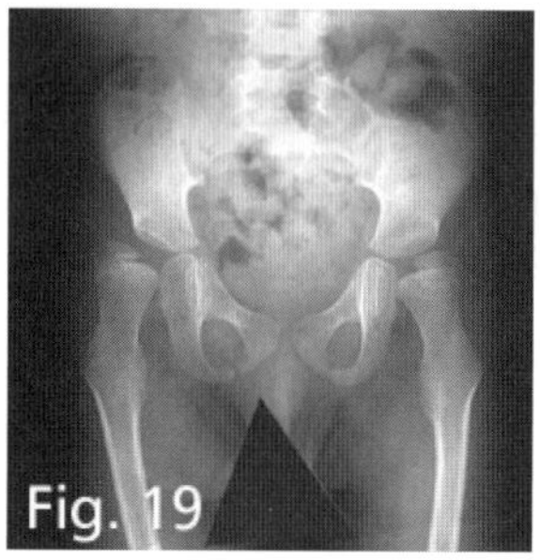

PREFERRED RESPONSE: 5

DISCUSSION: The natural history of the patient's hips, if left untreated, is gradual progression to dislocation. To prevent future pain, prevention of dislocation is often helpful. The patient is too old for soft-tissue releases alone. Therefore, the treatment of choice is medial release of both hips to obtain 45° or better of hip abduction in conjunction with psoas tenotomy and bilateral femoral varus osteotomies.

REFERENCES: Presedo A, Oh CW, Dabney KY, et al: Soft-tissue releases to treat spastic hip subluxation in children with cerebral palsy. *J Bone Joint Surg Am* 2005;87:832-841.

Miller F, Bagg MR: Age and migration percentage as risk factors for progression in spastic hip disease. *Dev Med Child Neurol* 1995;37:449-455.

A-44: Figures 20A through 20C show the clinical photograph and radiographs of a 15-year-old boy who stubbed his toe 1 day ago while walking barefoot in the yard. Management should consist of

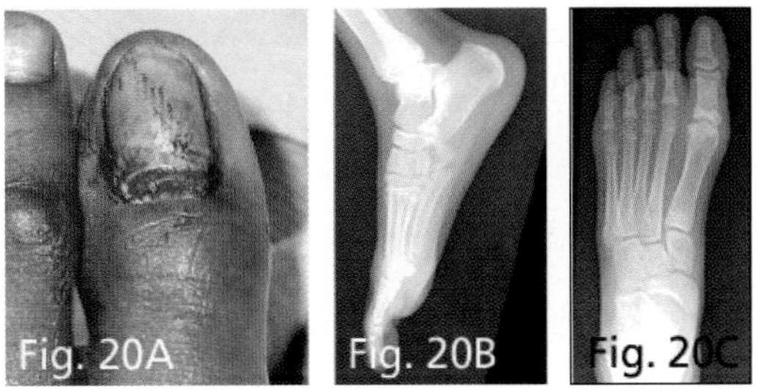

1. buddy taping of the great toe to the second toe for 3 weeks and use of a hard-soled shoe.
2. buddy taping of the great toe to the second toe for 3 weeks and application of a short leg cast.
3. buddy taping of the great toe to the second toe for 3 weeks, use of a hard-soled shoe, and a short course of antibiotics.
4. nail removal in the emergency department, buddy taping of the great toe to the second toe for 3 weeks, and use of a hard-soled shoe.
5. irrigation and open reduction, with or without fixation, and a short course of antibiotics.

PREFERRED RESPONSE: 5

DISCUSSION: The patient has an open fracture of the physis of the distal phalanx with a portion of the nail bed interposed in the physis. Seymour initially described this injury in the distal phalanges of fingers. Optimal treatment consists of removing the interposed tissue, irrigating the fracture, and a short course of antibiotics. The nail should be preserved to provide stability.

REFERENCES: Kensinger DR, Guille JT, Horn BD, et al: The stubbed great toe: Importance of early recognition and treatment of open fractures of the distal phalanx. *J Pediatr Orthop* 2001;21:31-34.

Pinckney LE, Currarino G, Kennedy LA: The stubbed great toe: A cause of occult compound fracture and infection. *Radiology* 1981;138:375-377.

Seymour N: Juxta-epiphysial fracture of the terminal phalanx of the finger. *J Bone Joint Surg Br* 1966;48:347-349.

A-45: A newborn girl is referred for evaluation of suspected hip instability. What information from her history would place her in the highest risk category?

1. History of maternal diabetes mellitus
2. Frank breech presentation
3. Female sex
4. Concomitant metatarsus adductus
5. Twin gestation

PREFERRED RESPONSE: 2

DISCUSSION: Breech positioning has been noted as the risk factor that most increases the relative risk of developmental dysplasia of the hip in multiple series and meta-analysis. All the other factors also increase the risk but to a lesser magnitude.

REFERENCES: Lehmann HP, Hinton R, Morello P, et al: Developmental dysplasia of the hip practice guideline: Technical report. Committee on Quality Improvement, and Subcommittee on Developmental Dysplasia of the Hip. *Pediatrics* 2000;105:E57.

Haynes RJ: Developmental dysplasia of the hip: Etiology, pathogenesis, and examination and physical findings in the newborn. *Instr Course Lect* 2001;50:535-540.

A-46: Figures 21A and 21B show the current radiographs of an 8-year-old girl who has had pain in the left thigh for the past 3 months. Hypothyroidism was recently diagnosed in this patient and she started treatment 1 week ago. Examination reveals a mild abductor deficiency limp on the left side. She lacks 30° internal rotation on the left hip compared with the right hip. Management should consist of

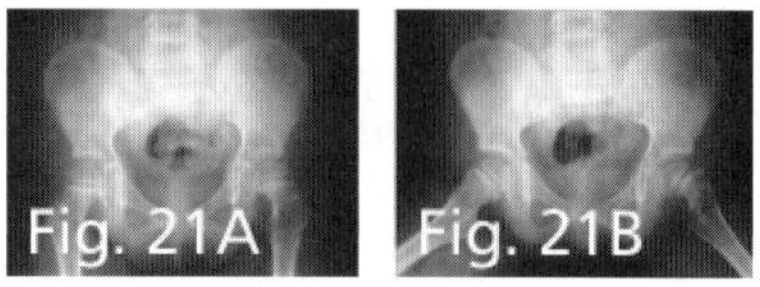

1. abductor muscle strengthening.
2. a left 1-½ hip spica cast.
3. closed reduction and pinning of the left hip.
4. symptomatic treatment with crutch walking and NSAIDs.
5. in situ pinning of both hips.

PREFERRED RESPONSE: 5

DISCUSSION: The radiographs confirm a slipped capital femoral epiphysis of the left hip, as well as a widened growth plate on the contralateral hip. This is considered a stable slip because the patient is able to walk. Treatment options for stable slips include in situ pinning, bone graft epiphysiodesis, and in some centers severe slips are treated with primary osteotomy and epiphyseal fixation. Percutaneous in situ fixation is the most popular and widely used method of treatment. This juvenile patient has an endocrine condition and a widened growth plate on the right side; therefore, strong consideration should be given to pinning the contralateral hip "preslip." Muscle strengthening, hip spica casting, and closed reduction have no place in the primary treatment of a stable slipped capital femoral epiphysis.

REFERENCES: Loder RT, Richards BS, Shapiro PS, et al: Acute slipped capital femoral epiphysis: The importance of physeal stability. *J Bone Joint Surg Am* 1993;75:1134-1140.

Loder R, Wittenberg B, DeSilva G: Slipped capital femoral epiphysis associated with endocrine disorders. *J Pediatr Orthop* 1995;15:349-356.

Aronson DD, Carlson WE: Slipped capital femoral epiphysis: A prospective study of fixation with a single screw. *J Bone Joint Surg Am* 1992;74:810-819.

A-47: A 3-year-old boy had been treated with serial casting for a right congenital idiopathic clubfoot deformity. The parents are concerned because the child now walks on the lateral border of the right foot. Examination shows that the foot passively achieves a plantigrade position with neutral heel valgus and ankle dorsiflexion to 15°. The forefoot inverts during active ankle dorsiflexion. Mild residual metatarsus adductus is present. Management should now consist of

1. additional serial casting.
2. a floor-reaction ankle-foot orthosis.
3. closing wedge cuboid osteotomy.
4. lateral transfer of the anterior tibialis tendon.
5. posterior tibial tendon transfer through the interosseous membrane to the third metatarsal.

PREFERRED RESPONSE: 4

DISCUSSION: Dynamic midfoot supination that is the result of peroneal weakness is a common residual problem after cast correction or surgical reconstruction of a congenital idiopathic clubfoot. Dynamic supination is unlikely to resolve spontaneously. Most parents do not want to use brace support forever. Transfer of the posterior tibialis to the dorsum of the foot has shown poor results in clubfeet. Preferred

(continued on next page)

(A-47: *continued*)

treatments include: (1) transfer of the entire anterior tibialis tendon to the lateral cuneiform, or (2) split transfer of the anterior tibialis tendon to the cuboid or to the peroneus brevis tendon.

REFERENCES: Kuo KN, Hennigan SP, Hastings ME: Anterior tibial tendon transfer in residual dynamic clubfoot deformity. *J Pediatr Orthop* 2001;21:35-41.

Garceau GJ: Anterior tibial tendon transfer for recurrent clubfoot. *Clin Orthop* 1972;84:61-65.

Miller GM, Hsu JD, Hoffer MM, et al: Posterior tibial tendon transfer: A review of the literature and analysis of 74 procedures. *J Pediatr Orthop* 1982;2:363-370.

A-48: A 12-month-old boy has right congenital fibular intercalary hemimelia with a normal contralateral limb. A radiograph of the lower extremities shows a limb-length discrepancy of 2 cm. All of the shortening is in the right tibia. Assuming that no treatment is rendered prior to skeletal maturity, the limb-length discrepancy will most likely

1. remain 2 cm at maturity.
2. decrease slowly until the limb lengths equalize.
3. increase at a constant rate of 2 cm per year.
4. increase markedly because of complete failure of tibial growth.
5. increase slowly, with the right lower extremity remaining in proportion to the left lower extremity.

PREFERRED RESPONSE: 5

DISCUSSION: Many congenital limb deficiencies and bowing deformities result in growth retardation. If unilateral, a gradually progressive limb-length discrepancy will result; however, the proportional lengths of the lower extremities will remain at a relatively constant ratio. For example, if the right foot is at the level of the left knee at birth, this will still be true at maturity. This concept can be useful for early prediction of limb-length discrepancy by using a multiplier method, as described by Paley and associates. This method can facilitate early treatment decisions, such as the need for amputation, without having to wait for serial scanography measurements.

REFERENCES: Paley D, Bhave A, Herzenberg JE, et al: Multiplier method for predicting limb-length discrepancy. *J Bone Joint Surg Am* 2000;82:1432-1446.

Moseley CF: A straight-line graph for leg length discrepancies. *Clin Orthop* 1978;136:33-40.

A-49: What zone of the physis is widened in rickets?

1. Reserve
2. Proliferative
3. Hypertrophic
4. Maturation
5. Primary spongiosa

PREFERRED RESPONSE: 3

DISCUSSION: Rickets causes widening of the hypertrophic layer of the physis because of the failure of mineralization and vascular invasion. The other zones of the physis may be altered in other disease conditions but remain relatively unchanged in rickets.

REFERENCES: Hunziker EB, Schenk RK, Cruz-Orive LM: Quantitation of chondrocyte performance in growth-plate cartilage during longitudinal bone growth. *J Bone Joint Surg Am* 1987;69:162-173.

Iannotti JP: Growth plate physiology and pathology. *Orthop Clin North Am* 1990;21:1-17.

A-50: A 7-year-old boy has had low back pain for the past 3 weeks. Radiographs reveal apparent disk space narrowing at L4-5. The patient is afebrile. Laboratory studies show a white blood cell count of 9,000/mm^3 and a C-reactive protein level of 10 mg/L. A lumbar MRI scan confirms the loss of disk height at L4-5 and reveals a small perivertebral abscess at that level. To achieve the most rapid improvement and to lessen the chances of recurrence, management should consist of

1. oral antibiotics.
2. intravenous antibiotics.
3. surgical drainage of the perivertebral abscess and intravenous antibiotics.
4. bed rest.
5. cast immobilization.

PREFERRED RESPONSE: 2

DISCUSSION: The patient has diskitis. Administration of intravenous antibiotics speeds resolution and minimizes recurrence. Bed rest and cast immobilization have been successfully used to treat this disorder but can be associated with prolonged recovery and frequent recurrence, even when oral antibiotics are administered. A perivertebral abscess seen in association with this condition usually resolves without surgery.

REFERENCES: Ring D, Johnston CE II, Wenger DR: Pyogenic infectious spondylitis in children: The convergence of discitis and vertebral osteomyelitis. *J Pediatr Orthop* 1995;15:652-660.

Crawford AH, Kucharzyk DW, Ruda R, et al: Diskitis in children. *Clin Orthop* 1991;266:70-79.

Spine

Q-1: During a retroperitoneal approach to the L4-5 disk, what structure must be ligated to safely mobilize the common iliac vessels toward the midline laterally and gain exposure?

1. Obturator vein
2. Iliolumbar vein
3. External iliac vein
4. Middle sacral artery
5. Hypogastric artery

Q-2: The injection shown in Figures 1A and 1B would most benefit a patient who reports which of the following symptoms?

1. Dorsal foot pain extending into the great toe
2. Foot pain extending along the lateral border of the foot
3. Pain extending into the foot in a stocking distribution
4. Anterior thigh and shin pain ending at the ankle
5. Lateral foot paresthesias

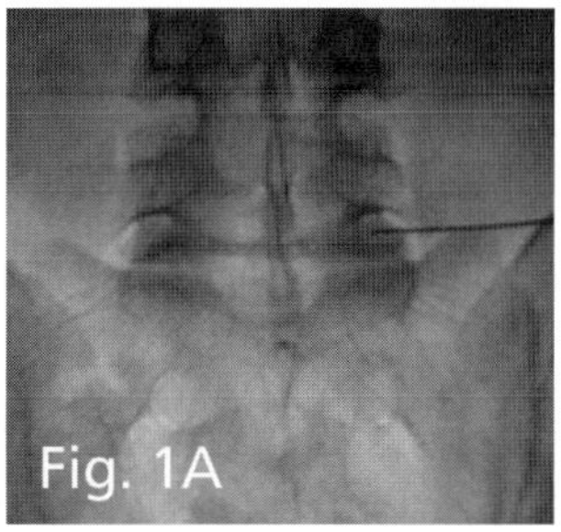
Fig. 1A

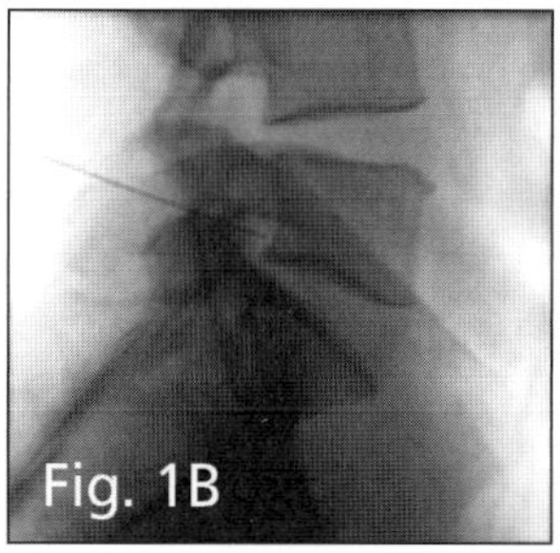
Fig. 1B

Q-3: If a surgeon inadvertently burrs through the midlateral wall of C5 during a anterior corpectomy, what structure is at greatest risk for injury?

1. C5 root
2. C6 root
3. Internal carotid artery
4. Vertebral artery
5. Vagus nerve

Q-4: What structure is located at the tip of the arrow in Figure 2?

1. Left L3 nerve root
2. Right L3 nerve root
3. Right L4 segmental artery
4. Right L4 nerve root
5. Left lateral disk herniation

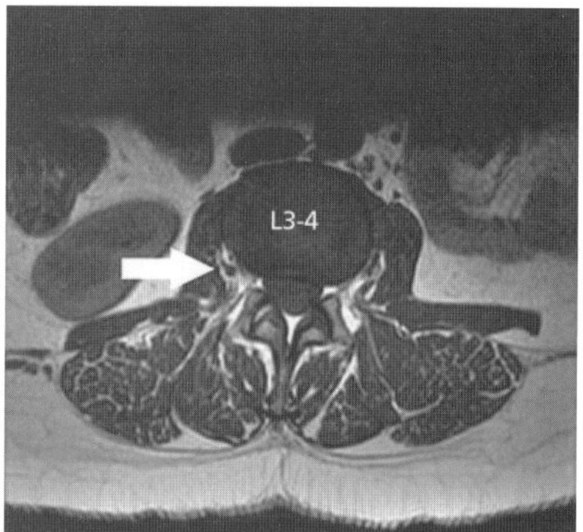

Fig. 2

Q-5: What structure is most at risk for injury from a retractor against the tracheoesophageal junction during an anterior approach to the cervical spine?

1. Esophagus
2. Trachea
3. Superior laryngeal nerve
4. Recurrent laryngeal nerve
5. Sympathetic chain

Q-6: A patient with a left-sided C6-7 herniated nucleous pulposus would likely have which of the following constellation of findings?

1. Pain into the thumb, triceps weakness, and loss of triceps reflex
2. Middle finger numbness, wrist extensor weakness, and diminished brachioradialis reflex
3. Thumb numbness, wrist extensor weakness, and diminished brachioradialis reflex
4. Middle finger numbness, triceps weakness, and loss of biceps reflex
5. Middle finger numbness, triceps weakness, and loss of triceps reflex

Q-7: Figures 3A and 3B show the sagittal T2- and T1-weighted MRI scans of a 25-year-old patient who is an intravenous drug abuser and who has low back pain that is increasing in intensity. Laboratory studies show a white blood cell count of 10,000/mm^3 and an erythrocyte sedimentation rate of 80 mm/hour. Blood culture is negative. Initial management consist of

1. CT-guided closed biopsy.
2. open surgical biopsy.
3. antibiotic coverage for *Staphylococcus aureus*.
4. broad-spectrum antibiotic coverage.
5. a follow-up MRI scan in 8 weeks.

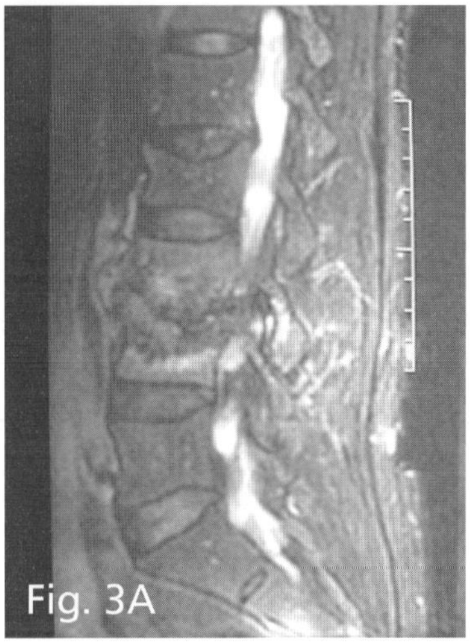
Fig. 3A

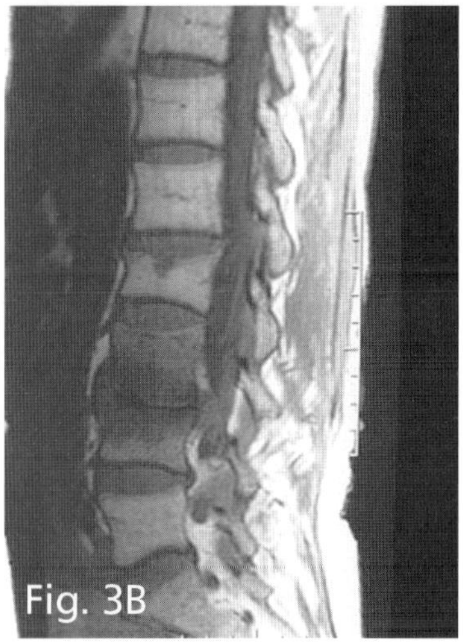
Fig. 3B

Q-8: A 27-year-old man sustained a gunshot wound to the lumbar spine and undergoes an exploratory laparotomy. An injury to the cecum is identified and treated. Management should now include

1. no antibiotics.
2. oral broad-spectrum antibiotics for 7 days.
3. intravenous broad-spectrum antibiotics for 48 hours.
4. intravenous broad-spectrum antibiotics for 7 days.
5. intravenous antibiotics specific for *Staphylococcus* for 7 days.

Q-9: A Trendelenburg gait is most likely to be seen in association with

1. a central disk herniation at L3-L4.
2. an ipsilateral paracentral disk herniation at L3-L4.
3. an ipsilateral paracentral disk herniation at L4-L5.
4. an ipsilateral paracentral disk herniation at L5-S1.
5. an ipsilateral far lateral disk herniation at L4-L5.

Spine: Questions

Q-10: Figure 4 shows the radiograph of a 64-year-old man who has neck pain and weakness of the upper and lower extremities following a motor vehicle accident. Examination reveals 3/5 quadriceps muscle strength and 4/5 hip flexors strength but no ankle dorsiflexion or plantar flexion. He has 1/5 intrinsic muscle strength and 3/5 finger flexors strength. He is awake, alert, and cooperative. Management should consist of

1. halo vest immobilization.
2. MRI.
3. Gardner-Wells tongs and closed reduction.
4. posterior open reduction and fusion.
5. observation until the patient's general medical status improves, followed by closed reduction via Gardner-Wells tongs.

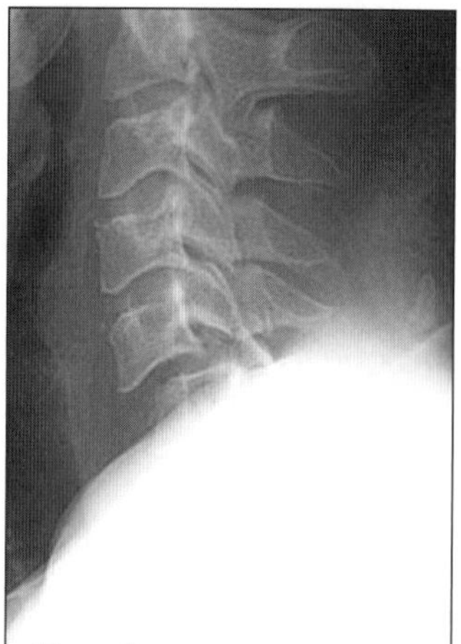

Fig. 4

Q-11: In a retroperitoneal approach to the lumbar spine, what structure runs along the medial aspect of the psoas and along the lateral border of the spine?

1. Ilioinguinal nerve
2. Genitofemoral nerve
3. Sympathetic trunk
4. Ureter
5. Aorta

Q-12: Flexion-distraction injuries of the thoracolumbar spine are most frequently associated with injury to what organ system?

1. Neurologic
2. Pulmonary
3. Gastrointestinal
4. Vascular
5. Lymphatic

Q-13: What is the most common adverse postoperative complication of laminaplasty for multilevel cervical spondylotic myelopathy?

1. Loss of cervical range of motion
2. Inadvertent closure of the laminaplasty postoperatively
3. Progressive cervical kyphosis
4. C5 nerve root palsy
5. Inadequate decompression of the spinal cord

Q-14: A patient who underwent an L5-S1 diskectomy 18 months ago has persistent pain in the left leg. Figures 5A and 5B show postoperative axial T1-weighted MRI scans at the L5-S1 level without and with gadolinium. What is the most likely diagnosis?

1. Epidural abscess
2. Neurilemmoma of the left S1 root
3. L5-S1 diskitis
4. Recurrent left L5-S1 disk herniation
5. Left S1 perineural fibrosis

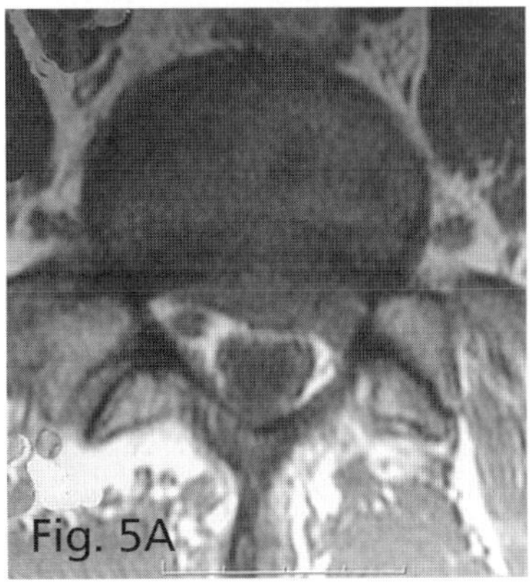

Fig. 5A

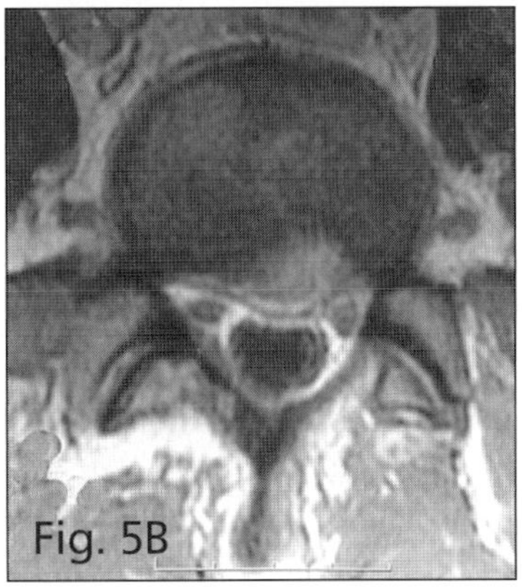

Fig. 5B

Q-15: If a laminectomy for spinal stenosis is performed, which of the following is an indication for concomitant arthrodesis at that level?

1. Prior laminectomy at an adjacent level
2. Ten degrees of degenerative scoliosis
3. Removal of 25% of each facet joint at surgery
4. Degenerative spondylolisthesis at the level of the laminectomy
5. Foraminal stenosis at the level of the laminectomy

Q-16: A previously healthy 30-year-old woman has neck pain and bilateral hand and lower extremity tingling with weakness after falling down stairs. She is alert and oriented. Examination reveals incomplete quadriplegia at the C6 level that remains unchanged throughout her evaluation and initial treatment. Radiographs show a bilateral facet dislocation of C6 on C7 without fracture. Attempts at reduction with halo cervical traction up to her body weight are unsuccessful. What is the most appropriate next step?

1. Posterior open reduction and fusion with fixation
2. Anterior open reduction and fusion with fixation
3. Technetium Tc-99m bone scan
4. Closed manipulation
5. MRI

Q-17: In a patient who has undergone fusion with instrumentation from T4 to the sacrum for adult scoliosis, at which site is a pseudarthrosis most likely to be discovered?

1. T4-T5
2. T7-T8
3. L2-L3
4. L4-L5
5. L5-S1

Q-18: When posterior fusion with instrumentation to the sacrum is used to treat adult scoliosis, what instrumentation technique best increases the chance of a successful lumbosacral fusion?

1. Addition of sublaminar wires to the midlumbar spine
2. Cross-linking of the longitudinal rods
3. Use of multiple claw-hook fixation in the upper thoracic spine
4. Use of large-diameter rods and pedicle screws
5. Fixation into both the ilium and the sacrum

Q-19: Which of the following complications is uniquely associated with an anterior approach to the lumbosacral junction?

1. Nerve root injury
2. Erectile dysfunction
3. Dural tear
4. Pulmonary embolism
5. Retrograde ejaculation

Spine: Questions

Q-20: An 18-year-old man sustained a knife injury to his midback, with the entry wound 2 cm to the left of the midline. Hemicord transection has been diagnosed. Neurologic examination will most likely reveal left-sided loss of

1. vibratory and light touch sensation and motor function, and right-sided loss of pain and temperature sensation.
2. pain and temperature sensation and motor function, and right-sided loss of vibratory and light touch sensation.
3. pain, temperature, vibratory, and light touch sensation and motor function.
4. motor function, and right-sided loss of pain, temperature, vibratory, and light touch sensation.
5. light touch and pain sensation and motor function, and right-sided loss of vibratory and temperature sensation.

Q-21: A 40-year-old woman has had sciatic pain on the left side for the past 8 weeks. She reports that the pain radiates to her posterior thigh, lateral calf, and into the dorsum of her left foot. Neurologic examination shows weakness of the left extensor hallucis longus. Axial T2-weighted MRI scans through L4-L5 are shown in Figure 6. Management should consist of

1. CT-guided needle biopsy at L4-L5.
2. a bone survey.
3. anterior interbody fusion.
4. left L4-L5 microdiskectomy.
5. left L4-L5 hemilaminectomy and partial facetectomy.

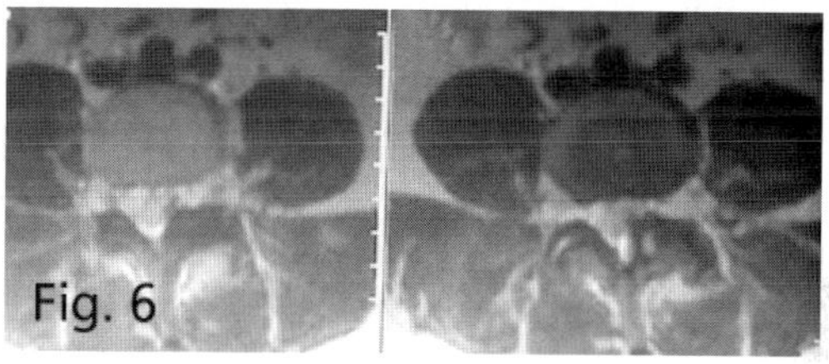
Fig. 6

Q-22: A collegiate football player who sustained an injury to his neck has significant neck pain and weakness in his extremities. Following immobilization, which of the following steps should be taken prior to transport?

1. His helmet should be removed.
2. His helmet and shoulder pads should be removed.
3. His face mask should be removed.
4. All equipment should be removed.
5. No equipment should be removed.

Q-23: Figure 7 shows the radiograph of a 56-year-old man who has neck pain after a rollover accident on his lawnmower. The injury appears to be isolated, and he is neurologically intact. Management of the fracture should consist of

1. posterior C1-2 fusion.
2. anterior C2-3 fusion.
3. Gardner-Wells traction for 6 weeks, followed by 6 weeks of halo vest immobilization.
4. halo vest immobilization.
5. a hard collar.

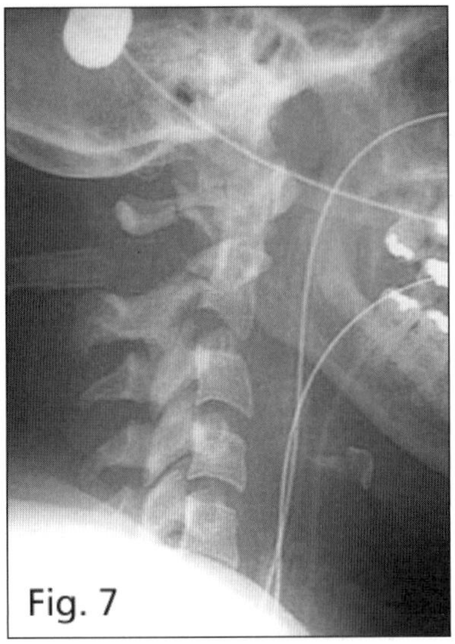

Fig. 7

Q-24: Degenerative spondylolisthesis of the cervical spine is most commonly seen at which of the following levels?

1. C1-2
2. C3-4
3. C5-6
4. C6-7
5. C7-T1

Q-25: When treating thoracic disk herniations, which of the following surgical approaches has the highest reported rate of neurologic complications?

1. Video-assisted thoracoscopic approach (VATS)
2. Posterior
3. Posterior-lateral
4. Transthoracic
5. Transpedicular

Q-26: When harvesting iliac crest bone graft during a posterior spinal decompression and fusion, injury to what structure can result in painful neuromas or numbness over the skin of the buttocks?

1. Ilioinguinal nerve
2. Superior gluteal nerve
3. Superior cluneal nerves
4. Iliohypogastric nerves
5. Lateral femoral cutaneous nerve

Q-27: A 42-year-old man sustained a burst fracture at L2 in a motor vehicle accident. Examination reveals that he is neurologically intact. Figure 8 shows a cross-sectional CT scan through the fracture. If the fracture is managed nonsurgically for the next 2 years, the retained fragments can be expected to

1. remain essentially unchanged in size.
2. result in neurologic deterioration.
3. gradually resorb and widen the spinal canal.
4. potentially migrate within the spinal canal.
5. increase the risk of further injury to the adjacent dural sac.

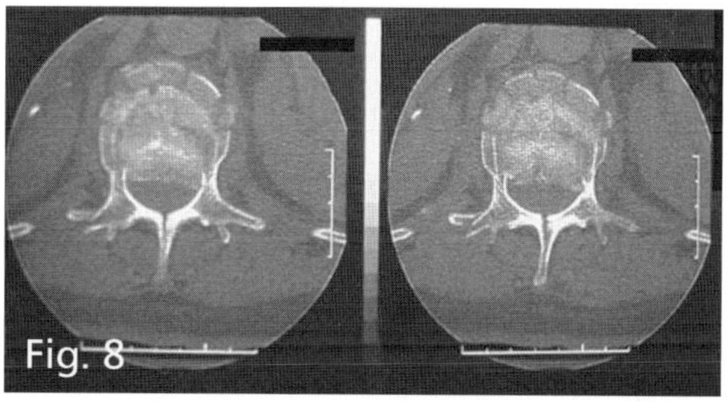
Fig. 8

Q-28: A 50-year-old man reports the onset of back pain and incapacitating pain radiating down his left leg posterolaterally and into the first dorsal web space of his foot 1 day after doing some yard work. He denies any history of trauma. Examination reveals ipsilateral extensor hallucis longus weakness. MRI scans are shown in Figures 9A through 9C. What nerve root is affected?

1. Left L4
2. Right L4
3. Left L5
4. Right L5
5. Left S1

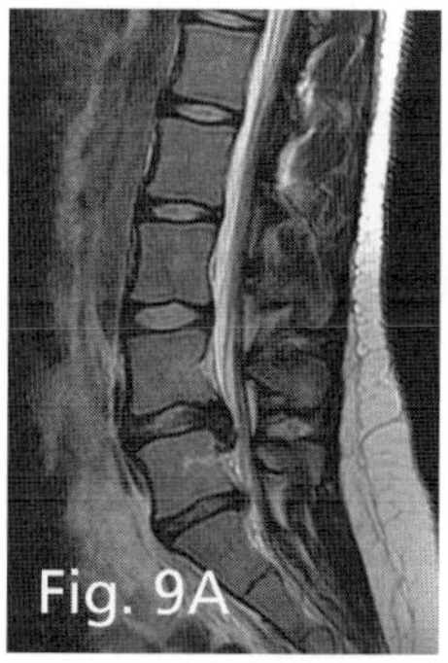
Fig. 9A

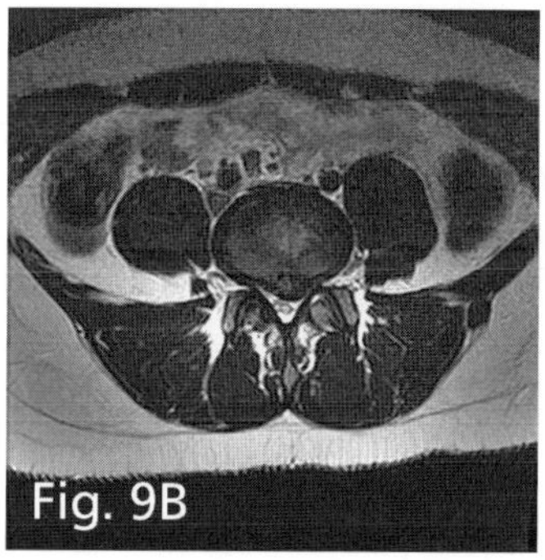
Fig. 9B

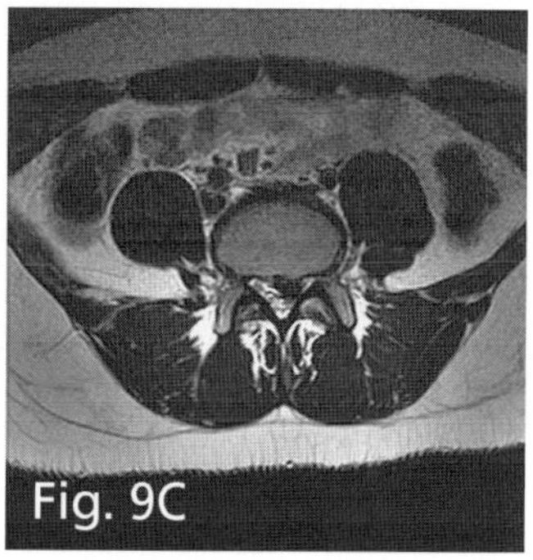
Fig. 9C

Q-29: What region of the spine is most susceptible to changes in the vascular supply to the spinal cord during an anterior approach?

1. C7-T1
2. T1-T3
3. T4-T7
4. T8-T12
5. L1-L3

Q-30: What is the most common presenting sign or symptom in an adult with lumbar pyogenic infection?

1. Fever
2. Night sweats
3. Unexplained weight loss
4. Foot drop
5. Back pain

Q-31: The natural history of cervical spondylotic myelopathy is best described as

1. slow, steady deterioration.
2. rapid deterioration.
3. stable over time.
4. stable for long periods with stepwise deterioration.
5. substantial improvement after an initial episode of severe symptoms.

Q-32: A 35-year-old woman undergoes an L4-5 anterior fusion via a left retroperitoneal approach. Postoperative examination reveals that her right foot is cool and pale. Her neurologic examination is normal, and her pedal pulses are asymmetric. What is the most likely reason for the right foot finding?

1. Injury to the lumbar sympathetic chain
2. Injury to the parasympathetic nerve
3. Immune response to the allograft bone
4. Occlusion of the left iliac vein
5. Prolonged retraction of the left iliac artery

Q-33: A 30-year-old man has had a 3-day history of severe, incapacitating low back pain without radiation. He reports improvement with rest. He denies any history of trauma, has no constitutional symptoms, and his neurologic examination is normal. What is the best course of action?

1. Facet injections
2. Epidural steroid injection
3. MRI of the lumbar spine
4. Bed rest for 2 weeks with continued restrictions
5. Early return to activities as his symptoms allow

Q-34: Which of the following patient factors is associated with recurrent radicular pain following lumbar diskectomy for sciatica?

1. Initial symptoms of more than 3 months' duration
2. Large annular defects seen intraoperatively
3. Large sequestered disk herniations
4. Initial treatment with lumbar epidural steroid injections prior to diskectomy
5. Preoperative reproduction of sciatica with straight leg raising (SLR)

Q-35: A 65-year-old woman has substantial neck pain after falling and striking her head. A radiograph and sagittal CT scan are shown in Figures 10A and 10B. What is the most likely diagnosis?

1. Degenerative spondylolisthesis
2. Superior facet fracture
3. Inferior facet fracture
4. Perched unilateral facet dislocation
5. Bilateral facet dislocation

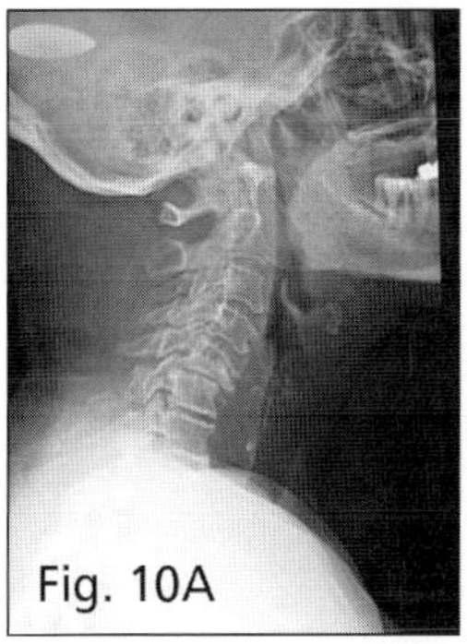
Fig. 10A

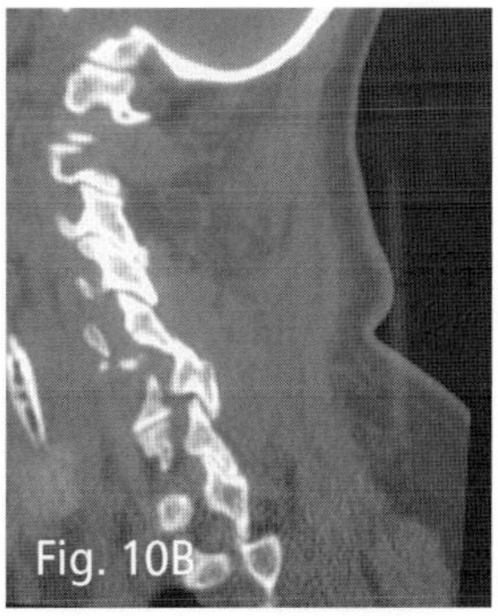
Fig. 10B

Q-36: Immediately after undergoing lumbar instrumentation, a patient reports severe right leg pain and has 4+/5 weakness. Figure 11 shows an axial CT scan of L5. Exploratory surgery will most likely reveal

1. transection of the L5 root.
2. displacement of the L5 root.
3. partial laceration of the L5 root.
4. segmental artery injury.
5. spinal fluid leakage.

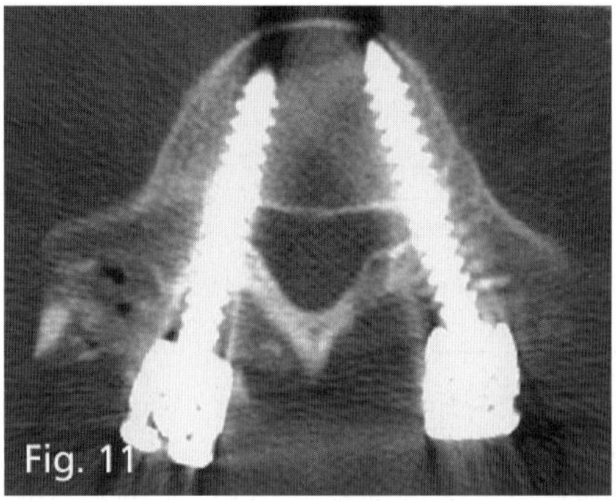
Fig. 11

Q-37: A 17-year-old boy who plays high school football is seen for follow-up after sustaining an injury 3 days ago. He reports that he tackled a player, felt numbness throughout his body, and could not move for approximately 15 seconds. A spinal cord injury protocol was initiated on the field. Evaluation in the emergency department revealed a normal neurologic examination and full painless neck motion. He states that he has no history of a similar injury. An MRI scan of the cervical spine is normal. During counseling, the patient and his family should be informed that he has sustained

1. a spinal cord injury and he cannot participate in contact sports.
2. no obvious injury and can return to all sports without risk of recurrence.
3. no obvious injury, but he is at a high risk for breaking his neck in athletic competition.
4. transient quadriplegia only, but this places him at greater risk for future spinal cord injury and he should refrain from all contact sports.
5. transient quadriplegia and that there is no evidence of increased risk of permanent spinal cord injury should he return to contact sports.

Q-38: Figures 12A through 12C show the MRI scans of a 30-year-old woman who weighs 290 lb and has low back and left leg pain. She also reports frequent urinary dribbling, which her gynecologist has advised her may be related to obesity. Examination will most likely reveal

1. ipsilateral weakness of the tibialis anterior.
2. ipsilateral weakness of the peroneus longus and brevis.
3. ipsilateral weakness of the extensor hallucis longus.
4. a positive Beevor sign.
5. a positive ipsilateral Gaenslen sign.

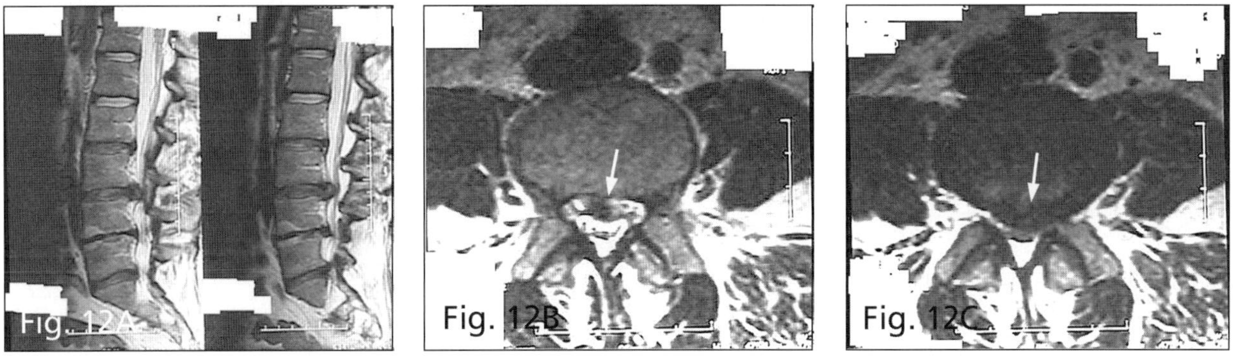

Q-39: Which of the following statements regarding conus medullaris syndrome is most accurate?

1. Conus medullaris syndrome most commonly accompanies injuries at the T12-L2 region.
2. Conus medullaris injury is a lower motor neuron injury, resulting in an excellent prognosis for recovery of bowel and bladder dysfunction.
3. The conus medullaris houses the motor cell bodies for the lumbar roots.
4. Lower extremity weakness is a common sign of conus medullaris syndrome.
5. Autonomic dysreflexia is common.

Q-40: Which of the following factors has the greatest effect on the pull-out strength of a lumbar pedicle screw?

1. Depth of vertebral body penetration
2. Percentage of pedicle filled by the screw
3. Bone mineral density
4. Tapping of the pedicle
5. Screw diameter

Q-41: An inverted radial reflex is associated with

1. spinal cord compression with myelopathy.
2. acute cervical radiculopathy.
3. chronic cervical radiculopathy.
4. Parsonage-Turner syndrome.
5. peripheral neuropathy.

Q-42: Figures 13A and 13B show the radiograph and CT scan of a 48-year-old man who has diffuse spinal pain. What is the most likely diagnosis?

1. Rheumatoid arthritis
2. Diffuse idiopathic skeletal hyperostosis (DISH)
3. Normal findings
4. Ankylosing spondylitis
5. Osteopetrosis

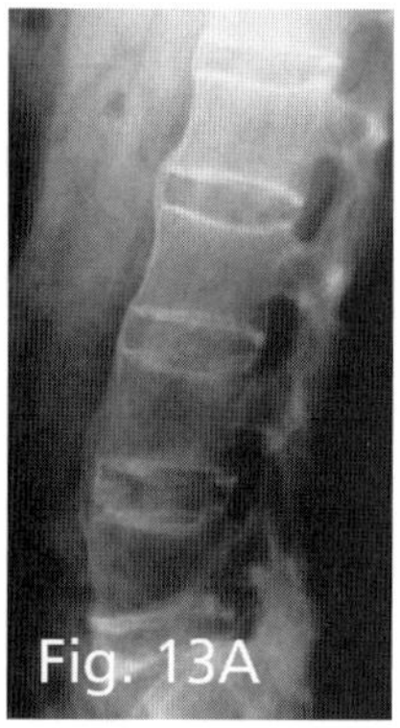
Fig. 13A

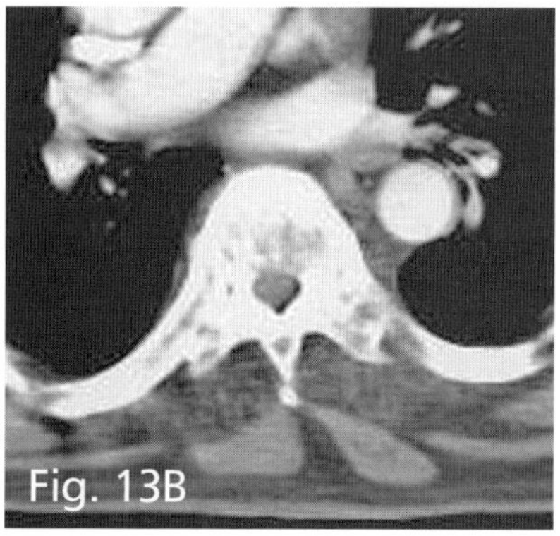
Fig. 13B

Q-43: The cervical disk herniation shown in the MRI scans in Figures 14A and 14B will most likely create which of the following constellations of symptoms?

1. Right thumb and index finger numbness and triceps weakness
2. Right thumb and index finger numbness and wrist extensor weakness
3. Right wrist extensor weakness and diminished triceps reflex
4. Right middle finger numbness and diminished brachioradialis reflex
5. Right little and ring finger numbness and diminished brachioradialis reflex

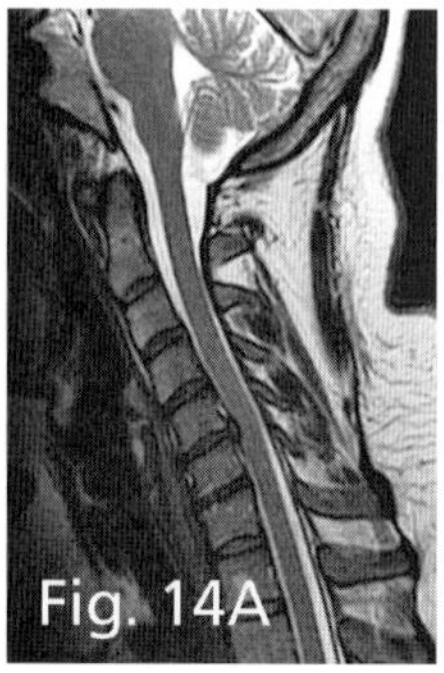
Fig. 14A

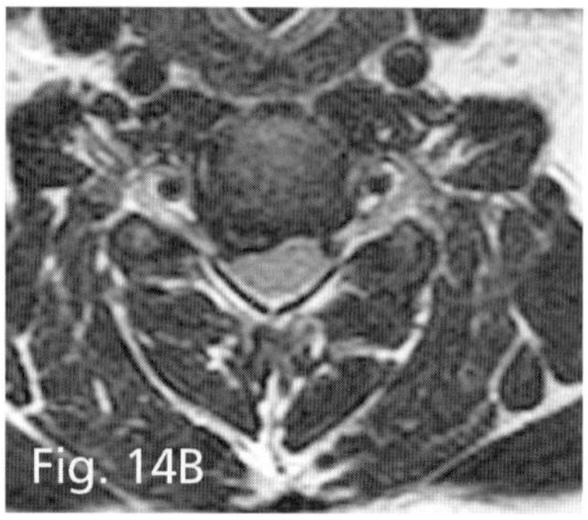
Fig. 14B

Q-44: A 21-year-old man has had posterior neck discomfort for the past 6 months. A whole-body bone scan and a cervical single-photon emission CT reveal increased activity at the C7 spinous process. MRI reveals multifocal involvement of the spinous process lamina and facet of C7. A CT-directed needle biopsy reveals osteoblastoma. What is the best course of action?

1. Observation
2. Radiation therapy
3. Curettage
4. En bloc excision with stabilization
5. En bloc excision followed by radiation therapy

Q-45: What is the most likely consequence of a vertebral compression fracture associated with osteoporosis?

1. The fractured vertebral body gradually becomes more stiff than before the fracture.
2. Scoliosis develops.
3. There is an increased risk of more vertebral fractures.
4. Overall sagittal alignment remains stable because the adjacent segments of the spine are able to compensate.
5. The extensor musculature will often hypertrophy in an attempt to stabilize the painful fracture.

Q-46: What is the most appropriate treatment for a chordoma involving the sacrum?

1. Chemotherapy
2. External beam radiation therapy
3. En bloc surgical resection with negative margins
4. Intralesional resection followed by radiation therapy
5. Intralesional resection followed by chemotherapy

Q-47: Which of the following is NOT considered a risk factor for nonunion of a type II odontoid fracture?

1. More than 6 mm of initial displacement
2. Patient age older than 60 years
3. Smoking
4. Inability to achieve reduction
5. Obesity

Q-48: A 27-year-old woman has a bilateral C5-C6 facet dislocation and quadriparesis after being involved in a motor vehicle accident. Initial management consisted of reduction with traction, but she remains a Frankel A quadriplegic. To facilitate rehabilitation, surgical stabilization and fusion is planned. From a biomechanical point of view, which of the following techniques is the LEAST stable method of fixation?

1. Anterior cervical plating with interbody bone graft
2. Posterior cervical plating with lateral mass screw fixation
3. Posterior sublaminar wiring
4. Simple posterior interspinous wiring
5. Bohlman interspinous wiring

A-1: During a retroperitoneal approach to the L4-5 disk, what structure must be ligated to safely mobilize the common iliac vessels toward the midline laterally and gain exposure?

1. Obturator vein
2. Iliolumbar vein
3. External iliac vein
4. Middle sacral artery
5. Hypogastric artery

PREFERRED RESPONSE: 2

DISCUSSION: To mobilize the common iliac vessels across the midline, the iliolumbar vein must be ligated. It has a short trunk and can be torn if mobilization is attempted without ligation. It is the only branch off the common iliac vessels (there are no arterial branches) prior to the terminal branches, and the internal (hypogastric) and external iliac vessels. The middle sacral vessels run distally from the axilla of the bifurcation and are a factor when accessing the L5-S1 disk.

REFERENCES: Baker JK, Reardon PR, Reardon MJ, et al: Vascular injury in anterior lumbar surgery. *Spine (Phila Pa 1976)* 1993;18:2227-2230.

Lewis WH: *Gray's Anatomy of the Human Body: The Veins of the Lower Extremity, Abdomen, and Pelvis*, ed 20. Philadelphia, PA, Lea & Febiger, 2000.

A-2: The injection shown in Figures 1A and 1B would most benefit a patient who reports which of the following symptoms?

1. Dorsal foot pain extending into the great toe
2. Foot pain extending along the lateral border of the foot
3. Pain extending into the foot in a stocking distribution
4. Anterior thigh and shin pain ending at the ankle
5. Lateral foot paresthesias

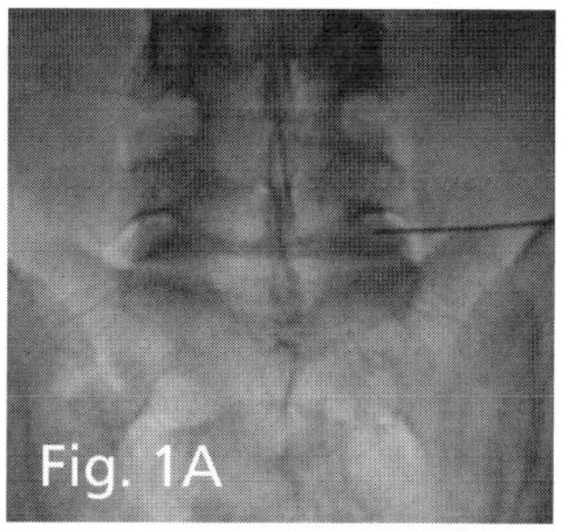
Fig. 1A

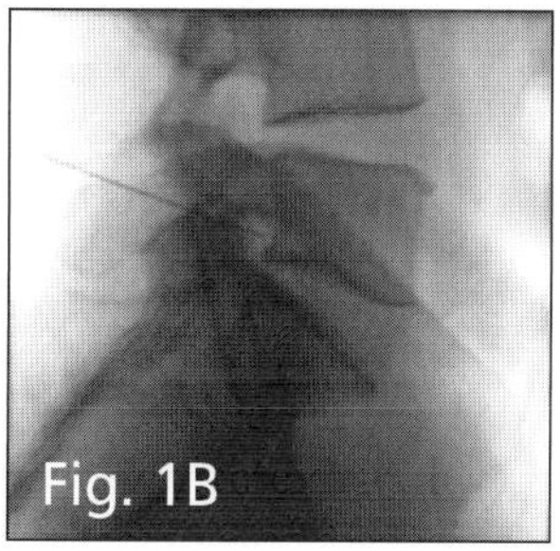
Fig. 1B

PREFERRED RESPONSE: 1

DISCUSSION: The images demonstrate an L5 selective root block as it exits the L5-S1 foramen. This root block best helps relieve pain or paresthesias in the L5 distribution, which is the dorsal first web space and the great toe. The lateral foot is an S1 distribution and would need to be blocked through the posterior first sacral foramen. The anterior shin and thigh represent the L4 root, which exits a level above this at the L4-5 foramen. A stocking distribution is nonanatomic and not indicative of a specific root.

REFERENCES: Magee D: Principles and concepts, in *Orthopaedic Physical Assessment*, ed 3. Philadelphia, PA, WB Saunders, 1997, pp 1-18.

Aeschbach A, Mekhail NA: Common nerve blocks in chronic pain management. *Anesthesiol Clin North Am* 2000;18:429-459.

A-3: If a surgeon inadvertently burrs through the midlateral wall of C5 during a anterior corpectomy, what structure is at greatest risk for injury?

1. C5 root
2. C6 root
3. Internal carotid artery
4. Vertebral artery
5. Vagus nerve

PREFERRED RESPONSE: 4

DISCUSSION: The vertebral artery is contained within the vertebral foramen and thus tethered alongside the vertebral body, making it vulnerable to injury if a drill penetrates the lateral wall. The C5 root passes over the C5 pedicle and is not in the vicinity. The C6 root passes under the C5 pedicle but is posterior to the vertebral artery and is only vulnerable at the very posterior-inferior corner. The carotid artery and the vagus nerve are both within the carotid sheath and well anterior.

REFERENCES: Pfeifer BA, Freidberg SR, Jewell ER: Repair of injured vertebral artery in anterior cervical procedures. *Spine (Phila Pa 1976)* 1994;19:1471-1474.

Gerszten PC, Welch WC, King JT: Quality of life assessment in patients undergoing nucleoplasty-based percutaneous discectomy. *J Neurosurg Spine* 2006;4:36-42.

A-4: What structure is located at the tip of the arrow in Figure 2?

1. Left L3 nerve root
2. Right L3 nerve root
3. Right L4 segmental artery
4. Right L4 nerve root
5. Left lateral disk herniation

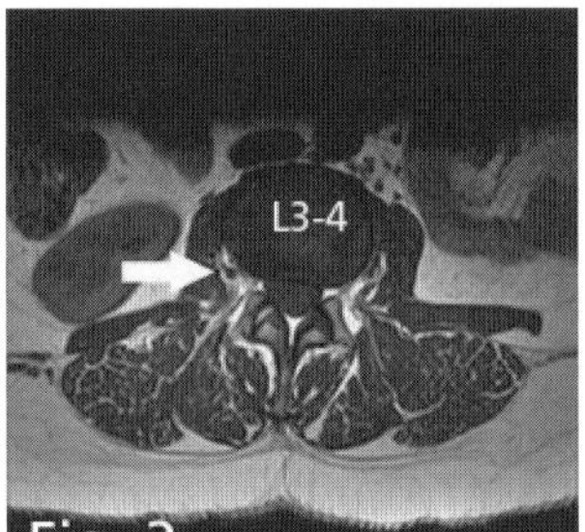

Fig. 2

PREFERRED RESPONSE: 2

DISCUSSION: The structure shown is the exiting nerve root at the L3-4 disk, which is the right L3 root.

REFERENCE: An H: Diagnostic imaging of the spine, in *Principles and Techniques of Spine Surgery*. Baltimore, MD, Lippincott Williams & Wilkins, 1998, pp 102-125.

A-5: What structure is most at risk for injury from a retractor against the tracheoesophageal junction during an anterior approach to the cervical spine?

1. Esophagus
2. Trachea
3. Superior laryngeal nerve
4. Recurrent laryngeal nerve
5. Sympathetic chain

(continued on next page)

(A-5: *continued*)

PREFERRED RESPONSE: 4

DISCUSSION: Although any of these structures can be injured by pressure from the medial blade of a self-retaining retractor, the recurrent laryngeal nerve runs cephalad in the interval between the esophagus and trachea and is vulnerable to pressure if caught between the retractor and an inflated endotracheal tube balloon.

REFERENCES: Ebraheim NA, Lu J, Skie M, et al: Vulnerability of the recurrent laryngeal nerve in the anterior approach to the lower cervical spine. *Spine (Phila Pa 1976)* 1997;22:2664-2667.

Kilburg C, Sullivan HG, Mathiason MA: Effect of approach side during anterior cervical discectomy and fusion on the incidence of recurrent laryngeal nerve injury. *J Neurosurg Spine* 2006;4:273-277.

A-6: A patient with a left-sided C6-7 herniated nucleous pulposus would likely have which of the following constellation of findings?

1. Pain into the thumb, triceps weakness, and loss of triceps reflex
2. Middle finger numbness, wrist extensor weakness, and diminished brachioradialis reflex
3. Thumb numbness, wrist extensor weakness, and diminished brachioradialis reflex
4. Middle finger numbness, triceps weakness, and loss of biceps reflex
5. Middle finger numbness, triceps weakness, and loss of triceps reflex

PREFERRED RESPONSE: 5

DISCUSSION: A C6-7 herniation affects the C7 root. The C7 root has the middle finger as its predominant sensory distribution. Its motor function is the triceps, wrist extension, and finger metacarpophalangeal extension. The reflex is the triceps.

REFERENCES: Magee D: Principles and concepts, in *Orthopedic Physical Assessment*, ed 3. Philadelphia, PA, WB Saunders, 1997, pp 1-18.

An H: History and physical examination of the spine, in *Principles and Techniques of Spine Surgery*. Baltimore, MD, Lippincott Williams & Wilkins, 1998, pp 91-101.

A-7: Figures 3A and 3B show the sagittal T2- and T1-weighted MRI scans of a 25-year-old patient who is an intravenous drug abuser and who has low back pain that is increasing in intensity. Laboratory studies show a white blood cell count of 10,000/mm^3 and an erythrocyte sedimentation rate of 80 mm/hour. Blood culture is negative. Initial management consist of

1. CT-guided closed biopsy.
2. open surgical biopsy.
3. antibiotic coverage for *Staphylococcus aureus*.
4. broad-spectrum antibiotic coverage.
5. a follow-up MRI scan in 8 weeks.

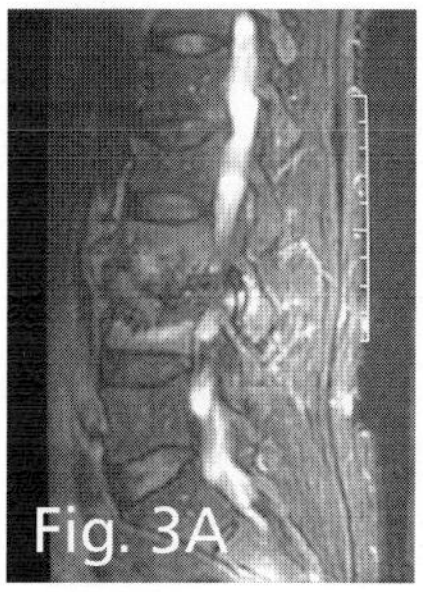
Fig. 3A

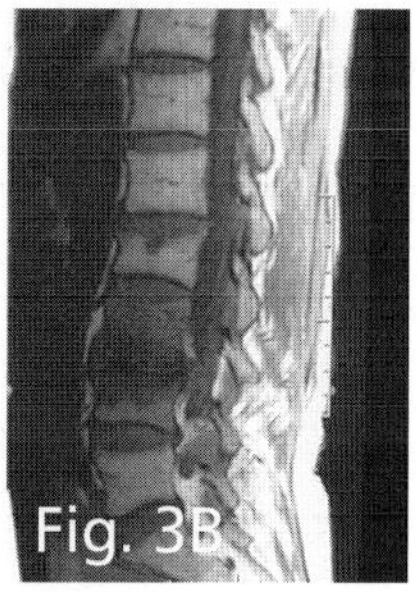
Fig. 3B

PREFERRED RESPONSE: 1

(continued on next page)

(A-7: *continued*)

DISCUSSION: The MRI scans show vertebral diskitis/osteomyelitis. The treatment of spinal infection in adults should be organism specific; therefore, initial management should consist of CT-guided closed biopsy prior to administration of antibiotic coverage. An open biopsy is indicated for a failed closed biopsy or failure of nonsurgical management. Although *Staphylococcus aureus* is the most common bacteria, a history of intravenous drug abuse raises suspicion for other organisms, including *Pseudomonas*.

REFERENCES: Tay BK, Deckey J, Hu SS: Spinal Infections. *J Am Acad Orthop Surg* 2002;10:188-197.

Jacofsky D, Currier BL: Infections of the spine, in Garfin SR, Fardon DF, Abitbol J, et al, eds: *Orthopaedic Knowledge Update: Spine*, ed 2. Rosemont, IL, American Academy of Orthopaedic Surgeons, 1997, pp 431-439.

A-8: A 27-year-old man sustained a gunshot wound to the lumbar spine and undergoes an exploratory laparotomy. An injury to the cecum is identified and treated. Management should now include

1. no antibiotics.
2. oral broad-spectrum antibiotics for 7 days.
3. intravenous broad-spectrum antibiotics for 48 hours.
4. intravenous broad-spectrum antibiotics for 7 days.
5. intravenous antibiotics specific for *Staphylococcus* for 7 days.

PREFERRED RESPONSE: 4

DISCUSSION: Gunshot wounds to the spine present relatively little risk of infection in most cases. When there has been an injury to the colon, the risk of infection can be minimized with a 7-day course of broad-spectrum antibiotics. Fragment removal is not indicated.

REFERENCES: Roffi RP, Waters RL, Adkins RH: Gunshot wounds to the spine associated with a perforated viscus. *Spine (Phila Pa 1976)* 1989;14:808-811.

Velmahoos GC, Demetriades D: Gunshot wounds of the spine: Should retained bullets be removed to prevent infection? *Ann R Coll Surg Engl* 1976;94:85-87.

A-9: A Trendelenburg gait is most likely to be seen in association with

1. a central disk herniation at L3-L4.
2. an ipsilateral paracentral disk herniation at L3-L4.
3. an ipsilateral paracentral disk herniation at L4-L5.
4. an ipsilateral paracentral disk herniation at L5-S1.
5. an ipsilateral far lateral disk herniation at L4-L5.

PREFERRED RESPONSE: 3

DISCUSSION: A Trendelenburg gait results from weakness of the gluteus medius, which is innervated by the L5 nerve root. A paracentral disk herniation at L4-L5 most commonly results in an L5 radiculopathy and thus weakness of the gluteus medius. A paracentral herniation at L5-S1 most commonly affects the S1 nerve root. A paracentral herniation at L3-L4, a central herniation at L3-L4, and a far lateral herniation at L4-L5 all affect the L4 root.

(continued on next page)

(A-9: *continued*)

REFERENCES: Johnson MG, Errico TJ: Lumbar disk herniation, in Fardon DF, Garfin SR, Abitbol J, et al, eds: *Orthopedic Knowledge Update: Spine*, ed 2. Rosemont, IL, American Academy of Orthopaedic Surgeons, 2002, pp 323-332.

Andersson GB, Deyo RA: History and physical examination in patients with herniated lumbar discs. *Spine (Phila Pa 1976)* 1996;21:10S-18S.

A-10: Figure 4 shows the radiograph of a 64-year-old man who has neck pain and weakness of the upper and lower extremities following a motor vehicle accident. Examination reveals 3/5 quadriceps muscle strength and 4/5 hip flexors strength but no ankle dorsiflexion or plantar flexion. He has 1/5 intrinsic muscle strength and 3/5 finger flexors strength. He is awake, alert, and cooperative. Management should consist of

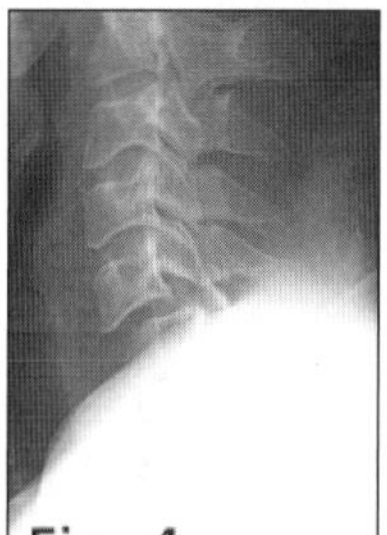
Fig. 4

1. halo vest immobilization.
2. MRI.
3. Gardner-Wells tongs and closed reduction.
4. posterior open reduction and fusion.
5. observation until the patient's general medical status improves, followed by closed reduction via Gardner-Wells tongs.

PREFERRED RESPONSE: 3

DISCUSSION: In patients with facet dislocations and an incomplete neurologic deficit, early decompression of the canal via reduction of the dislocation generally is considered safe if the patient is alert and can cooperate. However, patients who cannot cooperate with serial neurologic examinations during the reduction are at risk for increased deficit secondary to herniated nucleus pulposus, and MRI should be performed prior to either closed or open reduction.

REFERENCES: Star AM, Jones AA, Cotler JM, et al: Immediate closed reduction of cervical spine dislocations using traction. *Spine (Phila Pa 1976)* 1990;15:1068-1072.

Cotler JM, Herbison GJ, Nasuti JF, et al: Closed reduction of traumatic cervical spine dislocations using traction weight up to 140 pounds. *Spine (Phila Pa 1976)* 1993;18:386-390.

A-11: In a retroperitoneal approach to the lumbar spine, what structure runs along the medial aspect of the psoas and along the lateral border of the spine?

1. Ilioinguinal nerve
2. Genitofemoral nerve
3. Sympathetic trunk
4. Ureter
5. Aorta

PREFERRED RESPONSE: 3

DISCUSSION: The sympathetic trunk runs longitudinally along the medial border of the psoas. The ilioinguinal nerve emerges along the upper lateral border of the psoas and travels to the quadratus lumbori-

(continued on next page)

(A-11: *continued*)

um, and the genitofemoral nerve lies more laterally on the psoas. The ureter is adherent to the posterior peritoneum and falls away from the psoas and the spine in the dissection, as does the aorta.

REFERENCES: Watkins RG, ed: *Surgical Approaches to the Spine*. New York, NY, Springer-Verlag, 1983, p 107.

Johnson R, Murphy M, Sourthwick W: Surgical approaches to the spine, in Herkowitz HH, ed: *The Spine*, ed 4. Philadelphia, PA, WB Saunders, 1992, p 1559.

A-12: Flexion-distraction injuries of the thoracolumbar spine are most frequently associated with injury to what organ system?

1. Neurologic
2. Pulmonary
3. Gastrointestinal
4. Vascular
5. Lymphatic

PREFERRED RESPONSE: 3

DISCUSSION: In patients with flexion-distraction injuries of the thoracolumbar spine, 50% have associated, potentially life-threatening, visceral injuries that occasionally are diagnosed hours or even days after admission. Based on these findings, consultation with a general surgeon is recommended. Blunt and penetrating injuries to the cardiopulmonary system or aorta sometimes can be seen with this type of injury, but they are no more common than with other types of thoracolumbar fractures because of the relatively mild bony injury anteriorly. Neurologic trauma with this type of fracture is also somewhat rare.

REFERENCES: Burkus JK: Fractures of the thoracolumbar junction, in Levine AM, ed: *Orthopaedic Knowledge Update: Trauma*. Rosemont, IL, American Academy of Orthopaedic Surgeons, 1996, pp 351-360.

Inaba K, Kirkpatrick AW, Finkelstein J, et al: Blunt abdominal aortic trauma in association with thoracolumbar spine fractures. *Injury* 2001;32:201-207.

A-13: What is the most common adverse postoperative complication of laminaplasty for multilevel cervical spondylotic myelopathy?

1. Loss of cervical range of motion
2. Inadvertent closure of the laminaplasty postoperatively
3. Progressive cervical kyphosis
4. C5 nerve root palsy
5. Inadequate decompression of the spinal cord

PREFERRED RESPONSE: 1

DISCUSSION: A 30% to 50% loss of cervical range of motion is reported postoperatively in most patients following cervical laminaplasty. Inadvertent closure of the laminaplasty does occur but is rare.

(continued on next page)

(A-13: *continued*)

Laminaplasty is advocated in lieu of laminectomy to prevent progressive kyphosis and can effectively decompress the spinal cord. C5 nerve root palsies are a poorly understood but rare complication of surgical decompression for cervical spondylotic myelopathy.

REFERENCES: Emery SE: Cervical spondylotic myelopathy: Diagnosis and treatment. *J Am Acad Orthop Surg* 2001;9:376-388.

Edwards CC II, Riew KD, Anderson PA, et al: Cervical myelopathy: Current diagnostic and treatment strategies. *Spine J* 2003;3:68-81.

A-14: A patient who underwent an L5-S1 diskectomy 18 months ago has persistent pain in the left leg. Figures 5A and 5B show postoperative axial T1-weighted MRI scans at the L5-S1 level without and with gadolinium. What is the most likely diagnosis?

1. Epidural abscess
2. Neurilemmoma of the left S1 root
3. L5-S1 diskitis
4. Recurrent left L5-S1 disk herniation
5. Left S1 perineural fibrosis

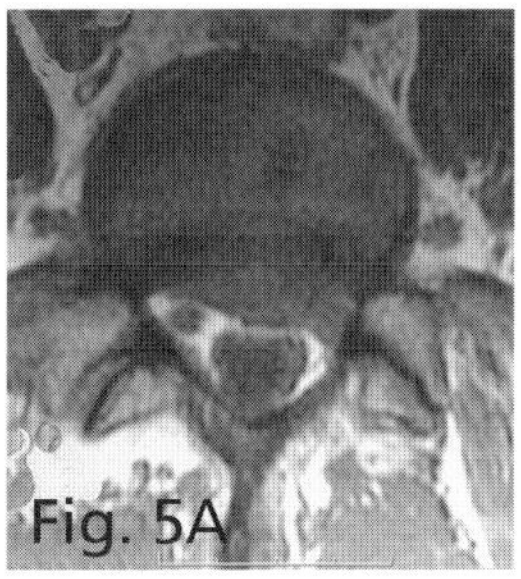

Fig. 5A

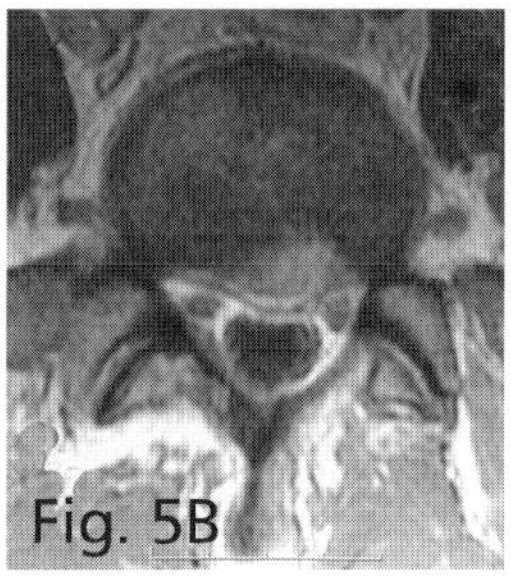

Fig. 5B

PREFERRED RESPONSE: 5

DISCUSSION: Persistent or recurrent symptoms after lumbar diskectomy are troublesome and can be difficult to assess. Gadolinium-enhanced MRI scans may be helpful. The images show enhancement about the left S1 root, a finding that is most consistent with perineural (epidural) fibrosis. The root itself does not enhance. Root enhancement has been associated with compressive radicular symptoms. A disk herniation does not enhance with gadolinium. A neurilemmoma enhances with gadolinium, but the involved root would be enlarged. There is no evidence of a fluid collection, which would be consistent with an epidural abscess.

REFERENCES: Babar S, Saifuddin A: MRI of the post-discectomy lumbar spine. *Clin Radiol* 2002;57:969-981.

Kikkawa I, Sugimoto H, Saita K, et al: The role of Gd-enhanced three-dimensional MRI fast low-angle shot (FLASH) in the evaluation of symptomatic lumbosacral nerve roots. *J Orthop Sci* 2001;6:101-109.

Vroomen PC, Van Hapert SJ, Van Acker RE, et al: The clinical significance of gadolinium enhancement of lumbar disc herniations and nerve roots on preoperative MRI. *Neuroradiology* 1998;40:800-806.

A-15: If a laminectomy for spinal stenosis is performed, which of the following is an indication for concomitant arthrodesis at that level?

1. Prior laminectomy at an adjacent level
2. Ten degrees of degenerative scoliosis
3. Removal of 25% of each facet joint at surgery
4. Degenerative spondylolisthesis at the level of the laminectomy
5. Foraminal stenosis at the level of the laminectomy

(continued on next page)

(A-15: *continued*)

PREFERRED RESPONSE: 4

DISCUSSION: A prospective randomized study of patients with degenerative spondylolisthesis and spinal stenosis by Herkowitz and Kurz showed significantly improved clinical outcomes in patients who also received a lumbar arthrodesis. Patients with a laminectomy at an adjacent level do not have improved outcomes with an arthrodesis. Minimal lumbar scoliosis does not require arthrodesis. Arthrodesis is indicated in cases where there is removal of more than 50% of the facets bilaterally but not with an associated foraminal stenosis.

REFERENCES: Herkowitz HN, Kurz LT: Degenerative lumbar spondylolisthesis with spinal stenosis: A prospective study comparing decompression with decompression and intertransverse process arthrodesis. *J Bone Joint Surg Am* 1991;73:802-807.

Garfin SR, Rauschning W: Spinal stenosis. *Instr Course Lect* 2001;50:145-152.

A-16: A previously healthy 30-year-old woman has neck pain and bilateral hand and lower extremity tingling with weakness after falling down stairs. She is alert and oriented. Examination reveals incomplete quadriplegia at the C6 level that remains unchanged throughout her evaluation and initial treatment. Radiographs show a bilateral facet dislocation of C6 on C7 without fracture. Attempts at reduction with halo cervical traction up to her body weight are unsuccessful. What is the most appropriate next step?

1. Posterior open reduction and fusion with fixation
2. Anterior open reduction and fusion with fixation
3. Technetium Tc-99m bone scan
4. Closed manipulation
5. MRI

PREFERRED RESPONSE: 5

DISCUSSION: A facet dislocation that cannot be reduced in an alert, awake patient with some preservation of cord function requires MRI to evaluate the disk prior to a reduction under anesthesia. The presence or absence of a disk herniation must be assessed, as this factor may influence the method of reduction.

REFERENCES: Vaccaro AR, Falatyn SP, Flanders AE, et al: Magnetic resonance evaluation of the intervertebral disc, spinal ligaments, and spinal cord before and after closed traction reduction of cervical spine dislocations. *Spine (Phila Pa 1976)* 1999;24:1210-1217.

Tay B K-B, Eismont F: Cervical spine fractures and dislocations, in Fardon DF, Garfin SR, Abitbol J, eds: *Orthopaedic Knowledge Update: Spine*, ed 2. Rosemont, IL, American Academy of Orthopaedic Surgeons, 2002, pp 247-262.

Eismont FJ, Arena MJ, Green BA: Extrusion of an intervertebral disc associated with traumatic subluxation or dislocation of cervical facets. *J Bone Joint Surg Am* 1991;73:1555-1560.

Cotler JM, Herbison GJ, Nasuti JF, et al: Closed reduction of traumatic cervical spine dislocation using traction weights up to 140 pounds. *Spine (Phila Pa 1976)* 1993;18:386-390.

A-17: In a patient who has undergone fusion with instrumentation from T4 to the sacrum for adult scoliosis, at which site is a pseudarthrosis most likely to be discovered?

1. T4-T5
2. T7-T8
3. L2-L3
4. L4-L5
5. L5-S1

PREFERRED RESPONSE: 5

DISCUSSION: Although pseudarthrosis can be found anywhere within the spine that has been fused using long multisegmental fixation to the sacrum, it most commonly occurs at the lumbosacral junction. The thoracolumbar junction is another common site of potential pseudarthrosis. In this location, the anatomy changes from lumbar transverse processes to thoracic through the transition zone, and overlying instrumentation often makes it difficult to obtain enough sound bone on decorticated bone to achieve a successful fusion.

REFERENCES: Saer EH III, Winter RB, Lonstein JE: Long scoliosis fusion to the sacrum in adults with nonparalytic scoliosis: An improved method. *Spine (Phila Pa 1976)* 1990;15;650-653.

Kostuik JP, Hall BB: Spinal fusions to the sacrum in adults with scoliosis. *Spine (Phila Pa 1976)* 1983;8:489-500.

Balderston RA, Winter RB, Moe JH, et al: Fusion to the sacrum for nonparalytic scoliosis in the adult. *Spine (Phila Pa 1976)* 1986;11:824-829.

A-18: When posterior fusion with instrumentation to the sacrum is used to treat adult scoliosis, what instrumentation technique best increases the chance of a successful lumbosacral fusion?

1. Addition of sublaminar wires to the midlumbar spine
2. Cross-linking of the longitudinal rods
3. Use of multiple claw-hook fixation in the upper thoracic spine
4. Use of large-diameter rods and pedicle screws
5. Fixation into both the ilium and the sacrum

PREFERRED RESPONSE: 5

DISCUSSION: As the chance of success of lumbosacral fusion increases with the stiffness and rigidity of the construct, fixation and stiffness improve with fixation into both the upper sacrum and the ilium. In a review of individuals treated with long constructs to the pelvis for adult scoliosis, Islam and associates reported that the rate of pseudarthrosis was significantly lower with sacral and iliac fixation compared with sacral fixation alone or iliac fixation alone. Iliac screws provide significant fixation anterior to the instantaneous axis of rotation for flexion and extension, as well as provides resistance to lateral bending and rotational forces. Numerous biomechanical studies support the concept of increasing biomechanical stabilization with increased fixation from the sacrum to the ilium.

REFERENCES: Islam NC, Wood KB, Transfeldt EE, et al: Extension of fusions to the pelvis in idiopathic scoliosis. *Spine (Phila Pa 1976)* 2001;26:166-173.

(continued on next page)

(A-18: *continued*)

O'Brien N, et al: Sacral pelvic fixation and spinal deformity, in DeWald RL, ed: *Spinal Deformities: A Comprehensive Text*. New York, NY, Thieme, 2003, pp 601-614.

McCord DH, Cunningham BW, Shono Y, et al: Biomechanical analysis of lumbosacral fixation. *Spine (Phila Pa 1976)* 1992;17:S235-S243.

A-19: Which of the following complications is uniquely associated with an anterior approach to the lumbosacral junction?

1. Nerve root injury
2. Erectile dysfunction
3. Dural tear
4. Pulmonary embolism
5. Retrograde ejaculation

PREFERRED RESPONSE: 5

DISCUSSION: Retrograde ejaculation is a sequela of injury to the superior hypogastric plexus. The structure needs protection, especially during anterior exposure of the lumbosacral junction. The use of monopolar electrocautery should be avoided in this region. The ideal exposure starts with blunt dissection just to the medial aspect of the left common iliac vein, sweeping the prevertebral tissues toward the patient's right side. Although erectile dysfunction can be seen after spinal surgery, it is not typically related to the surgical exposure because erectile function is regulated by parasympathetic fibers derived from the second, third, and fourth sacral segments that are deep in the pelvis and are not at risk with the anterior approach. The other choices are complications of spinal surgery but are not uniquely associated with an anterior L5-S1 exposure.

REFERENCES: Flynn JC, Price CT: Sexual complications of anterior fusion of the lumbar spine. *Spine (Phila Pa 1976)* 1984;9:489-492.

Watkins RG, ed: *Surgical Approaches to the Spine*. New York, NY, Springer-Verlag, 1983, p 107.

An HS, Riley LH III: *An Atlas of Surgery of the Spine*. New York, NY, Lippincott Raven, 1998, p 263.

A-20: An 18-year-old man sustained a knife injury to his midback, with the entry wound 2 cm to the left of the midline. Hemicord transection has been diagnosed. Neurologic examination will most likely reveal left-sided loss of

1. vibratory and light touch sensation and motor function, and right-sided loss of pain and temperature sensation.
2. pain and temperature sensation and motor function, and right-sided loss of vibratory and light touch sensation.
3. pain, temperature, vibratory, and light touch sensation and motor function.
4. motor function, and right-sided loss of pain, temperature, vibratory, and light touch sensation.
5. light touch and pain sensation and motor function, and right-sided loss of vibratory and temperature sensation.

(continued on next page)

(A-20: *continued*)

PREFERRED RESPONSE: 1

DISCUSSION: Brown-Séquard syndrome results from an injury to one half of the spinal cord and is characteristically seen in penetrating injuries. The spinothalamic fibers cross the midline below the level of the lesion, resulting in contralateral loss of pain and temperature sensation. The posterior columns and corticospinal tracts carry vibratory, position, and light touch sensation, as well as motor function from the ipsilateral side of the body. This results in the characteristic neurologic findings seen with Brown-Séquard syndrome.

REFERENCES: Northrup BE, Evaluation and early treatment of acute injuries to the spine and spinal cord, in Clark CR, ed: *The Cervical Spine*, ed 3. Philadelphia, PA, Lippincott Raven, 1998, pp 541-549.

Collins RD: *Illustrated Manual of Neurologic Diagnosis*. Philadelphia, PA, JB Lippincott, 1962, p 71.

A-21: A 40-year-old woman has had sciatic pain on the left side for the past 8 weeks. She reports that the pain radiates to her posterior thigh, lateral calf, and into the dorsum of her left foot. Neurologic examination shows weakness of the left extensor hallucis longus. Axial T2-weighted MRI scans through L4-L5 are shown in Figure 6. Management should consist of

1. CT-guided needle biopsy at L4-L5.
2. a bone survey.
3. anterior interbody fusion.
4. left L4-L5 microdiskectomy.
5. left L4-L5 hemilaminectomy and partial facetectomy.

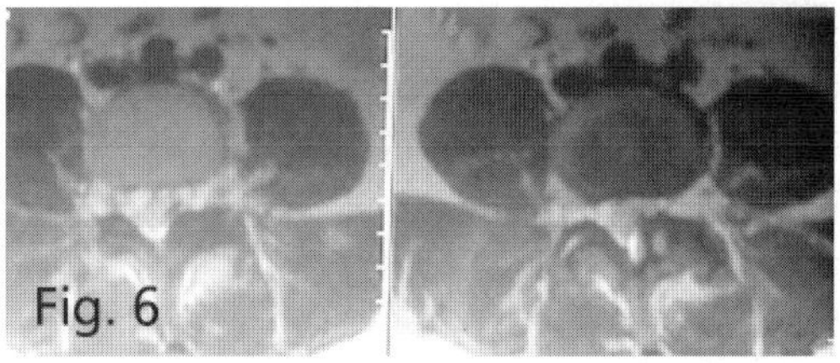
Fig. 6

PREFERRED RESPONSE: 5

DISCUSSION: The MRI scans show hypertrophy of the left L4-L5 facet joint and ligamentum flavum, with a synovial cyst. Appropriate surgical management consists of a hemilaminectomy and direct decompression of the neural elements. Fusion, in addition to the decompression, may be considered, particularly in patients with an associated spondylolisthesis.

REFERENCES: Epstein NE: Lumbar laminectomy for the resection of synovial cysts and coexisting lumbar spinal stenosis or degenerative spondylolisthesis: An outcome study. *Spine (Phila Pa 1976)* 2004;29:1049-1055.

Shah RV, Lutz GE: Lumbar intraspinal synovial cysts: Conservative management and review of the world's literature. *Spine J* 2003;3:479-488.

A-22: A collegiate football player who sustained an injury to his neck has significant neck pain and weakness in his extremities. Following immobilization, which of the following steps should be taken prior to transport?

1. His helmet should be removed.
2. His helmet and shoulder pads should be removed.
3. His face mask should be removed.
4. All equipment should be removed.
5. No equipment should be removed.

(continued on next page)

(A-22: *continued*)

PREFERRED RESPONSE: 3

DISCUSSION: Prior to transport, the face mask should be removed so that the airway can be easily accessible. If serious injury is suspected, the helmet and shoulder pads should be left in place until the patient is assessed at the hospital and radiographs are obtained. Leaving the helmet and shoulder pads in place helps to keep the spine in the most neutral alignment. Removal of the helmet will result in extension of the neck, whereas removal of the shoulder pads will most likely result in flexion of the neck.

REFERENCES: Clark CR, ed: *The Cervical Spine*, ed 3. Philadelphia, PA, Lippincott Williams & Wilkins, 1998, p 376. Thomas B, McCullen GM, Yuan HA: Cervical spine injuries in football players. *J Am Acad Orthop Surg* 1999;7:338-347.

Waninger KN, Richards JG, Pan WT, et al: An evaluation of head movement in backboard-immobilized helmeted football, lacrosse, and ice hockey players. *Clin J Sport Med* 2001;11:82-86.

Donaldson WF III, Lauerman WC, Heil B, et al: Helmet and shoulder pad removal from a player with suspected cervical spine injury: A cadaveric model. *Spine (Phila Pa 1976)* 1998;23:1729-1732.

Peris MD, Donaldson WF III, Towers J, et al: Helmet and shoulder pad removal in suspected cervical spine injury: Human control model. *Spine (Phila Pa 1976)* 2002;27:995-998.

A-23: Figure 7 shows the radiograph of a 56-year-old man who has neck pain after a rollover accident on his lawnmower. The injury appears to be isolated, and he is neurologically intact. Management of the fracture should consist of

1. posterior C1-2 fusion.
2. anterior C2-3 fusion.
3. Gardner-Wells traction for 6 weeks, followed by 6 weeks of halo vest immobilization.
4. halo vest immobilization.
5. a hard collar.

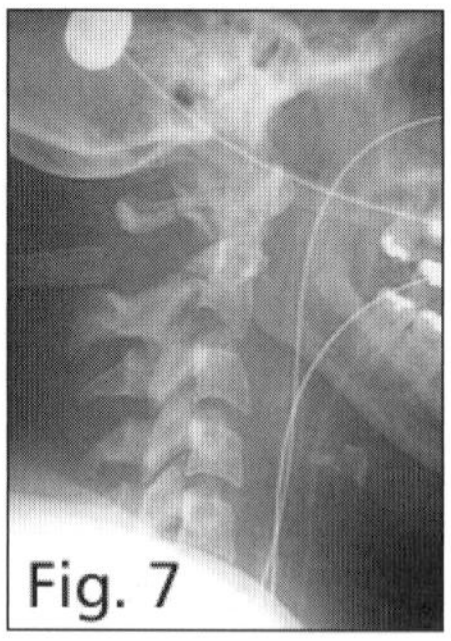

Fig. 7

PREFERRED RESPONSE: 4

DISCUSSION: The radiograph shows a type IIa hangman's fracture, and the classic treatment is halo vest immobilization. Traction should be avoided in type IIa injuries because of the risk of overdistraction. A lesser form of immobilization such as a hard collar or a Minerva jacket can be used for nondisplaced (type I) fractures. Surgery generally is reserved for type III fractures (includes C2-3 facet dislocation), or extenuating circumstances such as multiple trauma or other fractures of the cervical spine that require surgical stabilization.

REFERENCES: Levine AM, Edwards CC: The management of traumatic spondylolisthesis of the axis. *J Bone Joint Surg Am* 1985;67:217-226.

Jackson RS, Banit DM, Rhyne AL III, et al: Upper cervical spine injuries. *J Am Acad Orthop Surg* 2002;10:271-280.

Spine: Answers

A-24: Degenerative spondylolisthesis of the cervical spine is most commonly seen at which of the following levels?

1. C1-2
2. C3-4
3. C5-6
4. C6-7
5. C7-T1

PREFERRED RESPONSE: 2

DISCUSSION: Degenerative spondylolisthesis of the cervical spine is seen almost exclusively at C3-4 and C4-5; this is in contrast to degenerative changes, which are most commonly seen at C5-6 and C6-7.

REFERENCES: Tani T, Kawasaki M, Taniguchi S, et al: Functional importance of degenerative spondylolisthesis in cervical spondylotic myelopathy in the elderly. *Spine (Phila Pa 1976)* 2003;28:1128-1134.

Heller JG: Surgical treatment of degenerative cervical disc disease, in Fardon DF, Garfin SR, Abitbol J, et al, eds: *Orthopaedic Knowledge Update: Spine,* ed 2. Rosemont, IL, American Academy of Orthopaedic Surgeons, 2002, pp 299-309.

A-25: When treating thoracic disk herniations, which of the following surgical approaches has the highest reported rate of neurologic complications?

1. Video-assisted thoracoscopic approach (VATS)
2. Posterior
3. Posterior-lateral
4. Transthoracic
5. Transpedicular

PREFERRED RESPONSE: 2

DISCUSSION: Numerous surgical approaches have been used for thoracic diskectomy, including the most recent VATS. One of the first approaches described, posterior laminectomy, involves manipulation of the spinal cord, which the other approaches avoid. The posterior approach had dismal results, including further neurologic deterioration and even paralysis.

REFERENCES: Belanger TA, Emery SE: Thoracic disc disease and myelopathy, in Frymoyer JW, Wiesel SW, eds: *The Adult and Pediatric Spine.* Philadelphia, PA, Lippincott Williams and Wilkins, 2004, pp 855-864.

Benjamin V: Diagnosis and management of thoracic disc disease. *Clin Neurosurg* 1983;30:577-605.

Russell T: Thoracic intervertebral disc protrusion: Experience of 67 cases and review of the literature. *Br J Neurosurg* 1989;3:153-160.

Fessler RG, Sturgill M: Review: Complications of surgery for thoracic disc disease. *Surg Neurol* 1998;49:609-618.

A-26: When harvesting iliac crest bone graft during a posterior spinal decompression and fusion, injury to what structure can result in painful neuromas or numbness over the skin of the buttocks?

1. Ilioinguinal nerve
2. Superior gluteal nerve
3. Superior cluneal nerves
4. Iliohypogastric nerves
5. Lateral femoral cutaneous nerve

PREFERRED RESPONSE: 3

DISCUSSION: The superior cluneal nerves (L1, L2, and L3) are most at risk when harvesting iliac crest bone graft during a posterior decompression and fusion. These nerves pierce the lumbodorsal fascia and cross the posterior iliac crest, beginning 8 cm lateral to the posterior superior iliac spine. The ilioinguinal nerve is more at risk during exposure of the anterior ilium during retraction of the iliacus and abdominal wall muscles. Iliohypogastric nerve injury may arise in a manner similar to that of ilioinguinal neuralgia. The lateral femoral cutaneous nerve lies in close proximity to the anterior superior iliac spine and is also at risk with anterior iliac crest bone graft harvesting. The superior gluteal nerve courses through the sciatic notch and supplies motor branches to the gluteus medius, minimus, and tensor fascia lata muscles. Injury results in hip abduction weakness.

REFERENCES: An HS: *Principles and Techniques of Spine Surgery*. Baltimore, MD, Williams and Wilkins 1998, pp 770-773.

Kurz LT, Garfin SR, Booth RE Jr: Harvesting autogenous iliac bone grafts: A review of complications and techniques. *Spine (Phila Pa 1976)* 1989;14:1324-1331.

Mrazik J, Amato C, Leban S, et al: The ilium as a source of autogenous bone grafting: Clinical considerations. *J Oral Surg* 1980;38:29-32.

A-27: A 42-year-old man sustained a burst fracture at L2 in a motor vehicle accident. Examination reveals that he is neurologically intact. Figure 8 shows a cross-sectional CT scan through the fracture. If the fracture is managed nonsurgically for the next 2 years, the retained fragments can be expected to

1. remain essentially unchanged in size.
2. result in neurologic deterioration.
3. gradually resorb and widen the spinal canal.
4. potentially migrate within the spinal canal.
5. increase the risk of further injury to the adjacent dural sac.

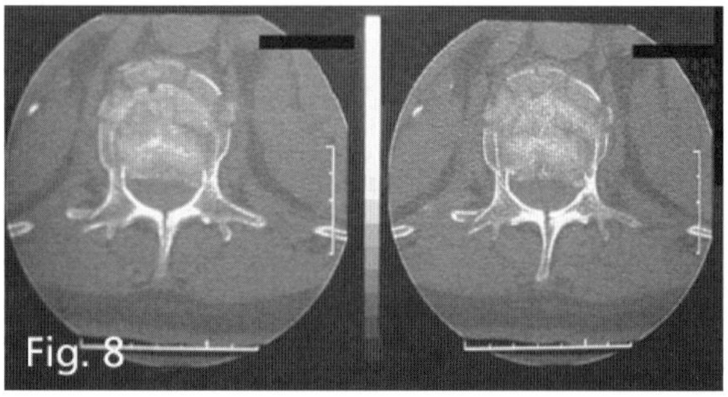
Fig. 8

PREFERRED RESPONSE: 3

DISCUSSION: Numerous articles have reported that both surgical and nonsurgical management of burst fractures are associated with resolution of impingement at long-term follow-up. If the patient is neurologically intact and appropriately treated at the time of injury, neurologic deterioration is not expected nor is there a risk of injury to the dural sac. The retained fragments can be expected to gradually resorb and widen the spinal canal.

(continued on next page)

(A-27: *continued*)

REFERENCES: Mumford J, Weinstein JN, Spratt KF, et al: Thoracolumbar burst fractures: The clinical efficacy and outcome of nonoperative management. *Spine (Phila Pa 1976)* 1993;18:955-970.

Wood KB, Butterman G, Mehbod A, et al: Operative compared with nonoperative treatment of a thoracolumbar burst fracture without neurologic deficit: A prospective, randomized study. *J Bone Joint Surg Am* 2003;85:773-781.

A-28: A 50-year-old man reports the onset of back pain and incapacitating pain radiating down his left leg posterolaterally and into the first dorsal web space of his foot 1 day after doing some yard work. He denies any history of trauma. Examination reveals ipsilateral extensor hallucis longus weakness. MRI scans are shown in Figures 9A through 9C. What nerve root is affected?

1. Left L4
2. Right L4
3. Left L5
4. Right L5
5. Left S1

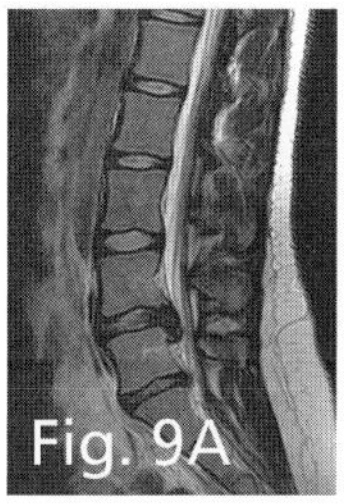
Fig. 9A

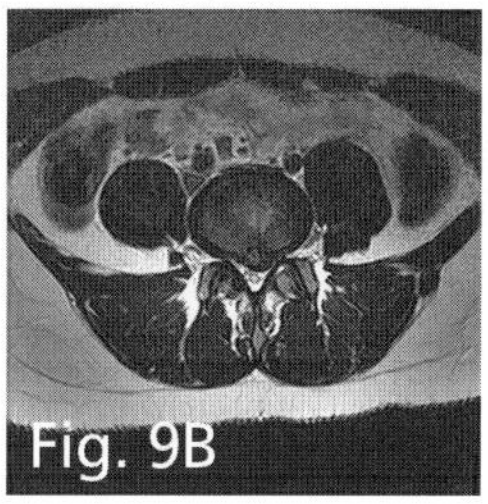
Fig. 9B

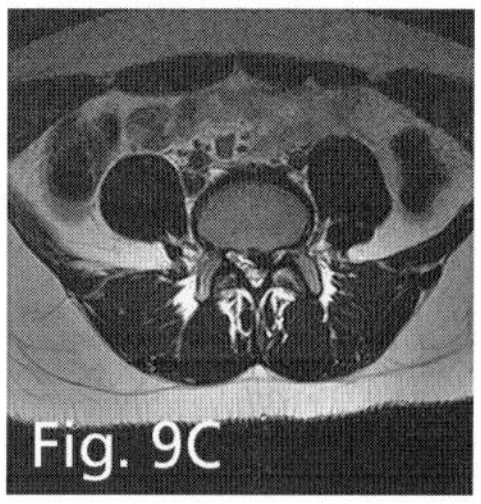
Fig. 9C

PREFERRED RESPONSE: 3

DISCUSSION: The MRI scans clearly show an extruded L4-5 disk that is affecting the L5 root on the left side. In addition, the L5 root has a cutaneous distribution in the first dorsal web space. S1 affects the lateral foot, and L4 affects the medial calf.

REFERENCES: An HS: *Principles and Techniques of Spine Surgery*. Baltimore, MD, Williams and Wilkins, 1998, pp 98-100.

Hoppenfeld S: *Orthopaedic Neurology*. Philadelphia, PA, JB Lippincott, 1977, pp 7-49.

A-29: What region of the spine is most susceptible to changes in the vascular supply to the spinal cord during an anterior approach?

1. C7-T1
2. T1-T3
3. T4-T7
4. T8-T12
5. L1-L3

PREFERRED RESPONSE: 4

DISCUSSION: The thoracic spinal cord is characterized by a variable and, at times, complicated blood supply. The artery of Adamkiewicz, also known as the great anterior medullary artery, most typically arises off the left side of the aorta between T8 and T12. It represents the sole medullary blood supply to the thoracic spine. When this artery is divided or injured, the blood supply to the thoracic cord may be interrupted. It is important to avoid electocautery of blood vessels within or near the thoracic foramen because this is a site of important, albeit limited, collateral circulation.

(continued on next page)

(A-29: *continued*)

REFERENCES: Sharma M, Anderson FC: Spinal vascular lesions, in Frymoyer JW, Wiesel SW, eds: *The Adult and Pediatric Spine*. Philadelphia, PA, Lippincott Williams and Wilkins, 2004, pp 301-306.

Alleyne CH, Cawley CM, Shenglaia GC, et al: Microsurgical anatomy of Adamkiewicz's artery. *J Neurosurg* 1998;89:791-795.

A-30: What is the most common presenting sign or symptom in an adult with lumbar pyogenic infection?

1. Fever
2. Night sweats
3. Unexplained weight loss
4. Foot drop
5. Back pain

PREFERRED RESPONSE: 5

DISCUSSION: Pain is very common but is often nonspecific; therefore, the diagnosis of spinal infection is often delayed. Fever and sepsis can occur but are not common. Neurologic manifestations also can occur but are absent in most patients. In findings reported by Carragee, the urinary tract is a common source for hematogenous spinal infection, but the source was found in only 27% of 111 patients. Direct inoculation during spinal surgery is uncommon.

REFERENCES: Carragee EJ: Pyogenic vertebral osteomyelitis. *J Bone Joint Surg Am* 1997;79:874-880.

Frazier DD, Campbell DR, Garvey TA, et al: Fungal infections of the spine: Report of eleven patients with long-term follow-up. *J Bone Joint Surg Am* 2001;83:560-565.

Hadjipavlou AG, Mader JT, Necessary JT, et al: Hematogenous pyogenic spinal infections and their surgical management. *Spine (Phila Pa 1976)* 2000;25:1668-1679.

A-31: The natural history of cervical spondylotic myelopathy is best described as

1. slow, steady deterioration.
2. rapid deterioration.
3. stable over time.
4. stable for long periods with stepwise deterioration.
5. substantial improvement after an initial episode of severe symptoms.

PREFERRED RESPONSE: 4

DISCUSSION: The natural history of cervical myelopathy has been described by Lees and Turner as exacerbations of symptoms followed by often long periods of static or deteriorating function (or very rarely improvement). This stepwise pattern of decreasing function has been corroborated by Clarke and Robinson. These authors described long periods of stable neurologic function, sometimes lasting for

(continued on next page)

(A-31: *continued*)

years, in about 75% of their patients. In the majority of the patients, however, the condition deteriorated between quiescent streaks. About 20% of their patients showed a slow, steady progression of symptoms and signs without a stable period, and 5% had rapid deterioration of neurologic function.

REFERENCES: Emery SF: Cervical spondylotic myelopathy: Diagnosis and treatment. *J Am Acad Orthop Surg* 2001;9:376-388.

Lees F, Turner JA: The natural history and prognosis of cervical spondylosis. *Br Med J* 1963;2:1607-1610.

Clarke E, Robinson PK: Cervical myelopathy: A complication of cervical spondylosis. *Brain* 1956;79:486-510.

A-32: A 35-year-old woman undergoes an L4-5 anterior fusion via a left retroperitoneal approach. Postoperative examination reveals that her right foot is cool and pale. Her neurologic examination is normal, and her pedal pulses are asymmetric. What is the most likely reason for the right foot finding?

1. Injury to the lumbar sympathetic chain
2. Injury to the parasympathetic nerve
3. Immune response to the allograft bone
4. Occlusion of the left iliac vein
5. Prolonged retraction of the left iliac artery

PREFERRED RESPONSE: 1

DISCUSSION: The lower extremity symptoms are consistent with a sympathectomy that is the result of an injury to the sympathetic chain, ipsilateral to the approach along the anterior border of the lumbar spine. This results in a warm, red foot, which creates the appearance that the normal cooler foot may have compromised circulation. The latter generally attracts greater attention because of the risks associated with limb ischemia. The condition usually is self-limited and does not require any specific treatment.

REFERENCES: Rothman RH, Simeone FA, eds: *The Spine*, ed 4. Philadelphia PA, WB Saunders, 1999, p1550.

Benzel EC, ed: *Spine Surgery Techniques, Complication Avoidance and Management*. New York, NY, Churchill Livingstone, 1999, p 190.

A-33: A 30-year-old man has had a 3-day history of severe, incapacitating low back pain without radiation. He reports improvement with rest. He denies any history of trauma, has no constitutional symptoms, and his neurologic examination is normal. What is the best course of action?

1. Facet injections
2. Epidural steroid injection
3. MRI of the lumbar spine
4. Bed rest for 2 weeks with continued restrictions
5. Early return to activities as his symptoms allow

(continued on next page)

(A-33: *continued*)

PREFERRED RESPONSE: 5

DISCUSSION: There are no red flags in the history or examination to warrant MRI. Limited bed rest (less than 3 days) has been shown to be more beneficial to early recovery compared with prolonged bed rest (more than 7 days). No data support the use of epidural or facet steroid injections for acute low back pain.

REFERENCE: Deyo RA, Diehl AK, Rosenthal M: How many days of bed rest for acute low back pain? A randomized clinical trial. *N Engl J Med* 1986;315:1064-1070.

A-34: Which of the following patient factors is associated with recurrent radicular pain following lumbar diskectomy for sciatica?

1. Initial symptoms of more than 3 months' duration
2. Large annular defects seen intraoperatively
3. Large sequestered disk herniations
4. Initial treatment with lumbar epidural steroid injections prior to diskectomy
5. Preoperative reproduction of sciatica with straight leg raising (SLR)

PREFERRED RESPONSE: 2

DISCUSSION: A large annular defect at the site of a lumbar disk herniation is associated with persistent radicular pain postoperatively. Large sequestered herniations and a positive SLR preoperatively correlate with good outcomes after diskectomy. Neither symptoms of more than 3 months' duration nor preoperative epidural steroid injections correlate with postoperative results after diskectomy.

REFERENCES: Carragee EJ, Han MY, Suen PW, et al: Clinical outcomes after lumbar discectomy for sciatica: The effects of fragment type and anular competence. *J Bone Joint Surg Am* 2003;85:102-108.

Johnson MG, Errico TJ: Lumbar disc herniation, in Fardon DF, Garfin SR, Abitbol J, et al, eds: *Orthopedic Knowledge Update Spine*, ed 2. Rosemont, IL, American Academy of Orthopaedic Surgeons, 2002, pp 323-332.

A-35: A 65-year-old woman has substantial neck pain after falling and striking her head. A radiograph and sagittal CT scan are shown in Figures 10A and 10B. What is the most likely diagnosis?

1. Degenerative spondylolisthesis
2. Superior facet fracture
3. Inferior facet fracture
4. Perched unilateral facet dislocation
5. Bilateral facet dislocation

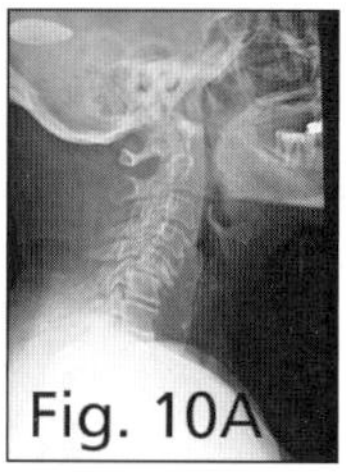
Fig. 10A

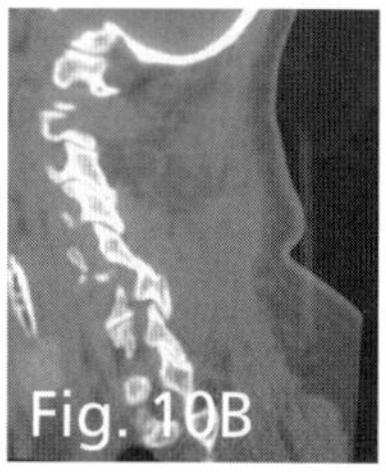
Fig. 10B

PREFERRED RESPONSE: 4

DISCUSSION: The radiograph shows a displacement of C5 on C6 of approximately 25%. The CT scan shows a perched facet at C5-6. There is no evidence of a facet fracture. A bilateral facet dislocation

(continued on next page)

(A-35: *continued*)

would show a displacement of more than 50%.

REFERENCES: Rothman RH, Simeone FA, eds: *The Spine*, ed 4. Philadelphia PA, WB Saunders, 1999, pp 927-937.

Vaccaro AR, Betz RR, Zeidman SM, eds: *Principles and Practice of Spine Surgery*. St Louis, MO, Mosby, 2003, pp 455-458.

A-36: Immediately after undergoing lumbar instrumentation, a patient reports severe right leg pain and has 4+/5 weakness. Figure 11 shows an axial CT scan of L5. Exploratory surgery will most likely reveal

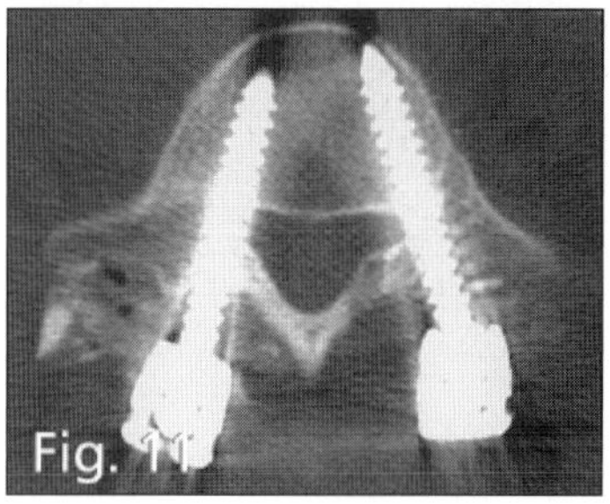
Fig. 11

1. transection of the L5 root.
2. displacement of the L5 root.
3. partial laceration of the L5 root.
4. segmental artery injury.
5. spinal fluid leakage.

PREFERRED RESPONSE: 2

DISCUSSION: The most common finding at exploration of an inappropriately placed pedicle screw is displacement of the nerve. Pedicle breach is common, ranging from 2% to 20%, but most are asymptomatic. All of the choices are possible, but in a large series conducted by Lonstein and associates, the authors reported that displacement of the root, most often medial, was the most common finding. Laceration, contusion, or transfixion usually was not seen. Spinal fluid leakage occurs less frequently and is not expected in the minimal breach illustrated.

REFERENCES: Esses SI, Sachs BL, Dreyzin V: Complications associated with the technique of pedicle screw fixation: A selected survey of ABS members. *Spine (Phila Pa 1976)* 1993;18:2231-2238.

Laine T, Lund T, Ylikoski M, et al: Accuracy of pedicle screw insertion with and without computer assistance: A randomised controlled clinical study in 100 consecutive patients. *Eur Spine J* 2000;9:235-240.

Lonstein JE, Denis F, Perra JH, et al: Complications associated with pedicle screws. *J Bone Joint Surg Am* 1999;81:1519-1528.

A-37: A 17-year-old boy who plays high school football is seen for follow-up after sustaining an injury 3 days ago. He reports that he tackled a player, felt numbness throughout his body, and could not move for approximately 15 seconds. A spinal cord injury protocol was initiated on the field. Evaluation in the emergency department revealed a normal neurologic examination and full painless neck motion. He states that he has no history of a similar injury. An MRI scan of the cervical spine is normal. During counseling, the patient and his family should be informed that he has sustained

1. a spinal cord injury and he cannot participate in contact sports.
2. no obvious injury and can return to all sports without risk of recurrence.
3. no obvious injury, but he is at a high risk for breaking his neck in athletic competition.
4. transient quadriplegia only, but this places him at greater risk for future spinal cord injury and he should refrain from all contact sports.
5. transient quadriplegia and that there is no evidence of increased risk of permanent spinal cord injury should he return to contact sports.

(continued on next page)

(A-37: *continued*)

PREFERRED RESPONSE: 5

DISCUSSION: The long-term effect of transient quadriplegia is unknown. Based on a history of one brief episode of transient quadriplegia and normal examination and MRI findings, the risk of permanent spinal cord injury with a return to play is low. There is a risk of recurrent episodes of transient quadriplegia after the initial episode.

REFERENCES: Morganti C, Sweeney CA, Albanese SA, et al: Return to play after cervical spine injury. *Spine (Phila Pa 1976)* 2001;26:1131-1136.

Odor JM, Watkins RG, Dillin WH, et al: Incidence of cervical spinal stenosis in professional and rookie football players. *Am J Sports Med* 1990;18:507-509.

Torg JS, Naranja RJ Jr, Palov H, et al: The relationship of developmental narrowing of the cervical spinal canal to reversible and irreversible injury of the cervical spinal cord in football players. *J Bone Joint Surg Am* 1996;78:1308-1314.

Vaccaro AR, Watkins B, Albert TJ, et al: Cervical spine injuries in athletes: Current return-to-play criteria. *Orthopedics* 2001;24:699-703.

A-38: Figures 12A through 12C show the MRI scans of a 30-year-old woman who weighs 290 lb and has low back and left leg pain. She also reports frequent urinary dribbling, which her gynecologist has advised her may be related to obesity. Examination will most likely reveal

1. ipsilateral weakness of the tibialis anterior.
2. ipsilateral weakness of the peroneus longus and brevis.
3. ipsilateral weakness of the extensor hallucis longus.
4. a positive Beevor sign.
5. a positive ipsilateral Gaenslen sign.

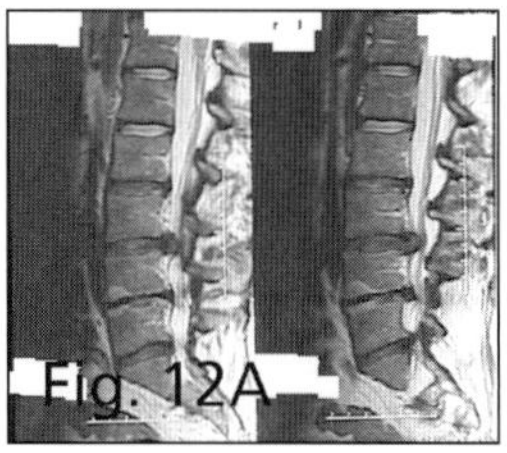
Fig. 12A

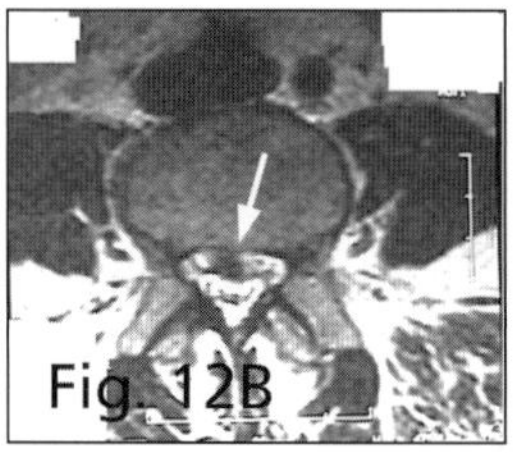
Fig. 12B

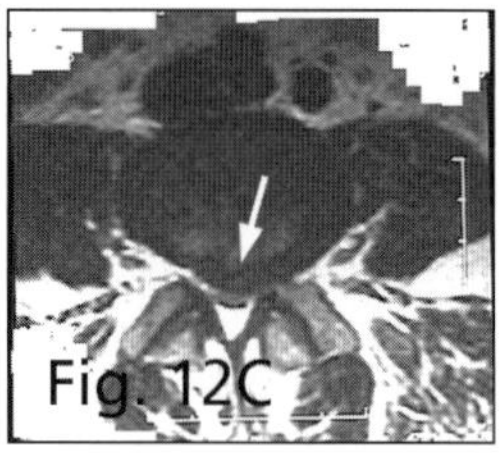
Fig. 12C

PREFERRED RESPONSE: 1

DISCUSSION: The patient will most likely exhibit ipsilateral weakness of the tibialis anterior. Gaenslen sign is designed to detect sacroiliac inflammation as a source of low back pain. Beevor sign tests the innervation of the rectus abdominus and paraspinal musculature (L1 innervation). The extensor hallucis longus is predominantly innervated by L5. The peroneals are predominantly innervated by S1.

REFERENCES: Hoppenfeld S: *Physical Examination of the Spine and Extremities*. Appleton, WI, Century-Crofts, 1976.
Hollinshead WH, ed: *Anatomy for Surgeons: The Back and the Limbs*, ed 3. Philadelphia, PA, Harper & Rowe, 1982.

A-39: Which of the following statements regarding conus medullaris syndrome is most accurate?

1. Conus medullaris syndrome most commonly accompanies injuries at the T12-L2 region.
2. Conus medullaris injury is a lower motor neuron injury, resulting in an excellent prognosis for recovery of bowel and bladder dysfunction.
3. The conus medullaris houses the motor cell bodies for the lumbar roots.
4. Lower extremity weakness is a common sign of conus medullaris syndrome.
5. Autonomic dysreflexia is common.

PREFERRED RESPONSE: 1

DISCUSSION: Conus medullaris syndrome most frequently occurs as a result of trauma or with a disk herniation at L1, resulting in a lower motor neuron syndrome but with a poor prognosis for recovery of bowel and bladder dysfunction. The conus region, as the termination of the spinal cord, contains the motor cell bodies of the sacral roots. The syndrome is usually a sacral level neural injury; therefore, lower extremity weakness is uncommon.

REFERENCES: Haher TR, Felmly WT, O'Brien M: Thoracic and lumbar fractures: Diagnosis and management, in Bridwell KH, Dewald RL, Hammerberg KW, et al, eds: *The Textbook of Spinal Surgery*, ed 2. New York, NY, Lippincott Williams & Wilkins, 1977, pp 1773-1778.

Reitman CA, ed: *Management of Thoracolumbar Fractures*. Rosemont, IL, American Academy of Orthopaedic Surgeons, 2004, pp 35-45.

A-40: Which of the following factors has the greatest effect on the pull-out strength of a lumbar pedicle screw?

1. Depth of vertebral body penetration
2. Percentage of pedicle filled by the screw
3. Bone mineral density
4. Tapping of the pedicle
5. Screw diameter

PREFERRED RESPONSE: 3

DISCUSSION: All of the factors listed contribute to some extent to the pull-out strength of lumbar pedicle screws, but bone mineral density correlates most precisely.

REFERENCES: Wittenberg RH, Shea M, Swartz DE, et al: Importance of bone mineral density in instrumented spine fusions. *Spine (Phila Pa 1976)* 1991;16:647-652.

Zindrick MR, Wiltse LL, Widell EH, et al: A biomechanical study of intrapeduncular screw fixation in the lumbosacral spine. *Clin Orthop* 1986;203:99-112.

A-41: An inverted radial reflex is associated with

1. spinal cord compression with myelopathy.
2. acute cervical radiculopathy.
3. chronic cervical radiculopathy.
4. Parsonage-Turner syndrome.
5. peripheral neuropathy.

PREFERRED RESPONSE: 1

DISCUSSION: An inverted radial reflex is a hypoactive brachioradialis reflex in combination with involuntary finger flexion. It is a spinal cord "release" sign and is associated with upper motor neuron pathology as seen in cervical stenosis with myelopathy. Radiculopathy is characterized by a diminished reflex but no finger flexion. Peripheral neuropathy is not associated with any reflex change. Parsonage-Turner syndrome is an idiopathic brachial neuritis.

REFERENCES: Clark CR, ed: *The Cervical Spine*, ed 3. Philadelphia, PA, Lippincott Williams & Wilkins, 1998, p 762. Vaccaro AR, Betz RR, Zeidman SM, eds: *Principles and Practice of Spine Surgery*. St Louis, MO, Mosby, 2002, p 323.

A-42: Figures 13A and 13B show the radiograph and CT scan of a 48-year-old man who has diffuse spinal pain. What is the most likely diagnosis?

1. Rheumatoid arthritis
2. Diffuse idiopathic skeletal hyperostosis (DISH)
3. Normal findings
4. Ankylosing spondylitis
5. Osteopetrosis

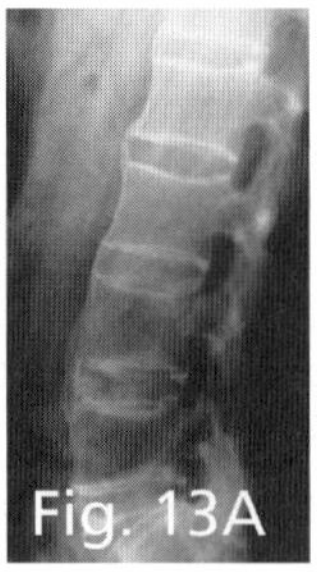
Fig. 13A

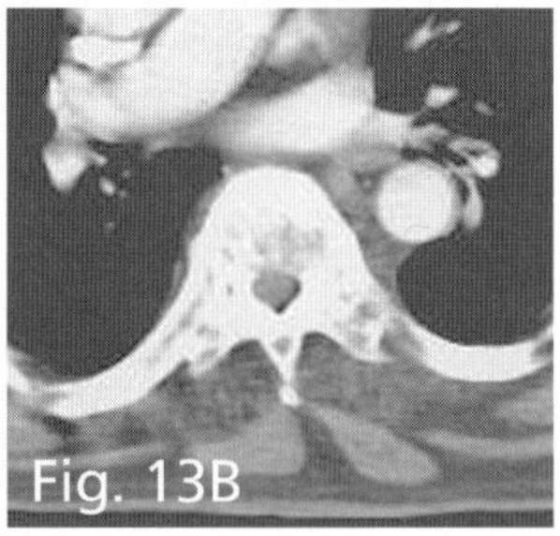
Fig. 13B

PREFERRED RESPONSE: 4

DISCUSSION: The studies show marginal syndesmophyte formation characteristic of ankylosing spondylitis. These patients typically have diffuse ossification of the disk space without large osteophyte formation. DISH typically presents with large osteophytes, referred to as nonmarginal syndesmophytes. In this patient, the zygoapophyseal joints are fused rather than degenerative as would be seen in rheumatoid arthritis, and the costovertebral joints are also fused. Osteopetrosis does not normally ankylose the disk space.

REFERENCES: McCullough JA, Transfeldt EE: *Macnab's Backache*, ed 3. Baltimore, MD, Williams and Wilkins, 1997, pp 190-194.

Frymoyer JW, Wiesel SW, eds: *The Adult and Pediatric Spine*, ed 3. Philadelphia, PA, Lippincott, Williams and Wilkins, 2003, pp 141-151.

A-43: The cervical disk herniation shown in the MRI scans in Figures 14A and 14B will most likely create which of the following constellations of symptoms?

1. Right thumb and index finger numbness and triceps weakness
2. Right thumb and index finger numbness and wrist extensor weakness
3. Right wrist extensor weakness and diminished triceps reflex
4. Right middle finger numbness and diminished brachioradialis reflex
5. Right little and ring finger numbness and diminished brachioradialis reflex

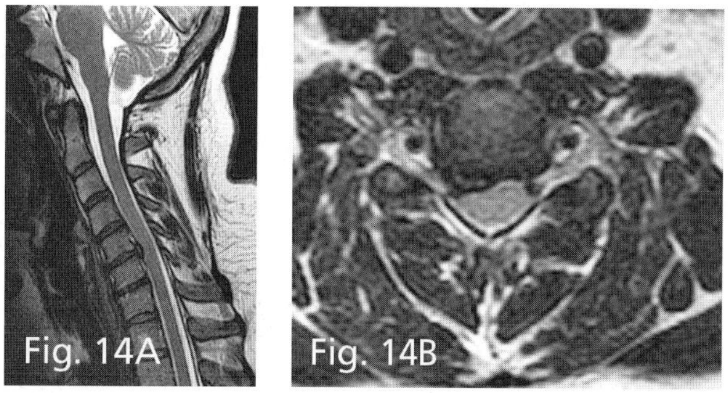

PREFERRED RESPONSE: 2

DISCUSSION: The MRI scans reveal a right-sided C5-6 herniated nucleus pulposus. A disk herniation in this region encroaches on the C6 root and is accompanied by a sensory change along the thumb and index finger, alterations in the brachioradialis reflex, and possible wrist extension weakness. Although the nerve root associated with the vertebral body passes above the pedicles such that the C6 root passes above the C6 pedicle, it is still the C6 root that is encroached on because the herniation affects the exiting root rather than the traversing root as seen in the lumbar spine.

REFERENCES: Klein JD, Garfin SR: Clinical evaluation of patients with suspected spine problems, in Frymoyer JW, ed: *Adult Spine: Principles and Practice*, ed 2. Philadephia, PA, Lippincott-Raven, 1997, pp 319-330.

Hoppenfeld S: *Orthopaedic Neurology*. Philadelphia, PA, JB Lippincott, 1977, pp 7-49.

A-44: A 21-year-old man has had posterior neck discomfort for the past 6 months. A whole-body bone scan and a cervical single-photon emission CT reveal increased activity at the C7 spinous process. MRI reveals multifocal involvement of the spinous process lamina and facet of C7. A CT-directed needle biopsy reveals osteoblastoma. What is the best course of action?

1. Observation
2. Radiation therapy
3. Curettage
4. En bloc excision with stabilization
5. En bloc excision followed by radiation therapy

PREFERRED RESPONSE: 4

DISCUSSION: En bloc excision is the recommended treatment of osteoblastoma. Treatment should consist of en bloc removal of the lamina, facet, and spinous process. Facet removal would necessitate fusion. Radiation therapy is not recommended. Intralesional curettage has a high rate of recurrence.

REFERENCES: Bridwell KH, Ogilvie JW: Primary tumors of the spine, in Bridwell KH, DeWald RL, eds: *The Textbook of Spinal Surgery*. Philadelphia, PA, JB Lippincott, 1991, vol 2, pp 1143-1174.

Ozaki T, Liljenquist U, Hillmann A, et al: Osteoid osteoma and osteoblastoma of the spine: Experience with 22 patients. *Clin Orthop* 2002;397:394-402.

Spine: Answers

A-45: What is the most likely consequence of a vertebral compression fracture associated with osteoporosis?

1. The fractured vertebral body gradually becomes more stiff than before the fracture.
2. Scoliosis develops.
3. There is an increased risk of more vertebral fractures.
4. Overall sagittal alignment remains stable because the adjacent segments of the spine are able to compensate.
5. The extensor musculature will often hypertrophy in an attempt to stabilize the painful fracture.

PREFERRED RESPONSE: 3

DISCUSSION: After an osteoporotic vertebral compression fracture, the risk of subsequent fractures at adjacent levels increases. This is thought to be the result of a shifting of the sagittal alignment more anteriorly, putting more stress on the osteopenic vertebral bodies and their anterior cortices. Pain generally resolves with rest, but this may take weeks or months. It has been demonstrated experimentally that osteoporotic vertebral bodies are actually less stiff and weaker after a compression fracture; therefore, deformity predisposes to further deformity. The extensor musculature often fatigues over time and usually does not hypertrophy. Frontal plane deformity is a rare development.

REFERENCES: Heaney RP: The natural history of vertebral osteoporosis: Is low bone mass an epiphenomenon? *Bone* 1992;13:S23-S26.

Tohmeh AG, Mathias JM, Fenton DC, et al: Biomechanical efficacy of unipedicular versus bipedicular vertebroplasty for the management of osteoporotic compression fractures. *Spine (Phila Pa 1976)* 1999;24:1772-1776.

A-46: What is the most appropriate treatment for a chordoma involving the sacrum?

1. Chemotherapy
2. External beam radiation therapy
3. En bloc surgical resection with negative margins
4. Intralesional resection followed by radiation therapy
5. Intralesional resection followed by chemotherapy

PREFERRED RESPONSE: 3

DISCUSSION: Chordomas are very resistant to radiotherapy and chemotherapy; therefore, en bloc resection with a negative margin is the preferred treatment. Lesions at or below S3 can be resected without compromising pelvis stability, and continence usually is maintained. The mean survival rate for patients with sacral chordomas is approximately 7 years. Patients with chordoma of the mobile (cervical, thoracic, or lumbar) spine have a mean survival rate of approximately 5 years. This difference is most likely the result of an earlier diagnosis.

REFERENCES: Zigler JE, Strausser DW: The aging spine, in Fardon DF, Garfin SR, Abitbol J, et al, eds: *Orthopaedic Knowledge Update: Spine*, ed 2. Rosemont, IL, American Academy of Orthopaedic Surgeons, 2002, pp 123-133.

Stener B, Gunterberg B: High amputation of the sacrum for extirpation of tumors: Principles and technique. *Spine (Phila Pa 1976)* 1978;3:351-366.

Stener B: Resection of the sacrum for tumors. *Chir Organi Mov* 1990;75:S108-S110.

A-47: Which of the following is NOT considered a risk factor for nonunion of a type II odontoid fracture?

1. More than 6 mm of initial displacement
2. Patient age older than 60 years
3. Smoking
4. Inability to achieve reduction
5. Obesity

PREFERRED RESPONSE: 5

DISCUSSION: Although obesity can make brace or halo wear difficult, it has not been associated with an increased risk for nonunion.

REFERENCES: Carson GD, Heller JG, Abitbol JJ, et al: Odontoid fractures, in Levine AM, Eismont FJ, Garfin SR, et al, eds: *Spine Trauma*. Philadelphia, PA, WB Saunders, 1998, pp 235-238.

Tay B K-B, Eismont F: Cevical spine fractures and dislocations, in Fardon DF, Garfin SR, Abitbol J, et al, eds: *Orthopaedic Knowledge Update: Spine*, ed 2. Rosemont, IL, American Academy of Orthopaedic Surgeons, 2002, pp 247-262.

A-48: A 27-year-old woman has a bilateral C5-C6 facet dislocation and quadriparesis after being involved in a motor vehicle accident. Initial management consisted of reduction with traction, but she remains a Frankel A quadriplegic. To facilitate rehabilitation, surgical stabilization and fusion is planned. From a biomechanical point of view, which of the following techniques is the LEAST stable method of fixation?

1. Anterior cervical plating with interbody bone graft
2. Posterior cervical plating with lateral mass screw fixation
3. Posterior sublaminar wiring
4. Simple posterior interspinous wiring
5. Bohlman interspinous wiring

PREFERRED RESPONSE: 1

DISCUSSION: In two different biomechanical studies performed in both bovine and human cadaver spines, all posterior techniques of stabilization were found to be superior to anterior plating in flexion-distraction injuries of the cervical spine. These injuries usually have an intact anterior longitudinal ligament that allows posterior fixation to function as a tension band. Anterior plating with grafting destroys this last remaining stabilizing structure and does not allow for a tension band effect because all of the posterior stabilizing structures have been destroyed with the injury. In clinical practice, however, anterior plating can be effective in the treatment of this injury with appropriate postoperative orthotic management.

REFERENCES: Sutterlin CE III, McAfee PC, Warden KE, et al: A biomechanical evaluation of cervical spine stabilization methods in a bovine model: Static and cyclical loading. *Spine (Phila Pa 1976)* 1988;13:795-802.

Coe JD, Warden KE, Sutterlin CE III, et al: Biomechanical evaluation of cervical spine stabilization methods in a human cadaveric model. *Spine (Phila Pa 1976)* 1989;14:1122-1131.

Shoulder and Elbow

Q-1: In Figure 1, which of the following structures is the primary stabilizer in preventing valgus instability of the elbow?

1. A
2. B
3. C
4. D
5. E

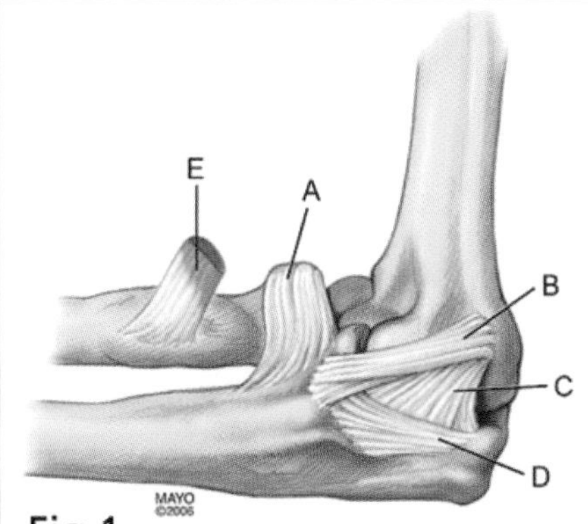

Fig.1

Q-2: Figure 2A shows the radiograph of a 20-year-old man who has an injury to the right shoulder. Figure 2B shows an arthroscopic view (posterior portal). The arrow points to a

1. rotator cuff tear.
2. bare area.
3. Hill-Sachs defect.
4. Bankart tear.
5. glenoid fracture.

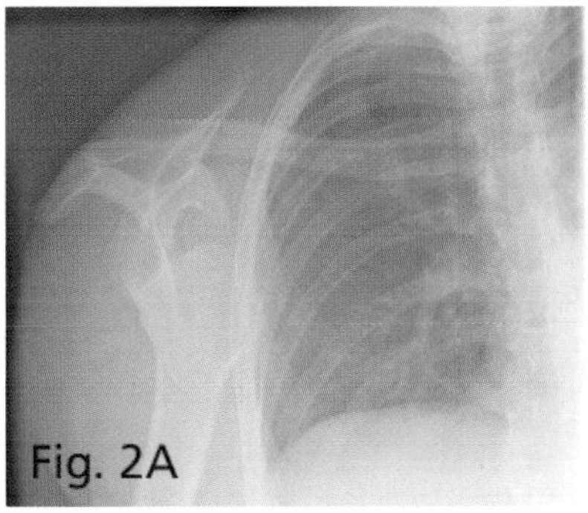
Fig. 2A

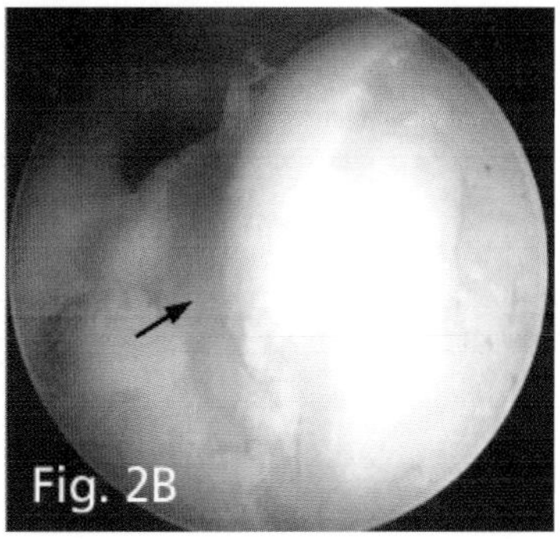
Fig. 2B

Q-3: A previously asymptomatic 40-year-old man injures his shoulder in a fall. Examination shows that he is unable to lift the hand away from his back while maximally internally rotated. An axial MRI scan of the shoulder is shown in Figure 3. What is the most likely diagnosis?

1. Pectoralis major tendon rupture
2. Supraspinatus rupture
3. Subscapularis rupture
4. Bankart tear
5. Humeral avulsion of the inferior glenohumeral ligament

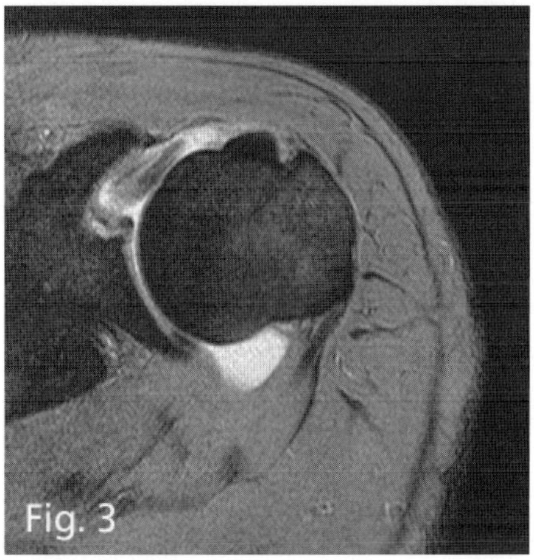
Fig. 3

Q-4: Figure 4 shows an arthroscopic view of a right shoulder in the lateral position through a posterior portal. What is the area between structure B (biceps) and SS (subscapularis tendon)?

1. Inferior glenohumeral ligament
2. Superior glenohumeral ligament
3. Rotator cuff interval
4. Subscapularis recess
5. Interior recess

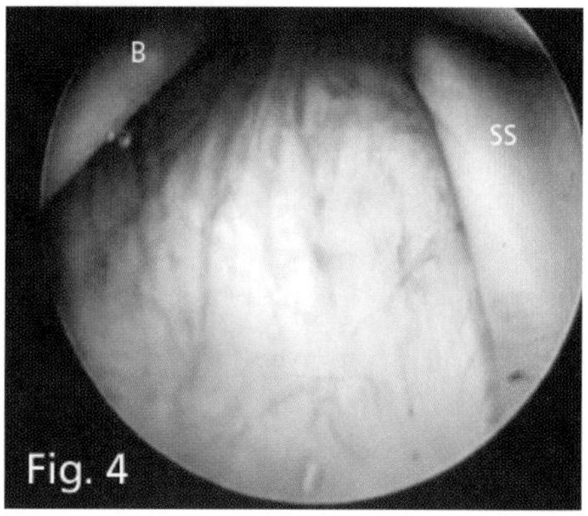

Fig. 4

Q-5: In recurrent posterior shoulder instability, what is the recommended approach to the posterior capsule?

1. A teres minor-splitting approach
2. An infraspinatus-splitting approach
3. Between the infraspinatus and teres minor
4. Between the supraspinatus and infraspinatus
5. In the rotator interval

Q-6: Figure 5 shows the MRI scan of a 38-year-old patient who is a weightlifter. What does the arrow on the MRI scan indicate?

1. Biceps tear
2. Pectoralis minor tear
3. Pectoralis major tear
4. Subscapularis tear
5. Abscess formation

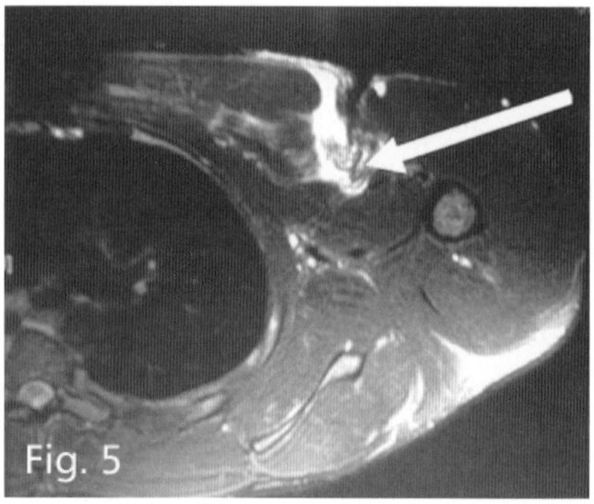
Fig. 5

Q-7: Which of the following muscle tendons inserts just lateral to the long head of the biceps tendon on the proximal humerus?

1. Teres major
2. Latissimus dorsi
3. Short head of the biceps
4. Pectoralis major
5. Subscapularis

Q-8: A 68-year-old man had a 3-year history of shoulder pain that failed to respond to nonsurgical management. Examination reveals forward elevation to 120° and external rotation to 30°. True AP and axillary radiographs and an axial CT scan are shown in Figures 6A through 6C. What management option would lead to the best long-term results?

1. Hemiarthroplasty
2. Total shoulder arthroplasty
3. Reverse total shoulder arthroplasty
4. Arthroscopic débridement
5. Glenoid osteotomy and interposition arthroplasty

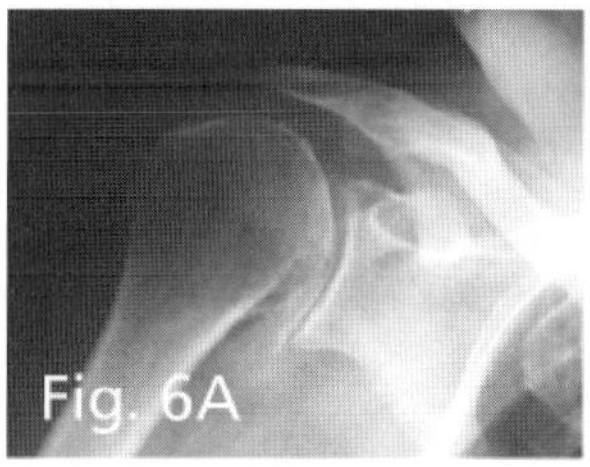
Fig. 6A

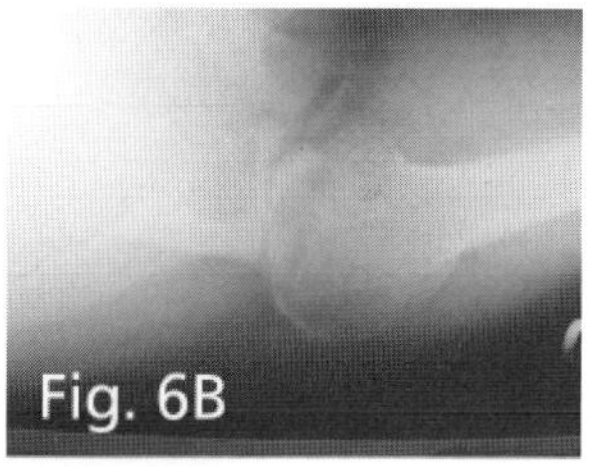
Fig. 6B

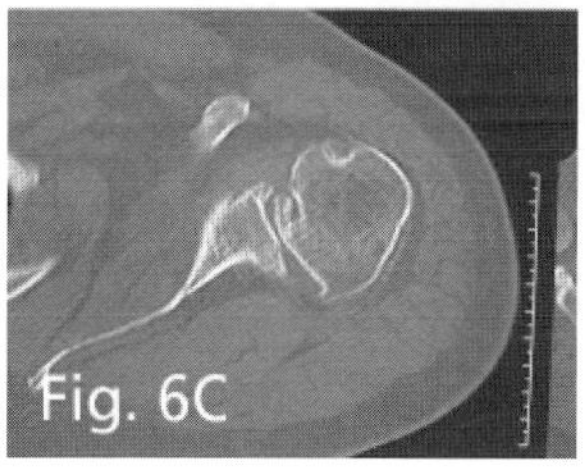
Fig. 6C

Q-9: A 66-year-old woman who previously underwent hemiarthroplasty 2 years ago for a fracture continues to have severe pain and loss of motion despite undergoing physical therapy. A radiograph is shown in Figure 7. What is the most likely reason that this patient has failed to improve her motion?

1. She was noncompliant in physical therapy.
2. The original surgery should have included resurfacing the glenoid.
3. The humeral head was too large.
4. The humeral component was placed too proud.
5. The tuberosities are malpositioned.

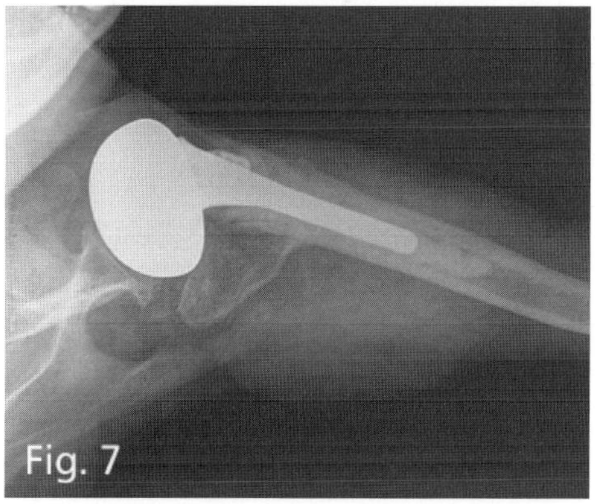
Fig. 7

Q-10: A 40-year-old woman underwent an arthroscopic acromioplasty and mini-open rotator cuff repair 4 weeks ago. At follow-up examination, the incision is painful, erythematous, and draining fluid. The patient is febrile and has an elevated white blood cell count. What infectious organism should be under high suspicion of causing this outcome?

1. *Escherichia coli*
2. *Streptococcus viridans*
3. *Oxalophagus oxalicus*
4. *Propionibacterium acnes*
5. *Enterococcus faecalis*

Q-11: A patient reports persistent anterior shoulder pain following a forceful external rotation injury to the shoulder. An MRI scan is shown in Figure 8. The patient remains symptomatic despite 3 months of nonsurgical management. Treatment should now consist of

1. repair of the superior labrum.
2. isolated supraspinatus repair.
3. biceps recentering.
4. subscapularis repair and biceps tenodesis.
5. subscapularis repair and recentering of the biceps tendon.

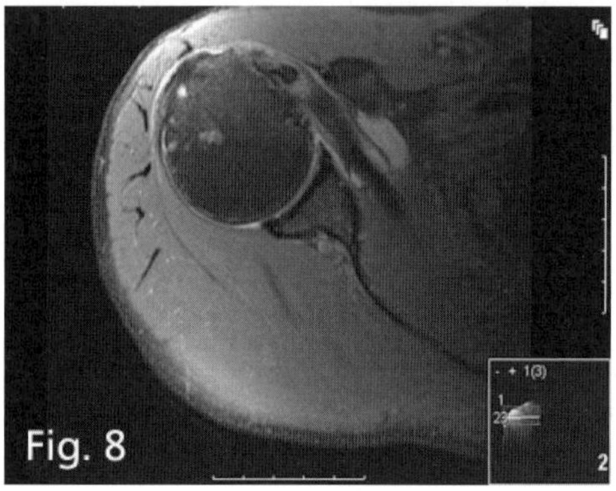
Fig. 8

Q-12: A 78-year-old woman falls onto her nondominant left elbow and sustains the injury shown in Figure 9. What treatment option allows her the shortest recovery time and highest likelihood of good function and range of motion?

1. Total elbow arthroplasty
2. Open reduction and internal fixation
3. Radial head arthroplasty
4. Sling and swathe
5. Bone stimulator

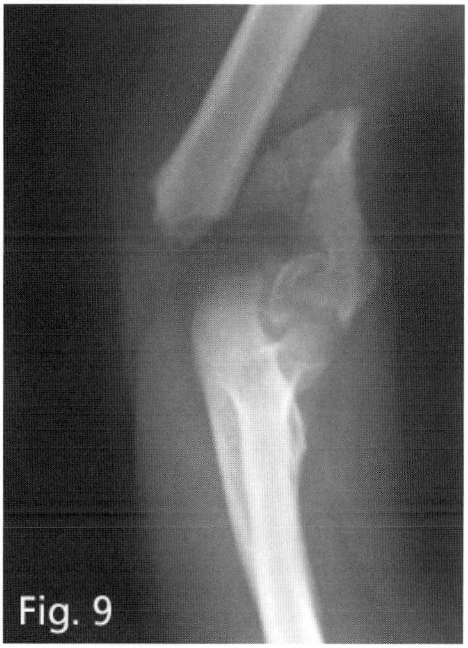

Fig. 9

Q-13: A 45-year-old woman awakens with the acute onset of burning left shoulder pain that radiates toward the axilla. She denies any history of trauma. On examination, she is unable to abduct her arm but has full passive shoulder motion. Her sensation is intact. Cervical spine examination reveals full range of motion and a negative Spurling test. Radiographs and MRI studies are normal for the cervical spine and shoulder. What is the most likely diagnosis?

1. Cervical C6-7 radiculopathy
2. Impingement
3. Rotator cuff tear
4. Brachial neuritis
5. Adhesive capsulitis

Q-14: A 72-year-old man who underwent total shoulder arthroplasty 2 years ago slipped on ice and fell on his shoulder 3 weeks ago. Immediately after falling he was unable to elevate his arm. Motor examination reveals deltoid 5-/5, subscapularis 5-/5, external rotation 4-/5, and supraspinatus 2/5. Radiographs are shown in Figures 10A and 10B. What is the most likely diagnosis?

1. Anterior shoulder dislocation
2. Humeral component loosening
3. Glenoid component loosening
4. Glenoid component catastrophic fracture
5. Rotator cuff tear

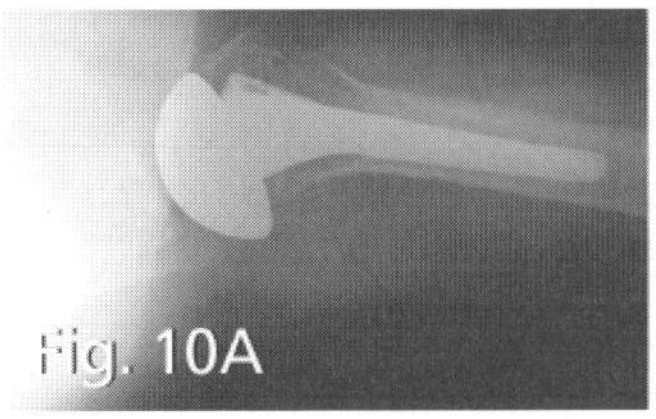
Fig. 10A

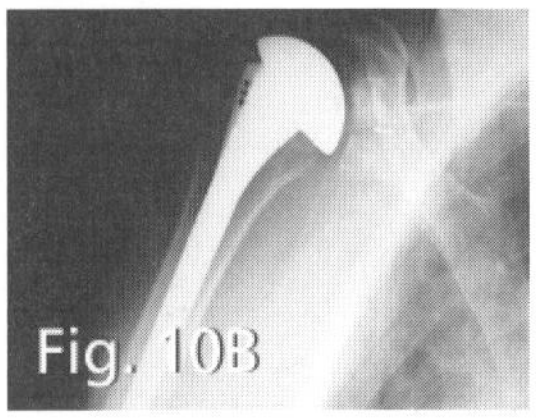
Fig. 10B

Q-15: A 39-year-old man has had persistent right shoulder pain for the past 6 months. A formal physical therapy program has failed to provide relief, and an injection several months ago provided only short-term relief. Examination reveals a positive Neer and Hawkins test. There is no instability and the neurovascular examination is normal. Arthroscopy reveals a partial rotator cuff tear on the bursal side measuring 60% of the tendon thickness. What is the next most appropriate step in management?

1. Arthroscopic débridement alone of the partial rotator cuff tear
2. Repair of the partial rotator cuff tear and subacromial decompression
3. Arthroscopic débridement combined with subacromial decompression
4. Arthroscopic subacromial decompression
5. Biceps tenotomy

Q-16: Figures 11A and 11B show the radiographs of a 47-year-old man who reports pain in both shoulders. He has a history of leukemia that was treated with chemotherapy and high-dose cortisone. What is the most reliable treatment option for pain relief in this patient?

1. Arthroscopic débridement
2. Arthrodesis
3. Resection arthroplasty
4. Hemiarthroplasty
5. Cortisone injection

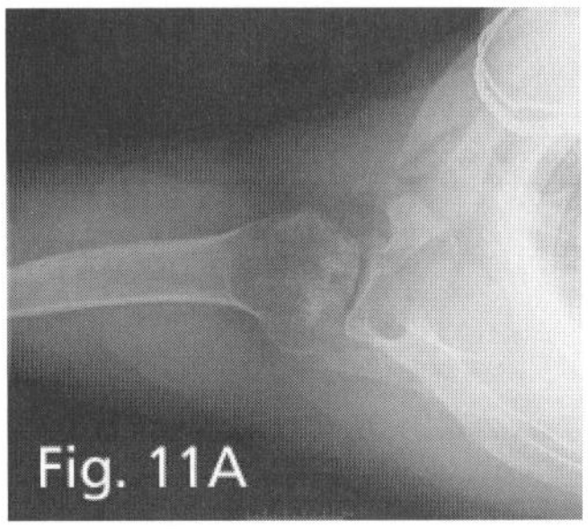
Fig. 11A

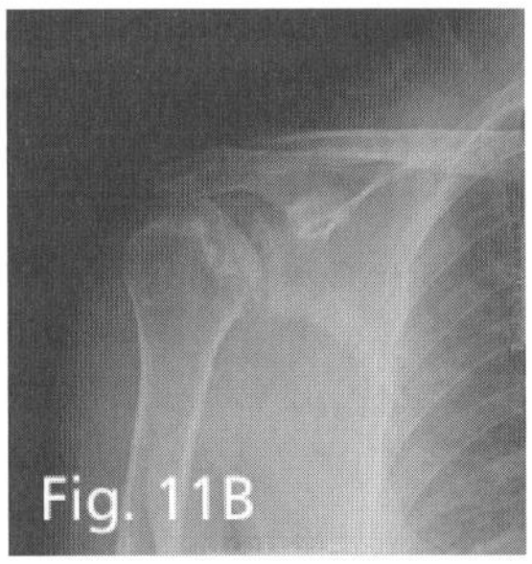
Fig. 11B

Q-17: Figure 12A shows the clinical photograph of a 36-year-old man who has left shoulder pain and dysfunction after undergoing a lymph node biopsy 2 years ago. The appearance of the shoulder during abduction and a wall push-up maneuver is shown in Figures 12B and 12C, respectively. Which of the following procedures provides the best pain relief and function?

1. Direct nerve repair
2. Sural nerve graft
3. Pectoralis major transfer
4. Levator scapula and rhomboid transfer
5. Scapulothoracic fusion

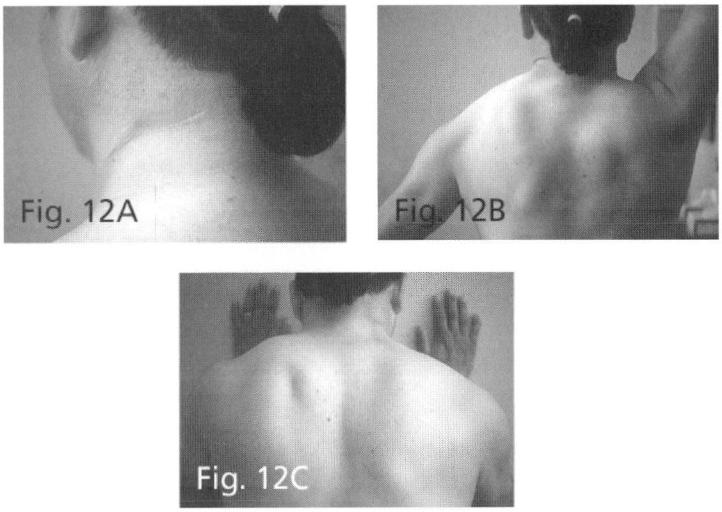

Q-18: What is the most common cause of poor outcomes in patients who undergo total shoulder arthroplasty?

1. Loosening of the humeral component
2. Loosening of the glenoid component
3. Infection
4. Brachial plexus injury
5. Rotator cuff tear

Q-19: A 49-year-old woman with serologically proven rheumatoid arthritis has Larsen grade II radiographic changes in the elbow. Examination reveals a preoperative arc of flexion of less than 90° and there is no instability. Nonsurgical management has failed to provide relief. What is the best treatment option?

1. Semiconstrained total elbow arthroplasty
2. Unlinked total elbow arthroplasty
3. Fascial arthroplasty
4. Open synovectomy
5. Arthroscopic synovectomy

Shoulder and Elbow: Questions

Q-20: A 68-year-old woman with serologically proven rheumatoid arthritis underwent an open synovectomy and radial head resection 10 years ago. She now has severe pain that has failed to respond to nonsurgical management. Examination reveals a flexion arc of greater than 90°. Radiographs are shown in Figures 13A and 13B. What is the most appropriate management?

1. Semiconstrained total elbow arthroplasty
2. Unconstrained total elbow arthroplasty
3. Fascial arthroplasty
4. Open synovectomy
5. Arthroscopic synovectomy

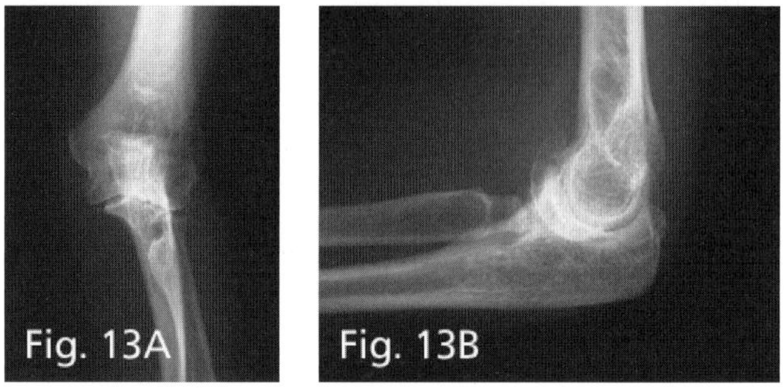

Fig. 13A Fig. 13B

Q-21: A football player sustains a traumatic anterior-inferior dislocation of the shoulder during the last game of the season. It is reduced 20 minutes later in the locker room. The patient is neurologically intact and has regained motion. If the patient undergoes arthroscopic evaluation, what finding is seen most consistently?

1. Superior labral detachment
2. Engaging Hill-Sachs lesion
3. Large glenoid rim fracture
4. Avulsion of the inferior glenohumeral ligament from the humerus
5. Avulsion of the anterior inferior glenoid labrum

Q-22: A 42-year-old patient undergoes resection of the medial clavicle for painful sternoclavicular degenerative joint disease. The postoperative course is complicated by an increase in symptoms, a medial bump, and subjective tingling in the digits. A clinical photograph and radiograph are shown in Figures 14A and 14B. What is the most appropriate procedure at this time?

1. Semitendinosus figure-of-8 graft
2. Subclavius tendon transfer
3. Medial clavicular osteotomy
4. Medial clavicular resection
5. Sternoclavicular arthrodesis

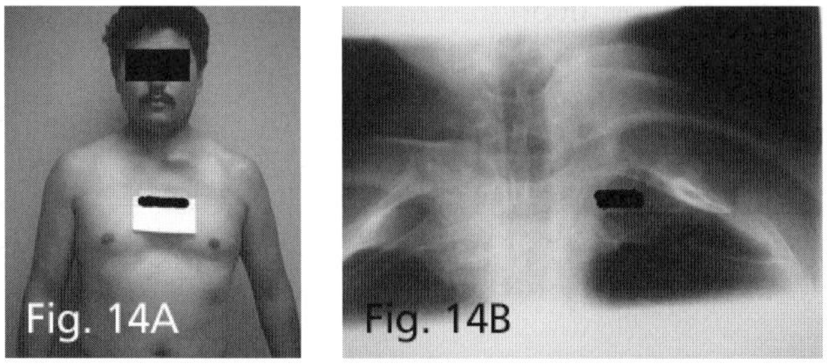

Fig. 14A Fig. 14B

Q-23: A 32-year-old woman sustained an elbow dislocation, and management consisted of early range of motion. Examination at the 3-month follow-up appointment reveals that she has regained elbow motion but has a weak pinch. A clinical photograph is shown in Figure 15. What is the most likely diagnosis?

1. Flexor pollicis longus rupture
2. Median nerve palsy
3. Ulnar nerve palsy
4. Anterior interosseous nerve palsy
5. Posterior interosseous nerve palsy

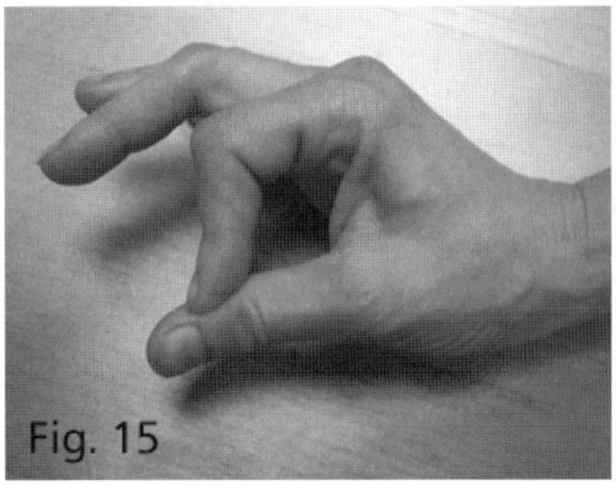
Fig. 15

Q-24: What are the proposed biomechanical advantages of the Grammont reverse total shoulder arthroplasty when compared to a standard shoulder arthroplasty?

1. Lateralization of the center of rotation, lengthening the deltoid, and decreasing the deltoid moment arm
2. Lateralization of the center of rotation, shortening the deltoid, and decreasing acromial stress
3. Lateralization of the center of rotation, lengthening the deltoid, and increasing the transverse force couple
4. Medialization of the center of rotation, lengthening the deltoid, and increasing the deltoid moment arm
5. Medialization of the center of rotation, shortening the deltoid, and decreasing acromial stress

Q-25: A 74-year-old woman with rheumatoid arthritis reports shoulder pain that has failed to respond to nonsurgical management. AP and axillary radiographs are shown in Figures 16A and 16B. Examination reveals active forward elevation to 120° and external rotation to 30°. What treatment option results in the most predictable pain relief and function?

1. Hemiarthroplasty
2. Arthroscopic débridement
3. Total shoulder arthroplasty with a cemented all-polyethylene glenoid component
4. Reverse total shoulder arthroplasty
5. Total shoulder arthroplasty with a metal-backed glenoid component

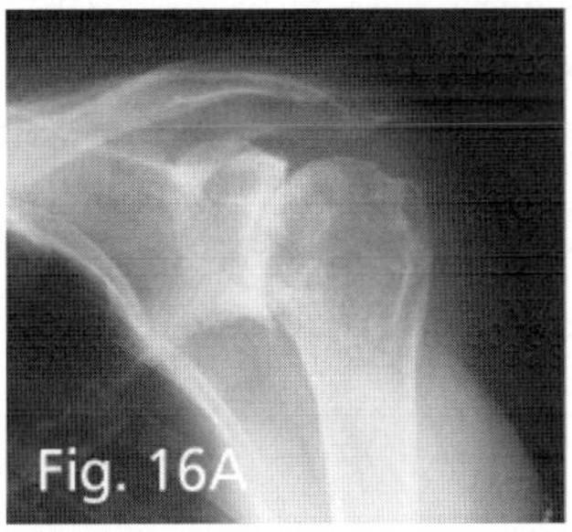
Fig. 16A

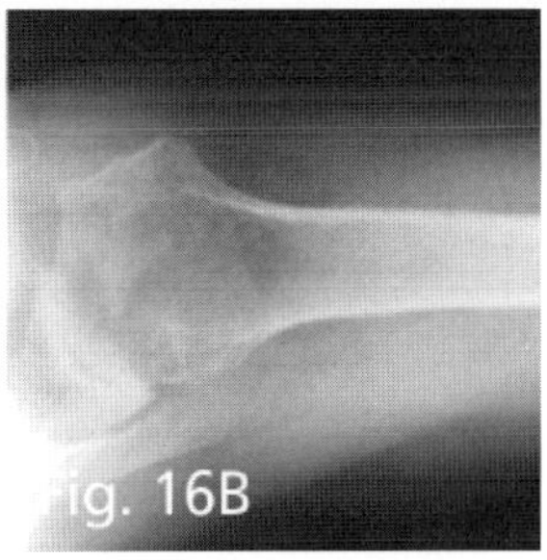
Fig. 16B

Q-26: A 69-year-old woman has just undergone an uncomplicated total shoulder arthroplasty for glenohumeral osteoarthritis. A press-fit humeral stem and a cemented all-polyethylene glenoid component were placed. At this point, what is the postoperative rehabilitation plan?

1. Maintain sling immobilization for 6 weeks, and then begin a global range-of-motion program.
2. Maintain sling immobilization for 3 weeks, and then begin a global range-of-motion program.
3. Immediately begin an active assisted range-of-motion program emphasizing forward elevation and external rotation to the side.
4. Immediately begin a passive range-of-motion program for forward elevation only; no external rotation is allowed for 6 weeks.
5. Immediately begin active range of motion in forward elevation and external rotation to the side with a progression to full rotator cuff strengthening in 3 weeks.

Q-27: A 22-year-old man who is right-handed fell off his motorcycle onto the tip of his right shoulder 2 weeks ago and now reports pain and difficulty raising his right arm. Examination reveals tenderness and gross movement over the lateral scapular spine and severe weakness during resisted abduction. A radiograph and three-dimensional CT scan are shown in Figures 17A and 17B. What is the next most appropriate step in management?

1. Open reduction and internal fixation
2. External bone stimulator
3. 90° abduction splint
4. Arthroscopic acromioplasty
5. Fragment excision

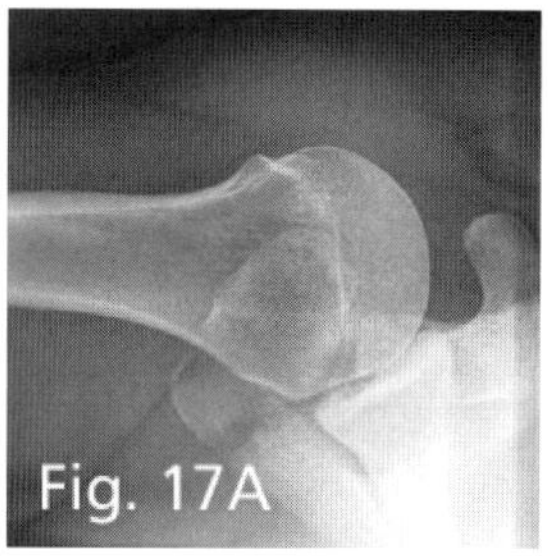
Fig. 17A

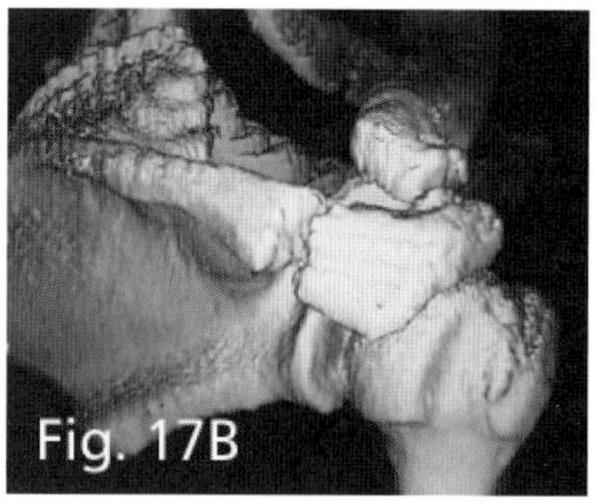
Fig. 17B

Q-28: A 20-year-old man who plays minor league baseball has a symptomatic torn ulnar collateral ligament (UCL) in his pitching elbow. Nonsurgical management consisting of rest and physical therapy aimed at elbow strengthening has failed to provide relief. He has concomitant cubital tunnel symptoms that worsen while throwing. What is his best surgical option?

1. UCL repair and nighttime elbow extension splinting
2. UCL repair with ulnar nerve decompression in situ
3. Allograft UCL reconstruction with interference screws
4. Autograft UCL reconstruction with ulnar nerve transposition
5. Autograft UCL reconstruction using a docking technique

Q-29: A patient who underwent open reduction and internal fixation of an olecranon fracture 2 months ago now reports painless limitation of motion. Examination reveals a well-healed incision and a flexion-extension arc from 40° to 80°. The patient has been performing home exercises. Radiographs are shown in Figures 18A and 18B. What is the most appropriate treatment?

1. Continued observation and home therapy
2. Radiation therapy, followed by aggressive range-of-motion exercises
3. Formal physical therapy and static progressive splinting
4. Revision open reduction and internal fixation and capsular release
5. Manipulation under anesthesia

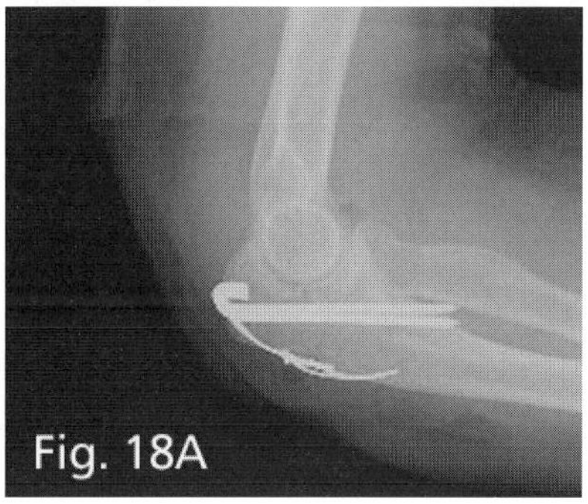
Fig. 18A

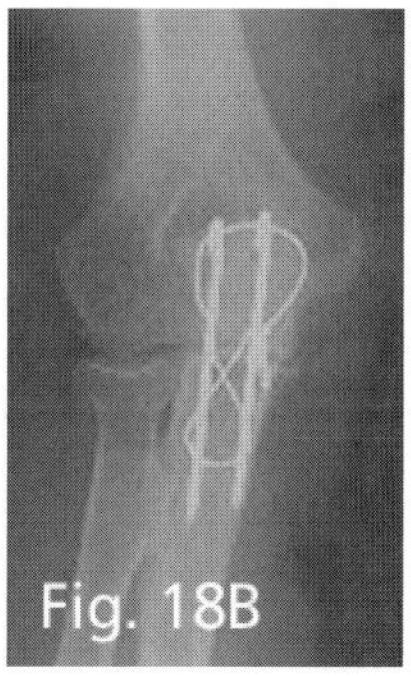
Fig. 18B

Q-30: A 23-year-old patient who is a professional baseball pitcher reports shoulder pain and decreased velocity while pitching. Physical examination reveals a side-to-side internal rotation deficit of 25°. The O'Brien sign is negative; Neer and Hawkins signs are negative. Rotator cuff strength is full. Radiographs are unremarkable. What is the next step in management?

1. MRI-arthrogram to evaluate the rotator cuff
2. Rotator cuff strengthening program
3. Posterior capsular stretching program
4. Shoulder arthroscopy with superior labrum anterior to posterior repair
5. Shoulder arthroscopy with posterior capsular release

Q-31: A 72-year-old woman who is right-handed has severe pain in the right shoulder that has failed to respond to nonsurgical management. She reports night pain and significant disability. Examination reveals 30° of active forward elevation. An AP radiograph is shown in Figure 19. Which of the following treatment options will provide the best functional improvement?

1. Arthroscopic débridement
2. Arthroscopic rotator cuff repair
3. Hemiarthroplasty with rotator cuff repair
4. Total shoulder arthroplasty
5. Reverse shoulder arthroplasty

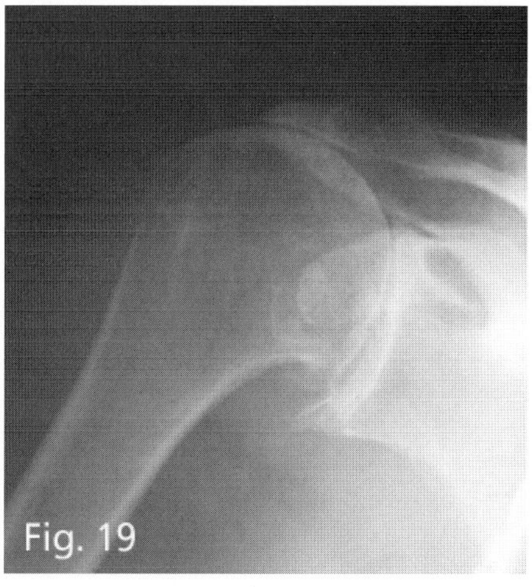
Fig. 19

Q-32: A 64-year-old man who was involved in a high-speed motor vehicle accident 6 weeks ago has been in the intensive care unit with a closed head injury. Examination reveals that his range of motion for external rotation to the side is –30°. Radiographs are shown in Figures 20A and 20B. What is the most likely diagnosis?

1. Adhesive capsulitis
2. Calcific tendinitis
3. Anterior shoulder dislocation
4. Posterior shoulder dislocation
5. Glenohumeral osteoarthritis

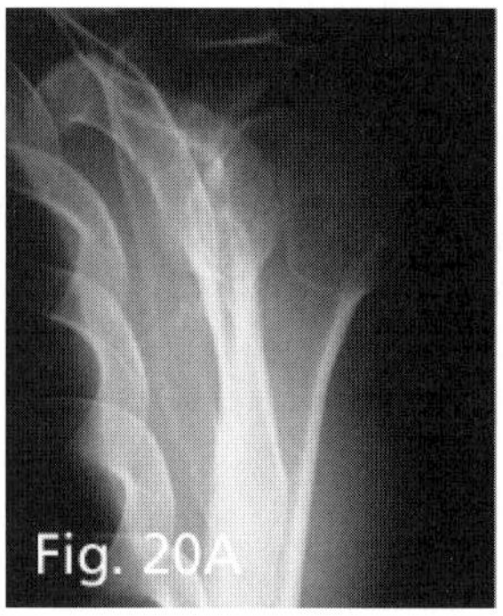
Fig. 20A

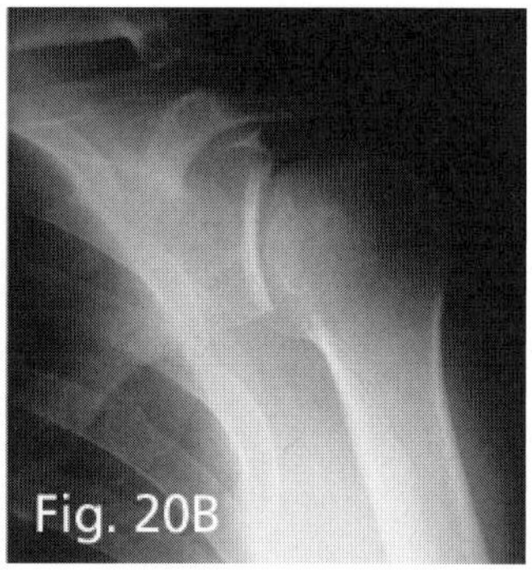
Fig. 20B

Q-33: A football lineman who sustained a traumatic injury while blocking during a game now reports that his shoulder is slipping while pass blocking. Examination reveals no apprehension in abduction and external rotation; however, he reports pain with posterior translation of the shoulder. He has full strength in external rotation, internal rotation, and supraspinatus testing. What is the pathology most likely responsible for his symptoms?

1. Anterior glenoid rim fracture tear
2. Anterior inferior labral tear
3. Posterior labral tear
4. Total capsular laxity
5. Osteochondral defect of the humeral head

Q-34: A 17-year-old girl has multidirectional instability of the shoulder. What is the most appropriate initial management?

1. Immobilization in a sling and swathe
2. Open capsular shift
3. Arthroscopic capsular plication
4. Thermal capsulorrhaphy
5. Physical therapy and home exercises

Q-35: A previously healthy 65-year-old woman has a closed fracture of the right clavicle after falling down the basement stairs. Examination reveals good capillary refill in the digits of her right hand. Radial and ulnar pulses are 1+ at the right wrist compared with 2+ on the opposite side. In the arteriogram shown in Figure 21, the arrow is pointing at which of the following arteries?

1. Brachiocephalic
2. Innominate
3. Subclavian
4. Axillary
5. Circumflex scapular

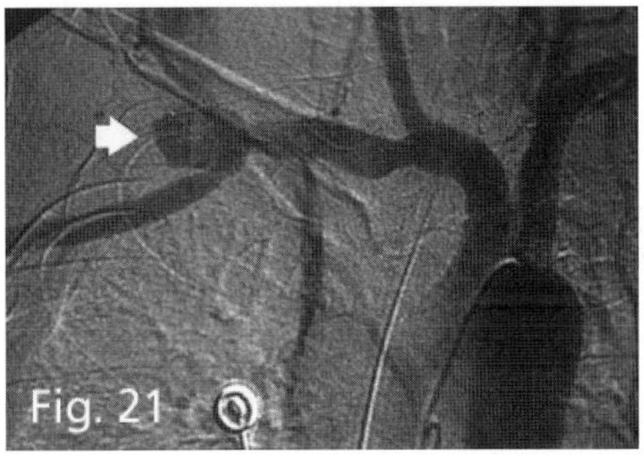
Fig. 21

Q-36: An adult patient has a closed humeral fracture that was treated nonsurgically and a concomitant radial nerve injury. Six weeks after injury, electromyography shows no evidence of recovery. Management should now consist of

1. exploration and neurolysis/repair.
2. MRI of the arm.
3. functional electrical stimulation.
4. radial nerve tendon transfers.
5. observation.

Q-37: A 55-year-old man who works as a carpenter reports chronic right anterior shoulder pain and weakness. Examination reveals 90° of external rotation (with the arm at the side) compared to 45° on the left side. His lift-off examination is positive, along with a positive belly press finding. An MRI scan reveals a chronic, retracted atrophied subscapularis tendon. What is the most appropriate management of his shoulder pain and weakness?

1. Shoulder fusion
2. Arthroscopic subscapularis repair
3. Intra-articular corticosteroid injection
4. Open subscapularis repair
5. Pectoralis major transfer

Q-38: With the arm abducted 90° and fully externally rotated, which of the following glenohumeral ligaments resists anterior translation of the humerus?

1. Coracohumeral
2. Superior glenohumeral
3. Middle glenohumeral
4. Anterior band of the inferior glenohumeral ligament complex
5. Posterior band of the inferior glenohumeral ligament complex

Q-39: Figure 22 shows the radiograph of a 75-year-old woman who has had right shoulder pain, difficulty sleeping on the affected arm, and difficulties performing activities of daily living for the past 6 weeks. Initial nonsurgical management includes analgesics, a subacromial cortisone injection, and gentle range-of-motion exercises. However, these modalities have failed to provide relief, and the patient reports that she is unable to elevate her arm. Her pain is worse and she would like the most reliable treatment method for pain relief and functional improvement. What is the best surgical treatment?

1. Reverse shoulder arthroplasty
2. Hemiarthroplasty
3. Resurfacing of the humeral head
4. Arthroscopic débridement
5. Shoulder fusion

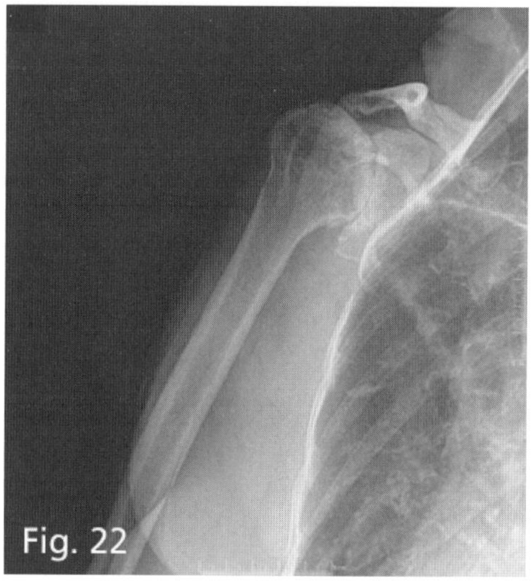
Fig. 22

Q-40: A 55-year-old man sustained an elbow dislocation during a fall. Postreduction radiographs are shown in Figures 23A and 23B. What is the best course of management?

1. Closed reduction and casting for 4 weeks
2. Closed reduction and bracing with immediate range of motion
3. Open reduction, lateral collateral ligament repair, and open reduction and internal fixation or metallic replacement of the radial head
4. Open reduction, radial head Silastic arthroplasty, and lateral collateral ligament repair
5. Open reduction, lateral collateral ligament repair, and radial head excision

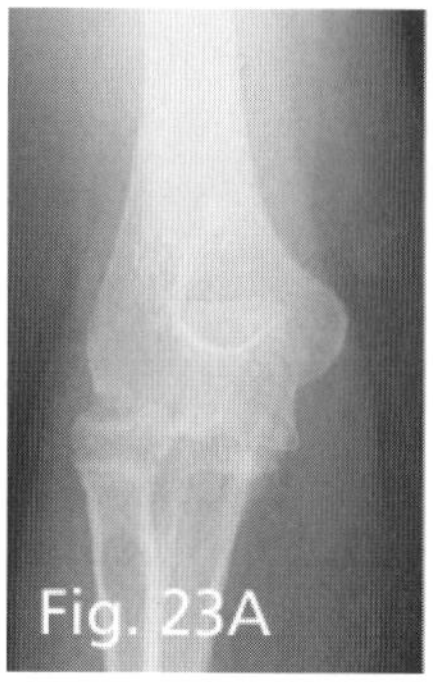
Fig. 23A

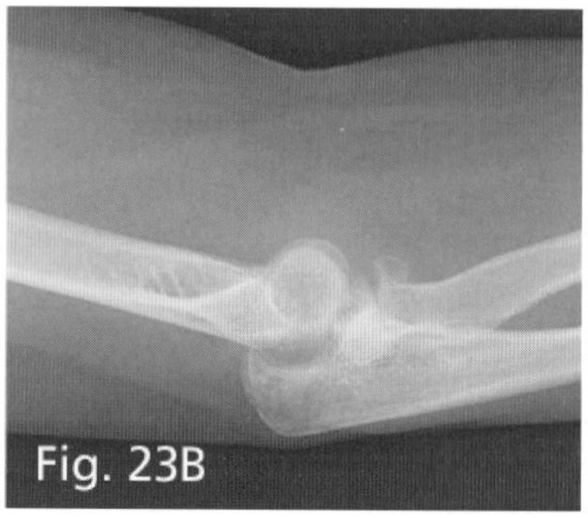
Fig. 23B

Q-41: Osteochondritis dissecans of the capitellum is a source of elbow pain and most commonly occurs in what patient population?

1. Swimmers and divers
2. Football lineman
3. Rugby players
4. Gymnasts and throwing athletes
5. Cyclists

Q-42: What are the two terminal branches of the lateral cord of the brachial plexus?

1. Musculocutaneous and median
2. Musculocutaneous and axillary
3. Median and axillary
4. Ulnar and median
5. Ulnar and medial pectoral

Q-43: A 32-year-old patient reports progressively increasing pain and stiffness after undergoing arthroscopic shoulder stabilization 1 year ago. The stabilization procedure was a Bankart repair with anchor fixation and supplemented with the heat probe. Radiographs are shown in Figures 24A and 24B. What is the most likely diagnosis?

1. Subscapularis failure
2. Frozen shoulder
3. Recurrent instability
4. Loose body
5. Chondrolysis

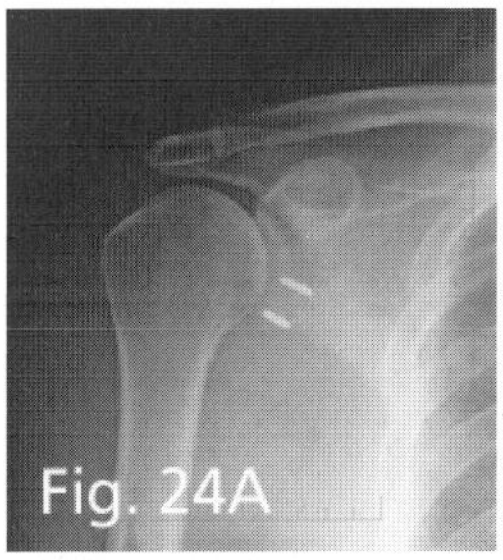

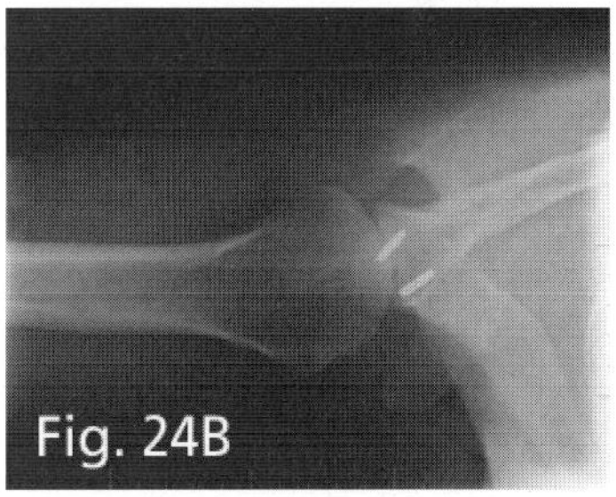

Q-44: Acute redislocation of the glenohumeral joint is a complication that occurs following a first-time dislocation. This is most often seen with

1. subglenoid dislocation.
2. subcoracoid dislocation.
3. fracture of the greater tuberosity.
4. fracture of the greater tuberosity and glenoid rim.
5. pediatric patients.

Q-45: A 51-year-old woman is seen for evaluation of chronic supraspinatus and infraspinatus tendon tears. Three years ago, in an attempted repair the surgeon was unable to repair the supraspinatus and infraspinatus tendon tears. Currently the patient has a marked amount of pain, reduced range of motion, and weakness. Examination reveals anterosuperior escape. Radiographs show no signs of arthritic changes. You are considering a latissimus dorsi tendon transfer. During the discussion, you mention that

1. she can expect to have good pain relief following surgery.
2. active forward elevation and external rotation are reliably obtained postoperatively.
3. with her current anterosuperior escape, she is likely to have a poor surgical result.
4. postoperatively, significant muscular atrophy in the latissimus dorsi commonly occurs.
5. no advancement in glenohumeral arthritic changes should occur following surgery.

Q-46: A 67-year-old woman is seen in the emergency department after falling at home. Radiographs before and after treatment are shown in Figures 25A and 25B, respectively. Which of the following best explains the 8-week postinjury clinical findings seen in Figure 25C?

1. Axillary nerve palsy
2. Spinal accessory nerve palsy
3. Deltoid avulsion
4. Rotator cuff tear
5. Unreduced posterior glenohumeral dislocation

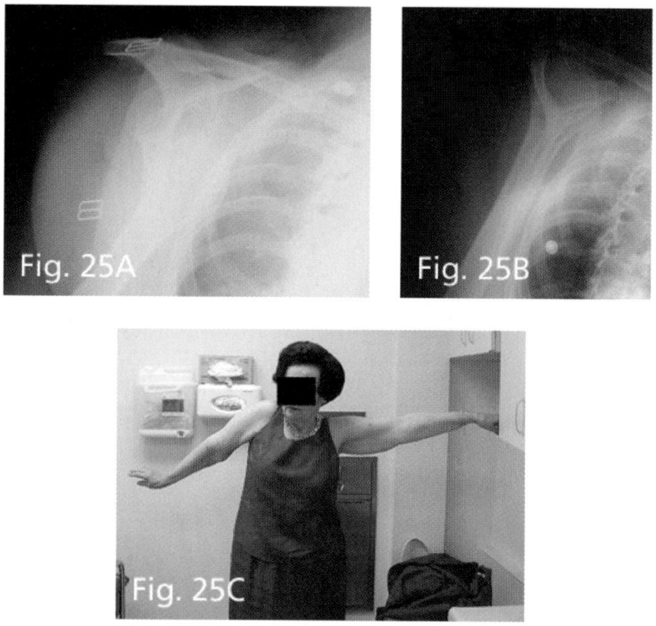

Fig. 25A Fig. 25B Fig. 25C

Q-47: Which of the following has been associated with a decreased rate of glenoid component radiolucent lines?

1. A curve-backed pegged cemented polyethylene glenoid component
2. A curve-backed keeled cemented polyethylene glenoid component design
3. A flat-backed keeled cemented polyethylene glenoid component
4. An oversized pegged cemented glenoid component
5. A superiorly placed pegged glenoid component

Q-48: Figure 26 shows the radiograph of a 42-year-old man who is a construction worker and who has pain and limited motion in his dominant elbow. Management consisting of NSAIDs and cortisone has failed to provide relief. What is the next most appropriate step in treatment?

1. Unlinked elbow arthroplasty
2. Linked elbow arthroplasty
3. Interposition arthroplasty
4. Arthroscopic or open débridement
5. Radial head excision

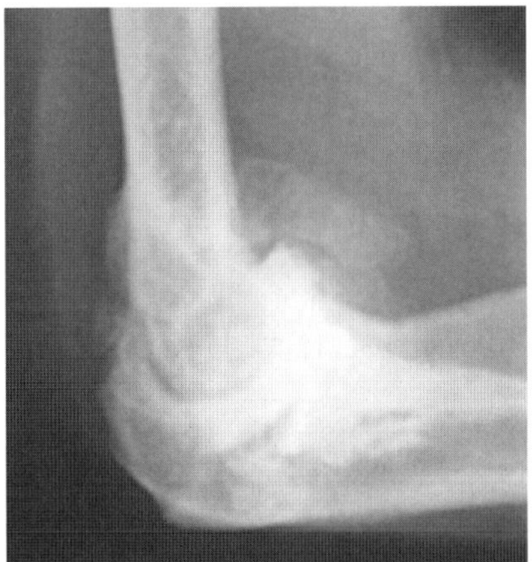
Fig. 26

Q-49: A 61-year-old woman with a long-standing history of rheumatoid arthritis reports progressive elbow pain for the past 12 months. She denies any recent trauma to the elbow; however, she notes increasing pain and decreased joint motion that are now compromising her function. Radiographs are shown in Figures 27A and 27B. What is the most appropriate treatment at this time?

1. Physical therapy for restoration of motion
2. Elbow arthroscopy, removal of loose bodies, excision of osteophytes, and capsular release (osteocapsulectomy)
3. Elbow arthroscopy and synovectomy
4. Constrained total elbow arthroplasty
5. Semiconstrained total elbow arthroplasty

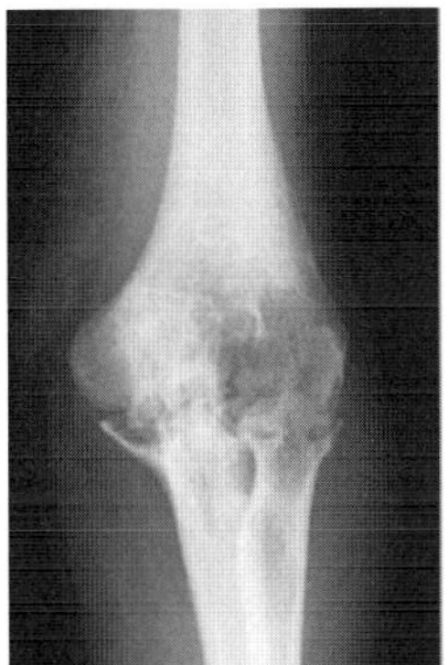
Fig. 27A

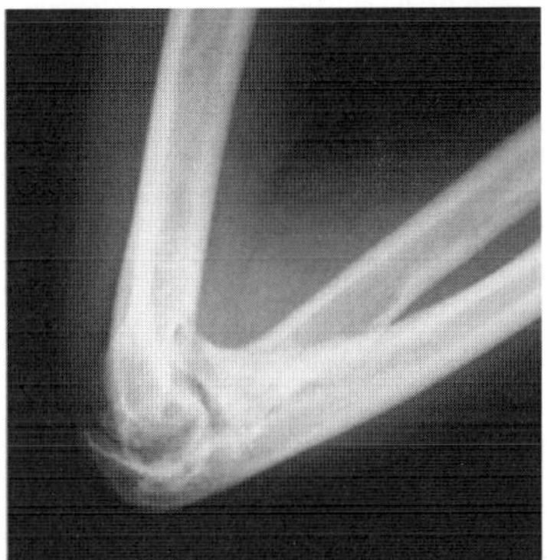
Fig. 27B

Q-50: What neurovascular structure is at greatest risk when creating a proximal anterolateral elbow arthroscopy portal?

1. Lateral antebrachial cutaneous nerve
2. Radial nerve
3. Posterior interosseous nerve
4. Median nerve
5. Brachial artery

A-1: In Figure 1, which of the following structures is the primary stabilizer in preventing valgus instability of the elbow?

1. A
2. B
3. C
4. D
5. E

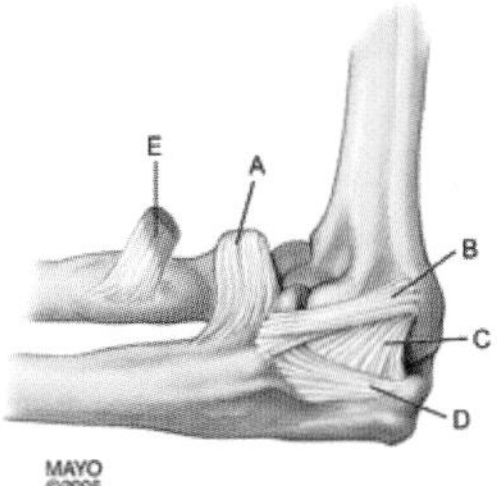

Fig.1

PREFERRED RESPONSE: 2

DISCUSSION: The anterior bundle of the medial collateral ligament is the prime stabilizer of the medial aspect of the elbow and is indicated by "B" in the figure. When intact, this anterior bundle of the medial collateral ligament is a restraint to valgus instability of the elbow. The posterior bundle is regarded as a secondary stabilizer of the medial elbow (C). The transverse bundle (D), annular ligament (A), and biceps tendon (E) do not play a role in valgus stability of the elbow.

REFERENCES: Jobe F, Elattrache N: Diagnosis and treatment of ulnar collateral ligament injuries in athletes, in Morrey B, ed: *The Elbow and Its Disorders*. Philadelphia, PA, WB Saunders, 1993, p 566.

Wilkins KE, Morrey BF, Jobe FW, et al: The elbow. *Instr Course Lect* 1991;40:1-87.

A-2: Figure 2A shows the radiograph of a 20-year-old man who has an injury to the right shoulder. Figure 2B shows an arthroscopic view (posterior portal). The arrow points to a

1. rotator cuff tear.
2. bare area.
3. Hill-Sachs defect.
4. Bankart tear.
5. glenoid fracture.

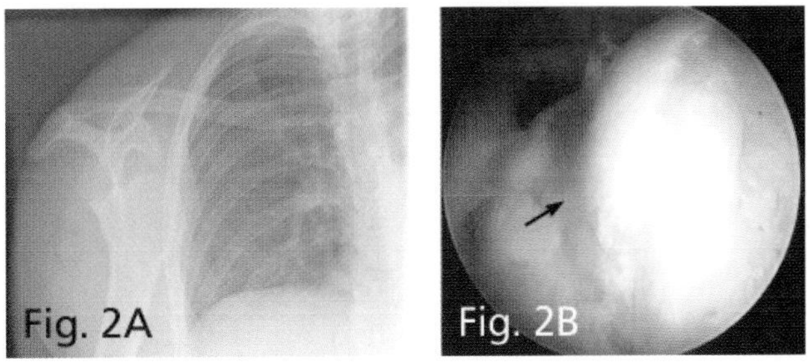
Fig. 2A Fig. 2B

PREFERRED RESPONSE: 3

DISCUSSION: The radiograph shows an anterior dislocation of the shoulder. A frequently encountered sequela of this is a compression fracture of the posterolateral humeral head, commonly referred to as a Hill-Sachs defect. The arthroscopic view of the glenohumeral joint visualizes the posterior aspect of the humeral head. In the image, the area devoid of cartilage to the right is the bare area. The indentation seen to the left is a Hill-Sachs defect.

REFERENCES: Matsen FA, Thomas SC, Rockwood CA, et al: Glenohumeral instability, in Rockwood CA, Matsen FA, eds: *The Shoulder*, ed 2. Philadelphia, PA, WB Saunders, 1998, pp 611-754.

Mazzocca AD, Noerdlinger M, Cole B, et al: Arthroscopy of the shoulder: Indications and general principals of techniques, in McGinty JB, ed: *Operative Arthroscopy*, ed 3. Philadelphia, PA, Lippincott Williams & Wilkins, 2003, pp 412-427.

A-3: A previously asymptomatic 40-year-old man injures his shoulder in a fall. Examination shows that he is unable to lift the hand away from his back while maximally internally rotated. An axial MRI scan of the shoulder is shown in Figure 3. What is the most likely diagnosis?

1. Pectoralis major tendon rupture
2. Supraspinatus rupture
3. Subscapularis rupture
4. Bankart tear
5. Humeral avulsion of the inferior glenohumeral ligament

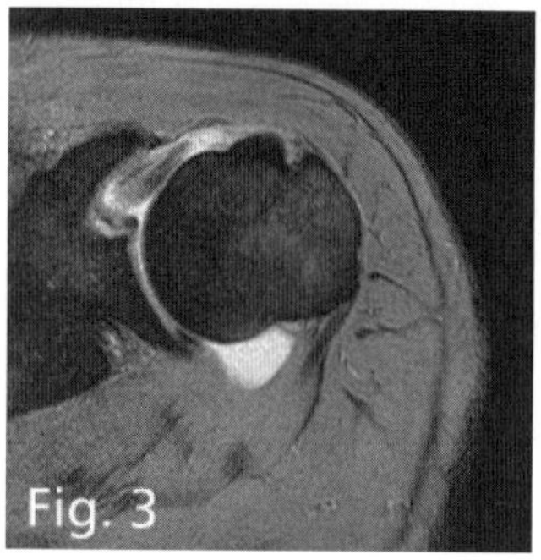
Fig. 3

PREFERRED RESPONSE: 3

DISCUSSION: The MRI scan shows detachment of the subscapularis from its insertion on the lesser tuberosity. The examination finding is consistent with a positive lift-off test, also indicating a tear of the subscapularis.

REFERENCES: Lyons RP, Green A: Subscapularis tendon tears. *J Am Acad Orthop Surg* 2005;13:353-363.

Warner JJ, Higgins L, Parsons IM, et al: Diagnosis and treatment of anterosuperior rotator cuff tears. *J Shoulder Elbow Surg* 2001;10:37-46.

A-4: Figure 4 shows an arthroscopic view of a right shoulder in the lateral position through a posterior portal. What is the area between structure B (biceps) and SS (subscapularis tendon)?

1. Inferior glenohumeral ligament
2. Superior glenohumeral ligament
3. Rotator cuff interval
4. Subscapularis recess
5. Interior recess

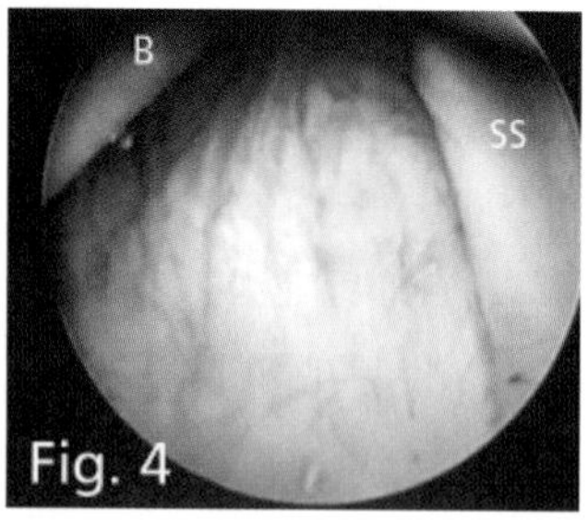

Fig. 4

PREFERRED RESPONSE: 3

DISCUSSION: The rotator cuff interval is located between the supraspinatus and subscapularis and the biceps tendon is deep to the interval. It is a triangular area where the base is the coracoid process and the apex is the transverse humeral ligament at the biceps sulcus. Closure or tightening of this area is often helpful in patients with shoulder instability. Conversely, this area is often contracted in patients with adhesive capsulitis and may need to be released.

REFERENCES: Selecky MT, Tibone JE, Yang BY, et al: Glenohumeral joint translation after arthroscopic thermal capsuloplasty of the rotator interval. *J Shoulder Elbow Surg* 2003;12:139-143.

Harryman DT, Sidles JA, Harris SL, et al: The role of the rotator interval capsule in passive motion and stability of the shoulder. *J Bone Joint Surg Am* 1992;74:53-66.

A-5: In recurrent posterior shoulder instability, what is the recommended approach to the posterior capsule?

1. A teres minor-splitting approach
2. An infraspinatus-splitting approach
3. Between the infraspinatus and teres minor
4. Between the supraspinatus and infraspinatus
5. In the rotator interval

PREFERRED RESPONSE: 2

DISCUSSION: Using an infraspinatus-splitting incision allows for excellent exposure of the posterior capsule and minimizes the risk of injury to the axillary nerve, which lies inferior to the teres minor in the quadrilateral space.

REFERENCES: Dreese J, D'Alessandro D: Posterior capsulorrhaphy through infraspinatus split for posterior instability. *Tech Shoulder Elbow Surg* 2005;6:199-207.

Shaffer BS, Conway J, Jobe FW, et al: Infraspinatus muscle-splitting incision in posterior shoulder surgery: An anatomic and electromyographic study. *Am J Sports Med* 1994;22:113-120.

Fuchs B, Jost B, Gerber C: Posterior-inferior capsular shift for the treatment of recurrent voluntary posterior subluxation of the shoulder. *J Bone Joint Surg Am* 2000;82:16-25.

A-6: Figure 5 shows the MRI scan of a 38-year-old weightlifter. What does the arrow on the MRI scan indicate?

1. Biceps tear
2. Pectoralis minor tear
3. Pectoralis major tear
4. Subscapularis tear
5. Abscess formation

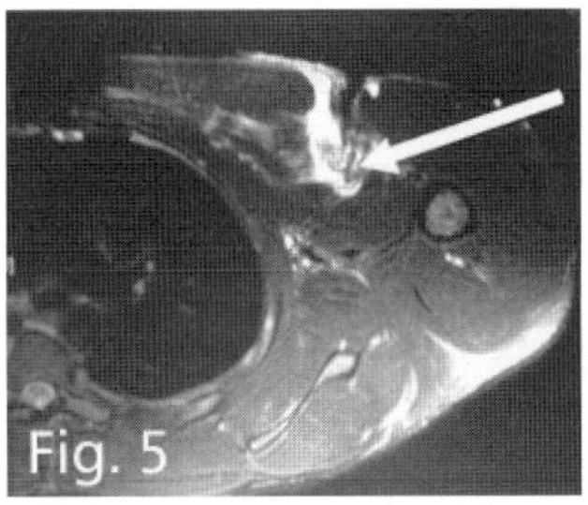
Fig. 5

PREFERRED RESPONSE: 3

DISCUSSION: Pectoralis major ruptures typically occur in avid weightlifters (often on supplements) and typically while bench-pressing. Clinically there is significant discoloration/bruising over the pectoralis and into the axilla. MRI helps confirm the diagnosis and may help determine if the tear is in the muscle belly or at the bone-tendon junction.

REFERENCES: Bal GK, Basamania CJ: Pectoralis major tendon ruptures: Diagnosis and treatment. *Tech Shoulder Elbow Surg* 2005;6:128-134.

Aarimaa V, Rantanen J, Heikkila J, et al: Ruptures of the pectoralis major muscle. *Am J Sports Med* 2004;32:1256-1262.

A-7: Which of the following muscle tendons inserts just lateral to the long head of the biceps tendon on the proximal humerus?

1. Teres major
2. Latissimus dorsi
3. Short head of the biceps
4. Pectoralis major
5. Subscapularis

PREFERRED RESPONSE: 4

DISCUSSION: The pectoralis major insertion is just lateral to the long head of the biceps tendon. Medial to the biceps is the insertion for the teres major and latissimus dorsi. The short head of the biceps originates on the coracoid process. The subscapularis inserts on the lesser tuberosity just medial to the biceps.

REFERENCE: Bal GK, Basamania CJ: Pectoralis major tendon ruptures: Diagnosis and treatment. *Tech Shoulder Elbow Surg* 2005;6:128-134.

A-8: A 68-year-old man had a 3-year history of shoulder pain that failed to respond to nonsurgical management. Examination reveals forward elevation to 120° and external rotation to 30°. True AP and axillary radiographs and an axial CT scan are shown in Figures 6A through 6C. What management option would lead to the best long-term results?

1. Hemiarthroplasty
2. Total shoulder arthroplasty
3. Reverse total shoulder arthroplasty
4. Arthroscopic débridement
5. Glenoid osteotomy and interposition arthroplasty

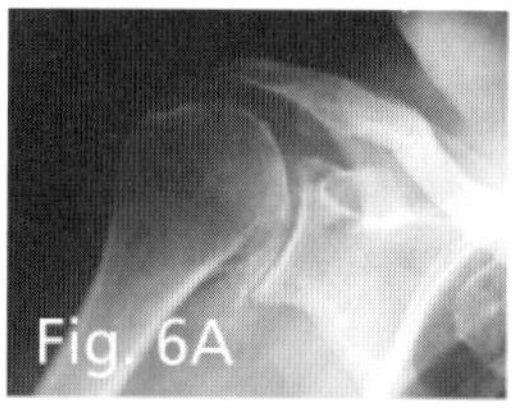
Fig. 6A

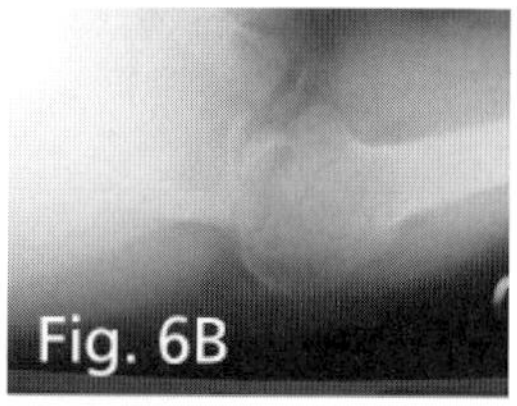
Fig. 6B

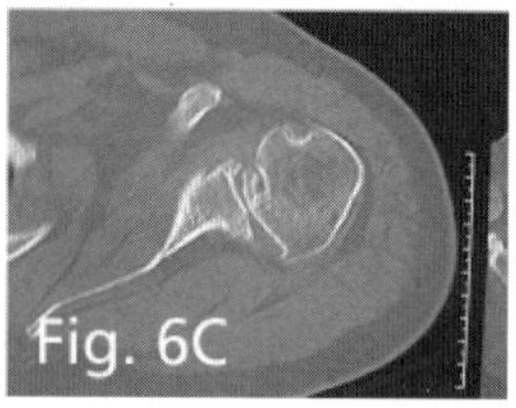
Fig. 6C

PREFERRED RESPONSE: 2

DISCUSSION: The radiographs and CT scan reveal osteoarthritis with posterior subluxation and posterior bone loss. Total shoulder arthroplasty with reaming of the high side to neutralize the glenoid surface has been shown to yield better results than hemiarthroplasty. The amount of bone loss in this patient does not require posterior glenoid augmentation. Reverse total shoulder arthroplasty is indicated for rotator cuff tear arthropathy; therefore, it is not applicable. Arthroscopic débridement has yielded poor results with advanced osteoarthritis and posterior subluxation. Results from glenoid osteotomy have been variable, and glenoid osteotomy is not indicated with associated osteoarthritis.

REFERENCES: Iannotti JP, Norris TR: Influence of preoperative factors on outcome of shoulder arthroplasty for glenohumeral osteoarthritis. *J Bone Joint Surg Am* 2003;85:251-258.

Rodosky MW, Bigliani LU: Indications for glenoid resurfacing in shoulder arthroplasty. *J Shoulder Elbow Surg* 1996;5:231-248.

A-9: A 66-year-old woman who previously underwent hemiarthroplasty 2 years ago for a fracture continues to have severe pain and loss of motion despite undergoing physical therapy. A radiograph is shown in Figure 7. What is the most likely reason that this patient has failed to improve her motion?

1. She was noncompliant in physical therapy.
2. The original surgery should have included resurfacing the glenoid.
3. The humeral head was too large.
4. The humeral component was placed too proud.
5. The tuberosities are malpositioned.

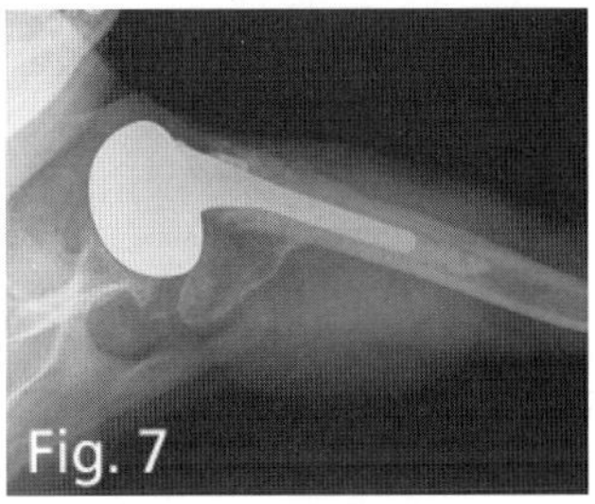
Fig. 7

PREFERRED RESPONSE: 5

DISCUSSION: The radiograph shows tuberosity malposition. The effect of improper prosthetic placement has also been associated with poor outcomes. However, the malposition of the tuberosity seen on the radiograph clearly explains loss of motion in this patient. It has been demonstrated that the functional results after hemiarthroplasty for three- and four-part proximal humeral fractures appear to be directly associated with tuberosity osteosynthesis. The most significant factor associated with poor and unsatisfactory postoperative functional results was malposition and/or migration of the tuberosities. Factors associated with a failure of tuberosity osteosynthesis in a recent study were poor initial position of the prosthesis, poor position of the greater tuberosity, and women older than 75 years (most likely with osteopenic bone). Greater tuberosity displacement has been identified by Tanner and Cofield as being the most common complication after prosthetic arthroplasty for proximal humeral fractures. Furthermore, Bigliani and associates examined the causes of failure after prosthetic replacement for proximal humeral fractures and found that although almost all failed cases had multiple causes, the most common single identifiable reason was greater tuberosity displacement.

REFERENCES: Bigliani LU, Flatow EL, McCluskey G, et al: Failed prosthetic replacement for displaced proximal humeral fractures. *Orthop Trans* 1991;15:747-748.

Boileau P, Krishnan SG, Tinsi L, et al: Tuberosity malposition and migration: Reasons for poor outcomes after hemiarthroplasty for displaced fractures of the proximal humerus. *J Shoulder Elbow Surg* 2002;11:401-412.

Tanner MW, Cofield RH: Prosthetic arthroplasty for fractures and fracture-dislocations of the proximal humerus. *Clin Orthop Relat Res* 1983;179:116-128.

A-10: A 40-year-old woman underwent an arthroscopic acromioplasty and mini-open rotator cuff repair 4 weeks ago. At follow-up examination, the incision is painful, erythematous, and draining fluid. The patient is febrile and has an elevated white blood cell count. What infectious organism should be under high suspicion of causing this outcome?

1. *Escherichia coli*
2. *Streptococcus viridans*
3. *Oxalophagus oxalicus*
4. *Propionibacterium acnes*
5. *Enterococcus faecalis*

PREFERRED RESPONSE: 4

(continued on next page)

(A-10: *continued*)

DISCUSSION: *Propionibacterium acnes* has been a leading cause of indolent shoulder infections. During shoulder arthroscopy, the arthroscopic fluid may actually dilute the shoulder preparation and lead to a higher rate of infection during subsequent mini-open rotator cuff repair surgery. The remaining bacteria listed are rarely associated with shoulder infections after arthroscopy.

REFERENCES: Herrera MF, Bauer G, Reynolds F, et al: Infection after mini-open rotator cuff repair. *J Shoulder Elbow Surg* 2002;11:605-608.

Nottage WM: Complications of arthroscopic shoulder surgery, in Norris TR, ed: *Orthopaedic Knowledge Update: Shoulder and Elbow*, ed 2. Rosemont, IL, American Academy of Orthopaedic Surgeons, 2002, pp 551-557.

A-11: A patient reports persistent anterior shoulder pain following a forceful external rotation injury to the shoulder. An MRI scan is shown in Figure 8. The patient remains symptomatic despite 3 months of nonsurgical management. Treatment should now consist of

1. repair of the superior labrum.
2. isolated supraspinatus repair.
3. biceps recentering.
4. subscapularis repair and biceps tenodesis.
5. subscapularis repair and recentering of the biceps tendon.

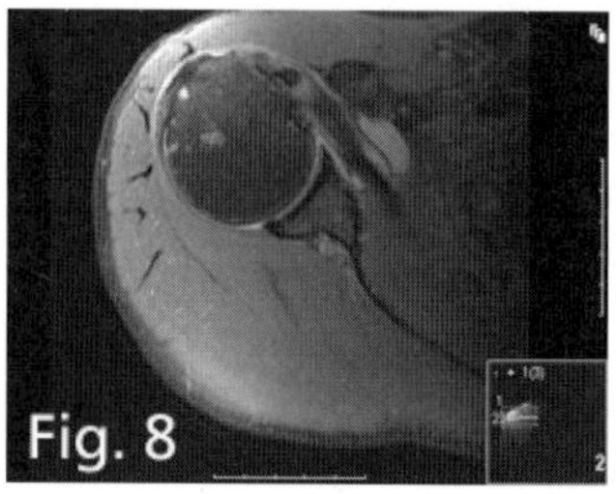

Fig. 8

PREFERRED RESPONSE: 4

DISCUSSION: The MRI scan reveals a subscapularis tear with a biceps that is out of the groove. Treatment in this patient is most predictable if the subscapularis is repaired. The biceps should either be tenodesed or tenotomized because it is unstable. Recentering of the biceps has been found to be unpredictable. Treatment of these lesions has been shown to have better results if the biceps is either released or tenodesed. This prevents recurrent biceps symptoms that can be source of surgical failure.

REFERENCES: Edwards TB, Walch G, Sirvenaux F, et al: Repair of tears of the subscapularis: Surgical technique. *J Bone Joint Surg Am* 2006;88:1-10.

Deutsch A, Altcheck DW, Veltri DM, et al: Traumatic tears of the subscapularis tendon: Clinical diagnosis, magnetic resonance imaging findings, and operative treatment. *Am J Sports Med* 1997;25:13-22.

Walch G, Nove-Josserand L, Boileau P, et al: Subluxations and dislocations of the tendon of the long head of the biceps. *J Shoulder Elbow Surg* 1998;7:100-108.

A-12: A 78-year-old woman falls onto her nondominant left elbow and sustains the injury shown in Figure 9. What treatment option allows her the shortest recovery time and highest likelihood of good function and range of motion?

1. Total elbow arthroplasty
2. Open reduction and internal fixation
3. Radial head arthroplasty
4. Sling and swathe
5. Bone stimulator

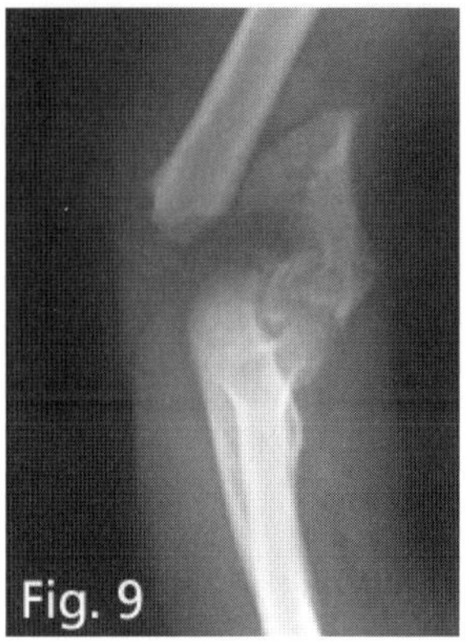

Fig. 9

PREFERRED RESPONSE: 1

DISCUSSION: Total elbow arthroplasty has become the treatment of choice for complex, comminuted distal humeral fractures in patients older than 70 years. It yields a faster recovery with more predictable functional outcomes, although limitations of lifting weight of more than 5 lb must be followed to avoid loosening.

REFERENCES: Kamineni S, Morrey BF: Distal humeral fractures treated with noncustom total elbow replacement. *J Bone Joint Surg Am* 2004;86:940-947.

Frankle MA, Herscovici D Jr, DiPasquale TG, et al: A comparison of open reduction and internal fixation and primary total elbow arthroplasty in the treatment of intra-articular distal humerus fractures in women older than age 65. *J Orthop Trauma* 2003;17:473-480.

A-13: A 45-year-old woman awakens with the acute onset of burning left shoulder pain that radiates toward the axilla. She denies any history of trauma. On examination, she is unable to abduct her arm but has full passive shoulder motion. Her sensation is intact. Cervical spine examination reveals full range of motion and a negative Spurling test. Radiographs and MRI studies are normal for the cervical spine and shoulder. What is the most likely diagnosis?

1. Cervical C6-7 radiculopathy
2. Impingement
3. Rotator cuff tear
4. Brachial neuritis
5. Adhesive capsulitis

PREFERRED RESPONSE: 4

DISCUSSION: The definition of brachial neuritis or Parsonage-Turner syndrome is a rare disorder of unknown etiology that causes pain or weakness of the shoulder and upper extremity. The loss of active motion excludes cervical C6-7 radiculopathy and impingement. A normal MRI scan and full passive motion exclude a rotator cuff tear and adhesive capsulitis, respectively.

REFERENCES: Misamore GW, Lehman DE: Parsonage-Turner syndrome (acute brachial neuritis). *J Bone Joint Surg Am* 1996;78:1405-1408.

McCarty EC, Tsairis P, Warren RF: Brachial neuritis. *Clin Orthop Relat Res* 1999;368:37-43.

A-14: A 72-year-old man who underwent total shoulder arthroplasty 2 years ago slipped on ice and fell on his shoulder 3 weeks ago. Immediately after falling he was unable to elevate his arm. Motor examination reveals deltoid 5-/5, subscapularis 5-/5, external rotation 4-/5, and supraspinatus 2/5. Radiographs are shown in Figures 10A and 10B. What is the most likely diagnosis?

1. Anterior shoulder dislocation
2. Humeral component loosening
3. Glenoid component loosening
4. Glenoid component catastrophic fracture
5. Rotator cuff tear

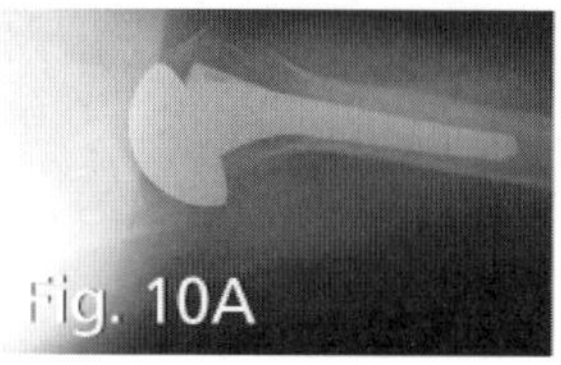
Fig. 10A

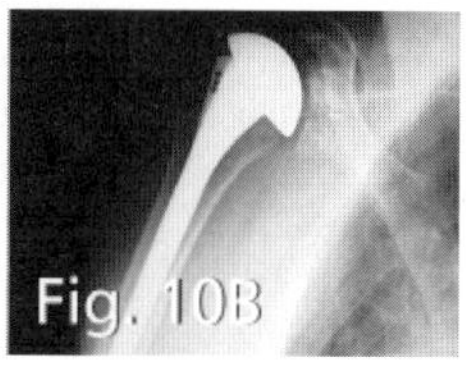
Fig. 10B

PREFERRED RESPONSE: 5

DISCUSSION: The patient has a traumatic rotator cuff tear. The history of the fall, the weakness on examination, and normal radiographic findings make a traumatic rotator cuff tear the most likely diagnosis. An MRI scan can be obtained to further evaluate the integrity of the rotator cuff. The axillary radiograph shows a reduced, nondislocated total shoulder arthroplasty. His radiographs show a well-seated humeral stem and no signs of loosening. The glenoid is a cemented all-polyethylene component with no evidence of radiolucent lines surrounding the cemented pegs. The polyethylene glenoid component is radiolucent; however, the space between the metallic humeral head and the glenoid bone is the thickness of the polyethylene glenoid component. If the humeral head were directly against the glenoid bone, then catastrophic fracture of the glenoid would be the working diagnosis.

REFERENCES: Hattrup SJ, Cofield RH, Cha SS: Rotator cuff repair after shoulder replacement. *J Shoulder Elbow Surg* 2006;15:78-83.

Sperling JW, Potter HG, Craig EV, et al: Magnetic resonance imaging of painful shoulder arthroplasty. *J Shoulder Elbow Surg* 2002;11:315-321.

A-15: A 39-year-old man has had persistent right shoulder pain for the past 6 months. A formal physical therapy program has failed to provide relief, and an injection several months ago provided only short-term relief. Examination reveals a positive Neer and Hawkins test. There is no instability and the neurovascular examination is normal. Arthroscopy reveals a partial rotator cuff tear on the bursal side measuring 60% of the tendon thickness. What is the next most appropriate step in management?

1. Arthroscopic débridement alone of the partial rotator cuff tear
2. Repair of the partial rotator cuff tear and subacromial decompression
3. Arthroscopic débridement combined with subacromial decompression
4. Arthroscopic subacromial decompression
5. Biceps tenotomy

PREFERRED RESPONSE: 2

DISCUSSION: Although arthroscopic débridement with or without subacromial decompression is a reasonable response, the patient has positive impingement signs. Several recent studies regarding the surgical treatment of partial rotator cuff tears have demonstrated good to excellent results after repair

(continued on next page)

(A-15: *continued*)

of tears involving more than 50% of the tendon thickness. This was shown specifically for bursal-sided tears and joint-side tears. Biceps tenotomy is not indicated in a young patient.

REFERENCES: Matava MJ, Purcell DB, Rudzki JR: Partial-thickness rotator cuff tears. *Am J Sports Med* 2005;33:1405-1417.

Fukuda H: The management of partial-thickness tears of the rotator cuff. *J Bone Joint Surg Br* 2003;85:3-11.

A-16: Figures 11A and 11B show the radiographs of a 47-year-old man who reports pain in both shoulders. He has a history of leukemia that was treated with chemotherapy and high-dose cortisone. What is the most reliable treatment option for pain relief in this patient?

1. Arthroscopic débridement
2. Arthrodesis
3. Resection arthroplasty
4. Hemiarthroplasty
5. Cortisone injection

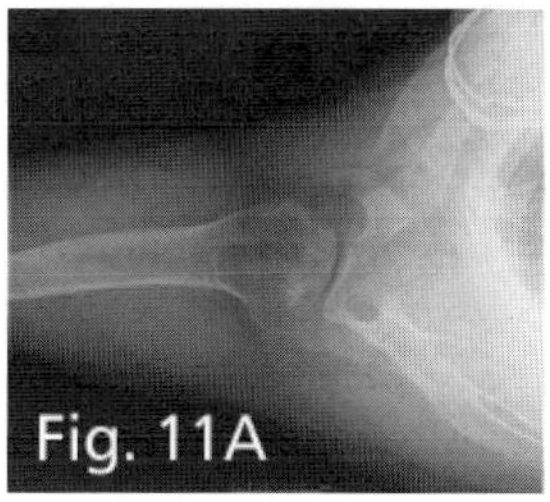
Fig. 11A

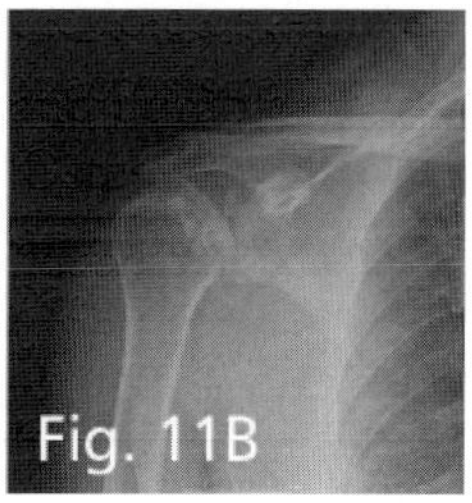
Fig. 11B

PREFERRED RESPONSE: 4

DISCUSSION: The radiographs reveal osteonecrosis with collapse. The most reliable and durable treatment for osteonecrosis of the humeral head remains prosthetic shoulder arthroplasty. Osteonecrosis of the humeral head may be seen after the use of steroids, and there is an increasing demand for shoulder arthroplasty in young people because of the use of high-dose steroids in chemotherapy regimens for the treatment of malignant tumors. The indications for most shoulder arthrodeses currently include post-traumatic brachial plexus injury, paralytic disorders in infancy, insufficiency of the deltoid muscle and rotator cuff, chronic infection, failed revision arthroplasty, severe refractory instability, and bone deficiency following resection of a tumor in the proximal aspect of the humerus. Clearly, the role of arthroscopy and related minimally invasive techniques in the treatment of humeral head osteonecrosis remains unknown.

REFERENCES: Hasan SS, Romeo AA: Nontraumatic osteonecrosis of the humeral head. *J Shoulder Elbow Surg* 2002; 11:281-298.

Hattrup SJ: Indications, technique, and results of shoulder arthroplasty in osteonecrosis. *Orthop Clin North Am* 1998;29:445-451.

Loebenberg MI, Plate AM, Zuckerman JD: Osteonecrosis of the humeral head. *Instr Course Lect* 1999;48:349-357.

A-17: Figure 12A shows the clinical photograph of a 36-year-old man who has left shoulder pain and dysfunction after undergoing a lymph node biopsy 2 years ago. The appearance of the shoulder during abduction and a wall push-up maneuver is shown in Figures 12B and 12C, respectively. Which of the following procedures provides the best pain relief and function?

1. Direct nerve repair
2. Sural nerve graft
3. Pectoralis major transfer
4. Levator scapula and rhomboid transfer
5. Scapulothoracic fusion

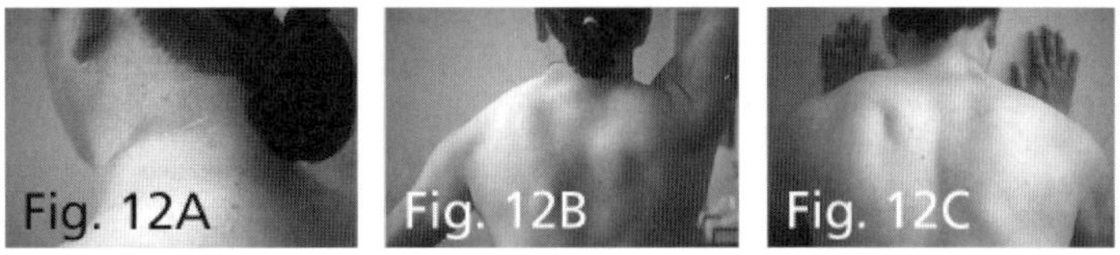
Fig. 12A Fig. 12B Fig. 12C

PREFERRED RESPONSE: 4

DISCUSSION: Injury to the spinal accessory nerve can occur after penetrating trauma to the shoulder. Blunt trauma may also cause loss of trapezius function. Most commonly, surgical dissection in the posterior triangle of the neck, such as lymph node biopsy, may expose the nerve to possible damage. Surgical repair of the nerve may be considered up to 1 year after injury; after this time muscle transfer is usually associated with a better functional outcome.

REFERENCES: Steinman SP, Spinner RJ: Nerve problems in the shoulder, in Rockwood CA, Matsen FA, Wirth MA, et al, eds: *The Shoulder*. Philadelphia, PA, WB Saunders, 2004, vol 2, pp 1013-1015.

Wiater JM, Bigliani LU: Spinal accessory nerve injury. *Clin Orthop Relat Res* 1999;368:5-16.

A-18: What is the most common cause of poor outcomes in patients who undergo total shoulder arthroplasty?

1. Loosening of the humeral component
2. Loosening of the glenoid component
3. Infection
4. Brachial plexus injury
5. Rotator cuff tear

PREFERRED RESPONSE: 5

DISCUSSION: In an article in the *Journal of Shoulder and Elbow Surgery*, 431 total shoulder arthroplasties were performed with a cemented all-polyethylene glenoid component between 1990 and 2000. Follow-up averaged 4.2 years. In total, 53 surgical complications occurred in 53 patients (12%). Of these, 32 were major complications (7.4%), with 17 of these requiring reoperation. Index complications in order of frequency included rotator cuff tearing, postoperative glenohumeral instability, and periprosthetic humeral fracture. Notably, glenoid and humeral component loosening requiring reoperation occurred in only one shoulder. Data from the contemporary patient group suggest that there are fewer complications of shoulder arthroplasty and less need for reoperation. Especially striking is the near-absence of component revision because of loosening or other mechanical factors. Complications involving the brachial plexus have been reported following total shoulder arthroplasty but are not as common of a cause for failure.

REFERENCES: Chin PY, Sperling JW, Cofield RH, et al: Complications of total shoulder arthroplasty: Are they fewer or different? *J Shoulder Elbow Surg* 2006;15:19-22.

Hasan SS, Leith JM, Campbell B, et al: Characteristics of unsatisfactory shoulder arthroplasties. J *Shoulder Elbow Surg* 2002;11:431-441.

A-19: A 49-year-old woman with serologically proven rheumatoid arthritis has Larsen grade II radiographic changes in the elbow. Examination reveals a preoperative arc of flexion of less than 90° and there is no instability. Nonsurgical management has failed to provide relief. What is the best treatment option?

1. Semiconstrained total elbow arthroplasty
2. Unlinked total elbow arthroplasty
3. Fascial arthroplasty
4. Open synovectomy
5. Arthroscopic synovectomy

PREFERRED RESPONSE: 5

DISCUSSION: Larsen grade I and II rheumatoid arthritis is best treated with synovectomy with arthroplasty reserved for later stages, especially in younger patients. Open synovectomy with or without a radial head excision has yielded good results for pain and function, with arthroscopic synovectomies yielding similar results. Arthroscopic synovectomy has been shown to be more effective in restoring function in patients with a flexion arc of less than 90°.

REFERENCES: Tanaka N, Sakahashi H, Hirose K, et al: Arthroscopic and open synovectomy of the elbow in rheumatoid arthritis. *J Bone Joint Surg Am* 2006;88:521-525.

Horiuchi K, Momohara S, Tomatsu T, et al: Arthroscopic synovectomy of the elbow in rheumatoid arthritis. *J Bone Joint Surg Am* 2002;84:342-347.

Maenpaa HM, Kuusela PP, Kaarela KK, et al: Reoperation rate after elbow synovectomy in rheumatoid arthritis. *J Shoulder Elbow Surg* 2003;12:480-483.

A-20: A 68-year-old woman with serologically proven rheumatoid arthritis underwent an open synovectomy and radial head resection 10 years ago. She now has severe pain that has failed to respond to nonsurgical management. Examination reveals a flexion arc of greater than 90°. Radiographs are shown in Figures 13A and 13B. What is the most appropriate management?

1. Semiconstrained total elbow arthroplasty
2. Unconstrained total elbow arthroplasty
3. Fascial arthroplasty
4. Open synovectomy
5. Arthroscopic synovectomy

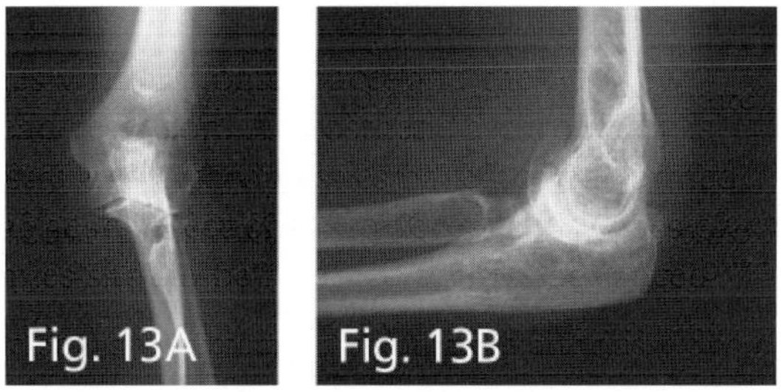
Fig. 13A Fig. 13B

PREFERRED RESPONSE: 1

DISCUSSION: The radiographs reveal severe arthritic changes with no joint space, and the AP view shows a progressive malalignment secondary to the radial head resection. A prosthetic arthroplasty is indicated given the severe arthritis (Larsen grade III). Unconstrained arthroplasties have not performed as well as semiconstrained arthroplasties after previous radial head resections. However, both types of arthroplasties performed better in native elbows. Synovectomies should be reserved for less advanced disease states.

REFERENCES: Whaley A, Morrey BF, Adams R: Total elbow arthroplasty after previous resection of the radial head and synovectomy. *J Bone Joint Surg Br* 2005;87:47-53.

(continued on next page)

(A-20: *continued*)

Maenpaa HM, Kuusela PP, Kaarela KK, et al: Reoperation rate after elbow synovectomy in rheumatoid arthritis. *J Shoulder Elbow Surg* 2003;12:480-483.

Schemitsch EH, Ewald FC, Thornhill TS: Results of total elbow arthroplasty after excision of the radial head and synovectomy in patients who had rheumatoid arthritis. *J Bone Joint Surg Am* 1996;78:1541-1547.

A-21: A football player sustains a traumatic anterior-inferior dislocation of the shoulder in the last game of the season. It is reduced 20 minutes later in the locker room. The patient is neurologically intact and has regained motion. If the patient undergoes arthroscopic evaluation, what finding is seen most consistently?

1. Superior labral detachment
2. Engaging Hill-Sachs lesion
3. Large glenoid rim fracture
4. Avulsion of the inferior glenohumeral ligament from the humerus
5. Avulsion of the anterior inferior glenoid labrum

PREFERRED RESPONSE: 5

DISCUSSION: In an acute first-time dislocation, arthroscopy has been shown to reveal a Bankart lesion in most shoulders. The classic finding of labral detachment from the anterior inferior glenoid along with occasional hemorrhage within the inferior glenohumeral ligament is the most common sequelae of a traumatic anterior inferior dislocation. Acute treatment, if chosen, is repair of the labral tissue back to the glenoid plus or minus any capsular plication to address potential plastic deformation of the glenohumeral ligament. Acute treatment of a patient sustaining a first-time dislocation remains controversial. The potential indications may be patients whose dislocation occurs at the end of a season and when the desire to minimize risk of future instability outweighs the risks of surgical intervention.

REFERENCES: Taylor DC, Arciero RA: Pathologic changes associated with shoulder dislocations: Arthroscopic and physical examination findings in first-time, traumatic anterior dislocations. *Am J Sports Med* 1997;25:306-311.

DeBerardino TM, Arciero RA, Taylor DC, et al: Prospective evaluation of arthroscopic stabilization of acute, initial anterior shoulder dislocations in young athletes: Two- to five-year follow-up. *Am J Sports Med* 2001;29:586-592.

Bottoni CR, Wilckens JH, DeBerardino TM, et al: A prospective, randomized evaluation of arthroscopic stabilization versus nonoperative treatment in patients with acute, traumatic, first-time shoulder dislocations. *Am J Sports Med* 2002;30:576-580.

A-22: A 42-year-old patient undergoes resection of the medial clavicle for painful sternoclavicular degenerative joint disease. The postoperative course is complicated by an increase in symptoms, a medial bump, and subjective tingling in the digits. A clinical photograph and radiograph are shown in Figures 14A and 14B. What is the most appropriate procedure at this time?

1. Semitendinosus figure-of-8 graft
2. Subclavius tendon transfer
3. Medial clavicular osteotomy
4. Medial clavicular resection
5. Sternoclavicular arthrodesis

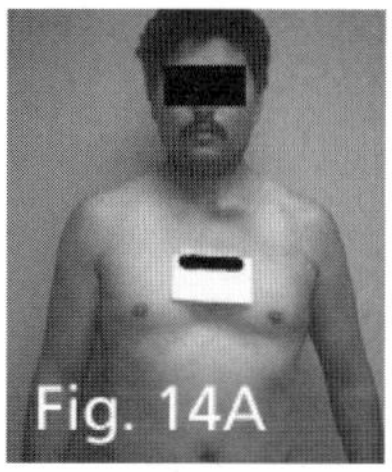
Fig. 14A

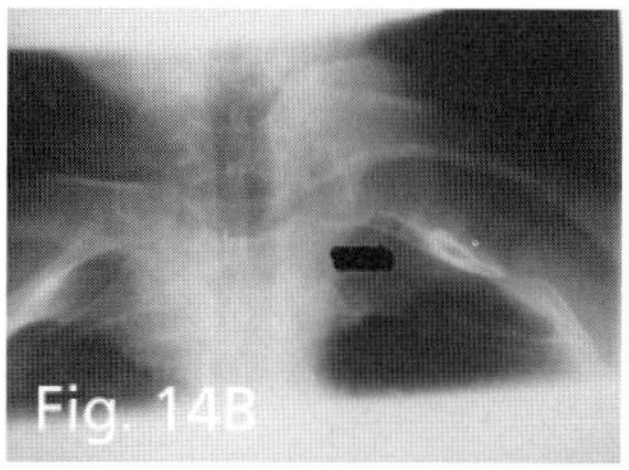
Fig. 14B

PREFERRED RESPONSE: 1

DISCUSSION: Improved peak-to-load failure data have been demonstrated by reconstruction of the sternoclavicular joint using a semitendinosis graft in a figure-of-8 pattern through the clavicle and manubrium. Resection of the medial clavicle, which compromises the integrity of the costoclavicular ligament, results in medial clavicular instability.

REFERENCES: Rockwood CA, Wirth MA: Disorders of the sternoclavicular joint, in Rockwood CA, Matsen FA, Wirth MA, et al, eds: *The Shoulder*. Philadelphia, PA, WB Saunders, 2004, vol 2, pp 608-609.

Spencer EE, Kuhn JE, Huston LJ, et al: Ligamentous restraints to anterior and posterior translation of the sternoclavicular joint. *J Shoulder Elbow Surg* 2002;11:43-47.

A-23: A 32-year-old woman sustained an elbow dislocation, and management consisted of early range of motion. Examination at the 3-month follow-up appointment reveals that she has regained elbow motion but has a weak pinch. A clinical photograph is shown in Figure 15. What is the most likely diagnosis?

1. Flexor pollicis longus rupture
2. Median nerve palsy
3. Ulnar nerve palsy
4. Anterior interosseous nerve palsy
5. Posterior interosseous nerve palsy

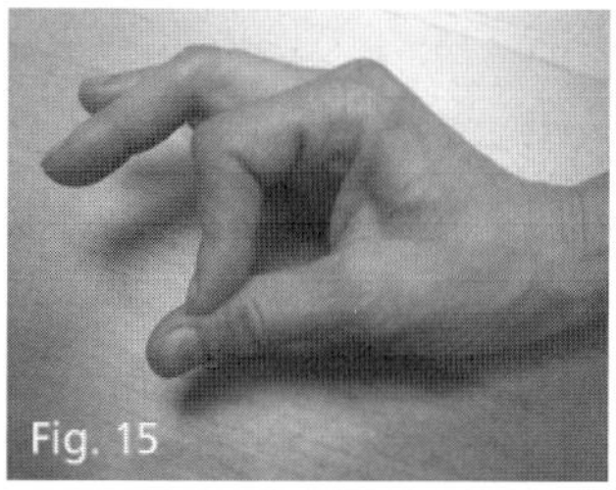
Fig. 15

PREFERRED RESPONSE: 4

DISCUSSION: The photograph shows the characteristic attitude of the hand when an anterior interosseous nerve palsy is present. The patient is unable to flex the interphalangeal joint to the joint of the thumb. Anterior interosseous nerve palsies are often misdiagnosed as tendon ruptures.

REFERENCES: Schantz K, Reigels-Nielsen P: The anterior interosseous nerve syndrome. *J Hand Surg Br* 1992;17: 510-512.

Seror P: Anterior interosseous nerve lesions: Clinical and electrophysiological features. *J Bone Joint Surg Br* 1996;78: 238-241.

A-24: What are the proposed biomechanical advantages of the Grammont reverse total shoulder arthroplasty when compared to a standard shoulder arthroplasty?

1. Lateralization of the center of rotation, lengthening the deltoid, and decreasing the deltoid moment arm
2. Lateralization of the center of rotation, shortening the deltoid, and decreasing acromial stress
3. Lateralization of the center of rotation, lengthening the deltoid, and increasing the transverse force couple
4. Medialization of the center of rotation, lengthening the deltoid, and increasing the deltoid moment arm
5. Medialization of the center of rotation, shortening the deltoid, and decreasing acromial stress

PREFERRED RESPONSE: 4

DISCUSSION: The Grammont reverse total shoulder arthroplasty is designed to medialize the center of rotation, thereby increasing the deltoid moment arm and lengthening the deltoid.

REFERENCES: Werner CM, Steinmann PA, Gilbert M: Treatment of painful pseudoparesis due to irreparable rotator cuff dysfunction with the Delta III reverse-ball-and-socket total shoulder prosthesis. *J Bone Joint Surg Am* 2005;87:z 1476-1486.

Rittmeister M, Kerschbaumer M: Grammont reverse total shoulder arthroplasty in patients with rheumatoid arthritis and nonreconstructible rotator cuff lesions. *J Shoulder Elbow Surg* 2001;10:17-22.

A-25: A 74-year-old woman with rheumatoid arthritis reports shoulder pain that has failed to respond to nonsurgical management. AP and axillary radiographs are shown in Figures 16A and 16B. Examination reveals active forward elevation to 120° and external rotation to 30°. What treatment option results in the most predictable pain relief and function?

1. Hemiarthroplasty
2. Arthroscopic débridement
3. Total shoulder arthroplasty with a cemented all-polyethylene glenoid component
4. Reverse total shoulder arthroplasty
5. Total shoulder arthroplasty with a metal-backed glenoid component

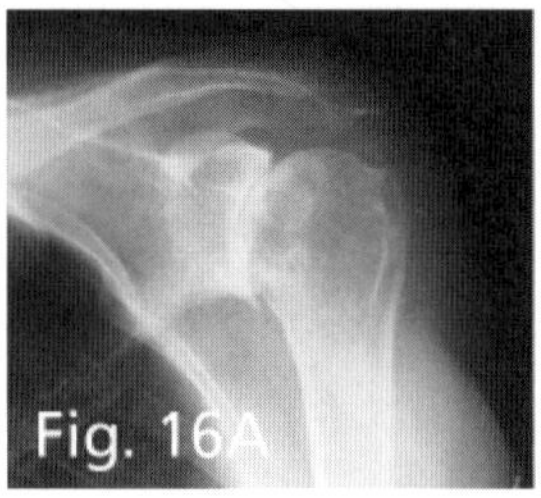
Fig. 16A

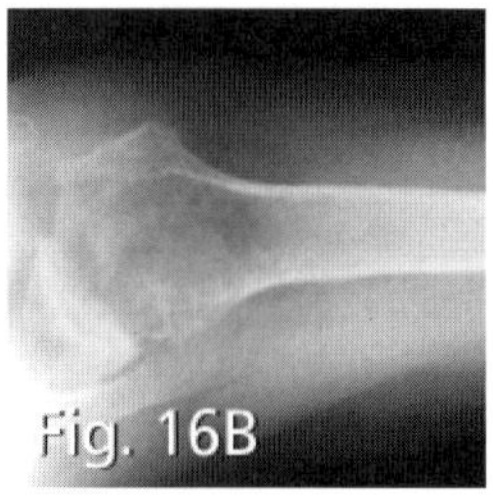
Fig. 16B

PREFERRED RESPONSE: 3

DISCUSSION: Most studies have shown that total shoulder arthroplasties yield better pain relief and improved forward elevation when compared to hemiarthroplasty in patients with rheumatoid arthritis. Although rotator cuff tears are more common in this patient population, this patient has good forward elevation and no significant superior migration of the humeral head; therefore, a reverse arthroplasty is not indicated. The arthritis is too advanced in this patient to consider arthroscopy, but in less advanced cases it can improve range of motion and decrease pain. Metal-backed glenoid components have shown higher rates of loosening.

(continued on next page)

(A-25: *continued*)

REFERENCES: Collin DN, Harryman DT II, Wirth MA: Shoulder arthroplasty for the treatment of inflammatory arthritis. *J Bone Joint Surg Am* 2004;86:2489-2496.

Baumgarten KM, Lashgari CM, Yamaguchi K: Glenoid resurfacing in shoulder arthroplasty: Indications and contraindications. *Instr Course Lect* 2004;53:3-11.

Martin SD, Zurakowski D, Thornhill TS: Uncemented glenoid component in total shoulder arthroplasty: Survivorship and outcomes. *J Bone Joint Surg Am* 2005;87:1284-1292.

A-26: A 69-year-old woman has just undergone an uncomplicated total shoulder arthroplasty for glenohumeral osteoarthritis. A press-fit humeral stem and a cemented all-polyethylene glenoid component were placed. At this point, what is the postoperative rehabilitation plan?

1. Maintain sling immobilization for 6 weeks, and then begin a global range-of-motion program.
2. Maintain sling immobilization for 3 weeks, and then begin a global range-of-motion program.
3. Immediately begin an active assisted range-of-motion program emphasizing forward elevation and external rotation to the side.
4. Immediately begin a passive range-of-motion program for forward elevation only; no external rotation is allowed for 6 weeks.
5. Immediately begin active range of motion in forward elevation and external rotation to the side with a progression to full rotator cuff strengthening in 3 weeks.

PREFERRED RESPONSE: 3

DISCUSSION: The patient needs to immediately begin an active assisted range-of-motion program emphasizing forward elevation and external rotation to the side. Sling immobilization without stretching for either 3 or 6 weeks will result in severe stiffness that will compromise her ultimate range of motion. Because she has a good-quality subscapularis tendon, there is no need to avoid beginning external rotation to the side. However, starting a strengthening program at 3 weeks risks tearing the subscapularis tendon repair. Active strengthening should not begin for 6 weeks postoperatively to allow the subscapularis tendon repair time to heal.

REFERENCES: Boardman ND III, Cofield RH, Bengston KA, et al: Rehabilitation after total shoulder arthroplasty. *J Arthroplasty* 2001;16:483-486.

Matsen FA III, Lippitt SB, Sidles JA, et al: *Practical Evaluation and Management of the Shoulder*. Philadelphia, PA, WB Saunders, 1994, pp 215-218.

A-27: A 22-year-old man who is right-handed fell off his motorcycle onto the tip of his right shoulder 2 weeks ago now and reports pain and difficulty raising his right arm. Examination reveals tenderness and gross movement over the lateral scapular spine and severe weakness during resisted abduction. A radiograph and three-dimensional CT scan are shown in Figures 17A and 17B. What is the next most appropriate step in management?

1. Open reduction and internal fixation
2. External bone stimulator
3. 90° abduction splint
4. Arthroscopic acromioplasty
5. Fragment excision

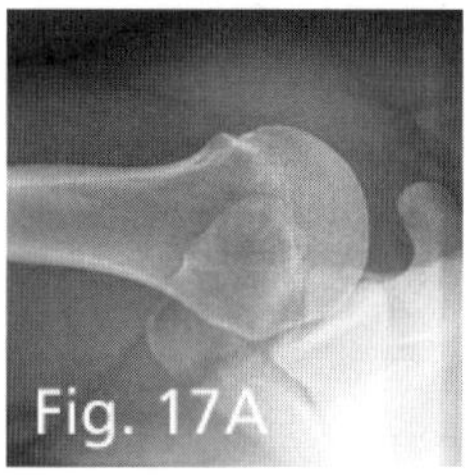
Fig. 17A

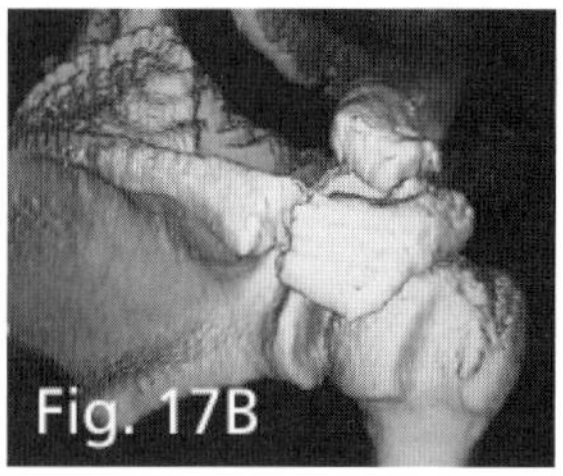
Fig. 17B

PREFERRED RESPONSE: 1

DISCUSSION: The patient has a displaced scapular spine fracture that has resulted in shoulder weakness from a poor deltoid lever arm. The downward tilt may lead to subacromial impingement and rotator cuff dysfunction. Open reduction and internal fixation would best allow normal deltoid and shoulder function. Bone stimulators and abduction bracing may lead to healing but in a malunited position. Arthroscopic acromioplasty and fragment excision should be avoided.

REFERENCES: Ogawa K, Naniwa T: Fractures of the acromion and the lateral scapular spine. *J Shoulder Elbow Surg* 1997;6:544-548.

Ada Jr, Miller ME: Scapular fractures: Analysis of 113 cases. *Clin Orthop Relat Res* 1991;269:174-180.

A-28: A 20-year-old man who plays minor league baseball has a symptomatic torn ulnar collateral ligament (UCL) in his pitching elbow. Nonsurgical management consisting of rest and physical therapy aimed at elbow strengthening has failed to provide relief. He has concomitant cubital tunnel symptoms that worsen while throwing. What is his best surgical option?

1. UCL repair and nighttime elbow extension splinting
2. UCL repair with ulnar nerve decompression in situ
3. Allograft UCL reconstruction with interference screws
4. Autograft UCL reconstruction with ulnar nerve transposition
5. Autograft UCL reconstruction using a docking technique

PREFERRED RESPONSE: 4

DISCUSSION: High-level pitchers with symptomatic UCL tears require reconstruction, with autograft being the best studied graft selection. With concomitant ulnar nerve symptoms, a simultaneous ulnar nerve transposition provides good results. Ligament "repairs" and allograft reconstructions have not shown good long-term results.

REFERENCES: Azar FM, Andrews JR, Wilk KE, et al: Operative treatment of ulnar collateral ligament injuries of the elbow in athletes. *Am J Sports Med* 2000;28:16-23.

Ciccotti MG, Jobe FW: Medial collateral ligament instability and ulnar neuritis in the athlete's elbow. *Instr Course Lect* 1999;48:383-391.

A-29: A patient who underwent open reduction and internal fixation of an olecranon fracture 2 months ago now reports painless limitation of motion. Examination reveals a well-healed incision and a flexion-extension arc from 40° to 80°. The patient has been performing home exercises. Radiographs are shown in Figures 18A and 18B. What is the most appropriate treatment?

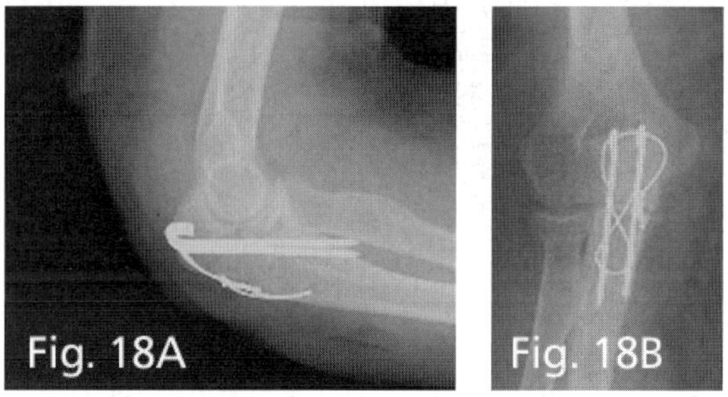

1. Continued observation and home therapy
2. Radiation therapy, followed by aggressive range-of-motion exercises
3. Formal physical therapy and static progressive splinting
4. Revision open reduction and internal fixation and capsular release
5. Manipulation under anesthesia

PREFERRED RESPONSE: 3

DISCUSSION: The radiographs do not show an articular malunion. Treatment is directed at the soft-tissue contracture and should begin with formal physical therapy and static progressive splinting. Radiation therapy is effective in the perioperative period and is indicated when ectopic bone formation is a concern.

REFERENCES: Morrey BF: The posttraumatic stiff elbow. *Clin Orthop Relat Res* 2005;431:26-35.

King GJ, Faber KJ: Posttraumatic elbow stiffness. *Orthop Clin North Am* 2000;31:129-143.

A-30: A 23-year-old patient who is a professional baseball pitcher reports shoulder pain and decreased velocity while pitching. Physical examination reveals a side-to-side internal rotation deficit of 25 degrees. The O'Brien sign is negative; Neer and Hawkins signs are negative. Rotator cuff strength is full. Radiographs are unremarkable. What is the next step in management?

1. MRI-arthrogram to evaluate the rotator cuff
2. Rotator cuff strengthening program
3. Posterior capsular stretching program
4. Shoulder arthroscopy with superior labrum anterior to posterior repair
5. Shoulder arthroscopy with posterior capsular release

PREFERRED RESPONSE: 3

DISCUSSION: Throwing athletes with symptomatic internal rotation deficits often benefit from an intensive posterior capsular stretching program. Patients who do not respond to nonsurgical management may benefit from an arthroscopic posterior capsular release.

REFERENCES: Wilk KE, Meister K, Andrews JR: Current concepts in rehabilitation of the overhead throwing athlete. *Am J Sports Med* 2002;30:136-151.

Myers JB, Laudner KG, Pasquale MR, et al: Glenohumeral range of motion deficits and posterior shoulder tightness in throwers with pathologic internal impingement. *Am J Sports Med* 2006;34:385-391.

A-31: A 72-year-old woman who is right-handed has severe pain in the right shoulder that has failed to respond to nonsurgical management. She reports night pain and significant disability. Examination reveals 30° of active forward elevation. An AP radiograph is shown in Figure 19. Which of the following treatment options will provide the best functional improvement?

1. Arthroscopic débridement
2. Arthroscopic rotator cuff repair
3. Hemiarthroplasty with rotator cuff repair
4. Total shoulder arthroplasty
5. Reverse shoulder arthroplasty

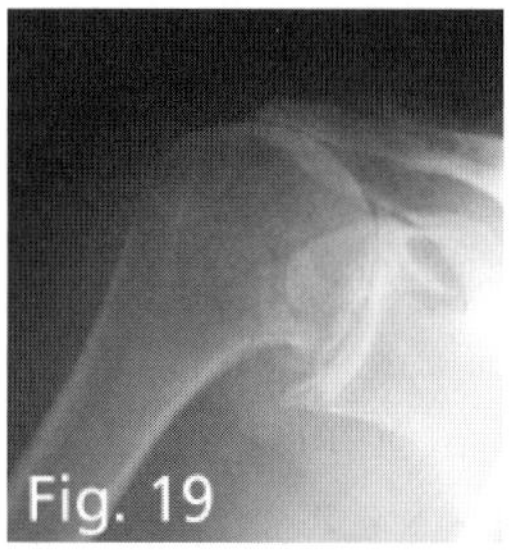
Fig. 19

PREFERRED RESPONSE: 5

DISCUSSION: The patient has end-stage rotator cuff tear arthropathy. The radiograph shows complete proximal humeral migration (acromiohumeral interval of 0 mm), severe glenohumeral arthritis, and acetabularization of the acromion. In addition, she has pseudoparalysis with active elevation of only 30°. Reverse shoulder arthroplasty affords her the best opportunity for pain relief and functional improvement. The other procedures have mixed results but typically are better for pain relief than they are for functional gains.

REFERENCES: Frankle M, Siegal S, Pupello D, et al: The reverse shoulder prosthesis for glenohumeral arthritis associated with severe rotator cuff deficiency: A minimum two-year follow-up study of sixty patients. *J Bone Joint Surg Am* 2005;87:1697-1705.

Werner CM, Steinmann PA, Gilbart M, et al: Treatment of painful pseudoparesis due to irreparable rotator cuff dysfunction with the Delta III reverse-ball-and-socket total shoulder prosthesis. *J Bone Joint Surg Am* 2005;87:1476-1486.

A-32: A 64-year-old man who was involved in a high-speed motor vehicle accident 6 weeks ago has been in the intensive care unit with a closed head injury. Examination reveals that his range of motion for external rotation to the side is –30°. Radiographs are shown in Figures 20A and 20B. What is the most likely diagnosis?

1. Adhesive capsulitis
2. Calcific tendinitis
3. Anterior shoulder dislocation
4. Posterior shoulder dislocation
5. Glenohumeral osteoarthritis

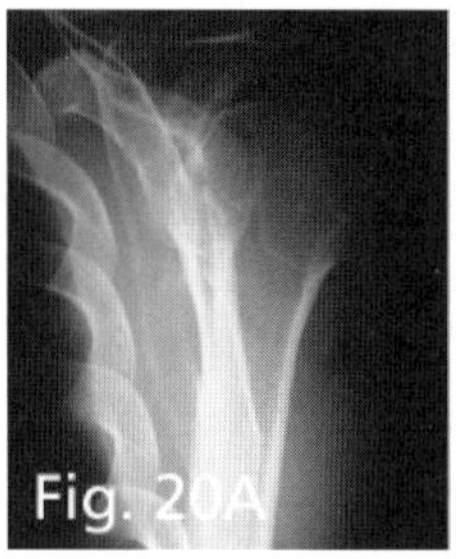
Fig. 20A

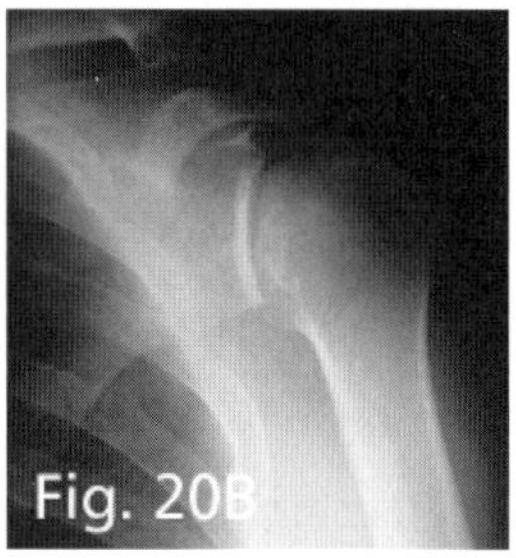
Fig. 20B

PREFERRED RESPONSE: 4

DISCUSSION: The patient has a posterior shoulder dislocation. The AP radiograph shows overlapping of the humeral head on the glenoid. The scapular Y view shows his humeral articular surface posterior to the glenoid. The posterior shoulder dislocation is frequently missed because the patient is comfortable in the "sling" position with the arm adducted and internally rotated across the abdomen. The marked restriction in external rotation on examination raises the suspicion of a posterior dislocation, adhesive capsulitis, or glenohumeral osteoarthritis. The posterior dislocation is diagnosed based on the radiographic findings. An axillary view or CT is recommended to better evaluate the dislocation.

REFERENCES: Robinson CM, Aderinto J: Posterior shoulder dislocations and fracture-dislocations. *J Bone Joint Surg Am* 2005;87:639-650.

Cicak N: Posterior dislocation of the shoulder. *J Bone Joint Surg Br* 2004;86:324-332.

A-33: A football lineman who sustained a traumatic injury while blocking during a game now reports that his shoulder is slipping while pass blocking. Examination reveals no apprehension in abduction and external rotation; however, he reports pain with posterior translation of the shoulder. He has full strength in external rotation, internal rotation, and supraspinatus testing. What is the pathology most likely responsible for his symptoms?

1. Anterior glenoid rim fracture tear
2. Anterior inferior labral tear
3. Posterior labral tear
4. Total capsular laxity
5. Osteochondral defect of the humeral head

PREFERRED RESPONSE: 3

DISCUSSION: Traumatic posterior instability is a common finding in football players, especially in the blocking positions as well as in the defensive linemen and linebackers. A traumatic blow to the outstretched arm results in posterior glenohumeral forces. Labral detachment at the glenoid rim is common. Patients report slipping or pain with posteriorly directed pressure. Rarely do these patients have true dislocations that require reduction; however, recurrent episodes of subluxation or pain are not uncommon. Posterior repair has been shown to be successful in the treatment of traumatic instability.

REFERENCES: Bottoni CR, Franks BR, Moore JH, et al: Operative stabilization of posterior shoulder instability. *Am J Sports Med* 2005;33:996-1002.

Williams RJ III, Strickland S, Cohen M, et al: Arthroscopic repair for traumatic posterior shoulder instability. *Am J Sports Med* 2003;31:203-209.

Kim SH, Ha KI, Park JH, et al: Arthroscopic posterior labral repair and capsular shift for traumatic unidirectional recurrent posterior subluxation of the shoulder. *J Bone Joint Surg Am* 2003;85:1479-1487.

A-34: A 17-year-old girl has multidirectional instability of the shoulder. What is the most appropriate initial management?

1. Immobilization in a sling and swathe
2. Open capsular shift
3. Arthroscopic capsular plication
4. Thermal capsulorrhaphy
5. Physical therapy and home exercises

PREFERRED RESPONSE: 5

DISCUSSION: Multidirectional instability of the shoulder is defined as symptomatic instability in two or more directions (anterior, posterior) but must include a component of inferior instability. Initial treatment should always include physical therapy and instruction in a home exercise program that emphasizes periscapular and rotator cuff strengthening to improve the dynamic stability of the glenohumeral joint. Immobilization has not been shown to be effective. Open capsular shift and arthroscopic capsular plication remain the surgical options when appropriate nonsurgical management fails (typically a minimum of 6 months of dedicated therapy and home program). Thermal capsulorrhaphy remains controversial but is not recommended by many clinicians because of reported complications including recurrent instability, axillary nerve injury, chondrolysis, and capsular injury.

(continued on next page)

(A-34: *continued*)

REFERENCES: Neer CS II, Foster CR: Inferior capsular shift for involuntary inferior and multidirectional instability of the shoulder: A preliminary report. *J Bone Joint Surg Am* 1980;62:897-908.

D'Alessandro DF, Bradley JP, Fleischli JE, et al: Prospective evaluation of thermal capsulorrhaphy for shoulder instability: Indications and results, two- to five-year follow-up. *Am J Sports Med* 2004;32:21-33.

Levine WN, Clark AM Jr, D'Alessandro DF, et al: Chondrolysis following arthroscopic thermal capsulorrhaphy to treat shoulder instability: A report of two cases. *J Bone Joint Surg Am* 2005;87:616-621.

Churchill RS, Matsen III FA: Shoulder instability, in Koval KJ, ed: *Orthopaedic Knowledge Update*, ed 7. Rosemont, IL, American Academy of Orthopaedic Surgeons, 2002, pp 278-279.

A-35: A previously healthy 65-year-old woman has a closed fracture of the right clavicle after falling down the basement stairs. Examination reveals good capillary refill in the digits of her right hand. Radial and ulnar pulses are 1+ at the right wrist compared with 2+ on the opposite side. In the arteriogram shown in Figure 21, the arrow is pointing at which of the following arteries?

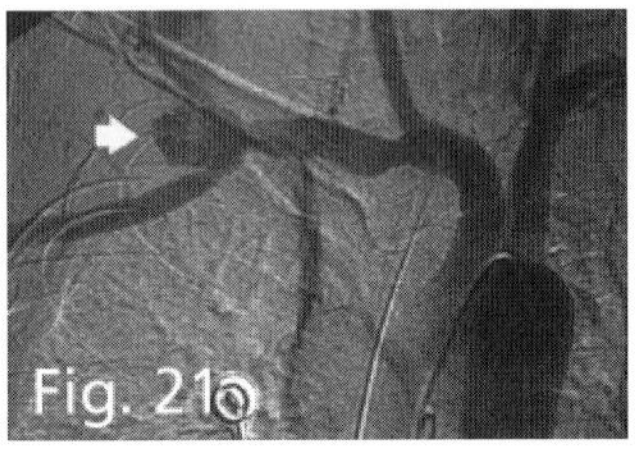
Fig. 21

1. Brachiocephalic
2. Innominate
3. Subclavian
4. Axillary
5. Circumflex scapular

PREFERRED RESPONSE: 4

DISCUSSION: The axillary artery commences at the first rib as a direct continuation of the subclavian artery and becomes the brachial artery at the lower border of the teres major. The arteriogram reveals a nonfilling defect in the third portion of the artery just distal to the subscapular artery. The complex arterial collateral circulation in this region often permits distal perfusion of the extremity despite injury.

REFERENCE: Radke HM: Arterial circulation of the upper extremity, in Strandness DE Jr, ed: *Collateral Circulation in Clinical Surgery*. Philadelphia, PA, WB Saunders, 1969, pp 294-307.

A-36: An adult patient has a closed humeral fracture that was treated nonsurgically and a concomitant radial nerve injury. Six weeks after injury, electromyography shows no evidence of recovery. Management should now consist of

1. exploration and neurolysis/repair.
2. MRI of the arm.
3. functional electrical stimulation.
4. radial nerve tendon transfers.
5. observation.

PREFERRED RESPONSE: 5

(continued on next page)

(A-36: *continued*)

DISCUSSION: In patients with radial nerve injuries with closed humeral fractures, it has been reported that 85% to 95% spontaneously recover. Based on this premise, most surgeons favor expectant management of these injuries. Even if there is no evidence of recovery at 6 weeks, repeat electromyography at 12 weeks is advocated. If there are no clinical or electromyographic signs of recovery at 6 months, exploration is recommended. If the nerve is in continuity at the time of exploration, nerve action potentials are useful in helping determine the need for neurolysis, excision, and grafting, or if excision and repair is the best option.

REFERENCES: Pollock FH, Drake D, Bovill EG, et al: Treatment of radial neuropathy associated with fractures of the humerus. *J Bone Joint Surg Am* 1981;63:239-243.

Mohler LR, Hanel DP: Closed fractures complicated by peripheral nerve injury. *J Am Acad Orthop Surg* 2006;14:32-37.

A-37: A 55-year-old man who works as a carpenter reports chronic right anterior shoulder pain and weakness. Examination reveals 90° of external rotation (with the arm at the side) compared to 45° on the left side. His lift-off examination is positive, along with a positive belly press finding. An MRI scan reveals a chronic, retracted atrophied subscapularis tendon. What is the most appropriate management of his shoulder pain and weakness?

1. Shoulder fusion
2. Arthroscopic subscapularis repair
3. Intra-articular corticosteroid injection
4. Open subscapularis repair
5. Pectoralis major transfer

PREFERRED RESPONSE: 5

DISCUSSION: Chronic subscapularis tendon ruptures preclude primary repair. In such instances, subcoracoid pectoralis major tendon transfers may improve function and diminish pain. The subcoracoid position of the transfer allows redirection of the pectoralis major in a direction re-creating the vector of the subscapularis tendon. Shoulder fusion is a salvage procedure, and corticosteroid injection may reduce pain but will not improve function.

REFERENCES: Jost B, Puskas GJ, Lustenberger A, et al: Outcome of pectoralis major transfer for the treatment of irreparable subscapularis tears. *J Bone Joint Surg Am* 2003;85:1944-1951.

Resch H, Povacz P, Ritter E, et al: Transfer of the pectoralis major muscle for the treatment of irreparable rupture of the subscapularis tendon. *J Bone Joint Surg Am* 2000;82:372-382.

A-38: With the arm abducted 90° and fully externally rotated, which of the following glenohumeral ligaments resists anterior translation of the humerus?

1. Coracohumeral
2. Superior glenohumeral
3. Middle glenohumeral
4. Anterior band of the inferior glenohumeral ligament complex
5. Posterior band of the inferior glenohumeral ligament complex

PREFERRED RESPONSE: 4

DISCUSSION: With the arm in the abducted, externally rotated position, the anterior band of the inferior glenohumeral ligament complex moves anteriorly, preventing anterior humeral head translation. Both the coracohumeral ligament and the superior glenohumeral ligament restrain the humeral head to inferior translation of the adducted arm, and to external rotation in the adducted position. The middle glenohumeral ligament is a primary stabilizer to anterior translation with the arm abducted to 45°. The posterior band of the inferior glenohumeral ligament complex resists posterior translation of the humeral head when the arm is internally rotated.

REFERENCES: Harryman DT II, Sidles JA, Harris SL, et al: The role of the rotator interval capsule in passive motion and stability of the shoulder. *J Bone Joint Surg Am* 1992;74:53-66.

Wang VM, Flatow EL: Pathomechanics of acquired shoulder instability: A basic science perspective. *J Shoulder Elbow Surg* 2005;14:2S-11S.

A-39: Figure 22 shows the radiograph of a 75-year-old woman who has had right shoulder pain, difficulty sleeping on the affected arm, and difficulties performing activities of daily living for the past 6 weeks. Initial nonsurgical management includes analgesics, a subacromial cortisone injection, and gentle range-of-motion exercises. However, these modalities have failed to provide relief, and the patient reports that she is unable to elevate her arm. Her pain is worse and she would like the most reliable treatment method for pain relief and functional improvement. What is the best surgical treatment?

1. Reverse shoulder arthroplasty
2. Hemiarthroplasty
3. Resurfacing of the humeral head
4. Arthroscopic debridement
5. Shoulder fusion

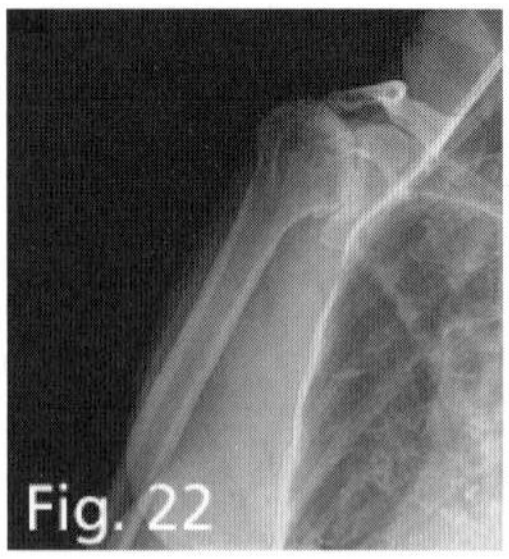

PREFERRED RESPONSE: 1

DISCUSSION: The authors of several studies conducted in Europe have reported promising results in the short- and medium-term with use of a reversed or inverted shoulder implant. The most recent investigation, a multicenter study in Europe in which 77 patients (80 shoulders) with glenohumeral osteoarthritis and a massive rupture of the rotator cuff were treated with the Delta III prosthesis, described an improvement in the mean constant score of 42 points, an increase of 65° in forward elevation, and minimal or no pain in 96% of the patients. Hemiarthroplasty, the "nonconstrained" option, has long been the standard of care for rotator cuff tear arthropathy. However, careful examination of the literature reveals that the results have not been uniform.

(continued on next page)

(A-39: *continued*)

REFERENCES: Favard L, Lautmann S, Sirveaux F, et al: Hemiarthroplasty versus reverse arthroplasty in the treatment of osteoarthritis with massive rotator cuff tear, in Walch G, Boileau P, Mole D, eds: *2000 Shoulder Prosthesis Two to Ten Year Follow-Up*. Montpellier, France, Sauramps Medical, 2001, pp 261-268.

Frankle M, Siegal S, Pupello D, et al: The reverse shoulder prosthesis for glenohumeral arthritis associated with severe rotator cuff deficiency: A minimum two-year follow-up study of sixty patients. *J Bone Joint Surg Am* 2005;87:1697-1705.

Werner CM, Steinmann PA, Gilbart M, et al: Treatment of painful pseudoparesis due to irreparable rotator cuff dysfunction with the Delta III reverse-ball-and-socket total shoulder prosthesis. *J Bone Joint Surg Am* 2005;87:1476-1486.

A-40: A 55-year-old man sustained an elbow dislocation during a fall. Postreduction radiographs are shown in Figures 23A and 23B. What is the best course of management?

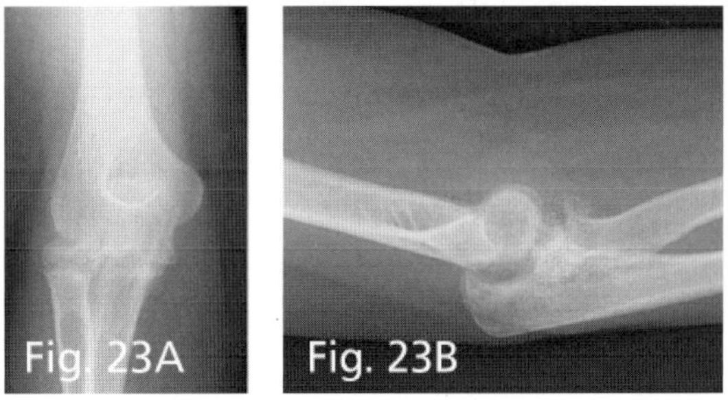
Fig. 23A Fig. 23B

1. Closed reduction and casting for 4 weeks
2. Closed reduction and bracing with immediate range of motion
3. Open reduction, lateral collateral ligament repair, and open reduction and internal fixation or metallic replacement of the radial head
4. Open reduction, radial head Silastic arthroplasty, and lateral collateral ligament repair
5. Open reduction, lateral collateral ligament repair, and radial head excision

PREFERRED RESPONSE: 3

DISCUSSION: The radiographs show an elbow dislocation associated with a comminuted radial head fracture. In the setting of comminution and instability, factures of the radial head are best managed with an arthroplasty rather than open reduction and internal fixation. Resection of the radial head will worsen the instability and is not recommended. Silastic radial head replacements are contraindicated.

REFERENCES: Hildebrand KA, Patterson SD, King GJ: Acute elbow dislocations: Simple and complex. *Orthop Clin North* Am 1999;30:63-79.

O'Driscoll SW, Jupiter JB, King GJ, et al: The unstable elbow. *Instr Course Lect* 2001;50:89-102.

A-41: Osteochondritis dissecans of the capitellum is a source of elbow pain and most commonly occurs in what patient population?

1. Swimmers and divers
2. Football lineman
3. Rugby players
4. Gymnasts and throwing athletes
5. Cyclists

(continued on next page)

(A-41: continued)

PREFERRED RESPONSE: 4

DISCUSSION: The etiology of osteochondritis dissecans of the capitellum is somewhat unclear. However, trauma has been implicated in this disease process. Gymnasts who load their upper extremities during tumbling, and throwing athletes with repetitive trauma during the throwing motion are common patient subgroups in which osteochondritis dissecans of the elbow is seen. This often occurs in the adolescent age population.

REFERENCES: Baumgarten TE, Andrews JR, Satterwhite YE: The arthroscopic classification and treatment of osteochondritis dissecans of the capitellum. *Am J Sports Med* 1998;26:520-523.

Takahara M, Ogino T, Fukushima S, et al: Nonoperative treatment of osteochondritis dissecans of the humeral capitellum. *Am J Sports Med* 1999;27:728-732.

A-42: What are the two terminal branches of the lateral cord of the brachial plexus?

1. Musculocutaneous and median
2. Musculocutaneous and axillary
3. Median and axillary
4. Ulnar and median
5. Ulnar and medial pectoral

PREFERRED RESPONSE: 1

DISCUSSION: The lateral cord divides into the musculocutaneous and median nerves. The posterior cord terminates into the axillary and radial nerves. The medial cord divides into the ulnar and median nerves.

REFERENCES: Hollinshead WH: *Anatomy for Surgeons*, ed 3. Philadelphia, PA, Harper and Row, 1982, pp 228-236. Shin AY, Spinner RJ, Steinmann SP, et al: Adult traumatic brachial plexus injuries. *J Am Acad Orthop Surg* 2005;13: 382-396.

A-43: A 32-year-old patient reports progressively increasing pain and stiffness after undergoing arthroscopic shoulder stabilization 1 year ago. The stabilization procedure was a Bankart repair with anchor fixation and supplemented with the heat probe. Radiographs are shown in Figures 24A and 24B. What is the most likely diagnosis?

1. Subscapularis failure
2. Frozen shoulder
3. Recurrent instability
4. Loose body
5. Chondrolysis

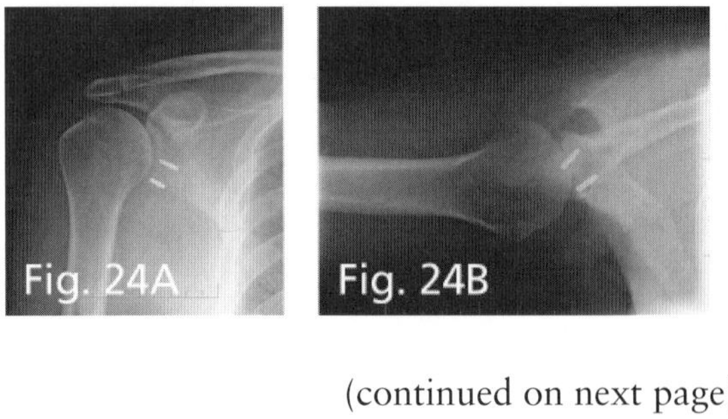

(continued on next page)

(A-43: *continued*)

PREFERRED RESPONSE: 5

DISCUSSION: Postshoulder stabilization chondrolysis is a rare but devastating complication. It has been implicated with the use of the radiofrequency heat probe in some patients.

REFERENCES: Levine WN, Clark AM Jr, D'Alessandro DF, et al: Chondrolysis following arthroscopic thermal capsulorrhaphy to treat shoulder instability: A report of two cases. *J Bone Joint Surg Am* 2005;87:616-621.

Petty DH, Jazrawi LM, Estrada LS, et al: Glenohumeral chondrolysis after shoulder arthroscopy: Case reports and review of the literature. *Am J Sports Med* 2004;32:509-515.

A-44: Acute redislocation of the glenohumeral joint is a complication that occurs following a first-time dislocation. This is most often seen with

1. subglenoid dislocation.
2. subcoracoid dislocation.
3. fracture of the greater tuberosity.
4. fracture of the greater tuberosity and glenoid rim.
5. pediatric patients.

PREFERRED RESPONSE: 4

DISCUSSION: Redislocation following acute dislocation occurs in approximately 3% of patients. This redislocation tends to occur in middle-aged and elderly patients. A higher incidence of redislocation occurs when there are accompanying fractures of the glenoid rim and the greater tuberosity.

REFERENCES: Robinson CM, Kelly M, Wakefield AE: Redislocation of the shoulder during the first six weeks after a primary anterior dislocation: Risk factors and results of treatment. *J Bone Joint Surg Am* 2002;84:1552-1559.

Bigliani LU, Newton PM, Steinmann SP, et al: Glenoid rim lesions associated with recurrent anterior dislocation of the shoulder. *J Sports Med* 1998;26:41-45.

A-45: A 51-year-old woman is seen for evaluation of chronic supraspinatus and infraspinatus tendon tears. Three years ago, in an attempted repair the surgeon was unable to repair the supraspinatus and infraspinatus tendon tears. Currently, the patient has a marked amount of pain, reduced range of motion, and weakness. Examination reveals anterosuperior escape. Radiographs show no signs of arthritic changes. You are considering a latissimus dorsi tendon transfer. During the discussion, you mention that

1. she can expect to have good pain relief following surgery.
2. active forward elevation and external rotation are reliably obtained postoperatively.
3. with her current anterosuperior escape, she is likely to have a poor surgical result.
4. postoperatively, significant muscular atrophy in the latissimus dorsi commonly occurs.
5. no advancement in glenohumeral arthritic changes should occur following surgery.

(continued on next page)

(A-45: *continued*)

PREFERRED RESPONSE: 3

DISCUSSION: Latissimus dorsi tendon transfer is considered a surgical option for treatment in patients with chronic supraspinatus and infraspinatus tendon tears. Preoperative subscapularis function is necessary for good clinical results. Additionally, men with active elevation to shoulder level and active external rotation to 20° have predictably good results. Women with active shoulder elevation limited to below chest level have poor results from this procedure and should not be considered candidates. Postoperatively they lack pain control, active elevation, and active external rotation. Muscular atrophy in the latissimus dorsi does not occur, and glenohumeral arthritic changes frequently develop postoperatively.

REFERENCES: Gerber C, Maquieira G, Espinosa N: Latissimus dorsi transfer for the treatment of irreparable rotator cuff tears: Factors affecting outcome. *J Bone Joint Surg Am* 2006;88:113-120.

Iannotti JP, Hennigan S, Herzog R, et al: Latissimus dorsi tendon transfer for irreparable posterosuperior rotator cuff tears. *J Bone Joint Surg Am* 2006;88:342-348.

A-46: A 67-year-old woman is seen in the emergency department after falling at home. Radiographs before and after treatment are shown in Figures 25A and 25B, respectively. Which of the following best explains the 8-week postinjury clinical findings seen in Figure 25C?

1. Axillary nerve palsy
2. Spinal accessory nerve palsy
3. Deltoid avulsion
4. Rotator cuff tear
5. Unreduced posterior glenohumeral dislocation

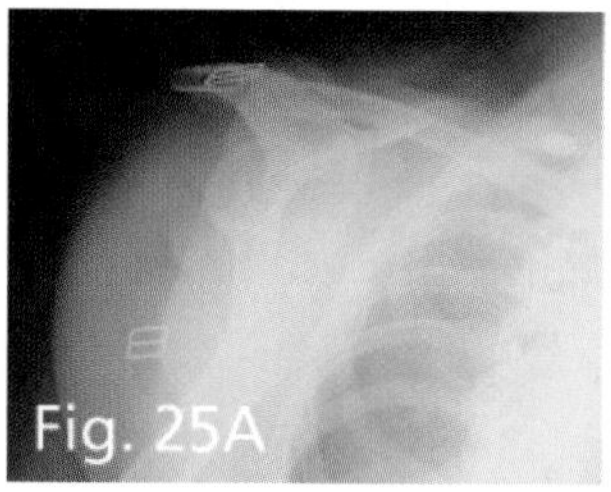
Fig. 25A

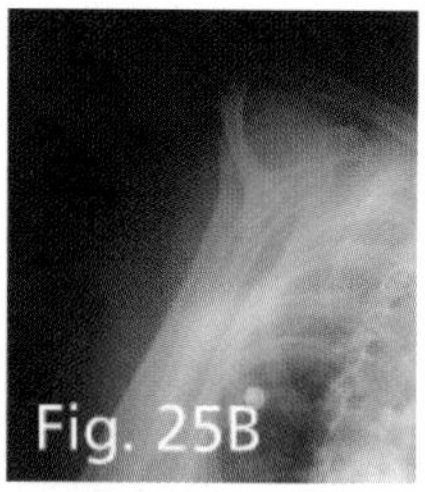
Fig. 25B

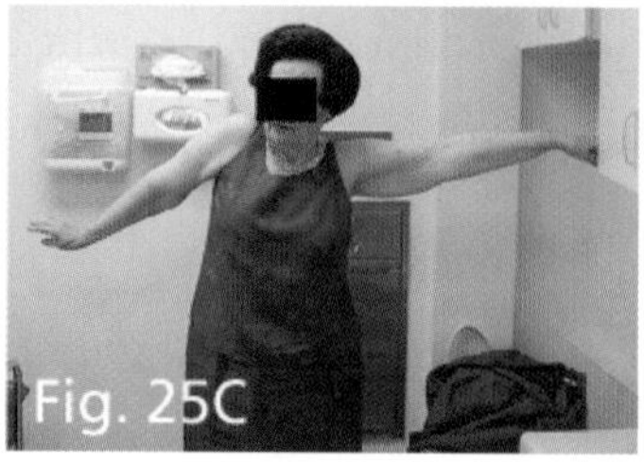
Fig. 25C

PREFERRED RESPONSE: 4

DISCUSSION: Patients older than 40 years at the time of initial anterior dislocation have low rates of redislocation; however, 15% of these patients experience a rotator cuff tear. Moreover, there is a dramatic increase (up to 40%) in the incidence of rotator cuff tears in patients older than 60 years. Axillary nerve injury may occur but is less common than rotator cuff tear.

REFERENCES: Churchill RS, Matsen III FA: Shoulder instability, in Koval KJ, ed: *Orthopaedic Knowledge Update*, ed 7. Rosemont, IL, American Academy of Orthopaedic Surgeons, 2002, pp 273-284.

Neviaser RJ, Neviaser TJ, Neviaser JS: Anterior dislocation of the shoulder and rotator cuff rupture. *Clin Orthop Relat Res* 1993;291:103-106.

A-47: Which of the following has been associated with a decreased rate of glenoid component radiolucent lines?

1. A curve-backed pegged cemented polyethylene glenoid component
2. A curve-backed keeled cemented polyethylene glenoid component design
3. A flat-backed keeled cemented polyethylene glenoid component
4. An oversized pegged cemented glenoid component
5. A superiorly placed pegged glenoid component

PREFERRED RESPONSE: 1

DISCUSSION: According to a recent study, cemented pegged glenoid components had fewer radiolucent lines initially and at 2-year follow-up when compared to a cemented keeled design. Curve-backed designs have also shown fewer radiolucent lines when compared to flat-backed designs. Oversizing the glenoid can lead to impaired rotator cuff function and decreased range of motion. An off-centered glenoid can lead to early loosening.

REFERENCES: Gartsman GM, Elkousy HA, Warnock KM, et al: Radiographic comparison of pegged and keeled glenoid components. *J Shoulder Elbow Surg* 2005;14:252-257.

Szabo I, Buscayret F, Edwards TB, et al: Radiographic comparison of flat-back and convex-back glenoid components in total shoulder arthroplasty. *J Shoulder Elbow Surg* 2005;14:636-642.

Mileti J, Boardman ND III, Sperling JW, et al: Radiographic analysis of polyethylene glenoid components using modern cementing techniques. *J Shoulder Elbow Surg* 2004;13:492-498.

A-48: Figure 26 shows the radiograph of a 42-year-old man who is a construction worker and who has pain and limited motion in his dominant elbow. Management consisting of NSAIDs and cortisone has failed to provide relief. What is the next most appropriate step in treatment?

1. Unlinked elbow arthroplasty
2. Linked elbow arthroplasty
3. Interposition arthroplasty
4. Arthroscopic or open débridement
5. Radial head excision

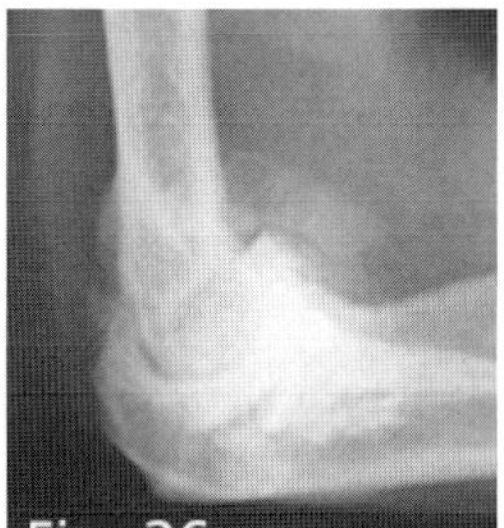
Fig. 26

PREFERRED RESPONSE: 4

DISCUSSION: The patient has symptomatic primary osteoarthritis of the elbow with multiple loose bodies. Given his age and occupation, an elbow arthroplasty is not an option. Arthroscopic débridement and removal of loose bodies has been shown to be effective for osteoarthritis of the elbow.

REFERENCES: Gramstad GD, Galatz LM: Management of elbow osteoarthritis. *J Bone Joint Surg Am* 2006;88:421-430.

Steinmann SP, King GJ, Savoie FH III, et al: Arthroscopic treatment of the arthritic elbow. *J Bone Joint Surg Am* 2005;87:2114-2121.

A-49: A 61-year-old woman with a long-standing history of rheumatoid arthritis reports progressive elbow pain for the past 12 months. She denies any recent trauma to the elbow; however, she notes increasing pain and decreased joint motion that are now compromising her function. Radiographs are shown in Figures 27A and 27B. What is the most appropriate treatment at this time?

1. Physical therapy for restoration of motion
2. Elbow arthroscopy, removal of loose bodies, excision of osteophytes, and capsular release (osteocapsulectomy)
3. Elbow arthroscopy and synovectomy
4. Constrained total elbow arthroplasty
5. Semiconstrained total elbow arthroplasty

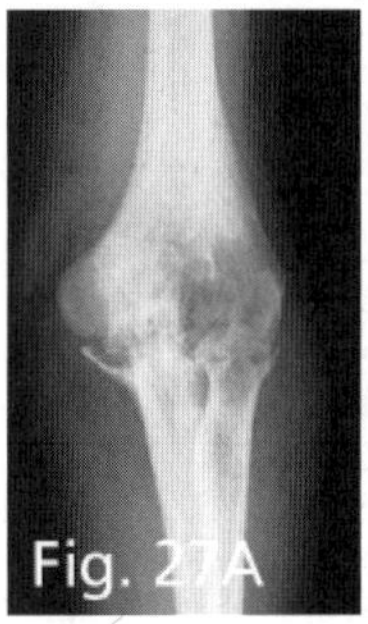

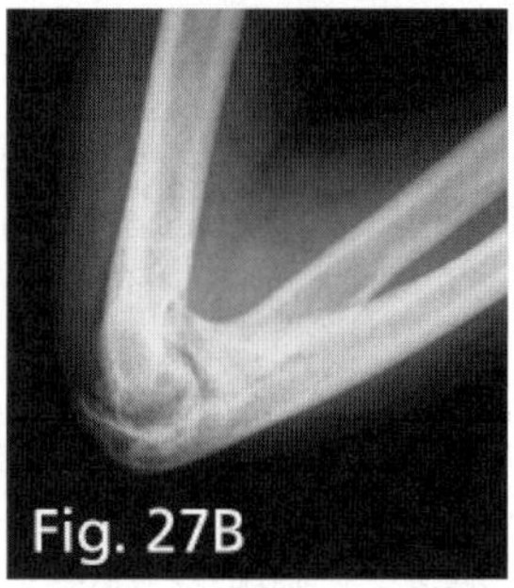

PREFERRED RESPONSE: 5

DISCUSSION: The patient has end-stage arthritis of the elbow with advanced joint destruction. At this point, nonsurgical management is unlikely to provide much relief of symptoms. Arthroscopic procedures can provide relief, but it is likely to be incomplete and unpredictable. The most reliable surgical option is total elbow arthroplasty. Currently, semiconstrained components are generally preferred because constrained components have been associated with a high rate of early prosthetic loosening.

REFERENCES: Little CP, Graham AJ, Karatzas G, et al: Outcomes of total elbow arthroplasty for rheumatoid arthritis: Comparative study of three implants. *J Bone Joint Surg Am* 2005;87:2439-2448.

Little CP, Graham AJ, Carr AJ: Total elbow arthroplasty: A systemic review of the literature in the English language until the end of 2003. *J Bone Joint Surg Br* 2005;87:437-444.

A-50: What neurovascular structure is at greatest risk when creating a proximal anterolateral elbow arthroscopy portal?

1. Lateral antebrachial cutaneous nerve
2. Radial nerve
3. Posterior interosseous nerve
4. Median nerve
5. Brachial artery

PREFERRED RESPONSE: 2

DISCUSSION: The radial nerve is 4 to 7 mm from the anterolateral portal, which is placed 1 cm anterior and 3 cm proximal to the lateral epicondyle. The posterior interosseous nerve can lie 1 to 14 mm from the portal site.

REFERENCES: Andrews JR, Carson WG: Arthroscopy of the elbow. *Arthroscopy* 1985;1:97-107.

Lynch G, Meyers JF, Whipple TL, et al: Neurovascular anatomy and elbow arthroscopy: Inherent risks. *Arthroscopy* 1986;2:190-197.

Hand and Wrist

Q-1: When performing surgical excision of the lesion shown in the MRI scan in Figure 1, what nerve is most likely at risk?

1. Deep branch of the ulnar nerve
2. Anterior interosseous branch of the median nerve
3. Recurrent branch of the median nerve
4. Recurrent branch of the ulnar nerve
5. Palmar cutaneous branch of the ulnar nerve

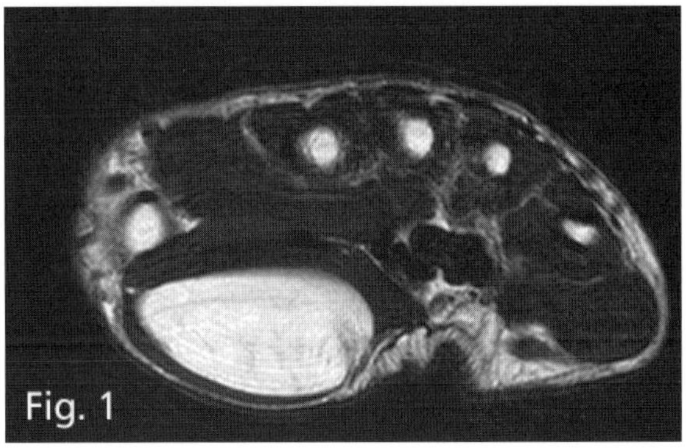

Fig. 1

Q-2: A 21-year-old man sustains multiple gunshot wounds to his right upper extremity. He cannot extend his digits or his thumb but can extend and radially deviate his wrist. An injury to the radial nerve or one of its branches has most likely occurred at which of the following locations?

1. Spiral groove of the humerus
2. Midshaft of the radius
3. Radial neck
4. Anatomic neck of the humerus
5. Surgical neck of the humerus

Q-3: The attachments of the transverse carpal ligament include which of the following structures?

1. Scaphoid and the ulna
2. Trapezium and the hook of the hamate
3. Trapezium and the triquetrum
4. Trapezoid and the hook of the hamate
5. Trapezoid and the pisiform

Q-4: A patient undergoes the procedure shown in Figure 2. An important part of this procedure is preservation of what wrist ligament?

1. Radioscaphocapitate
2. Scapholunate interosseous
3. Ulnotriquetral
4. Volar radioulnar
5. Deep proximal capitohamate

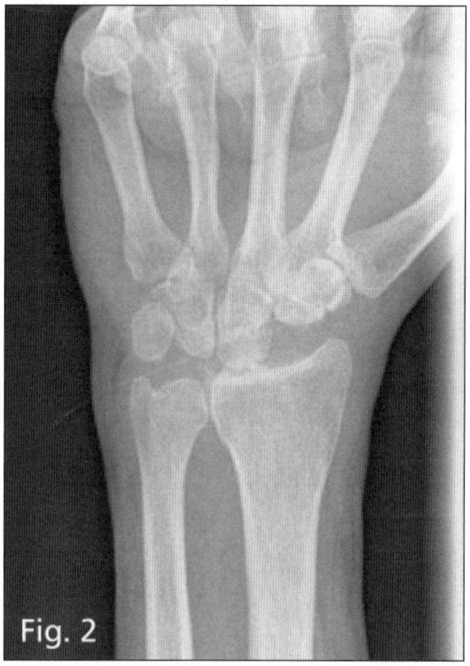

Fig. 2

Q-5: A 37-year-old patient with type I diabetes mellitus has a flexor tenosynovitis of the thumb flexor tendon sheath following a kitchen knife puncture wound to the volar aspect of the thumb. Left unattended, this infection will likely first spread proximally, creating an abscess in which of the following spaces of the palm?

1. Central space
2. Hypothenar space
3. Carpal tunnel
4. Posterior adductor space
5. Thenar space

Q-6: New painful paresthesias near the site of the incision after an ulnar nerve transposition is the result of injury to what nerve?

1. Medial antebrachial cutaneous
2. Lateral antebrachial cutaneous
3. Posterior antebrachial cutaneous
4. Medial brachial cutaneous
5. Dorsal antebrachial cutaneous

Q-7: Which of the following best describes the relationship of the median nerve to the flexor carpi radialis tendon just proximal to the carpal canal?

1. Median nerve is volar and ulnar
2. Median nerve is radial and volar
3. Median nerve is dorsal and ulnar
4. Median nerve is dorsal and radial
5. Median nerve is volar and radial

Q-8: Which of the following muscles has dual innervation?

1. Pronator teres
2. Flexor digitorum superficialis
3. Coracobrachialis
4. Latissimus dorsi
5. Brachialis

Q-9: A 21-year-old man who was injured in a snowboarding accident 18 months ago now reports wrist pain. An MRI scan is shown in Figure 3. Based on the image findings, what is the most likely diagnosis?

1. Preiser disease
2. Scaphoid nonunion and osteonecrosis
3. Kienbock disease
4. Intraosseous ganglion
5. Scapholunate dissociation

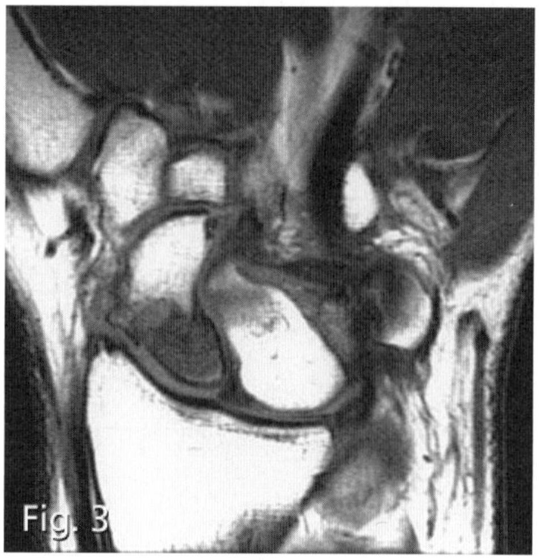
Fig. 3

Q-10: Which of the following tendons is found in the same dorsal compartment of the wrist as the posterior interosseous nerve?

1. Extensor digiti minimi
2. Extensor carpi radialis brevis
3. Extensor pollicis longus
4. Extensor indicis proprius
5. Abductor pollicis longus

Q-11: Which of the following describes the correct proximal to distal progression of the annular and cruciform pulleys of the digits?

1. A1, C1, A2, C2, A3, A4, C3
2. A1, A2, A3, C1, C2, C3, A4
3. A1, C1, C2, A2, A3, A4, C3
4. A1, A2, C1, A3, C2, A4, C3
5. A1, A2, A3, A4, C1, C2, C3

Q-12: In Dupuytren disease, the retrovascular cord typically displaces the radial proper digital nerve of the ring finger in what direction?

1. Palmarly and radially
2. Dorsally and ulnarly
3. Palmarly and ulnarly
4. Dorsally and radially
5. Directly dorsal

Q-13: Ganglion cysts about the wrist most commonly arise from what structure?

1. First carpometacarpal joint
2. Second carpometacarpal joint
3. Scapholunate interosseous ligament
4. Radioscaphocapitate ligament
5. Capitohamate interosseous ligament

Q-14: Spontaneous entrapment of the posterior interosseous nerve most commonly occurs in which of the following locations?

1. Lateral intermuscular septum
2. Extensor carpi radialis brevis
3. Arcade of Frohse
4. Midsubstance of the supinator
5. Leash of Henry

Q-15: What ligament is the primary stabilizer of the wrist following a proximal row carpectomy?

1. Dorsal radiocarpal
2. Dorsal intercarpal
3. Radioscaphocapitate
4. Ulnocapitate
5. Ulnotriquetral

Q-16: The condition shown in Figures 4A and 4B is most likely the result of

1. infection.
2. uric acid deposition.
3. trauma.
4. a virus.
5. severe cold exposure.

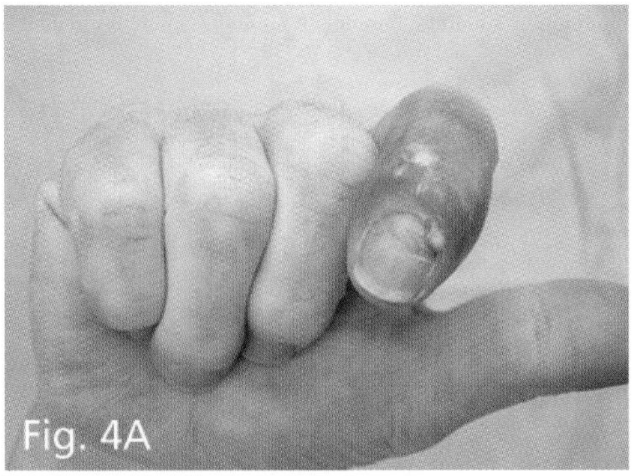
Fig. 4A

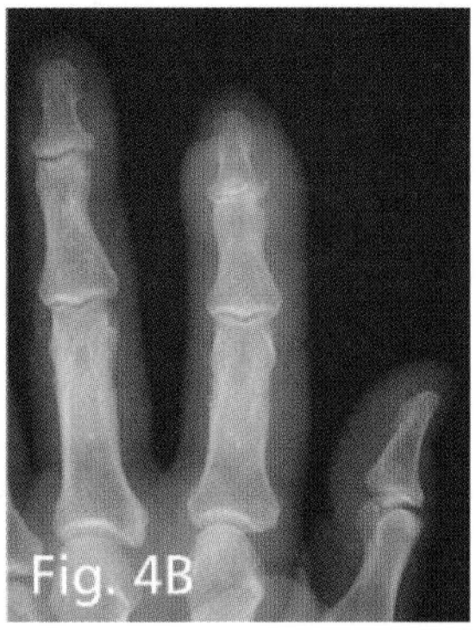
Fig. 4B

Q-17: A patient reports hyperesthesia over the base of the thenar eminence following volar locked plating of a distal radius fracture. A standard volar approach of Henry was used. What is the most likely cause of the hyperesthesia?

1. Complex regional pain syndrome
2. Wartenberg syndrome
3. Carpal tunnel syndrome
4. Palmar cutaneous nerve injury
5. C7 radiculopathy

Q-18: A patient sustained a sharp laceration to the base of his left, nondominant thumb 4 months ago. Examination reveals no active flexion but full passive motion of the interphalangeal joint. What is the best treatment option?

1. Interphalangeal joint fusion
2. Intercalary tendon graft
3. Silicone rod placement
4. Primary flexor pollicis longus repair
5. Flexor digitorum superficialis transfer

Q-19: A 17-year-old boy reports medial-sided elbow pain and diminished grip strength while throwing a javelin. He has decreased sensation in the little and ring fingers of his throwing hand only while throwing. The sensory deficits resolve at rest. Examination of the elbow reveals no instability and full motion. He has a positive Tinel sign over the cubital tunnel and a positive elbow flexion test. Radiographs are normal. What is the most appropriate next step in management?

1. Anterior ulnar nerve transposition
2. Cortisone injection
3. Nighttime elbow extension splinting
4. Medial collateral ligament reconstruction
5. Ulnar nerve decompression in situ

Q-20: What are the most likely symptoms and examination findings related to the mass in zone 2 of Guyon canal seen in Figure 5?

1. Numbness and tingling in the little finger and the ulnar side of the ring finger
2. Weakness and atrophy of the first dorsal interosseous
3. Hypothenar muscle atrophy
4. Dorsal ulnar hand numbness and tingling
5. Weakness of the interossei of the hand and numbness and tingling of the little finger and the ulnar side of the ring finger

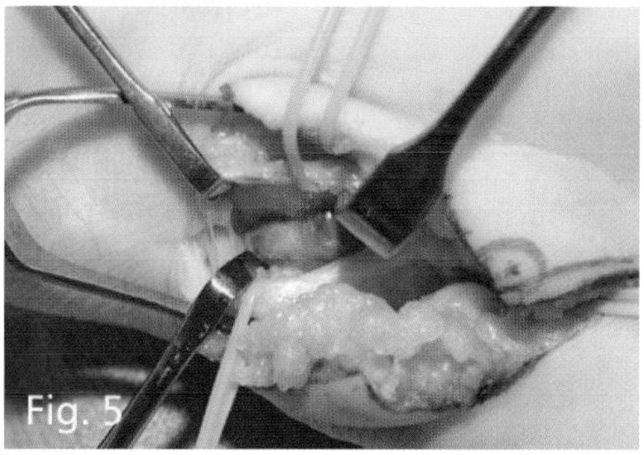

Q-21: Examination of a hand with compartment syndrome is most likely to reveal which of the following?

1. Clenched fist
2. Intrinsic minus posturing
3. Pain with passive stretch
4. Compression of the superficial arch
5. Pallor

Q-22: A 32-year-old woman sustained an elbow dislocation, and management consisted of early range of motion. Examination at the 3-month follow-up appointment reveals that she has regained elbow motion but has a weak pinch. A clinical photograph is shown in Figure 6. What is the most likely diagnosis?

1. Flexor pollicis longus rupture
2. Median nerve palsy
3. Ulnar nerve palsy
4. Anterior interosseous nerve palsy
5. Posterior interosseous nerve palsy

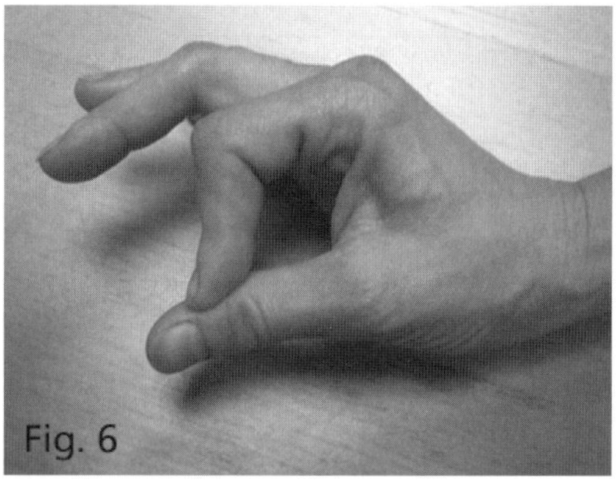

Fig. 6

Q-23: A 17-year-old boy reports wrist pain after being tackled while playing football. Radiographs are shown in Figures 7A through 7C. What is the recommended intervention?

1. Pedicled vascularized bone graft
2. Long arm thumb spica cast
3. Percutaneous screw fixation
4. Corticocancellous bone grafting via a volar approach (Matti-Russe)
5. Open reduction and differential pitch screw placement via a dorsal approach

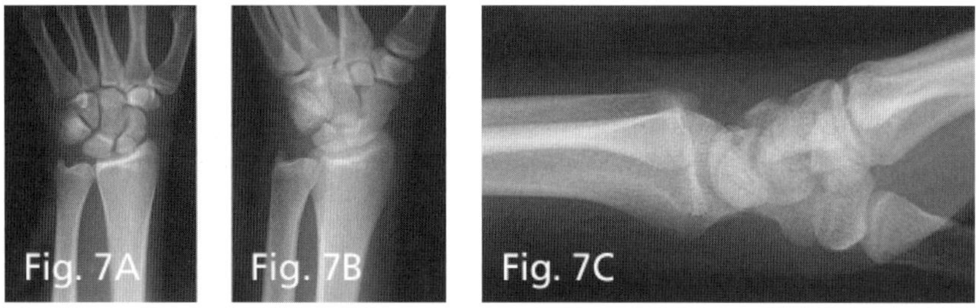

Fig. 7A Fig. 7B Fig. 7C

Q-24: A 27-year-old woman reports the acute atraumatic onset of burning pain in her right shoulder followed a week later by substantial weakness and the inability to abduct her shoulder. One week prior to this incident she had recovered from a flu-like syndrome. Examination reveals full passive motion of the shoulder and the inability to actively raise the arm. Sensation in the right upper extremity is normal. Cervical spine examination is normal. Radiographs of the shoulder and cervical spine are normal. What is the most likely diagnosis?

1. Calcific tendinitis
2. Poliomyelitis
3. Diskogenic cervical spine disease
4. Impingement
5. Brachial neuritis

Q-25: A 30-year-old man has pain in the left arm after a motor vehicle accident. His neurovascular examination is intact, and radiographs are shown in Figures 8A and 8B. What is the best course of management?

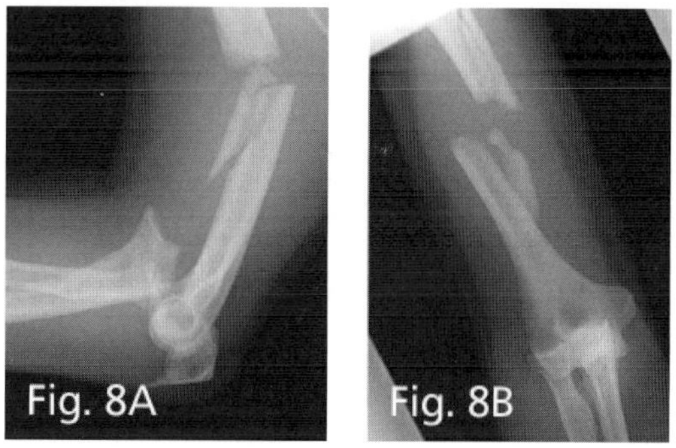

1. Closed reduction and cast immobilization for 4 weeks, followed by therapy directed at regaining motion
2. Open reduction and internal fixation of the olecranon fracture, functional bracing of the humeral fracture, and therapy directed at regaining motion initiated at 2 weeks after surgery
3. Open reduction and internal fixation of the olecranon and humeral fractures, followed by therapy directed at regaining motion
4. Open reduction and internal fixation of the olecranon and humeral fractures, and splint immobilization for 4 weeks followed by therapy directed at regaining motion
5. Open reduction and internal fixation of the olecranon fracture, functional bracing of the humeral fracture, and therapy directed at regaining motion initiated at 4 weeks after surgery

Q-26: A patient who underwent open reduction and internal fixation of an olecranon fracture 2 months ago now reports painless limitation of motion. Examination reveals a well-healed incision and a flexion-extension arc from 40° to 80°. The patient has been performing home exercises. Radiographs are shown in Figures 9A and 9B. What is the most appropriate treatment?

1. Continued observation and home therapy
2. Radiation therapy, followed by aggressive range-of-motion exercises
3. Formal physical therapy and static progressive splinting
4. Revision open reduction and internal fixation and capsular release
5. Manipulation under anesthesia

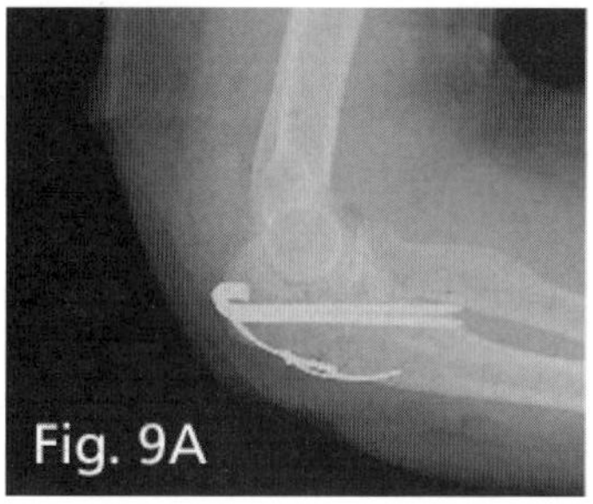
Fig. 9A

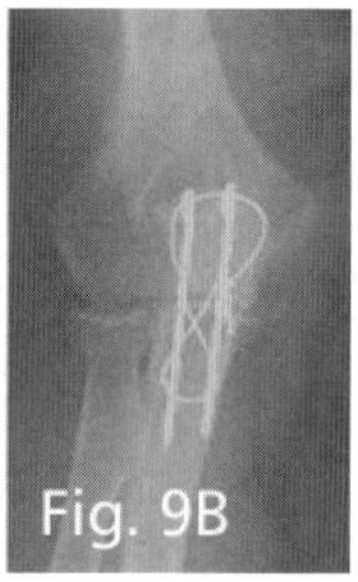
Fig. 9B

Q-27: A 17-year-old boy who plays high school football reports wrist pain 5 months after the conclusion of the football season. A radiograph and MRI scan are shown in Figures 10A and 10B. What is the recommended intervention?

1. Pedicled vascularized bone graft
2. Long arm thumb spica cast
3. Percutaneous screw fixation
4. Corticocancellous bone grating via a volar approach (Matti-Russe)
5. Open reduction and differential pitch screw placement via a dorsal approach

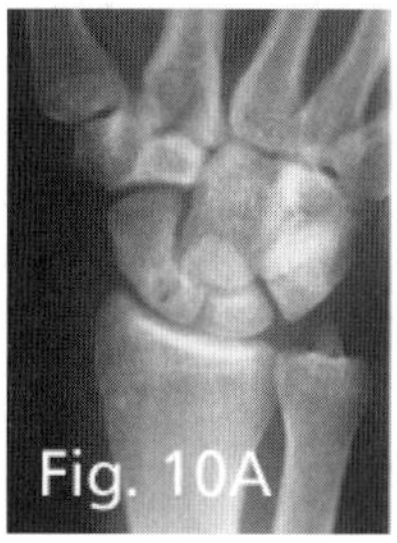
Fig. 10A

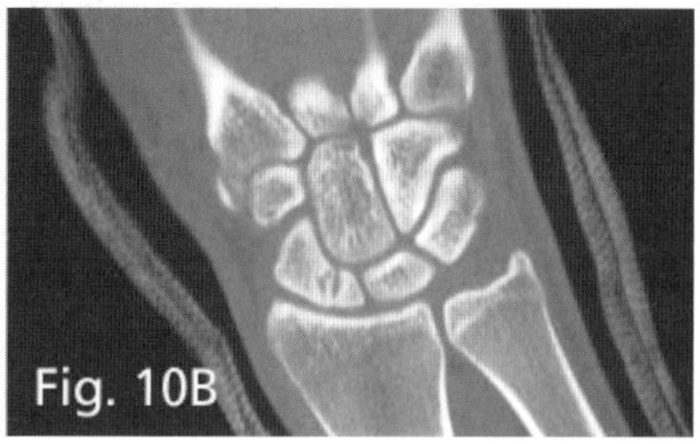
Fig. 10B

Q-28: A 34-year-old man underwent open reduction and internal fixation of a closed both-bones forearm fracture 11 months ago. The radiographs shown in Figures 11A and 11B reveal a 3-mm gap and loose screws. What is the best treatment option?

1. Vascularized fibular graft
2. Locked intramedullary rodding
3. Tricortical iliac crest grafting and compression plating
4. Cancellous autograft and plating
5. Bone morphogenetic protein-7

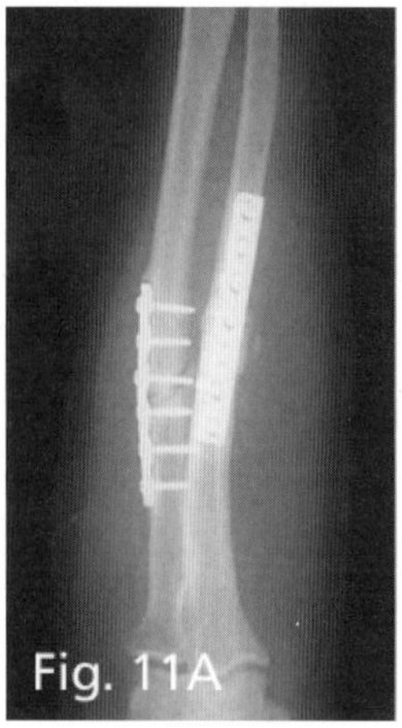
Fig. 11A

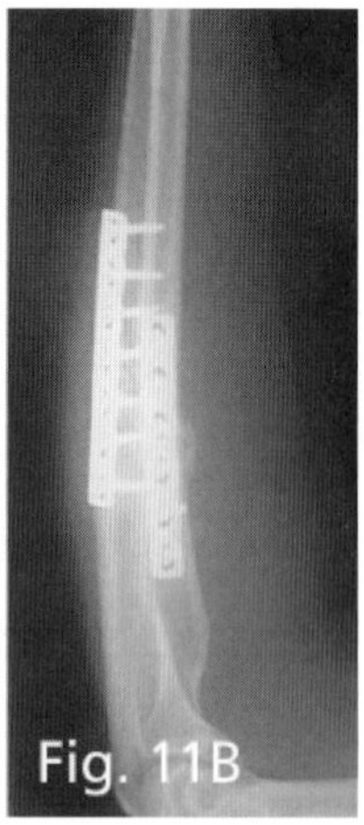
Fig. 11B

Q-29: In surgically treating hand and finger infections in patients with diabetes mellitus, what factor is associated with higher amputation rates?

1. Insulin dependence
2. Gram-positive organisms
3. Renal failure
4. Retinopathy
5. Peripheral neuropathy

Q-30: What is the primary indication for performing a total wrist arthroplasty in a patient with painful rheumatoid arthritis?

1. Ipsilateral total elbow arthroplasty
2. Contralateral wrist arthrodesis
3. Type III degenerative changes of the wrist
4. Age older than 55 years
5. Less than 30° of wrist flexion/extension

Q-31: What is the most common bacteria cultured from dog and cat bites to the upper extremity?

1. *Pasteurella*
2. *Streptococcus*
3. *Staphylococcus*
4. *Bacterioides*
5. *Moraxella*

Q-32: A previously healthy 65-year-old woman has a closed fracture of the right clavicle after falling down the basement stairs. Examination reveals good capillary refill in the digits of her right hand. Radial and ulnar pulses are 1+ at the right wrist compared with 2+ on the opposite side. In the arteriogram shown in Figure 12, the arrow is pointing to which of the following arteries?

1. Brachiocephalic
2. Innominate
3. Subclavian
4. Axillary
5. Circumflex scapular

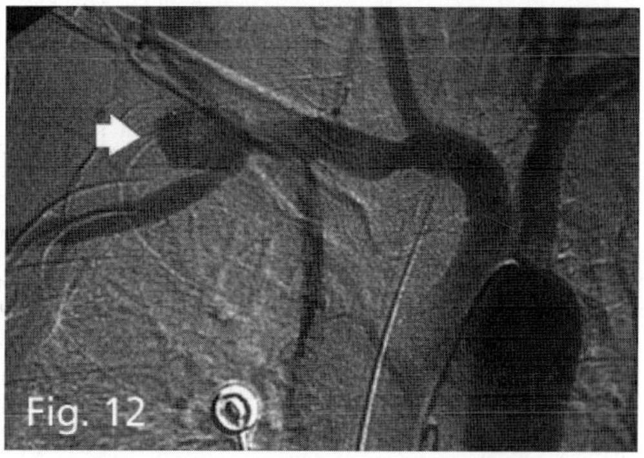
Fig. 12

Q-33: Which of the following structures may help maintain radial length after a radial head fracture?

1. Triangular fibrocartilage complex
2. Medial ulnar collateral ligament
3. Lateral ulnar collateral ligament
4. Annular ligament
5. Coronoid

Q-34: Outcome measures should have established psychometric properties of reliability, validity, and responsiveness. Reliability refers to which of the following?

1. The amount of change in the score over time
2. Sensitivity of the measure in evaluating a problem
3. The ability of the instruments to actually measure what it intends to measure
4. The measure of change over the course of treatment
5. The reproducibility of the measurements either between repeated tests or between observers

Q-35: Figure 13 shows a coronal T2-weighted MRI scan. The arrow is pointing to what torn structure?

1. Brachialis tendon
2. Biceps tendon
3. Flexor/pronator origin
4. Medial collateral ligament (MCL)
5. Lateral collateral ligament (LCL)

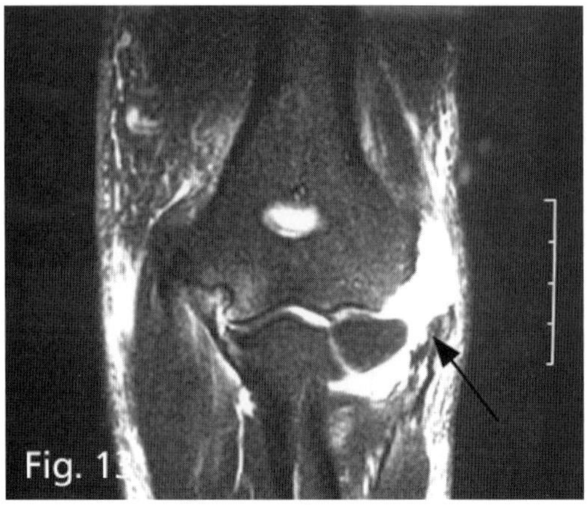

Q-36: Which of the following findings is a contraindication to isolated percutaneous pinning of a distal radius fracture?

1. Dorsal comminution
2. Volar comminution
3. Radial comminution
4. Intra-articular fracture
5. Physeal fracture

Q-37: A 55-year-old man sustained an elbow dislocation in a fall. Postreduction radiographs are shown in Figures 14A and 14B. What is the best course of management?

1. Closed reduction and casting for 4 weeks
2. Closed reduction and bracing with immediate range of motion
3. Open reduction, lateral collateral ligament repair, and open reduction and internal fixation or metallic replacement of the radial head
4. Open reduction, radial head Silastic arthroplasty, and lateral collateral ligament repair
5. Open reduction, lateral collateral ligament repair, and radial head excision

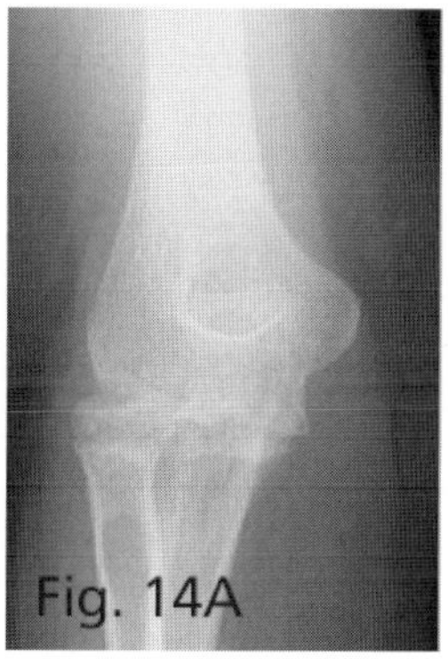

Fig. 14A

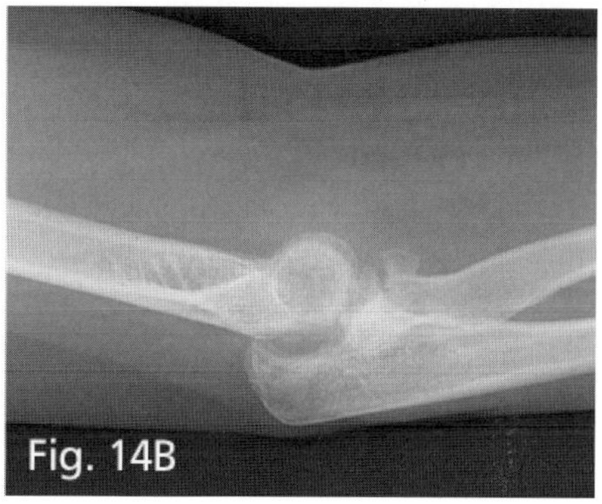

Fig. 14B

Q-38: In a patient with rheumatoid arthritis of the wrist, which of the following extensor tendons is most at risk of rupture?

1. Extensor digiti quinti
2. Abductor pollicis longus
3. Extensor pollicis longus
4. Extensor carpi radialis brevis
5. Extensor carpi ulnaris

Q-39: What is the most appropriate surgical treatment for a stage III symptomatic scapholunate advanced collapsed (SLAC) wrist?

1. Radioscapholunate arthrodesis
2. Scaphotrapeziotrapezoid arthrodesis
3. Scaphocapitate arthrodesis
4. Proximal row carpectomy
5. Scaphoid excision and capitate-lunate-triquetrum-hamate arthrodesis

Q-40: A 25-year-old man shot himself at the base of the right index finger while cleaning his handgun. Examination reveals that the finger is cool and cyanotic. A radiograph and clinical photograph are shown in Figures 15A and 15B. What is the recommended treatment?

1. Open reduction and internal fixation and arterial reconstruction
2. Crossed pinning with Kirschner wires
3. Open (guillotine) finger amputation
4. Index ray amputation
5. Application of an external fixator

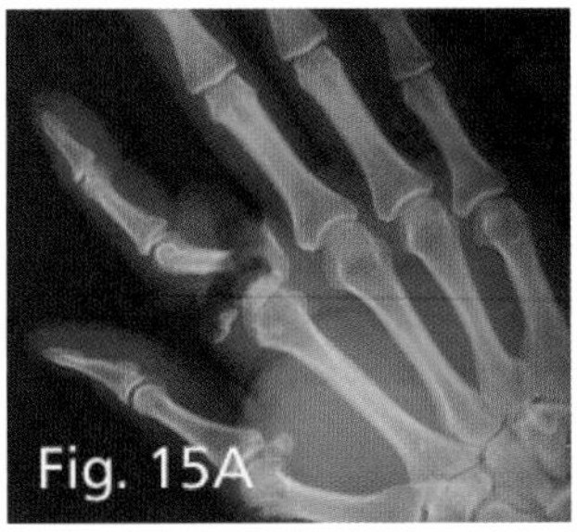
Fig. 15A

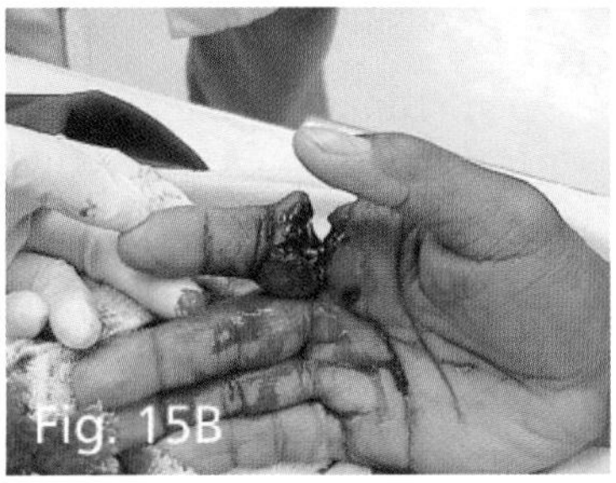
Fig. 15B

Q-41: What are the two terminal branches of the lateral cord of the brachial plexus?

1. Musculocutaneous and median
2. Musculocutaneous and axillary
3. Median and axillary
4. Ulnar and median
5. Ulnar and medial pectoral

Q-42: What is the most common complaint in patients with a developmental radial head dislocation?

1. Pain
2. Recurrent elbow subluxation
3. Limitation of extension
4. Cosmetic deformity
5. Locking

Q-43: A 35-year-old man sustained the closed injury shown in Figure 16 in his dominant extremity. Neurologic function is normal. Treatment should consist of

1. functional bracing.
2. a sling and swathe.
3. intramedullary nail fixation.
4. open reduction and internal fixation.
5. iliac crest bone graft.

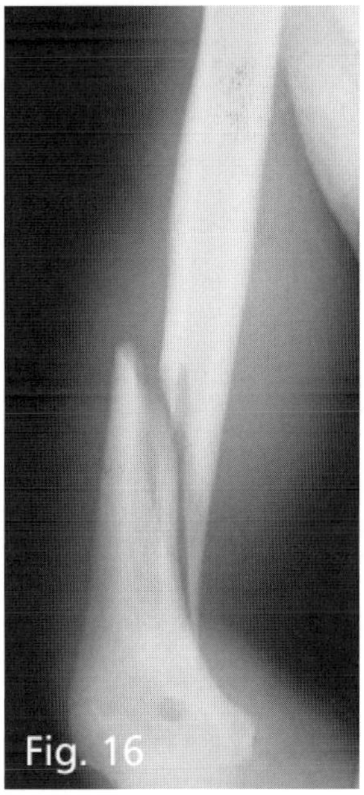

Fig. 16

Hand and Wrist: Questions

Q-44: The radiograph shown in Figure 17 reveals that the plate on the second metacarpal is acting in what manner?

1. Compression
2. Tension band
3. Bridge
4. Buttress
5. Spring

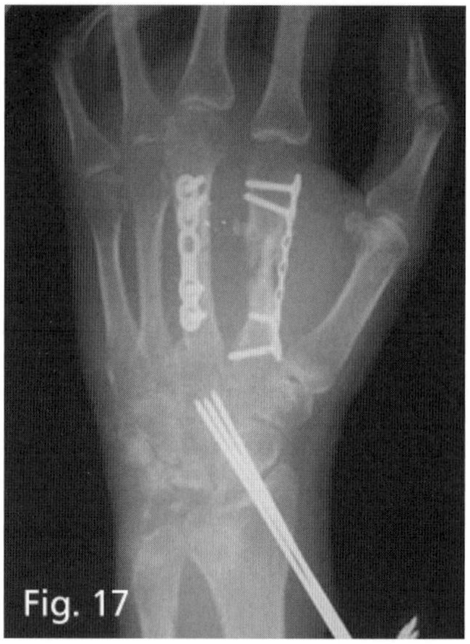

Fig. 17

Q-45: Figure 18 shows the radiograph of a 30-year-old man who sustained a closed comminuted fracture of the right clavicle. Examination reveals decreased sensation in the radial nerve distribution. Weakness is noted with shoulder abduction, internal rotation, and wrist extension. A displaced bone fragment is most likely pressing on what portion of the brachial plexus?

1. C5 and C6 spinal roots
2. Superior trunk
3. Anterior division of the inferior trunk
4. Posterior cord
5. Lateral and posterior cords

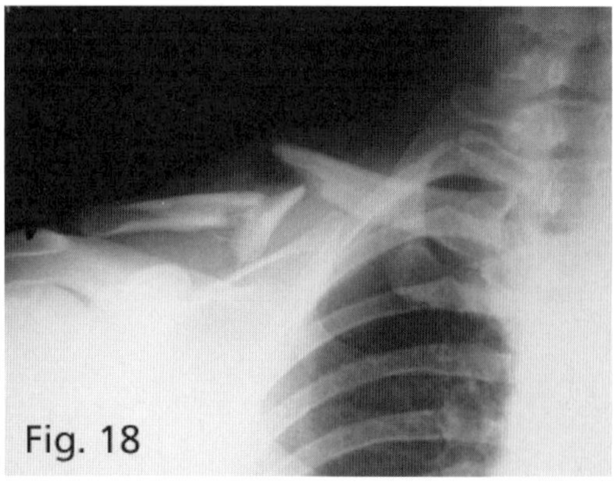

Fig. 18

Q-46: Which of the following is considered an important component in treating the lesion shown in Figure 19?

1. Excision of the skin in addition to the cyst
2. Resection of the nail plate
3. Excision of bony osteophytes from the distal interphalangeal (DIP) joint
4. Injection of corticosteroid into the DIP joint
5. Resection of part of the collateral ligament and extensor mechanism

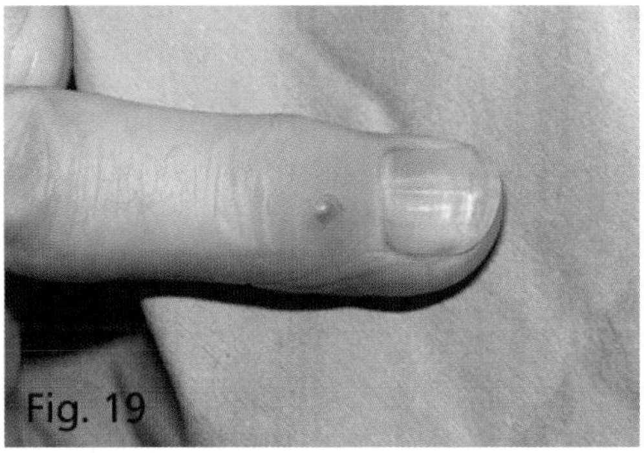
Fig. 19

Q-47: A patient with rheumatoid arthritis has a rupture of the extensor digitorum communis to the fourth and fifth metacarpals. You are planning to perform an extensor indicis proprius (EIP) tendon transfer. What effect will this have on index finger extension?

1. No effect
2. Index finger weakness
3. Index metacarpophalangeal hyperextension
4. Index metacarpophalangeal hyperflexion
5. Index metacarpophalangeal ulnar deviation

Q-48: A 22-year-old man is tackled while playing college football and sustains a reducible first carpometacarpal dislocation. What is the recommended treatment?

1. Closed reduction and casting
2. Closed reduction and percutaneous pinning
3. First carpometacarpal arthrodesis
4. Dorsal capsulodesis
5. Ligament reconstruction using tendon autograft

Q-49: What structure provides the most static stability for valgus restraint in the elbow?

1. Posterior band of the ulnar collateral ligament
2. Anterior band of the ulnar collateral ligament
3. Transverse band of the ulnar collateral ligament
4. Annular ligament
5. Flexor/pronator mass

A-1: When performing surgical excision of the lesion shown in the MRI scan in Figure 1, what nerve is most likely at risk?

1. Deep branch of the ulnar nerve
2. Anterior interosseous branch of the median nerve
3. Recurrent branch of the median nerve
4. Recurrent branch of the ulnar nerve
5. Palmar cutaneous branch of the ulnar nerve

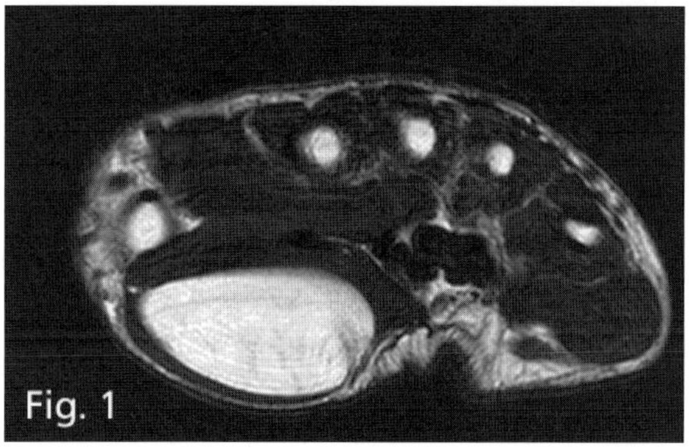
Fig. 1

PREFERRED RESPONSE: 3

DISCUSSION: The MRI scan shows a large mass (lipoma) in the thenar muscles of the palm. The recurrent motor branch of the median nerve innervates the thenar muscles. The anterior interosseous nerve (AIN) in the proximal forearm innervates the flexor pollicis longus, pronator quadratus, and flexor digitorum pollicis to the index and frequently the middle finger. The terminal branch of the AIN innervates only the wrist capsule. The palmar cutaneous branch of the ulnar nerve is a sensory structure to the hypothenar area. There is no commonly described recurrent branch of the ulnar nerve.

REFERENCE: Kozin SH: The anatomy of the recurrent branch of the median nerve. *J Hand Surg Am* 1998;23:852-858.

A-2: A 21-year-old man sustains multiple gunshot wounds to his right upper extremity. He cannot extend his digits or his thumb but can extend and radially deviate his wrist. An injury to the radial nerve or one of its branches has most likely occurred at which of the following locations?

1. Spiral groove of the humerus
2. Midshaft of the radius
3. Radial neck
4. Anatomic neck of the humerus
5. Surgical neck of the humerus

PREFERRED RESPONSE: 3

DISCUSSION: In this patient, the radial nerve is most likely injured at the level of the radial neck. The radial nerve emerges from the posterior cord of the brachial plexus and travels along the spiral groove of the humerus. At the level of the lateral humeral condyle, the radial nerve branches into the posterior interosseous nerve after giving off two cutaneous branches, the superficial radial and the posterior cutaneous. The posterior interosseous nerve travels through the supinator muscle and winds around the radial neck. At this level, the posterior interosseous nerve is vulnerable to injury, particularly following fracture or penetrating trauma.

REFERENCES: Netter F: *The Ciba Collection of Medical Illustrations: The Musculoskeletal System, Part 1. Anatomy, Physiology and Metabolic Disorders*. West Caldwell, NJ, Ciba-Geigy Corporation, 1987, vol 8, p 53.

Hollinshead W: *Anatomy for Surgeons: The Back and Limbs*, ed 3. Philadelphia, PA, Harper and Row, 1982, vol 3, pp 428-429.

A-3: The attachments of the transverse carpal ligament include which of the following structures?

1. Scaphoid and the ulna
2. Trapezium and the hook of the hamate
3. Trapezium and the triquetrum
4. Trapezoid and the hook of the hamate
5. Trapezoid and the pisiform

PREFERRED RESPONSE: 2

DISCUSSION: The transverse carpal ligament is the volar boundary of the carpal tunnel. It attaches to the scaphoid and trapezium radially and the pisiform and the hook of the hamate ulnarly. The ulna and trapezoid do not receive attachments of the transverse carpal ligament.

REFERENCES: Hollinshead W: *Anatomy for Surgeons: The Back and Limbs*, ed 3. Philadelphia, PA, Harper and Row, 1982, vol 3, pp 471-472.

Hoppenfeld S, deBoer P: *Surgical Exposures in Orthopaedics*, ed 2. Philadelphia, PA, Lippincott-Raven, 1994, pp 168-170.

A-4: A patient undergoes the procedure shown in Figure 2. An important part of this procedure is preservation of what wrist ligament?

1. Radioscaphocapitate
2. Scapholunate interosseous
3. Ulnotriquetral
4. Volar radioulnar
5. Deep proximal capitohamate

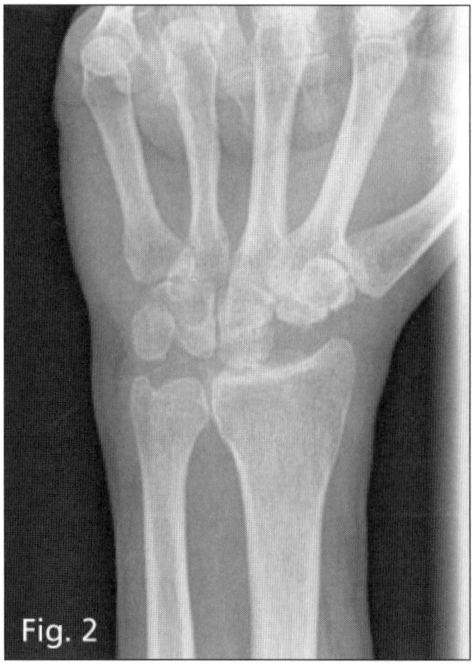

Fig. 2

PREFERRED RESPONSE: 1

DISCUSSION: Proximal row carpectomy is a salvage wrist procedure that yields a surprisingly stable construct. This has been attributed to two factors: (1) the congruency of the head of the capitate in the lunate fossa (this articulation is less congruent than the native lunate/lunate fossa relationship, but surprisingly stable), and (2) preservation of the radioscaphocapitate ligament, the most radial of the palmar extrinsic ligaments, which prevents ulnar subluxation after proximal row carpectomy.

REFERENCE: Jebson PJ, Engber WD: Proximal row carpectomy. *Tech Hand Up Extrem Surg* 1999;3:32-36.

A-5: A 37-year-old patient with type I diabetes mellitus has a flexor tenosynovitis of the thumb flexor tendon sheath following a kitchen knife puncture wound to the volar aspect of the thumb. Left unattended, this infection will likely first spread proximally, creating an abscess in which of the following spaces of the palm?

1. Central space
2. Hypothenar space
3. Carpal tunnel
4. Posterior adductor space
5. Thenar space

PREFERRED RESPONSE: 5

DISCUSSION: Flexor tenosynovitis of the thumb flexor tendon sheath can spread proximally and form an abscess within the thenar space of the palm. The flexor pollicis longus tendon does not pass through the central space of the palm or the hypothenar space of the palm. The flexor pollicis longus tendon does pass through the carpal tunnel, but this is not a palmar space. The three palmar spaces include the hypothenar space, the thenar space, and the central space. The posterior adductor space would likely only be involved secondarily after spread from a thenar space infection.

REFERENCES: Hollinshead W: *Anatomy for Surgeons: The Back and Limbs*, ed 3. Philadelphia, PA, Harper and Row, 1982, vol 3, pp 478-479.

Lee D, Ferlic R, Neviaser R: Hand infections, in Berger R, Weiss AP, eds: *Hand Surgery*. Philadelphia, PA, Lippincott Williams & Wilkins, 2004, pp 1784-1785.

A-6: New painful paresthesias near the site of the incision after an ulnar nerve transposition is the result of injury to what nerve?

1. Medial antebrachial cutaneous
2. Lateral antebrachial cutaneous
3. Posterior antebrachial cutaneous
4. Medial brachial cutaneous
5. Dorsal antebrachial cutaneous

PREFERRED RESPONSE: 1

DISCUSSION: Branches of the medial antebrachial cutaneous nerve can often be identified during routine ulnar nerve surgery crossing the medial aspect of the elbow. It should be preserved to avoid development of painful paresthesias.

REFERENCE: Dellon AL, Mackinnon SE: Injury to the medial antebrachial cutaneous nerve during cubital tunnel surgery. *J Hand Surg Br* 1985;10:33-36.

A-7: Which of the following best describes the relationship of the median nerve to the flexor carpi radialis tendon just proximal to the carpal canal?

1. Median nerve is volar and ulnar
2. Median nerve is radial and volar
3. Median nerve is dorsal and ulnar
4. Median nerve is dorsal and radial
5. Median nerve is volar and radial

PREFERRED RESPONSE: 3

DISCUSSION: The median nerve has an intimate association with the palmaris longus and the flexor carpi radialis at the proximal aspect of the carpal canal. The median nerve lies just ulnar and dorsal to the flexor carpi radialis tendon.

REFERENCES: Hoppenfeld S, deBoer P: *Surgical Exposures in Orthopaedics*, ed 2. Philadelphia, PA, Lippincott-Raven, 1994, pp 118-131.

Henry A: *Extensile Exposure*, ed 3. Edinburgh, UK, Churchill Livingstone, 1995, pp 100-107.

A-8: Which of the following muscles has dual innervation?

1. Pronator teres
2. Flexor digitorum superficialis
3. Coracobrachialis
4. Latissimus dorsi
5. Brachialis

PREFERRED RESPONSE: 5

DISCUSSION: The brachialis muscle typically receives dual innervation. The major portion is innervated by the musculocutaneous nerve. Its inferolateral portion is innervated by the radial nerve. The other muscles listed have single innervation. The anterior approach to the humerus, which requires splitting of the brachialis, capitalizes on this dual innervation.

REFERENCE: Mahakkanukrauh P, Somsarp V: Dual innervation of the brachialis muscle. *Clin Anat* 2002;15:206-209.

A-9: A 21-year-old man who was injured in a snowboarding accident 18 months ago now reports wrist pain. An MRI scan is shown in Figure 3. Based on the image findings, what is the most likely diagnosis?

1. Preiser disease
2. Scaphoid nonunion and osteonecrosis
3. Kienbock disease
4. Intraosseous ganglion
5. Scapholunate dissociation

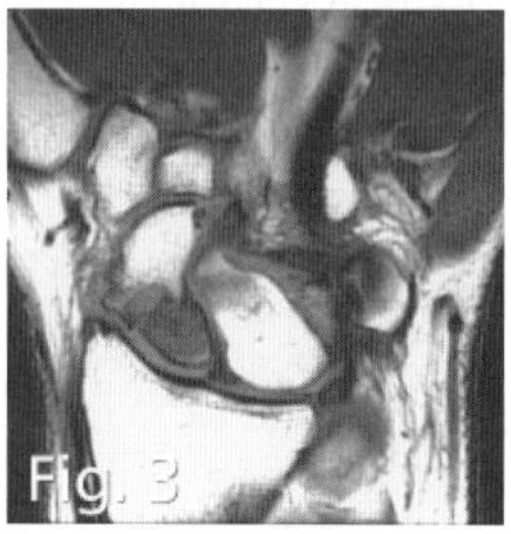

(continued on next page)

(A-9: *continued*)

PREFERRED RESPONSE: 2

DISCUSSION: The coronal MRI scan of the wrist shows the scaphoid. There is a subtle fracture line with a step-off at the radial surface consistent with a nonunion. The signal intensity is markedly different between the two fragments of the scaphoid. This strongly suggests osteonecrosis. Preiser disease is osteonecrosis typically involving most or all of the scaphoid. Kienbock disease involves the lunate. Intraosseous ganglia are easily diagnosed on MRI but typically have a fluid-filled area surrounded by denser bone in the periphery. Scapholunate dissociation can be seen on MRI as an injury to the scapholunate ligament and widening of the scapholunate interval, neither of which is seen on this image.

REFERENCE: Perlik PC, Guilford WB: Magnetic resonance imaging to assess vascularity of scaphoid nonunions. *J Hand Surg Am* 1991;16:479-484.

A-10: Which of the following tendons is found in the same dorsal compartment of the wrist as the posterior interosseous nerve?

1. Extensor digiti minimi
2. Extensor carpi radialis brevis
3. Extensor pollicis longus
4. Extensor indicis proprius
5. Abductor pollicis longus

PREFERRED RESPONSE: 4

DISCUSSION: The terminal branch of the posterior interosseous nerve is contained in the fourth dorsal compartment. The contents of the various dorsal wrist compartments are as follows:

First Compartment: Abductor pollicis longus, extensor pollis brevis

Second Compartment: Extensor carpi radialis brevis, extensor carpi radialis longus

Third Compartment: Extensor pollicis longus

Fourth Compartment: Extensor digitorum communis, extensor indicus proprius, posterior interosseous nerve

Fifth Compartment: Extensor digiti minimi

Sixth Compartment: Extensor carpi ulnaris

The extensor indicis proprius is also contained in the fourth dorsal compartment. The extensor digiti minimi is located in the fifth dorsal compartment. The extensor carpi radialis brevis is located in the second dorsal compartment. The extensor pollicis longus is located in the third dorsal compartment, and the abductor pollicis longus is located in the first dorsal compartment.

REFERENCES: Hoppenfeld S, deBoer P: *Surgical Exposures in Orthopaedics*, ed 2. Philadelphia, PA, Lippincott-Raven, 1994, pp 150-151.

Netter F: *The Ciba Collection of Medical Illustrations: The Musculoskeletal System, Part 1 Anatomy, Physiology and Metabolic Disorders*. West Caldwell, NJ, Ciba-Geigy Corporation, 1987, vol 8, p 60.

A-11: Which of the following describes the correct proximal to distal progression of the annular and cruciform pulleys of the digits?

1. A1, C1, A2, C2, A3, A4, C3
2. A1, A2, A3, C1, C2, C3, A4
3. A1, C1, C2, A2, A3, A4, C3
4. A1, A2, C1, A3, C2, A4, C3
5. A1, A2, A3, A4, C1, C2, C3

PREFERRED RESPONSE: 4

DISCUSSION: The correct progression of the annular and cruciform pulley in the digits is A1, A2, C1, A3, C2, A4, C3. The two cruciform pulleys are collapsible elements adjacent to the more rigid annular pulleys of the flexor tendon sheath. This arrangement enables unrestricted flexion of the proximal interphalangeal joint.

REFERENCES: Hoppenfeld S, deBoer P: *Surgical Exposures in Orthopaedics*, ed 2. Philadelphia, PA, Lippincott-Raven, 1994, pp 176-186.

Strickland J: Flexor tendon-acute injuries, in Green D, Hotchkiss R, Pederson W, eds: *Green's Operative Hand Surgery*, ed 4. New York, NY, Churchill Livingstone, 1999, pp 1853-1855.

A-12: In Dupuytren disease, the retrovascular cord typically displaces the radial proper digital nerve of the ring finger in what direction?

1. Palmarly and radially
2. Dorsally and ulnarly
3. Palmarly and ulnarly
4. Dorsally and radially
5. Directly dorsal

PREFERRED RESPONSE: 3

DISCUSSION: Retrovascular cords are common in Dupuytren disease and commonly require surgical treatment. Nerve injury during surgery to treat Dupuytren disease is an infrequent complication that occurs partly because the digital nerves can be displaced from their normal anatomic relationships by retrovascular cords. The nerves are displaced superficially, toward the center of the digit (palmarly and ulnarly). This displacement is typically seen at the level of the metacarpophalangeal joint.

REFERENCE: Rayan GM: Palmar fascial complex anatomy and pathology in Dupuytren's disease. *Hand Clin* 1999;15:73-86.

A-13: Ganglion cysts about the wrist most commonly arise from what structure?

1. First carpometacarpal joint
2. Second carpometacarpal joint
3. Scapholunate interosseous ligament
4. Radioscaphocapitate ligament
5. Capitohamate interosseous ligament

PREFERRED RESPONSE: 3

DISCUSSION: Ganglion cysts are the most common mass or mass-like lesions seen in the hand and wrist. They arise in a variety of locations, including synovial joints or tendon sheaths. The most common location is the dorsal/radial wrist arising from the dorsal scapholunate interosseous ligament.

REFERENCE: Thornburg LE: Ganglions of the hand and wrist. *J Am Acad Orthop Surg* 1999;7:231-238.

A-14: Spontaneous entrapment of the posterior interosseous nerve most commonly occurs in which of the following locations?

1. Lateral intermuscular septum
2. Extensor carpi radialis brevis
3. Arcade of Frohse
4. Midsubstance of the supinator
5. Leash of Henry

PREFERRED RESPONSE: 3

DISCUSSION: The extensor carpi radialis brevis, supinator muscle, arcade of Frohse, and leash of Henry are potential sites of compression for the posterior interosseous nerve. The most common location of spontaneous entrapment is the arcade of Frohse. The lateral intermuscular septum is a site of compression for the radial nerve.

REFERENCE: Spinner RJ, Spinner M: Nerve entrapment syndromes, in Morrey BF: *The Elbow and Its Disorders*, ed 3. Philadelphia, PA, WB Saunders, 2000, pp 839-862.

A-15: What ligament is the primary stabilizer of the wrist following a proximal row carpectomy?

1. Dorsal radiocarpal
2. Dorsal intercarpal
3. Radioscaphocapitate
4. Ulnocapitate
5. Ulnotriquetral

(continued on next page)

(A-15: *continued*)

PREFERRED RESPONSE: 3

DISCUSSION: The radioscaphocapitate ligament is the primary stabilizer between the radius and capitate, preventing ulnar translocation of the carpus. Its oblique orientation prevents the carpus from drifting ulnarly. This stout ligament must be protected when excising the scaphoid.

REFERENCES: Stern PJ, Agabegi SS, Kiefhaber TR, et al: Proximal row carpectomy. *J Bone Joint Surg Am* 2005;87: 166-174.

Wyrick JD: Proximal row carpectomy and intercarpal arthrodesis for the management of wrist arthritis. *J Am Acad Orthop Surg* 2003;11:227-281.

A-16: The condition shown in Figures 4A and 4B is most likely the result of

1. infection.
2. uric acid deposition.
3. trauma.
4. a virus.
5. severe cold exposure.

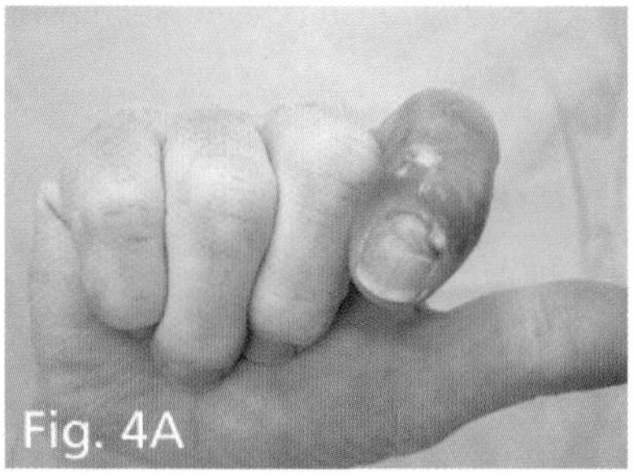
Fig. 4A

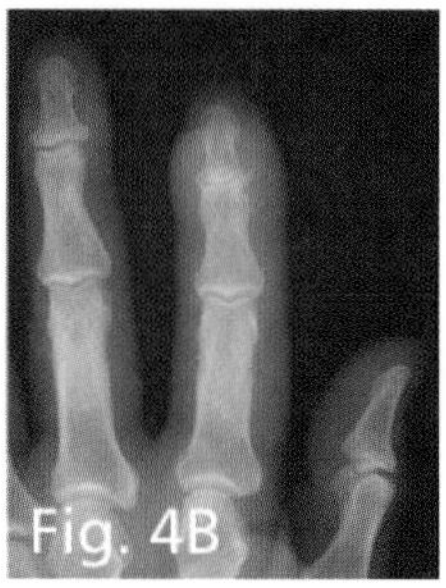
Fig. 4B

PREFERRED RESPONSE: 2

DISCUSSION: The clinical photograph and radiograph show gout, which is the result of urate deposition in the joint and soft tissues. Radiographs frequently reveal periarticular erosions. The crystals are intracellular and negatively birefringent under the polarized microscope. Treatment for acute flares include colchicine, indomethacin, and corticosteroids (including injections). Medications such as allopurinol help prevent recurrent flares. Tophi such as that seen in this patient are often confused with and associated with infection.

REFERENCES: Wortmann RL, Kelley WM: Crystal-induced inflammation: Gout and hyperuricemia, in Harris ED, Budd RC, Firestein GS, et al, eds: *Kelley's Textbook of Rheumatology*, ed 7. New York, NY, Elsevier Science, 2005, pp 1402-1429.

Trumble TE, ed: *Hand Surgery Update: Hand, Elbow, & Shoulder*, ed 3. Rosemont, IL, American Society for Surgery of the Hand, 2003, pp 433-457.

Louis DS, Jebson PJ: Mimickers of hand infections. *Hand Clin* 1998;14:519-529.

A-17: A patient reports hyperesthesia over the base of the thenar eminence following volar locked plating of a distal radius fracture. A standard volar approach of Henry was used. What is the most likely cause of the hyperesthesia?

1. Complex regional pain syndrome
2. Wartenberg syndrome
3. Carpal tunnel syndrome
4. Palmar cutaneous nerve injury
5. C7 radiculopathy

(continued on next page)

(A-17: *continued*)

PREFERRED RESPONSE: 4

DISCUSSION: The palmar cutaneous branch of the median nerve separates from the median nerve approximately 4 to 6 cm proximal to the wrist crease and travels between the median nerve and the flexor carpi radialis tendon. It supplies the skin of the thenar region. This nerve is at risk for injury with retraction of the digital flexor tendons in plating the distal radius. Wartenberg syndrome is compression of the superficial radial nerve, which innervates the dorsum of the thumb and the first dorsal web space. Carpal tunnel syndrome causes dysesthesias of the thumb, index, and/or middle fingers. C7 radiculopathy affects the index and middle fingers.

REFERENCES: Jupiter JB, Fernandez DL, Toh CL, et al: Operative treatment of volar intra-articular fractures of the distal end of the radius. *J Bone Joint Surg Am* 1996;78:1817-1828.

Hoppenfield S, deBoer P, eds: *Surgical Exposures in Orthopaedics: The Anatomic Approach*, ed 2. Philadelphia, PA, JB Lippincott, 1994, pp 156-176.

A-18: A patient sustained a sharp laceration to the base of his left, nondominant thumb 4 months ago. Examination reveals no active flexion but full passive motion of the interphalangeal joint. What is the best treatment option?

1. Interphalangeal joint fusion
2. Intercalary tendon graft
3. Silicone rod placement
4. Primary flexor pollicis longus repair
5. Flexor digitorum superficialis transfer

PREFERRED RESPONSE: 5

DISCUSSION: The patient has a chronic flexor tendon laceration. There are options to restore motion and strength; therefore, fusion is not necessary. Full range of motion is present so the soft tissues are suitable for a tendon transfer. A transfer of the flexor digitorum superficialis of the ring finger to the insertion of the flexor pollicis longus on the distal phalanx provides good results with a one-stage operation.

REFERENCES: Schneider LH, Wiltshire D: Restoration of flexor pollicis longus function by flexor digitorum superficialis transfer. *J Hand Surg Am* 1983;8:98-101.

Posner MA: Flexor superficialis tendon transfers to the thumb: An alternative to the free tendon graft for treatment of chronic injuries within the digital sheath. *J Hand Surg Am* 1983;8:876-881.

A-19: A 17-year-old boy reports medial-sided elbow pain and diminished grip strength while throwing a javelin. He has decreased sensation in the little and ring fingers of his throwing hand only while throwing. The sensory deficits resolve at rest. Examination of the elbow reveals no instability and full motion. He has a positive Tinel sign over the cubital tunnel and a positive elbow flexion test. Radiographs are normal. What is the most appropriate next step in management?

1. Anterior ulnar nerve transposition
2. Cortisone injection
3. Nighttime elbow extension splinting
4. Medial collateral ligament reconstruction
5. Ulnar nerve decompression in situ

PREFERRED RESPONSE: 3

DISCUSSION: The patient's symptoms and examination findings are consistent with ulnar neuritis/cubital tunnel syndrome, most probably exacerbated by javelin throwing. The first step includes rest and extension splinting. Surgical intervention should only be considered after failure of nonsurgical management.

REFERENCES: Posner MA: Compressive neuropathies of the ulnar nerve at the elbow and wrist. *Instr Course Lect* 2000;49:305-317.

Omer GE, Spinner M, Van Beek AL, eds: *Management of Peripheral Nerve Problems*, ed 2. Philadelphia, PA, WB Saunders, 1998, pp 65-69.

A-20: What are the most likely symptoms and examination findings related to the mass in zone 2 of Guyon canal seen in Figure 5?

1. Numbness and tingling in the little finger and the ulnar side of the ring finger
2. Weakness and atrophy of the first dorsal interosseous
3. Hypothenar muscle atrophy
4. Dorsal ulnar hand numbness and tingling
5. Weakness of the interossei of the hand and numbness and tingling of the little finger and the ulnar side of the ring finger

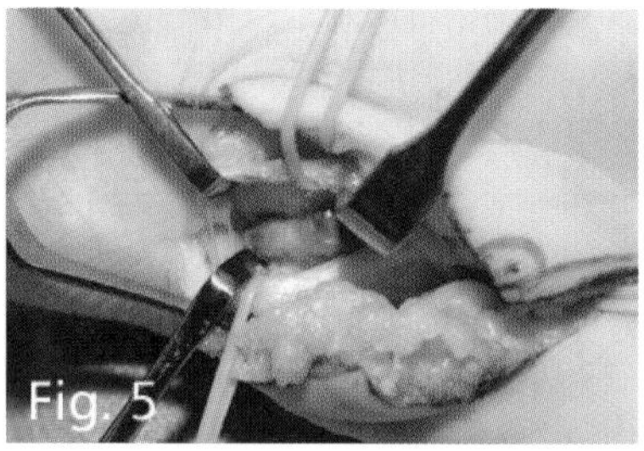

PREFERRED RESPONSE: 2

DISCUSSION: The lesion lies in zone II of the ulnar tunnel. In that zone the deep motor branch of the ulnar nerve is susceptible to compression. Distal to the hook of the hamate, the motor branch of the ulnar nerve dives deep to innervate the interossei as it begins to move from an ulnar to radial direction. Because of its course, it has little or no give in response to a mass effect from the floor of Guyon canal. Ganglions are the most common cause of ulnar nerve entrapment in the wrist. Lesions in zone I can affect both sensory and motor aspects of the ulnar nerve as well as the motor innervation of the hypothenar muscles. Lesions at the elbow or mid to proximal forearm are associated with dorsal hand numbness and tingling.

REFERENCES: Kuschner SH, Gelberman RH, Jennings C: Ulnar nerve compression at the wrist. *J Hand Surg Am* 1988;13:577-580.

Posner MA: Compressive neuropathies of the ulnar nerve at the elbow and wrist. *Instr Course Lect* 2000;49:305-317.

A-21: Examination of a hand with compartment syndrome is most likely to reveal which of the following?

1. Clenched fist
2. Intrinsic minus posturing
3. Pain with passive stretch
4. Compression of the superficial arch
5. Pallor

PREFERRED RESPONSE: 2

DISCUSSION: In a study of 19 patients with compartment syndrome of the hand, all had tense swollen hands with elevated compartment pressures. Most patients were neurologically compromised, so pain with passive stretch may be difficult to elicit. Arterial inflow is present in the arch and thus pallor is not present. The typical posture of the hand is not clenched, rather it is an intrinsic minus posture of metacarpophalangeal joint extension and flexion of the proximal and distal interphalangeal joints.

REFERENCES: Oullette EA, Kelly R: Compartment syndromes of the hand. *J Bone Joint Surg Am* 1996;78:1515-1522.

Dellaero DT, Levin LS: Compartment syndrome of the hand: Etiology, diagnosis, and treatment. *Am J Orthop* 1996;25:404-408.

A-22: A 32-year-old woman sustained an elbow dislocation, and management consisted of early range of motion. Examination at the 3-month follow-up appointment reveals that she has regained elbow motion but has a weak pinch. A clinical photograph is shown in Figure 6. What is the most likely diagnosis?

1. Flexor pollicis longus rupture
2. Median nerve palsy
3. Ulnar nerve palsy
4. Anterior interosseous nerve palsy
5. Posterior interosseous nerve palsy

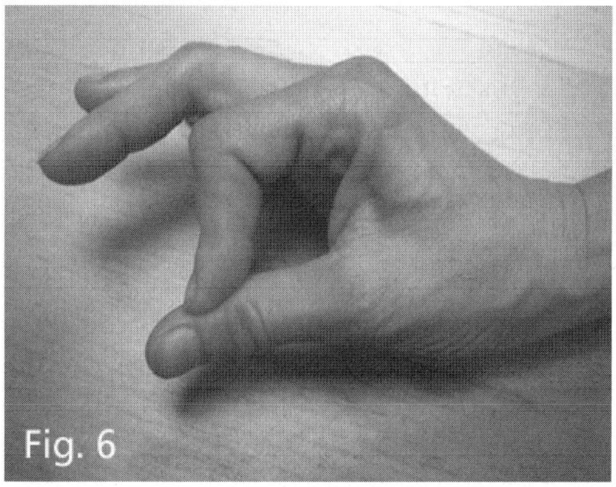
Fig. 6

PREFERRED RESPONSE: 4

DISCUSSION: The photograph shows the characteristic attitude of the hand when an anterior interosseous nerve palsy is present. The patient is unable to flex the interphalangeal joint to the joint of the thumb. Anterior interosseous nerve palsies are often misdiagnosed as tendon ruptures.

REFERENCES: Schantz K, Reigels-Nielsen P: The anterior interosseous nerve syndrome. *J Hand Surg Br* 1992;17:510-512.

Seror P: Anterior interosseous nerve lesions: Clinical and electrophysiological features. *J Bone Joint Surg Br* 1996;78:238-241.

Hand and Wrist: Answers

A-23: A 17-year-old high school football player reports wrist pain after being tackled. Radiographs are shown in Figures 7A through 7C. What is the recommended intervention?

1. Pedicled vascularized bone graft
2. Long arm thumb spica cast
3. Percutaneous screw fixation
4. Corticocancellous bone grafting via a volar approach (Matti-Russe)
5. Open reduction and differential pitch screw placement via a dorsal approach

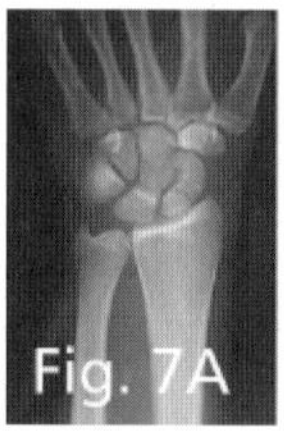
Fig. 7A

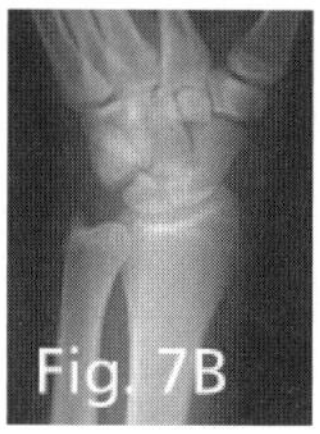
Fig. 7B

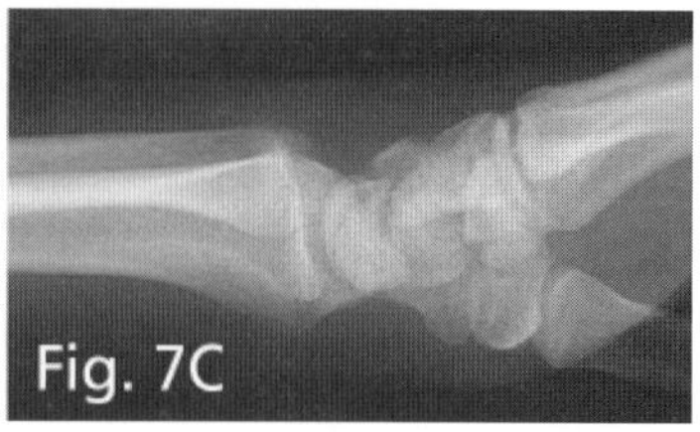
Fig. 7C

PREFERRED RESPONSE: 5

DISCUSSION: The patient has an acute fracture of the proximal pole. A 100% healing rate has been reported for open reduction and internal fixation of proximal pole fractures via a dorsal approach. This allows for direct viewing of the fracture line, facilitates reduction, and bone grafting can be done through the same incision if necessary. A vascularized or corticocancellous graft is reserved for nonunions. Proximal fractures are very slow to heal with a cast, if they heal at all. As a small fragment, percutaneous fixation is very difficult and has been reported for waist fractures.

REFERENCES: Rettig ME, Raskin KB: Retrograde compression screw fixation of acute proximal pole scaphoid fractures. *J Hand Surg Am* 1999;24:1206-1210.

Raskin KB, Parisi D, Baker J, et al: Dorsal open repair of proximal pole scaphoid fractures. *Hand Clin* 2001;17:601-610.

A-24: A 27-year-old woman reports the acute atraumatic onset of burning pain in her right shoulder followed a week later by significant weakness and the inability to abduct her shoulder. One week prior to this incident she had recovered from a flu-like syndrome. Examination reveals full passive motion of the shoulder and the inability to actively raise the arm. Sensation in the right upper extremity is normal. Cervical spine examination is normal. Radiographs of the shoulder and cervical spine are normal. What is the most likely diagnosis?

1. Calcific tendinitis
2. Poliomyelitis
3. Diskogenic cervical spine disease
4. Impingement
5. Brachial neuritis

PREFERRED RESPONSE: 5

DISCUSSION: The patient has symptoms and examination findings of acute brachial neuritis, which is often a diagnosis of exclusion. The recent viral flu-like symptoms have shown a correlation with the development of this disorder. The acute, severe shoulder weakness excludes calcific tendinitis, impingement, and poliomyelitis. A normal cervical spine examination makes cervical disk disease unlikely.

REFERENCES: Turner JW, Parsonage MJ: Neuralgic amyotrophy (paralytic brachial neuritis). *Lancet* 1957;2:209-212. Omer GE, Spinner M, Van Beek AL, eds: *Management of Peripheral Nerve Problems*, ed 2. Philadelphia, PA, WB Saunders, 1998, pp 101-104.

A-25: A 30-year-old man has pain in the left arm after a motor vehicle accident. His neurovascular examination is intact, and radiographs are shown in Figures 8A and 8B. What is the best course of management?

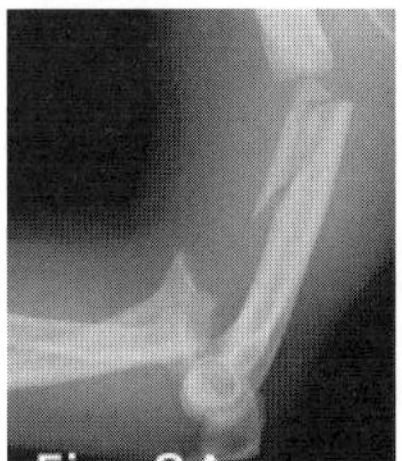

Fig. 8A

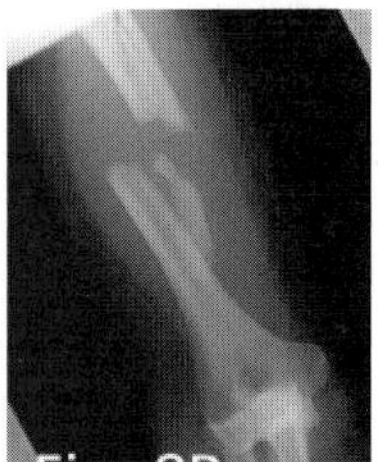

Fig. 8B

1. Closed reduction and cast immobilization for 4 weeks, followed by therapy directed at regaining motion
2. Open reduction and internal fixation of the olecranon fracture, functional bracing of the humeral fracture, and therapy directed at regaining motion initiated at 2 weeks after surgery
3. Open reduction and internal fixation of the olecranon and humeral fractures, followed by therapy directed at regaining motion
4. Open reduction and internal fixation of the olecranon and humeral fractures, and splint immobilization for 4 weeks followed by therapy directed at regaining motion
5. Open reduction and internal fixation of the olecranon fracture, functional bracing of the humeral fracture, and therapy directed at regaining motion initiated at 4 weeks after surgery

PREFERRED RESPONSE: 3

DISCUSSION: The floating elbow is best managed with early open reduction and internal fixation of the humeral and forearm fractures, followed by early range of motion. These fractures predispose the elbow to stiffness, and early range of motion is recommended.

REFERENCES: Solomon HB, Zadnik M, Eglseder WA: A review of outcomes in 18 patients with floating elbow. *J Orthop Trauma* 2003;17:563-570.

Yokoyama K, Itoman M, Kobayashi A, et al: Functional outcomes of "floating elbow" injuries in adult patients. *J Orthop Trauma* 1998;12:284-290.

A-26: A patient who underwent open reduction and internal fixation of an olecranon fracture 2 months ago now reports painless limitation of motion. Examination reveals a well-healed incision and a flexion-extension arc from 40° to 80° The patient has been performing home exercises. Radiographs are shown in Figures 9A and 9B. What is the most appropriate treatment?

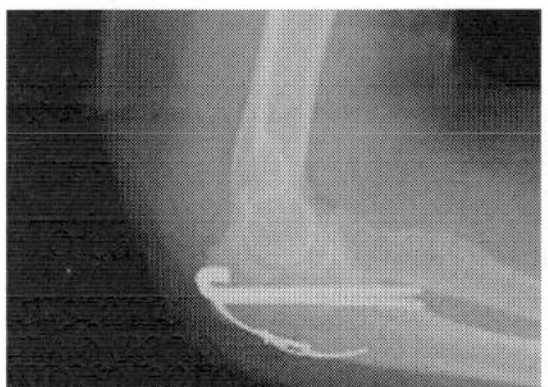

Fig. 9A

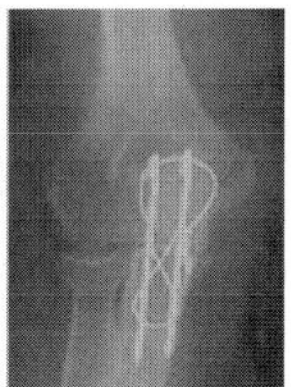

Fig. 9B

1. Continued observation and home therapy
2. Radiation therapy, followed by aggressive range-of-motion exercises
3. Formal physical therapy and static progressive splinting
4. Revision open reduction and internal fixation and capsular release
5. Manipulation under anesthesia

PREFERRED RESPONSE: 3

DISCUSSION: The radiographs do not show an articular malunion. Treatment is directed at the soft-tissue contracture and should begin with formal physical therapy and static progressive splinting. Radiation therapy is effective in the perioperative period and is indicated when ectopic bone formation is a concern.

REFERENCES: Morrey BF: The posttraumatic stiff elbow. *Clin Orthop Relat Res* 2005;431:26-35.

King GJ, Faber KJ: Posttraumatic elbow stiffness. *Orthop Clin North Am* 2000;31:129-143.

A-27: A 17-year-old high school football player reports wrist pain 5 months after the conclusion of the football season. A radiograph and MRI scan are shown in Figures 10A and 10B. What is the recommended intervention?

1. Pedicled vascularized bone graft
2. Long arm thumb spica cast
3. Percutaneous screw fixation
4. Corticocancellous bone grating via a volar approach (Matti-Russe)
5. Open reduction and differential pitch screw placement via a dorsal approach

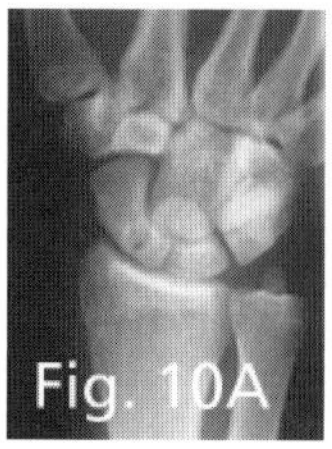
Fig. 10A

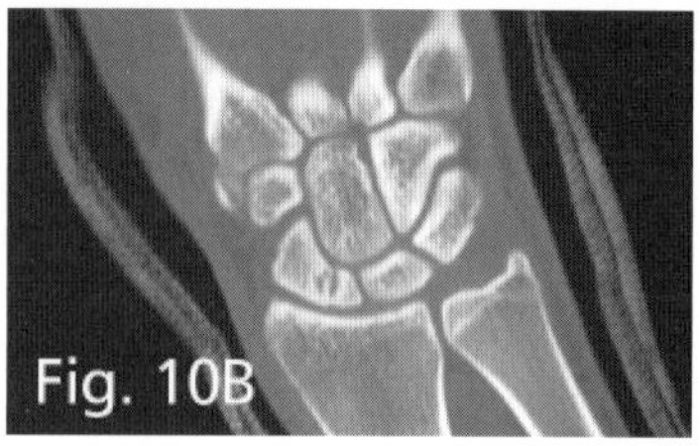
Fig. 10B

PREFERRED RESPONSE: 1

DISCUSSION: The patient has a nonunion of the proximal pole of the scaphoid. Acutely, this condition can be repaired with a screw alone, but as a nonunion the proximal pole has very poor healing potential. Vascularized bone grafts have been successful for these challenging nonunions, particularly in adolescents. A cast can be used for nondisplaced acute waist fractures, and corticocancellous grafts can be used for nonunions of the waist.

REFERENCES: Waters PM, Stewart SL: Surgical treatment of nonunion and avascular necrosis of the proximal part of the scaphoid in adolescents. *J Bone Joint Surg Am* 2002;84:915-920.

Steinmann SP, Bishop AT, Berger RA: Use of the 1,2 intercompartmental supraretinacular artery as a vascularized pedicle bone graft for difficult scaphoid nonunion. *J Hand Surg Am* 2002;27:391-401.

A-28: A 34-year-old man underwent open reduction and internal fixation of a closed both-bones forearm fracture 11 months ago. The radiographs shown in Figures 11A and 11B reveal a 3-mm gap and loose screws. What is the best treatment option?

1. Vascularized fibular graft
2. Locked intramedullary rodding
3. Tricortical iliac crest grafting and compression plating
4. Cancellous autograft and plating
5. Bone morphogenetic protein-7

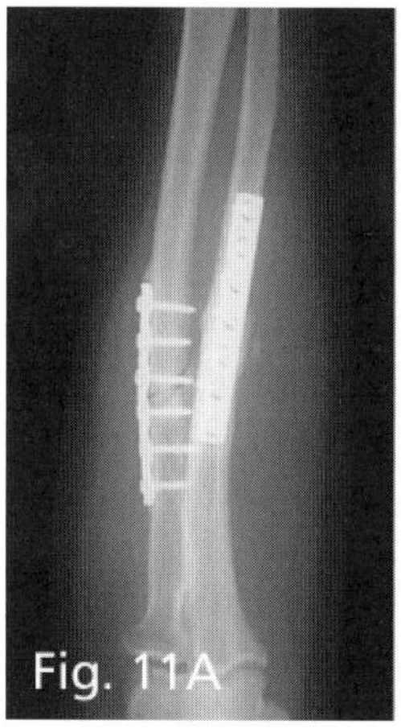
Fig. 11A

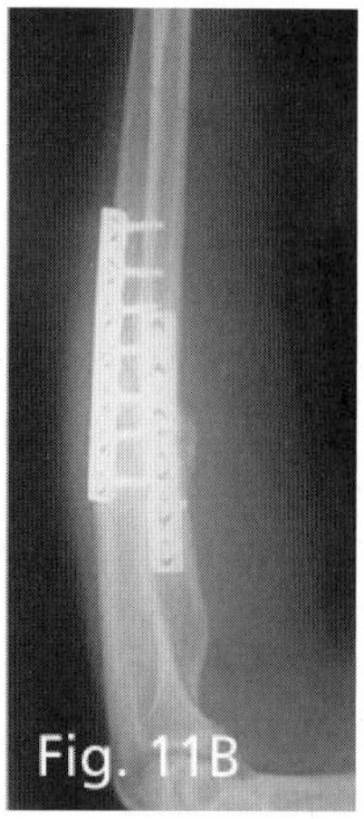
Fig. 11B

PREFERRED RESPONSE: 4

DISCUSSION: In an atrophic nonunion with a good soft-tissue envelope, adequate plating with cancellous bone graft can be used to span defects of up to 6 cm. Cortical graft from the fibula or iliac crest is not necessary. Bone morphogenetic protein-7 is a bone graft substitute and should not be used alone in this patient because the hardware is loose.

REFERENCE: Ring D, Allende C, Jafarnia K, et al: Ununited diaphyseal forearm fractures with segmental defects: Plate fixation and autogenous cancellous bone-grafting. *J Bone Joint Surg Am* 2004;86:2440-2445.

A-29: In surgically treating hand and finger infections in patients with diabetes mellitus, what factor is associated with higher amputation rates?

1. Insulin dependence
2. Gram-positive organisms
3. Renal failure
4. Retinopathy
5. Peripheral neuropathy

PREFERRED RESPONSE: 3

DISCUSSION: Patients with diabetes mellitus are prone to infection, and surgical treatment of their infections frequently requires multiple procedures. The triad of poor wound healing, chronic neuropathy, and vascular disease contributes to the increased infection rate. Studies have demonstrated increased amputation rates in patients with diabetes mellitus who have renal failure or deep polymicrobial or gram-negative infections.

REFERENCES: Gonzalez MH, Bochar S, Novotny J, et al: Upper extremity infections in patients with diabetes mellitus. *J Hand Surg Am* 1999;24:682-686. Trumble TE, ed: *Hand Surgery Update: Hand, Elbow, & Shoulder*, ed 3. Rosemont, IL, American Society for Surgery of the Hand, 2003, pp 433-457.

Kour AK, Looi KP, Phone MH, et al: Hand infections in patients with diabetes. *Clin Orthop Relat Res* 1996;331:238-244.

A-30: What is the primary indication for performing a total wrist arthroplasty in a patient with painful rheumatoid arthritis?

1. Ipsilateral total elbow arthroplasty
2. Contralateral wrist arthrodesis
3. Type III degenerative changes of the wrist
4. Age older than 55 years
5. Less than 30° of wrist flexion/extension

PREFERRED RESPONSE: 2

DISCUSSION: The most conservative indications for a total wrist arthroplasty are to spare motion on one side and to improve activities of daily living. Component loosening, dislocation, and wound problems are frequent. Suitable patients can be of various ages, and have various degrees of wrist motion and radiographic stages of arthritis. Ipsilateral total elbow arthroplasty, type III degenerative changes of the wrist, age older than 55 years, and limited range of motion are neither primary indications nor contraindications to a total wrist arthroplasty.

REFERENCES: Divelbiss BJ, Sollerman C, Adams BD: Early results of the universal total wrist arthroplasty in rheumatoid arthritis. *J Hand Surg Am* 2002;27:195-204.

Vicar AJ, Burton RI: Surgical management of rheumatoid wrist-fusion or arthroplasty. *J Hand Surg Am* 1986;11:790-797.

Carlson JR, Simmons BP: Total wrist arthroplasty. *J Am Acad Orthop Surg* 1998;6:308-315.

A-31: What is the most common bacteria cultured from dog and cat bites to the upper extremity?

1. *Pasteurella*
2. *Streptococcus*
3. *Staphylococcus*
4. *Bacteroides*
5. *Moraxella*

PREFERRED RESPONSE: 1

DISCUSSION: To define bacteria responsible for dog and cat bite infections, a prospective study yielded a median of five bacterial isolates per culture. *Pasteurella* is most common from both dog bites (50%) and cat bites (75%). *Pasteurella canis* was the most frequent pathogen of dog bites, and *Pasteurella multocida* was the most common isolate of cat bites. Other common aerobes included streptococci, staphylococci, *Moraxella*, and *Neisseria*.

REFERENCE: Talan DA, Citron DM, Abrahamian FM, et al: Bacteriologic analysis of infected dog and cat bites: Emergency Medicine Animal Bite Infection Study Group. *N Engl J Med* 1999;340:85-92.

A-32: A previously healthy 65-year-old woman has a closed fracture of the right clavicle after falling down the basement stairs. Examination reveals good capillary refill in the digits of her right hand. Radial and ulnar pulses are 1+ at the right wrist compared with 2+ on the opposite side. In the arteriogram shown in Figure 12, the arrow is pointing to which of the following arteries?

1. Brachiocephalic
2. Innominate
3. Subclavian
4. Axillary
5. Circumflex scapular

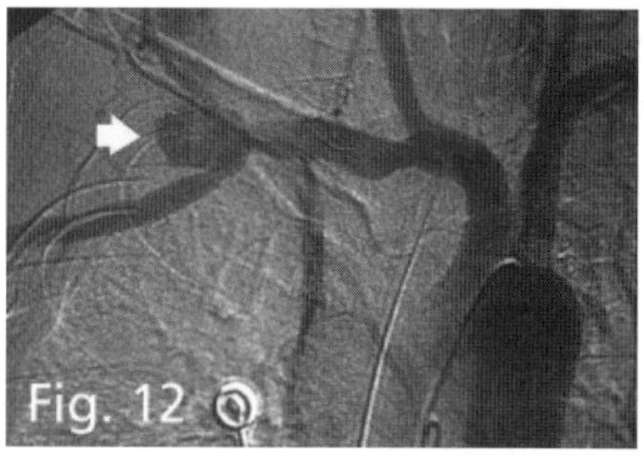

Fig. 12

PREFERRED RESPONSE: 4

DISCUSSION: The axillary artery commences at the first rib as a direct continuation of the subclavian artery and becomes the brachial artery at the lower border of the teres major. The arteriogram reveals a nonfilling defect in the third portion of the artery just distal to the subscapular artery. The complex arterial collateral circulation in this region often permits distal perfusion of the extremity despite injury.

REFERENCE: Radke HM: Arterial circulation of the upper extremity, in Strandness DE Jr, ed: *Collateral Circulation in Clinical Surgery*. Philadelphia, PA, WB Saunders, 1969, pp 294-307.

A-33: Which of the following structures may help maintain radial length after a radial head fracture?

1. Triangular fibrocartilage complex
2. Medial ulnar collateral ligament
3. Lateral ulnar collateral ligament
4. Annular ligament
5. Coronoid

PREFERRED RESPONSE: 1

DISCUSSION: Essex-Lopresti injuries affect axial stability of the forearm. Injury to the interosseous membrane or the triangular fibrocartilage complex can result in proximal migration of the radius.

REFERENCES: Morrey BF, Chao EY, Hui FC: Biomechanical study of the elbow following excision of the radial head. *J Bone Joint Surg Am* 1979;61:63-68.

Coleman DA, Blair WF, Shurr D: Resection of the radial head for fracture of the radial head: Long-term follow-up of seventeen cases. *J Bone Joint Surg Am* 1987;69:385-392.

A-34: Outcome measures should have established psychometric properties of reliability, validity, and responsiveness. Reliability refers to which of the following?

1. The amount of change in the score over time
2. Sensitivity of the measure in evaluating a problem
3. The ability of the instruments to actually measure what it intends to measure
4. The measure of change over the course of treatment
5. The reproducibility of the measurements either between repeated tests or between observers

PREFERRED RESPONSE: 5

DISCUSSION: The recent *J Bone Joint Surg Am* article by Kocher and associates defines the different psychometric properties that are used in outcome measures. Reliability is a measure of how reproducible a test is. This can be interobserver reliability (reliability between people), or intraobserver reliability (reliability for the same person doing the outcome measure at different occasions).

REFERENCE: Kocher MS, Horan MP, Briggs KK, et al: Reliability, validity, and responsiveness of the American Shoulder and Elbow Surgeons subjective shoulder scale in patients with shoulder instability, rotator cuff disease, and glenohumeral arthritis. *J Bone Joint Surg Am* 2005;87:2006-2011.

A-35: Figure 13 shows a coronal T2-weighted MRI scan. The arrow is pointing to what torn structure?

1. Brachialis tendon
2. Biceps tendon
3. Flexor/pronator origin
4. Medial collateral ligament (MCL)
5. Lateral collateral ligament (LCL)

PREFERRED RESPONSE: 5

DISCUSSION: The arrow is pointing to the LCL, and it is avulsed from the lateral humeral epicondyle. This is the most common site of injury for the LCL. The biceps and brachialis tendon insertions are not well visualized in this section. The MCL and flexor/pronator origins are intact.

REFERENCES: Potter HG, Weiland AJ, Schatz JA, et al: Posterolateral rotatory instability of the elbow: Usefulness of MR imaging in diagnosis. *Radiology* 1997;204:185-189.

King JC, Spencer EE: Lateral ligamentous instability: Techniques of repair and reconstruction. *Tech Orthop* 2000;8:93-104.

A-36: Which of the following findings is a contraindication to isolated percutaneous pinning of a distal radius fracture?

1. Dorsal comminution
2. Volar comminution
3. Radial comminution
4. Intra-articular fracture
5. Physeal fracture

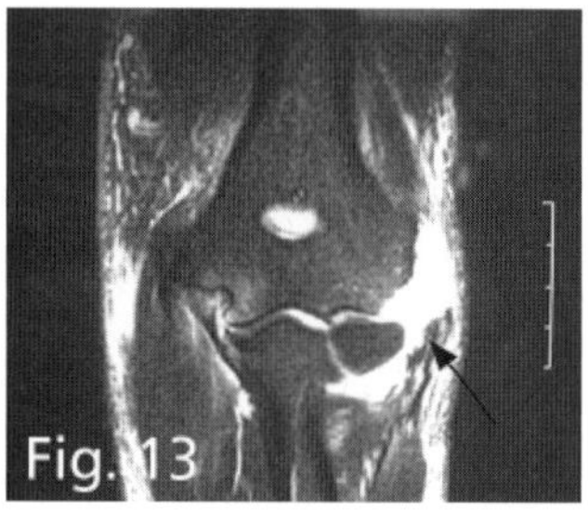

PREFERRED RESPONSE: 2

DISCUSSION: Intrafocal pinning allows the Kirschner wires to be placed through a site of comminution and then drilled through intact cortex. Generally Kapandji intrafocal pinning is done for dorsal comminuted extra-articular dorsal bending fractures, but it also may be used to elevate and buttress radial comminution. Simple intra-articular fractures can also be treated with pinning alone. Intrafocal pinning works best as a dorsal or radial buttress to prevent shortening. When there is volar comminution, the fracture is prone to shortening and supplemental external fixation or plating is recommended.

REFERENCES: Trumble TE, Wagner W, Hanel DP, et al: Intrafocal (Kapandji) pinning of distal radius fractures with and without external fixation. *J Hand Surg Am* 1998;23:381-394.

Choi KY, Chan WS, Lam TP, et al: Percutaneous Kirschner-wire pinning for severely displaced distal radial fractures in children: A report of 157 cases. *J Bone Joint Surg Br* 1995;77:797-801.

Weil WM, Trumble TE: Treatment of distal radius fractures with intrafocal (Kapandji) pinning and supplemental skeletal stabilization. *Hand Clin* 2005;21:317-328.

A-37: A 55-year-old man sustained an elbow dislocation in a fall. Postreduction radiographs are shown in Figures 14A and 14B. What is the best course of management?

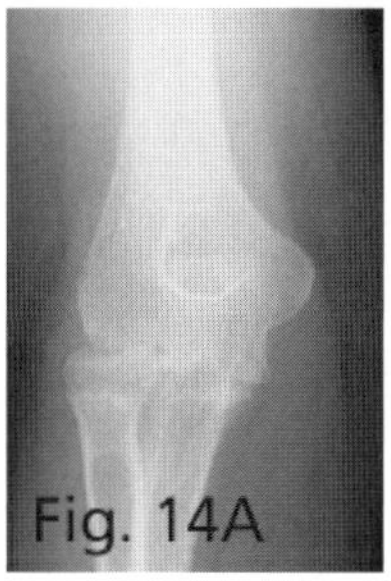

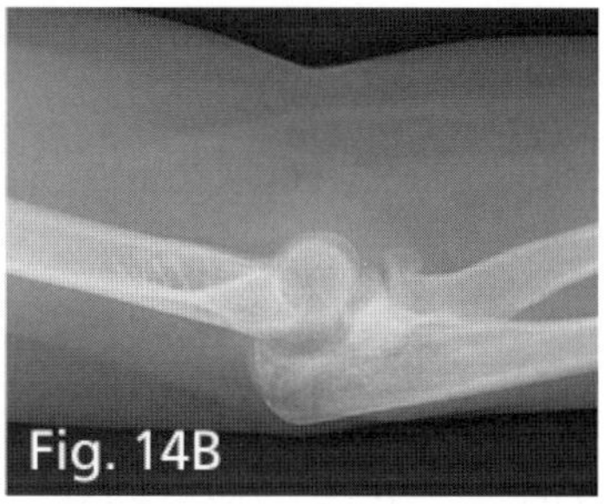

1. Closed reduction and casting for 4 weeks
2. Closed reduction and bracing with immediate range of motion
3. Open reduction, lateral collateral ligament repair, and open reduction and internal fixation or metallic replacement of the radial head
4. Open reduction, radial head Silastic arthroplasty, and lateral collateral ligament repair
5. Open reduction, lateral collateral ligament repair, and radial head excision

PREFERRED RESPONSE: 3

DISCUSSION: The radiographs show an elbow dislocation associated with a comminuted radial head fracture. In the setting of comminution and instability, factures of the radial head are best managed with an arthroplasty rather than open reduction and internal fixation. Resection of the radial head will worsen the instability and is not recommended. Silastic radial head replacements are contraindicated.

REFERENCES: Hildebrand KA, Patterson SD, King GJ: Acute elbow dislocations: Simple and complex. *Orthop Clin North Am* 1999;30:63-79.

O'Driscoll SW, Jupiter JB, King GJ, et al: The unstable elbow. *Instr Course Lect* 2001;50:89-102.

A-38: In a patient with rheumatoid arthritis of the wrist, which of the following extensor tendons is most at risk of rupture?

1. Extensor digiti quinti
2. Abductor pollicis longus
3. Extensor pollicis longus
4. Extensor carpi radialis brevis
5. Extensor carpi ulnaris

PREFERRED RESPONSE: 1

DISCUSSION: The tendon most prone to rupture in a patient with rheumatoid arthritis of the wrist is the extensor digiti quinti. It can be a silent injury because the extensor digitorum communis can provide extension to the fifth finger. The extensor digiti quinti is at high risk because it is overlying the ulnar head where it is prone to attritional rupture (Vaughan-Jackson syndrome).

REFERENCES: Vaughan-Jackson OJ: Rupture of extensor tendons by attrition at the inferior radioulnar joint: A report of two cases. *J Bone Joint Surg Br* 1948;30:528-530.

Papp SR, Athwal GS, Pichora DR: The rheumatoid wrist. *J Am Acad Orthop Surg* 2006;14:65-77.

A-39: What is the most appropriate surgical treatment for a stage III symptomatic scapholunate advanced collapsed (SLAC) wrist?

1. Radioscapholunate arthrodesis
2. Scaphotrapeziotrapezoid arthrodesis
3. Scaphocapitate arthrodesis
4. Proximal row carpectomy
5. Scaphoid excision and capitate-lunate-triquetrum-hamate arthrodesis

PREFERRED RESPONSE: 5

DISCUSSION: SLAC is the end result of chronic scapholunate instability. The arthritis follows a predictable pattern. Stage I disease involves cartilage loss between the waist of the scaphoid and the radial styloid. In stage II, the arthritis progresses to include the proximal pole of the scaphoid and the scaphoid fossa of the radius. Finally, stage III goes on to include arthritis of the capitolunate joint. The only treatment option that addresses all of the sites of arthritis is the scaphoid excision and four-corner fusion.

REFERENCES: Ashmead DT IV, Watson HK, Damon C, et al: Scapholunate advanced collapse wrist salvage. *J Hand Surg Am* 1994;19:741-750.

Sauerbier M, Trankle M, Linsner G, et al: Midcarpal arthrodesis with complete scaphoid excision and interposition bone graft in the treatment of advanced carpal collapse (SNAC/SLAC wrist): Operative technique and outcome assessment. *J Hand Surg Br* 2000;25:341-345.

A-40: A 25-year-old man shot himself at the base of the right index finger while cleaning his handgun. Examination reveals that the finger is cool and cyanotic. A radiograph and clinical photograph are shown in Figures 15A and 15B. What is the recommended treatment?

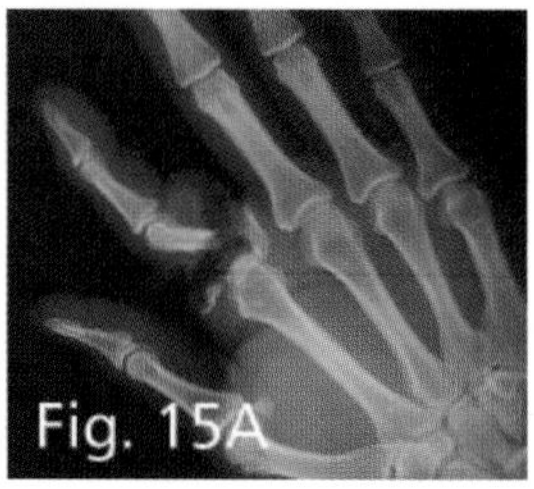
Fig. 15A

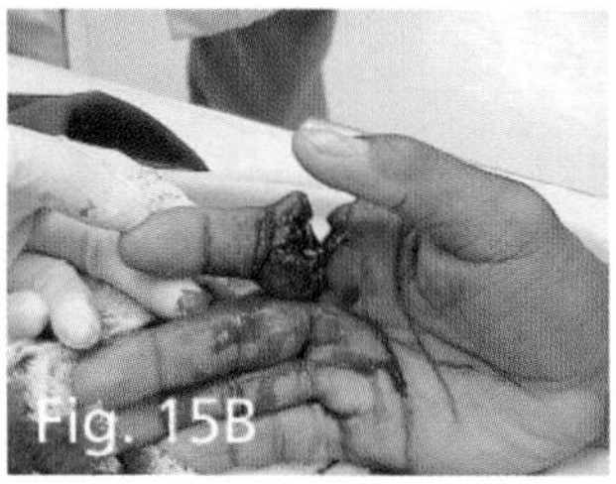
Fig. 15B

1. Open reduction and internal fixation and arterial reconstruction
2. Crossed pinning with Kirschner wires
3. Open (guillotine) finger amputation
4. Index ray amputation
5. Application of an external fixator

PREFERRED RESPONSE: 4

DISCUSSION: The gunshot wound has caused injury to multiple systems: bone, vascular, skin, and tendon; therefore, the treatment of choice is amputation. An immediate ray amputation allows for a more rapid return to activities and less time off work.

REFERENCES: Peimer CA, Wheeler DR, Barrett A, et al: Hand function following single ray amputation. *J Hand Surg Am* 1999;24:1245-1248.

Neumeister MW, Brown RE: Mutilating hand injuries: Principles and management. *Hand Clin* 2003;19:1-15.

A-41: What are the two terminal branches of the lateral cord of the brachial plexus?

1. Musculocutaneous and median
2. Musculocutaneous and axillary
3. Median and axillary
4. Ulnar and median
5. Ulnar and medial pectoral

PREFERRED RESPONSE: 1

DISCUSSION: The lateral cord divides into the musculocutaneous and median nerves. The posterior cord terminates into the axillary and radial nerves. The medial cord divides into the ulnar and median nerves.

REFERENCES: Hollinshead WH: *Anatomy for Surgeons*, ed 3. Philadelphia, PA, Harper and Row, 1982, pp 228-236.
Shin AY, Spinner RJ, Steinmann SP, et al: Adult traumatic brachial plexus injuries. *J Am Acad Orthop Surg* 2005;13: 382-396.

A-42: What is the most common complaint in patients with a developmental radial head dislocation?

1. Pain
2. Recurrent elbow subluxation
3. Limitation of extension
4. Cosmetic deformity
5. Locking

PREFERRED RESPONSE: 4

DISCUSSION: Developmental dislocation of the radial head most frequently presents as a painless mass over the posterior aspect of the elbow. Patients do not have feelings of elbow subluxation but may report pain or clicking. Limitation of motion is most frequently found in the pronation and supination arc rather than in flexion and extension.

REFERENCES: Lloyd-Roberts GC, Bucknill TM: Anterior dislocation of the radial head in children-etiology: Natural history and management. *J Bone Joint Surg Am* 1977;58:402.

Hamilton W, Parks JC II: Isolated dislocation of the radial head without fracture of the ulna. *Clin Orthop Relat Res* 1973;97:94-96.

A-43: A 35-year-old man sustained the closed injury shown in Figure 16 in his dominant extremity.

Neurologic function is normal. Treatment should consist of
1. functional bracing.
2. a sling and swathe.
3. intramedullary nail fixation.
4. open reduction and internal fixation.
5. iliac crest bone graft.

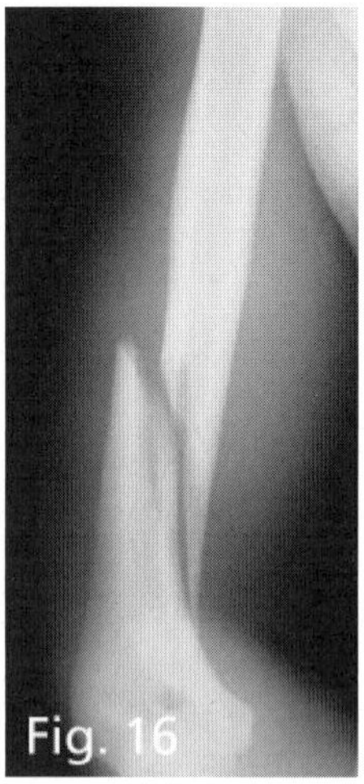

Fig. 16

PREFERRED RESPONSE: 1

DISCUSSION: Functional bracing has been demonstrated to have a very high rate of healing without any functional limitations in a large series of patients. Surgery is reserved for "floating elbows," open injuries, neurovascular injuries, and those fractures that go on to nonunion.

REFERENCES: Sarmiento A, Zagorski JB, Zych GA, et al: Functional bracing for the treatment of fractures of the humeral diaphysis. *J Bone Joint Surg Am* 2000;82:478-486.

Dirschl DR: Shoulder trauma: Bone, in Koval KJ, ed: *Orthopaedic Knowledge Update*, ed 7. Rosemont, IL, American Academy of Orthopaedic Surgeons, 2002, p 267.

A-44: The radiograph shown in Figure 17 reveals that the plate on the second metacarpal is acting in what manner?

1. Compression
2. Tension band
3. Bridge
4. Buttress
5. Spring

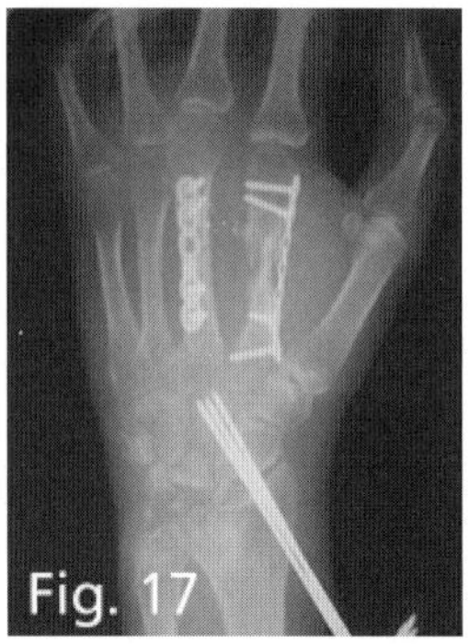

Fig. 17

PREFERRED RESPONSE: 3

DISCUSSION: There are four ways in which a plate acts: compression, tension band, bridge or spanning, and buttress. Because there is no cortical contact with the large span of comminution, this plate is acting as a bridge plate. A bridge plate is defined as one that is used as an extramedullary splint attached to the two main fragments, leaving the comminution untouched.

REFERENCE: Ruedi T, Murphy WM, eds: *AO Principles of Fracture Management*. New York, NY, Thieme, 2000, p 221.

A-45: Figure 18 shows the radiograph of a 30-year-old man who sustained a closed comminuted fracture of the right clavicle. Examination reveals decreased sensation in the radial nerve distribution. Weakness is noted with shoulder abduction, internal rotation, and wrist extension. A displaced bone fragment is most likely pressing on what portion of the brachial plexus?

1. C5 and C6 spinal roots
2. Superior trunk
3. Anterior division of the inferior trunk
4. Posterior cord
5. Lateral and posterior cords

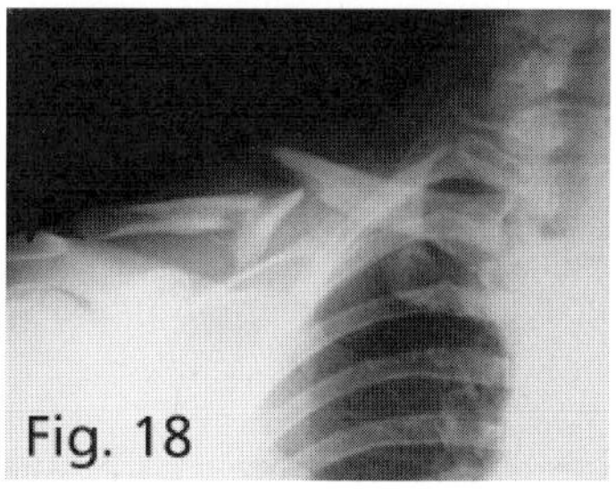
Fig. 18

PREFERRED RESPONSE: 4

DISCUSSION: Clavicular fractures are occasionally complicated by injury to the brachial plexus. A displaced bone fragment pressing on the posterior cord proximal to the upper subscapularis nerve would account for these findings.

REFERENCES: Jobe CM, Coen MJ: Gross anatomy of the shoulder, in Rockwood CA, Matsen FA, Wirth MA, et al, eds: *The Shoulder*. Philadelphia, PA, WB Saunders, 2004, vol 2, pp 1078-1079.

Barbier O, Malghem J, Delaere O, et al: Injury to the brachial plexus by a fragment of bone after fracture of the clavicle. *J Bone Joint Surg Br* 1997;79:534-536.

A-46: Which of the following is considered an important component in treating the lesion shown in Figure 19?

1. Excision of the skin in addition to the cyst
2. Resection of the nail plate
3. Excision of bony osteophytes from the distal interphalangeal (DIP) joint
4. Injection of corticosteroid into the DIP joint
5. Resection of part of the collateral ligament and extensor mechanism

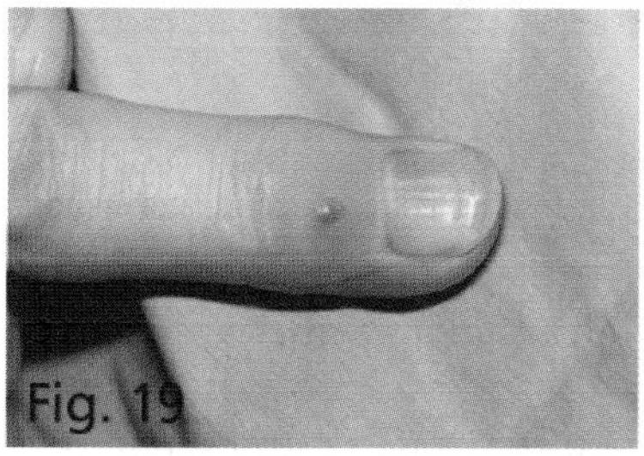
Fig. 19

PREFERRED RESPONSE: 3

DISCUSSION: Mucoid cysts are commonly associated with DIP joint arthritis. Two treatment options are commonly used: (1) aspiration/drainage and injection of corticosteroid and (2) surgical excision. When performing the surgery, excision of the bony osteophytes about the DIP joint is helpful in achieving a cure. There are no reports of significant benefit with nail removal or partial ligament or extensor tendon resection. Some authors have advocated skin excision and rotational flaps for wound coverage, but this is somewhat controversial.

REFERENCES: Rizzo M, Beckenbaugh RD: Treatment of mucous cysts of the fingers: Review of 134 cases with minimum 2-year follow-up evaluation. *J Hand Surg Am* 2003;28:519-524.

Eaton RG, Dobranski AI, Littler JW: Marginal osteophyte excision in treatment of mucous cysts. *J Bone Joint Surg Am* 1973;55:570-574.

A-47: A patient with rheumatoid arthritis has a rupture of the extensor digitorum communis to the fourth and fifth metacarpals. You are planning to perform an extensor indicis proprius (EIP) tendon transfer. What effect will this have on index finger extension?

1. No effect
2. Index finger weakness
3. Index metacarpophalangeal hyperextension
4. Index metacarpophalangeal hyperflexion
5. Index metacarpophalangeal ulnar deviation

PREFERRED RESPONSE: 1

DISCUSSION: EIP transfer results in no functional deficit. If the tendon is cut proximal to the sagittal band, there will be no extensor deficit.

REFERENCES: Browne EX, Teague MA, Snyder CC: Prevention of extensor lag after indicis proprius transfer. *J Hand Surg Am* 1979;4:168-172.

Moore JR, Weiland AJ, Valdata L: Independent index extension after extensor indicis proprius transfer. *J Hand Surg Am* 1987;12:232-236.

A-48: A 22-year-old man is tackled while playing college football and sustains a reducible first carpometacarpal dislocation. What is the recommended treatment?

1. Closed reduction and casting
2. Closed reduction and percutaneous pinning
3. First carpometacarpal arthrodesis
4. Dorsal capsulodesis
5. Ligament reconstruction using tendon autograft

PREFERRED RESPONSE: 5

DISCUSSION: When comparing closed reduction and pinning to ligament reconstruction, the reconstruction group had slightly better abduction and pinch strength. The volar oblique ligament usually tears off the first metacarpal in a subperiosteal fashion. In this young patient, motion-sparing procedures are preferred.

REFERENCES: Simonian PT, Trumble TE: Traumatic dislocation of the thumb carpometacarpal joint: Early ligamentous reconstruction versus closed reduction and pinning. *J Hand Surg Am* 1996;21;802-806.

Strauch RJ, Behrman MJ, Rosenwasser MP: Acute dislocation of the carpometacarpal joint of the thumb: An anatomic and cadaver study. *J Hand Surg Am* 1994;19:93-98.

A-49: What structure provides the most static stability for valgus restraint in the elbow?

1. Posterior band of the ulnar collateral ligament
2. Anterior band of the ulnar collateral ligament
3. Transverse band of the ulnar collateral ligament
4. Annular ligament
5. Flexor/pronator mass

PREFERRED RESPONSE: 2

DISCUSSION: The anterior band of the ulnar collateral ligament provides the greatest restraint to valgus stress in the elbow. The posterior band is taut in flexion and resists stress between 60° and full flexion. The annular ligament stabilizes the radial head. The flexor/pronator mass are important dynamic stabilizers of the medial elbow.

REFERENCES: Ahmad CS, ElAttrache NS: Elbow valgus instability in the throwing athlete. *J Am Acad Orthop Surg* 2006;14:693-700.

Regan WD, Korinek SL, Morrey BF, et al: Biomechanical study of ligaments around the elbow joint. *Clin Orthop Relat Res* 1991;271:170-179.

Safran M, Ahmad CS, ElAttrache NS: Ulnar collateral ligament of the elbow. *Arthroscopy* 2005;21:1381-1395.

Preservation, Arthroplasty, and Salvage Surgery of the Hip and Knee

Q-1: Which of the following radiographic images is best for detecting anterior acetabular deficiency in the dysplastic hip?

1. Pelvic inlet
2. Judet
3. AP pelvis
4. False profile
5. Frog lateral

Q-2: At the level of tibial bone resection in total knee arthroplasty, where does the common peroneal nerve lie?

1. Deep to the arcuate ligament
2. Closer to bone in larger legs
3. On the muscle belly of the popliteus
4. On the bony posterolateral corner of the tibia
5. Superficial to the lateral head of the gastrocnemius

Q-3: The anatomy of the sciatic nerve as it exits the pelvis is best described as exiting through the

1. greater sciatic notch and passing between the inferior gemellus and the obturator externus.
2. greater sciatic notch and passing between the piriformis and the superior gemellus.
3. obturator foramen and passing between the obturator internus and the obturator externus.
4. lesser sciatic notch and passing between the piriformis and the superior gemellus.
5. lesser sciatic notch and passing between the superior gemellus and the inferior gemellus.

Q-4: What complication is more likely following excessive medial retraction of the anterior covering structures during the anterolateral (Watson-Jones) approach to the hip?

1. Numbness over the anterolateral thigh
2. Ischemia to the leg
3. Quadriceps weakness
4. Abductor insufficiency
5. Foot drop

Q-5: A 40-year-old man has had hip pain with increased activity over the past year. Examination reveals restriction of motion and tenderness with combined hip flexion, adduction, and internal rotation. An AP radiograph is shown in Figure 1. What is the most likely diagnosis?

1. Developmental dysplasia of the hip
2. Osteonecrosis
3. Perthes disease
4. Pseudogout
5. Femoral acetabular impingement

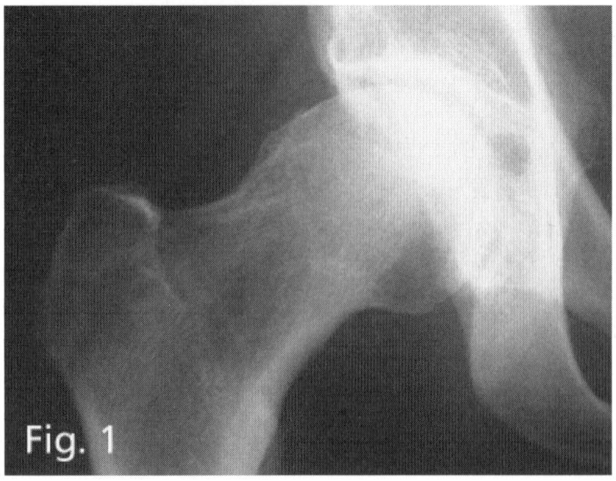
Fig. 1

Q-6: Bleeding is encountered while developing the internervous plane between the tensor fascia lata and the sartorius during the anterior approach to the hip. The most likely cause is injury to what artery?

1. Ascending branch of the lateral femoral circumflex
2. Superior gluteal
3. Femoral
4. Profunda femoris
5. Medial femoral circumflex

Q-7: When using the direct lateral (or Hardinge) approach for hip arthroplasty, three muscles are detached from the femur. In addition to the vastus lateralis, they include the

1. iliopsoas and sartorius.
2. piriformis and obturator internus.
3. gluteus maximus and tensor fascia lata.
4. gluteus minimus and rectus femoris.
5. gluteus medius and gluteus minimus.

Q-8: Figure 2 shows the radiograph of a patient who underwent a total knee revision with a posterior stabilized mobile-bearing prosthesis and who now has recurrent knee dislocations. What is the most likely cause?

1. Loose extension gap
2. Loose flexion gap
3. Malrotation of the tibial component
4. Malrotation of the femoral component
5. Poor prosthetic design

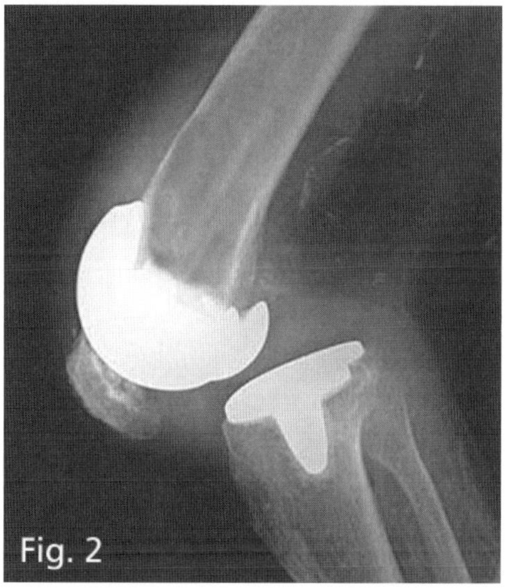
Fig. 2

Q-9: Figures 3A and 3B show the radiographs of a 72-year-old man with aseptic loosening of the tibial component of his total knee arthroplasty. Optimal management should include

1. tibial revision only, without stems or augmentations.
2. tibial revision only, with stems and augmentations.
3. revision of the tibial and femoral components, without stems or augmentations.
4. revision of the tibial and femoral components, with stems and augmentations.
5. primary arthrodesis.

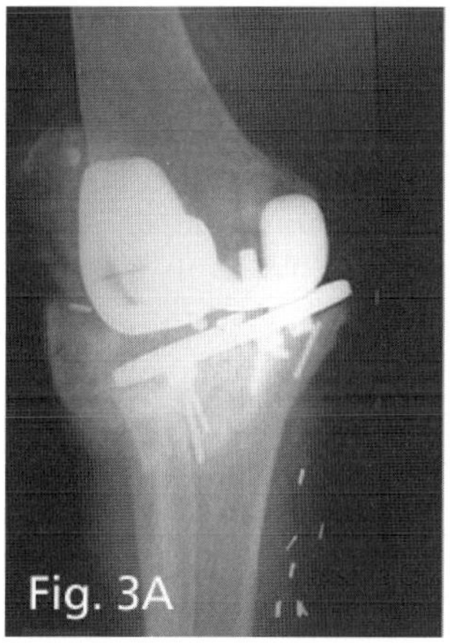
Fig. 3A

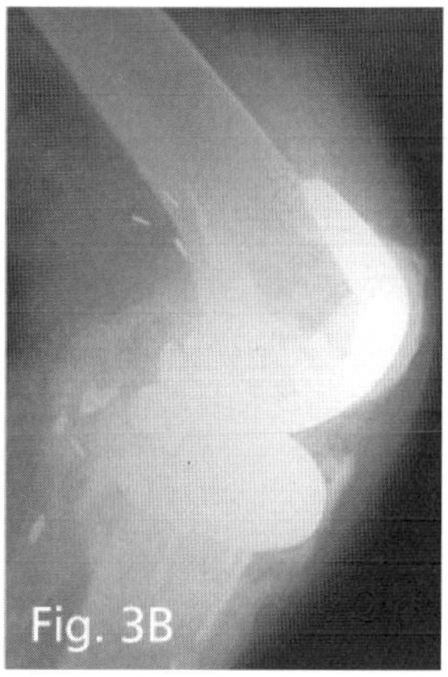
Fig. 3B

Q-10: Figure 4 shows the AP radiograph of a patient with diabetes mellitus who has knee pain. A semi-constrained knee prosthesis was used in this patient to prevent which of the following complications?

1. Infection
2. Instability
3. Stiffness
4. Bone loss
5. Malalignment

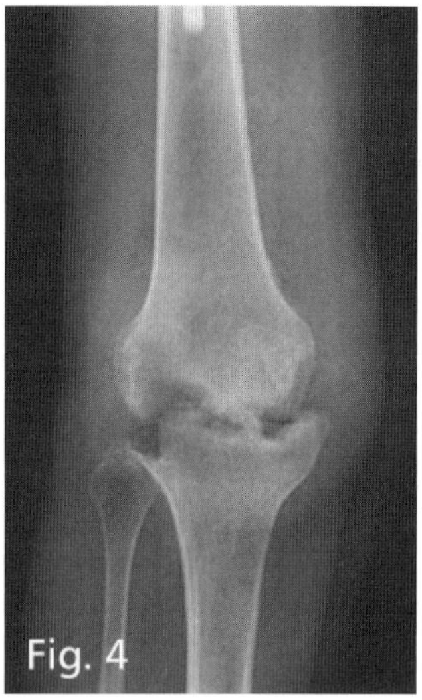
Fig. 4

Q-11: A 75-year-old woman who fell on her right knee now reports pain and is unable to bear weight. History reveals that she underwent total knee arthroplasty on the right knee 6 years ago. Radiographs are shown in Figure 5. Management should now consist of

1. closed reduction and casting for 6 weeks.
2. open reduction and internal fixation, using a locked intramedullary rod.
3. open reduction and internal fixation, using two cancellous screws.
4. open reduction and internal fixation, using a locked plate and screws.
5. open reduction and internal fixation and revision of the femoral component.

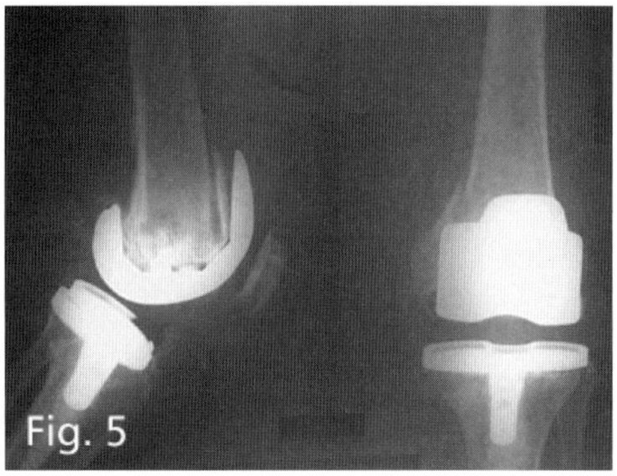
Fig. 5

Q-12: A 64-year-old man undergoes a primary total knee arthroplasty. Three months after surgery he reports persistent pain, weakness, and difficulty ambulating. Postoperative radiographs are shown in Figures 6A through 6C. What is the best course of action at this time?

1. Hinged knee brace
2. Patellar component revision with a tantalum implant and lateralization of the patella
3. Revision knee arthroplasty with greater internal rotation of the tibial component
4. Revision total knee arthroplasty with a lateral release and external rotation of the femoral component
5. Revision total knee arthroplasty with a lateral release and internal rotation of the femoral component

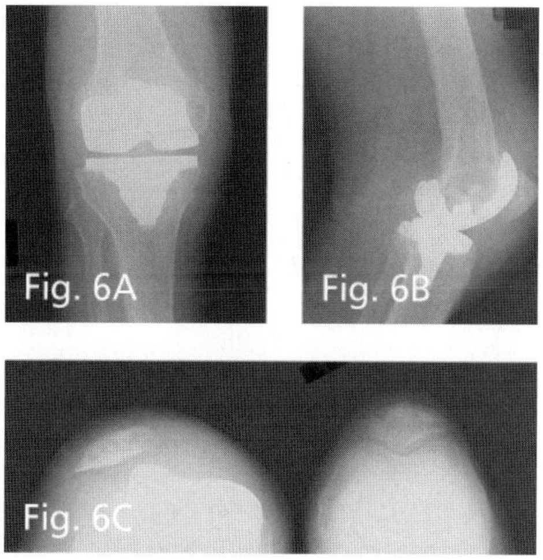

Q-13: Compared to metal-on-polyethylene total hip bearing surfaces, the debris particles generated by metal-on-metal articulations are

1. larger and less numerous.
2. larger and more numerous.
3. smaller and less numerous.
4. smaller and more numerous.
5. not detectable.

Q-14: A 60-year-old patient had the procedure shown in Figure 7 performed 5 years ago. During transition to a total knee arthroplasty (TKA), what patellar problem is commonly encountered intraoperatively?

1. Fracture
2. Patella baja
3. Patella alta
4. Osteonecrosis
5. Maltracking

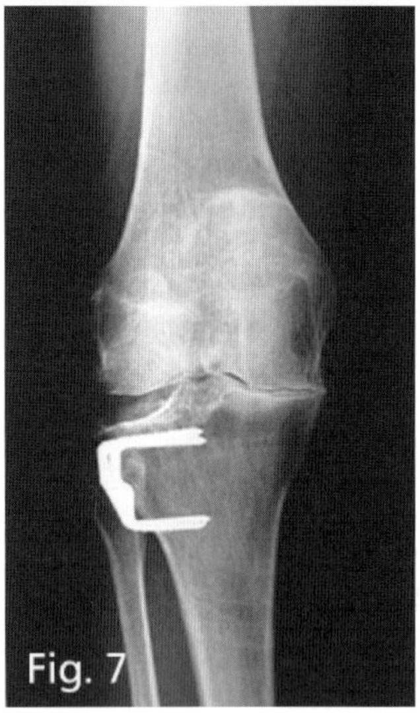
Fig. 7

Q-15: Figures 8A and 8B show the radiographs of a 75-year-old man who underwent a revision total knee arthroplasty with a long-stemmed tibial component. In rehabilitation, he reports fullness and tenderness in the proximal medial leg (at the knee). The strategy that would best limit this postoperative problem is use of

1. a base plate with an offset tibial stem attachment.
2. a bone ingrowth surface on the augment.
3. a nonstemmed tibial base plate.
4. allograft bone instead of metal augments.
5. bone cement to smooth the outline of the proximal medial tibia.

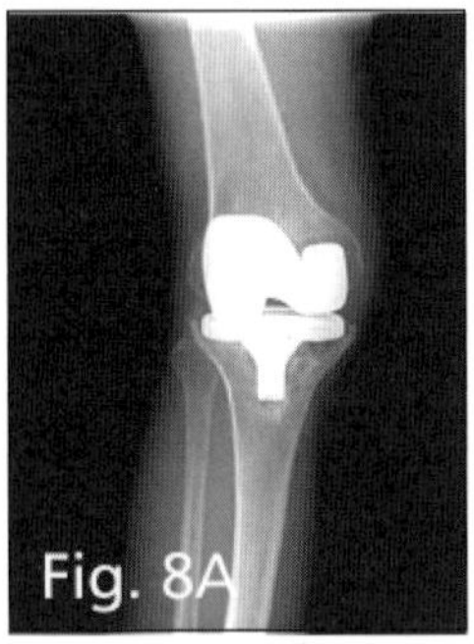
Fig. 8A

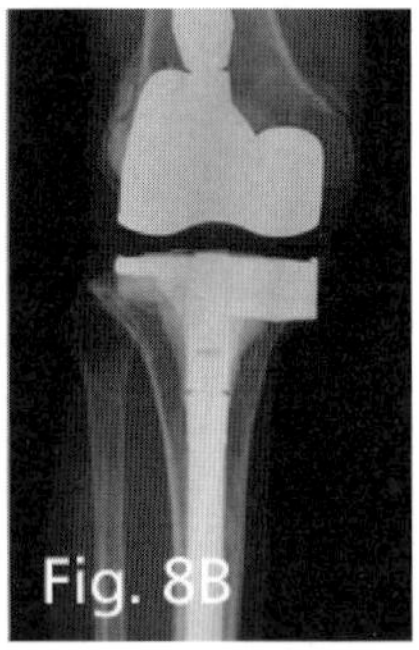
Fig. 8B

Q-16: Figure 9 shows the AP radiograph of an ambulatory 76-year-old patient. What is the most appropriate surgical treatment option for this patient?

1. Revision arthroplasty using a cemented femoral component
2. Impaction allografting of the femoral component
3. Proximal femoral replacement arthroplasty
4. Resection arthroplasty
5. Hip arthrodesis

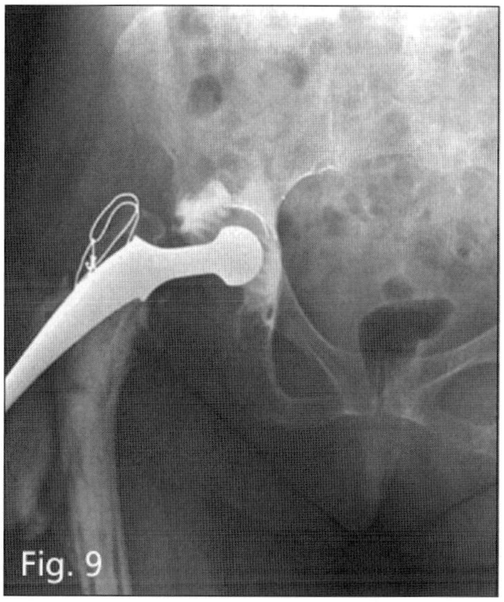

Fig. 9

Q-17: Increasing articular conformity of the tibial polyethylene insert of a fixed-bearing total knee arthroplasty (TKA) prosthesis will have which of the following biomechanical effects?

1. Decreased contact stress within the polyethylene
2. Decreased risk of patellofemoral instability
3. Decreased risk of mechanical loosening
4. Increased risk of subsurface polyethylene cracking
5. Increased tibial rollback during flexion

Q-18: A 63-year-old woman reports giving way of the knee and pain after undergoing primary total knee arthroplasty (TKA) 1 year ago. Examination reveals that the knee is stable in full extension but has gross anteroposterior instability at 90° of flexion. The patient can fully extend her knee with normal quadriceps strength. Studies for infection are negative. AP and lateral radiographs are shown in Figures 10A and 10B, respectively. What is the appropriate management?

1. Anti-inflammatory drugs
2. Knee brace
3. Physical therapy for quadriceps strengthening
4. Revision to a thicker polyethylene insert
5. Revision to a larger, posterior stabilized implant

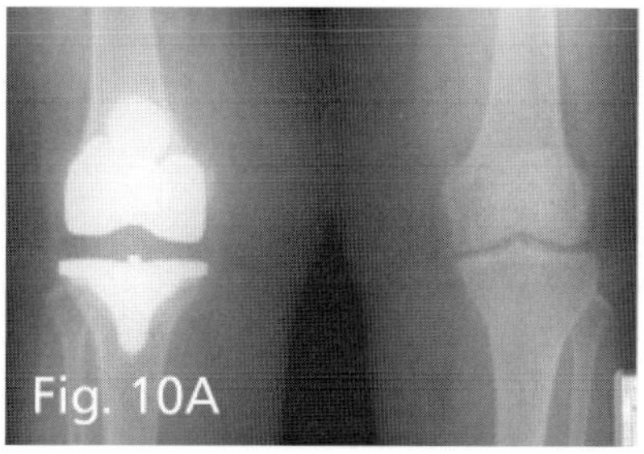

Fig. 10A

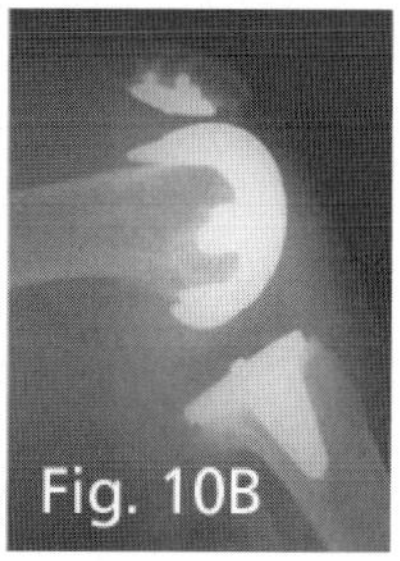

Fig. 10B

Q-19: Stiffness can occur following total knee arthroplasty. What is the most appropriate management for a patient who has deteriorating arc of motion after undergoing a revision knee arthroplasty 9 months ago?

1. Aggressive physical therapy
2. Manipulation under anesthesia
3. Investigation for periprosthetic infection
4. Revision knee arthroplasty
5. Resection arthroplasty

Q-20: A 59-year-old woman who underwent a total hip arthroplasty 5 years ago now has recurrent dislocation following bariatric surgery and a weight loss of 200 lb. An attempt at conversion to a larger head size and trochanteric advancement has failed. Her components are well aligned. What is the best course of action?

1. Resection arthroplasty
2. Hip abduction brace
3. Constrained acetabular liner
4. Thermal ablation of the posterior capsule
5. Conversion to a bipolar prosthesis

Q-21: Figure 11 shows the radiograph of an otherwise healthy 62-year-old woman who fell. Management should consist of

1. revision total hip arthroplasty with a cemented femoral component and adjuvant fracture fixation.
2. revision total hip arthroplasty with a cementless femoral component and adjuvant fracture fixation.
3. open reduction and internal fixation of the fracture and retention of the original components.
4. removal of the components, open reduction and internal fixation of the fracture, and delayed replantation of the components when the fracture is healed.
5. resection arthroplasty and internal fixation of the fracture.

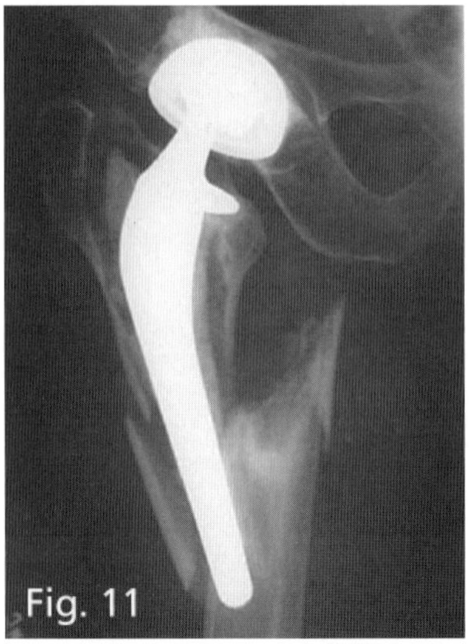

Fig. 11

Q-22: A 75-year-old woman undergoes hybrid total hip arthroplasty for osteoarthritis. A postoperative radiograph obtained in the recovery room is shown in Figure 12. Treatment should now consist of

1. open reduction and internal fixation with strut graft and cerclage wire.
2. open reduction and internal fixation with a plate, screws, and bone graft.
3. exchange of the femoral components with insertion of a long stem cementless implant.
4. cast immobilization.
5. minimal weight bearing and observation.

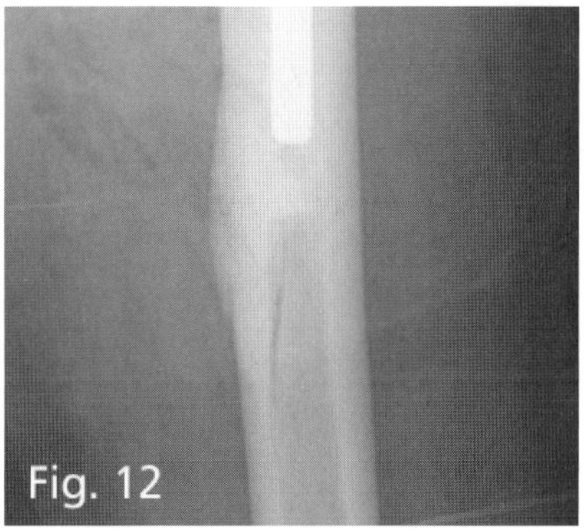
Fig. 12

Q-23: A 58-year-old man reports a 2-month onset of groin pain with no history of trauma. Examination reveals that range of motion of the hip is mildly restricted, and he has pain with both weight bearing and at rest. An MRI scan is shown in Figure 13. Treatment should consist of

1. protected weight bearing and anti-inflammatory drugs.
2. core decompression of the femoral head.
3. vascularized free fibular grafting to the femoral head.
4. bipolar hemiarthroplasty of the hip.
5. total hip arthroplasty.

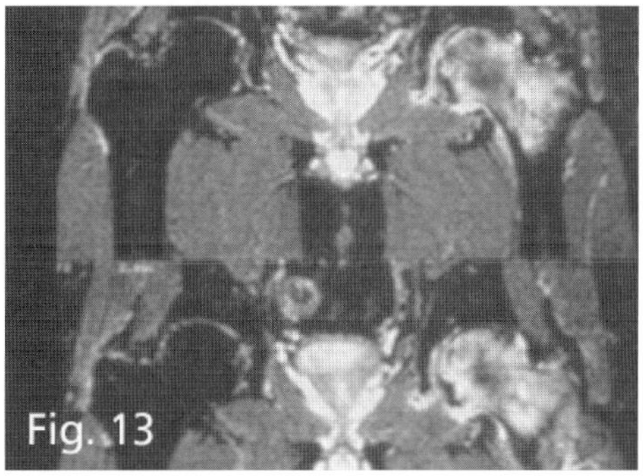
Fig. 13

Q-24: Figure 14 shows the radiograph of a 32-year-old patient with right hip pain that has failed to respond to nonsurgical management. What is the most appropriate surgical treatment at this time?

1. Femoral derotational osteotomy
2. Total hip arthroplasty
3. Arthrodesis
4. Surgical dislocation of the hip
5. Periacetabular osteotomy

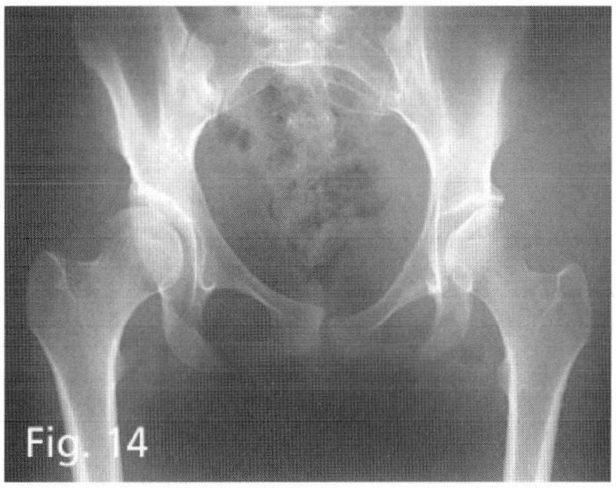
Fig. 14

Q-25: A patient reports pain in the hip with functional positioning. With the patient supine, pain in which of the following positions would be typical for femoral acetabular impingement?

1. Hip is internally rotated, passively flexed to 90°, and adducted
2. Hip is internally rotated, passively flexed to 90°, and abducted
3. Hip is externally rotated, maximally flexed to 90°, and adducted
4. Hip is externally rotated, passively flexed to 90°, and abducted
5. Hip is externally rotated, maximally flexed, and abducted

Q-26: A 38-year-old man who is an avid tennis player has had persistent pain over the medial aspect of his knee for the past 6 years. He notes that the pain occurs on a daily basis with any significant activity. NSAIDs have failed to provide relief. Radiographs are shown in Figures 15A and 15B. What is the best course of action?

1. Total knee arthroplasty
2. Unicompartmental arthroplasty
3. Insertion of a unispacer
4. Tibial osteotomy
5. Knee arthroscopy

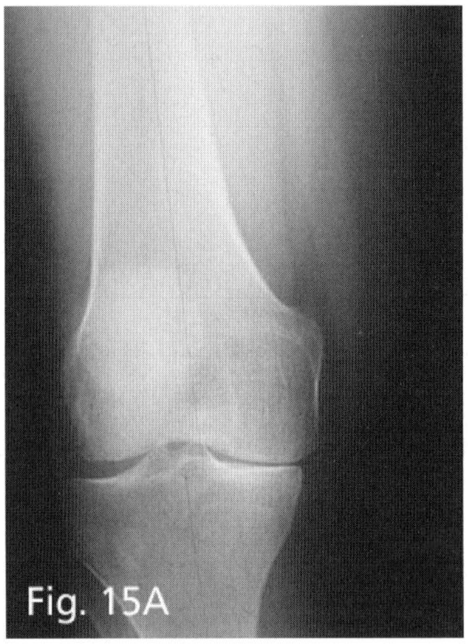
Fig. 15A

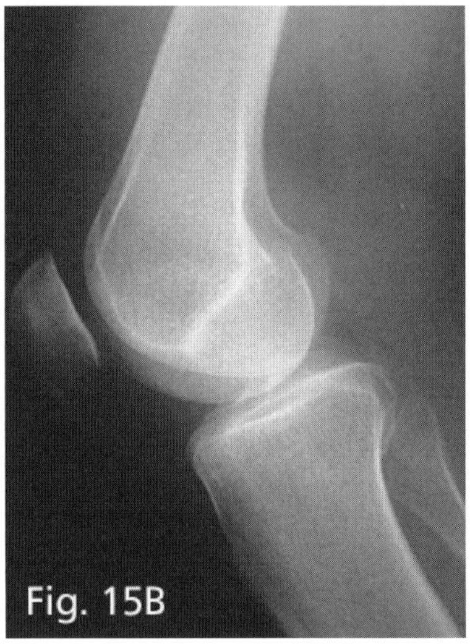
Fig. 15B

Q-27: Which of the following statements best describes the outcome of the routine use of continuous passive motion (CPM) machines after total knee arthroplasty (TKA)?

1. CPM is likely to improve early range of motion and final range of motion.
2. CPM may improve early range of motion but is unlikely to improve final range of motion.
3. CPM is likely to decrease postoperative pain.
4. CPM is likely to improve extension but not flexion.
5. CPM is likely to restore quicker ambulatory ability.

Q-28: When performing knee arthroplasty, which of the following procedures provides the most consistent fixation for the tibial component?

1. Cementless fixation of the tibial component
2. Augmenting cementless fixation of the tibial component with pegs or screws
3. Cementing the metaphyseal portion and press fitting the keel of the tibial component
4. Cementing the metaphyseal and keel portions of the tibial component
5. Cemented fixation of the tibial component with screws

Q-29: Figure 16 shows the radiograph of an 84-year-old woman who has pain and is unable to extend her knee. History reveals that she underwent total knee arthroplasty 8 years ago. Aspiration and studies for infection are negative. During revision surgery, management of the tibial bone loss should consist of

1. reconstruction with a metal augmented revision tibial implant.
2. reconstruction with a hinged prosthesis.
3. reconstruction with a structural allograft.
4. reconstruction with iliac crest bone graft.
5. filling the defect with cement.

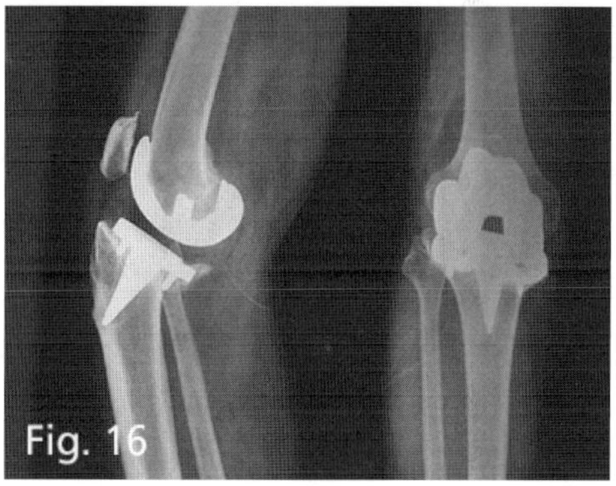
Fig. 16

Q-30: A 62-year-old woman with a bone mineral density (BMD) T-score of -2.0 sustained a subcapital fracture of her hip. She is an avid tennis player, and history reveals no previous fractures. What is the most appropriate follow-up care?

1. Antiresorptive bisphosphonate medication
2. A repeat dual-energy x-ray absorptiometry scan (DEXA) and treatment if the T-score is less than –2.5
3. A repeat DEXA scan and treatment if the T-score is greater than –1.5
4. No treatment because the BMD is not in osteoporotic range
5. Parathyroid hormone followed by surgery

Q-31: A 58-year-old patient who underwent bilateral hip arthroplasty 12 years ago now reports pain in his hips and difficulty with ambulation to the point where he now uses crutches. A radiograph of the hip and pelvis is shown in Figure 17. What is the best treatment option for this patient?

1. Revision hip arthroplasty with a bipolar implant
2. Revision hip arthroplasty with impaction grafting on the femoral and acetabular side
3. Revision hip arthroplasty with a cemented jumbo acetabular component
4. Revision hip arthroplasty with a cementless acetabular component
5. Acetabular component revision with a triflange protrusio ring

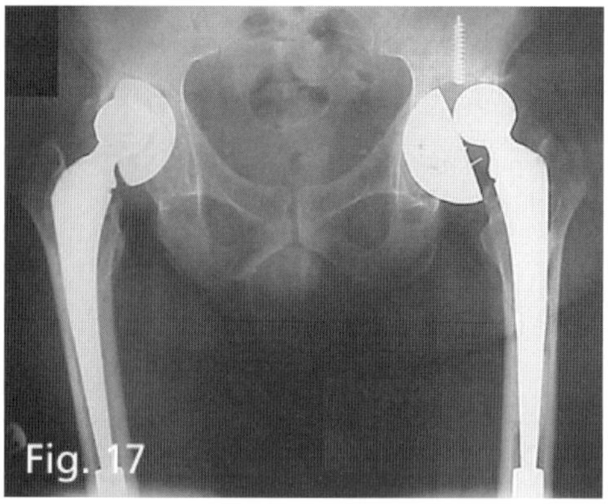
Fig. 17

Q-32: Embolic material (shown in Figure 18) generated during total knee arthroplasty (TKA) is composed of which of the following substances?

1. Fat only
2. Fat and air
3. Fat and marrow
4. Fat and cement
5. Fat and bone

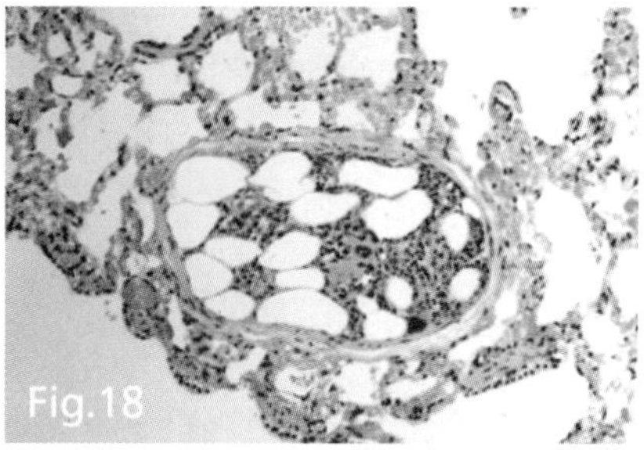
Fig.18

Q-33: A 30-year-old patient has had severe left hip pain and difficulty ambulating, necessitating the use of a cane, for the past 6 months. A photomicrograph of the femoral head sectioned at the time of surgery is shown in Figure 19. What is the most likely diagnosis?

1. Renal osteodystrophy
2. Pyogenic osteomyelitis
3. Osteoarthritis
4. Osteonecrosis
5. Tuberculosis osteomyelitis

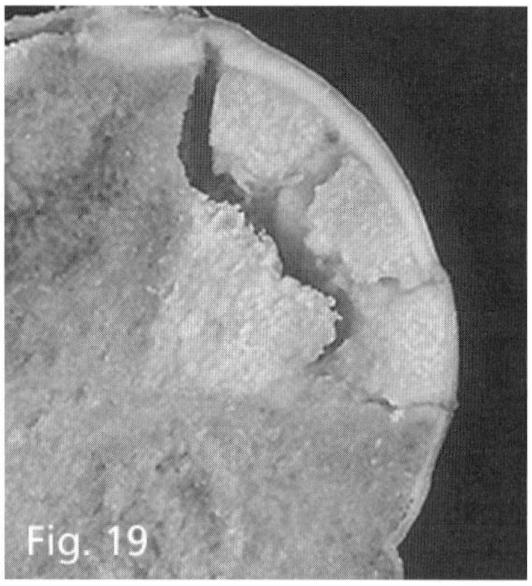
Fig. 19

Q-34: When comparing mobile-bearing total knee arthroplasty (TKA) to fixed-bearing total condylar arthroplasty, the mobile-bearing procedure provides

1. no improvement in survivorship.
2. approximately 15° greater flexion.
3. appreciable reduction in wear rates.
4. a faster recovery profile.
5. better quadriceps strength.

Q-35: Based on the type of articulation shown in Figure 20, wear is not affected by which of the following factors?

1. Radial mismatch of the femoral head to the acetabular component
2. Sphericity of the bearings
3. Surface finish of the articulation
4. Carbon content of the metal-on-metal bearing
5. Head-to-neck ratio

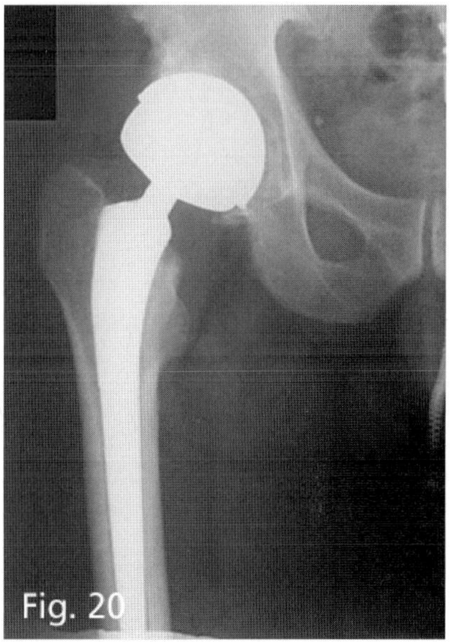
Fig. 20

Q-36: A 78-year-old patient undergoing revision total knee arthroplasty has bone loss throughout the knee at the time of revision. A distal femoral augment is used to restore the joint line. One month after surgery, the patient reports pain and is unable to ambulate. A lateral radiograph is shown in Figure 21. What is the most likely etiology of this problem?

1. Inadequate restoration of the joint line
2. Patellar tendon rupture
3. Excessive internal rotation of the tibial component
4. Flexion gap instability
5. Hyperextension of the femoral component

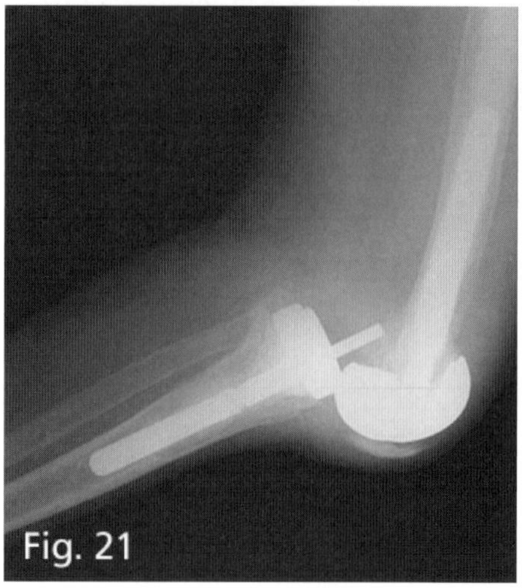

Fig. 21

Q-37: Figure 22 reveals a periprosthetic fracture around a cemented femoral stem in an 81-year-old patient with Paget disease and mild coagulopathy. What is the most appropriate reconstructive management on the femoral side?

1. Open reduction and internal fixation
2. Impaction allografting
3. Proximally coated femoral stem
4. Allograft prosthetic composite (APC)
5. Proximal femoral replacement (PFR)

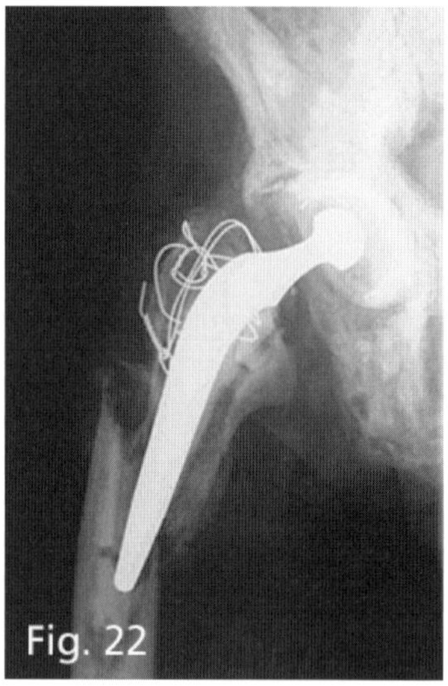

Fig. 22

Q-38: A patient with a documented allergy to nickel requires a total knee arthroplasty. Which of the following prostheses is most likely to provide long-term success in this individual?

1. All-polyethylene tibial component and pure titanium femoral component
2. All-polyethylene tibial component and cobalt-chromium alloy femoral component
3. Cobalt-chromium alloy tibial component and cobalt-chromium alloy femoral component
4. Modular titanium tibial component and pure titanium femoral component
5. Modular titanium tibial component and oxidized zirconium femoral component

Q-39: A 42-year-old man reports the recent onset of right hip pain. A radiograph and MRI scan are shown in Figures 23A and 23B. White blood cell count, erythrocyte sedimentation rate, and hip aspiration results are within normal limits. Management should now consist of

1. core decompression.
2. biopsy of the femoral head.
3. protected weight bearing and observation.
4. total hip arthroplasty.
5. percutaneous cannulated pin fixation of the femoral neck.

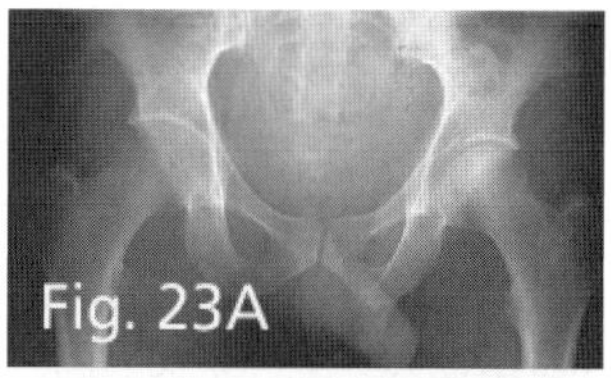
Fig. 23A

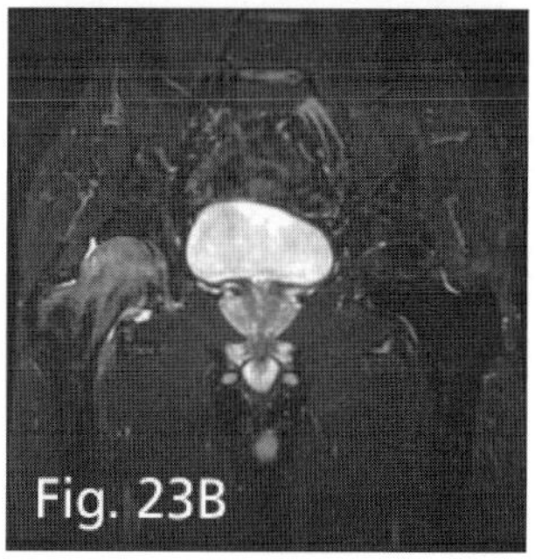
Fig. 23B

Q-40: During cemented total hip arthroplasty, peak pulmonary embolization of marrow contents occurs when the

1. hip is dislocated.
2. femoral neck is osteotomized.
3. acetabulum is prepared.
4. acetabular component is inserted.
5. femoral stem is inserted.

Q-41: What are the optimal conditions for leaving the acetabular shell in place, replacing the acetabular liner, and grafting the osteolytic defect shown in Figure 24?

1. Nonmodular implant
2. Instability
3. Well-designed, well-fixed modular implant
4. Complete radiolucency of the acetabular component
5. Migration of the acetabular component

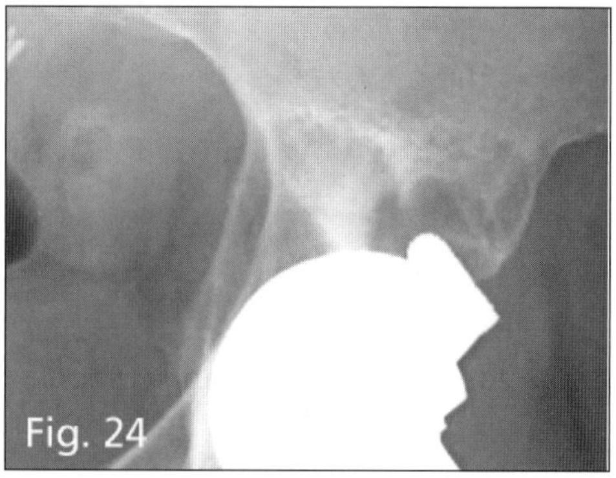
Fig. 24

Q-42: A 53-year-old patient is seen in the emergency department after sustaining a fall onto her left hip. A current radiograph is shown in Figure 25. What is the best treatment option?

1. Bed rest and weight bearing for 6 to 8 weeks
2. Component retention and open reduction and internal fixation
3. Proximal femoral replacement prosthesis
4. Revision arthroplasty with a long cemented stem
5. Revision arthroplasty with a long porous-coated cylindrical stem

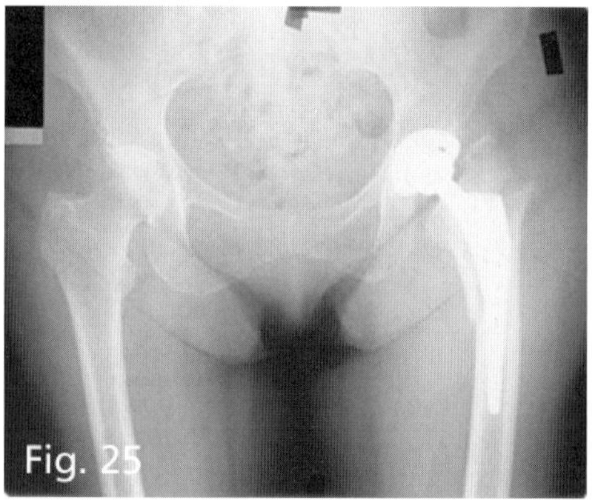
Fig. 25

Q-43: Figure 26 shows the radiograph of a 65-year-old man who underwent a revision arthroplasty to remove a loose, cemented femoral stem. When planning the postoperative restrictions, the surgeon should be aware that

1. the approach used reduces the torque-to-failure (fracture) of the construct to less than 50% of the intact femur.
2. the technique of repair can return the reconstructed prosthesis/bone composite to nearly the strength of the intact femur.
3. there is no relationship between the density of the native bone and the strength of the prosthesis/bone composite.
4. the addition of bone graft substitute or autograft has been shown to lessen the time to complete healing.
5. there is a one in five chance of fracture with this technique; therefore, the surgeon must carefully weigh the potential benefits versus this risk.

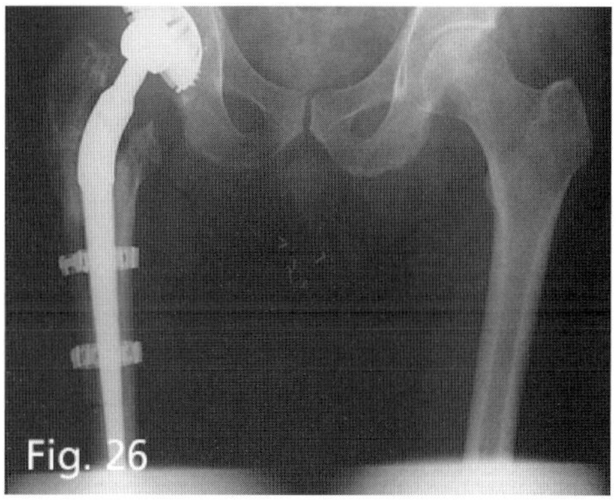
Fig. 26

Q-44: A 37-year-old man who works in a factory has isolated, lateral unicompartmental pain about his knee with activities. Nonsurgical management has failed to provide relief. The radiograph shown in Figure 27 reveals a tibiofemoral angle of approximately 15° that is clinically correctable to neutral. What is the best surgical option in this patient?

1. Unicompartmental arthroplasty
2. Total knee arthroplasty
3. Lateral closing wedge proximal tibial osteotomy
4. Medial opening wedge proximal tibial osteotomy
5. Medial closing wedge supracondylar femoral osteotomy

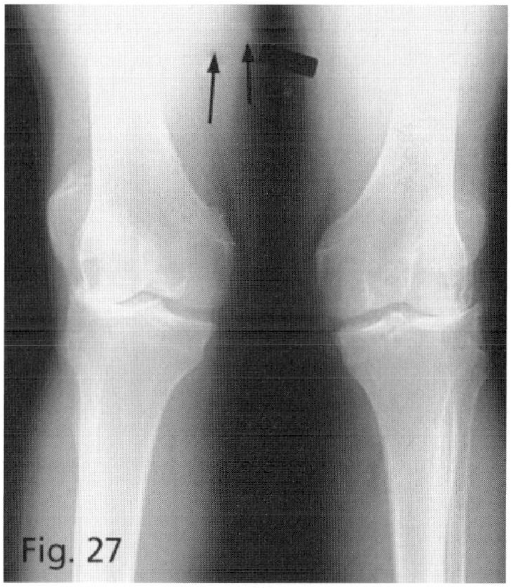
Fig. 27

Q-45: Figure 28 shows the AP radiograph of an active 80-year-old patient with an acetabular fracture. The fracture was initially managed nonsurgically; however, the patient is now scheduled to undergo total hip arthroplasty. What is the treatment of choice for the contained acetabular bone defect?

1. Bipolar femoral component
2. Acetabular cage
3. Large structural allograft
4. Use of the femoral head
5. Double-bubble acetabular cup

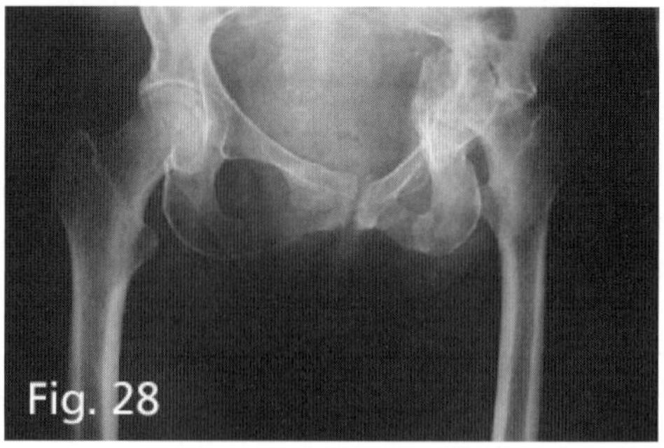
Fig. 28

Q-46: After trial placement of components in a primary total knee arthroplasty, the knee is unable to come to full extension, but the flexion gap is appropriately balanced. After adequate soft-tissue releases have been performed, what is the most appropriate next action to balance the reconstruction?

1. Use a larger femoral component
2. Use a thinner polyethylene insert
3. Add posterior femoral augments
4. Resect more proximal tibia
5. Resect additional distal femur

Q-47: During total knee arthroplasty, the patella is noted to subluxate laterally despite a lateral retinacular release. Which of the following methods is most likely to improve patellar stability?

1. Slight external rotation of the tibial component
2. Slight internal rotation of the femoral component
3. Slight anterior translation of the tibial component
4. Use of a fixed-bearing knee as opposed to a mobile-bearing knee
5. Use of a thicker patellar component

Q-48: A 73-year-old man has stiffness after undergoing primary posterior cruciate ligament-retaining total knee arthroplasty 18 months ago. Extensive physiotherapy, dynamic splinting, and manipulations under anesthesia have failed to result in improvement. Examination reveals range of motion from 30° to 60° of flexion. The components are well fixed, and the evaluation for infection is negative. In discussing the possibility of revision arthroplasty, the patient should be advised that

1. the success of improving range of motion to a functional range of 0° to 90° in the literature is between 75% to 80%.
2. the preoperative arc of motion will not influence the ultimate range of motion after formal component revision.
3. change from a posterior cruciate ligament-retaining to a posterior cruciate ligament-substituting design has a much greater chance of success.
4. manipulation under anesthesia will effectively improve range of motion if postoperative stiffness develops following revision.
5. the major postoperative focus will be to regain near-full extension.

Q-49: A 62-year-old patient is seen for routine follow-up after undergoing cementless total hip arthroplasty 2 years ago. The patient reports limited range of motion that severely affects daily activities. A radiograph is shown in Figure 29. Management should now consist of

1. observation only.
2. NSAIDs and protected weight bearing.
3. irradiation to the affected area.
4. surgical excision.
5. surgical excision and postoperative irradiation.

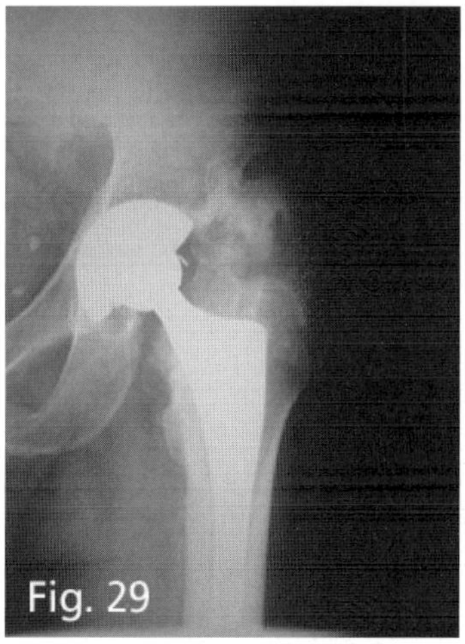

Fig. 29

Q-50: What bilateral surgical intervention is considered inappropriate based on the findings shown in the radiograph in Figure 30?

1. Vascularized fibular graft
2. Proximal femoral osteotomy
3. Core decompression
4. Hip arthrodesis
5. Femoral resurfacing

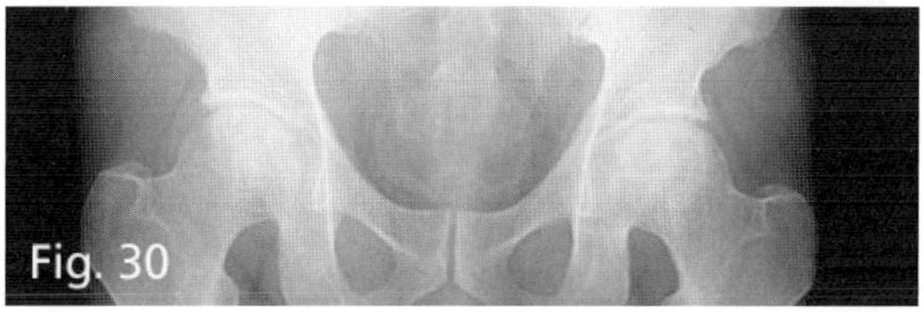

Fig. 30

A-1: Which of the following radiographic images is best for detecting anterior acetabular deficiency in the dysplastic hip?

1. Pelvic inlet
2. Judet
3. AP pelvis
4. False profile
5. Frog lateral

PREFERRED RESPONSE: 4

DISCUSSION: The false profile view of Lequesne and de Seze is obtained with the patient standing with the affected hip on the cassette, the ipsilateral foot parallel to the cassette, and the pelvis rotated 65° from the plane of the cassette. This view best assesses anterior coverage of the femoral head.

REFERENCES: Garbuz DS, Masri BA, Haddad F, et al: Clinical and radiographic assessment the young adult with symptomatic dysplasia. *Clin Orthop Relat Res* 2004;418:18-22.

Delauney S, Dussault RG, Kaplan PA, et al: Radiographic measurements of dysplastic adult hips. *Skel Radiol* 1997;26:75-81.

A-2: At the level of tibial bone resection in total knee arthroplasty, where does the common peroneal nerve lie?

1. Deep to the arcuate ligament
2. Closer to bone in larger legs
3. On the muscle belly of the popliteus
4. On the bony posterolateral corner of the tibia
5. Superficial to the lateral head of the gastrocnemius

PREFERRED RESPONSE: 5

DISCUSSION: At the level of tibial bone resection in total knee arthroplasty, the common peroneal nerve lies superficial to the lateral head of the gastrocnemius and is therefore protected by this structure. In an MRI study of 60 knees, the mean distance from the bony posterolateral corner of the tibia to the nerve was 1.49 cm, with no distance less than 0.9 cm. The distance from the bone to nerve was greater in larger legs.

REFERENCES: Clarke HD, Schwartz JB, Math KR, et al: Anatomic risk of peroneal nerve injury with the "pie crust" technique for valgus release in total knee arthroplasty. *J Arthroplasty* 2004;19:40-44.

Anderson JE: *Grant's Atlas of Anatomy*, ed 7. Baltimore, MD, Lippincott Williams & Wilkins, 1978, pp 4-52, 4-53.

A-3: The anatomy of the sciatic nerve as it exits the pelvis is best described as exiting through the

1. greater sciatic notch and passing between the inferior gemellus and the obturator externus.
2. greater sciatic notch and passing between the piriformis and the superior gemellus.
3. obturator foramen and passing between the obturator internus and the obturator externus.
4. lesser sciatic notch and passing between the piriformis and the superior gemellus.
5. lesser sciatic notch and passing between the superior gemellus and the inferior gemellus.

PREFERRED RESPONSE: 2

DISCUSSION: The sciatic nerve is formed by the roots of the lumbosacral plexus. It exits the pelvis through the greater sciatic notch and appears in the buttock anterior to the piriformus. From that point, the sciatic nerve passes posteriorly over the superior gemellus, obturator internus, inferior gemellus, and quadratus femoris before it passes deep to the biceps femoris. The tendon of the obturator internus passes through the lesser sciatic notch.

REFERENCES: Hoppenfeld S, deBoer P: *Surgical Exposures in Orthopaedics: The Anatomic Approach*. Philadelphia, PA, JB Lippincott, 1984, p 347.

Anderson JE: *Grant's Atlas of Anatomy*, ed 7. Baltimore, MD, Lippincott Williams & Wilkins, 1978, pp 4-34, 4-36.

Hollingshead WH: *Anatomy for Surgeons: The Back and Limbs*, ed 2. Hagerstown, MD, Harper & Row, 1969, pp 607-609.

A-4: What complication is more likely following excessive medial retraction of the anterior covering structures during the anterolateral (Watson-Jones) approach to the hip?

1. Numbness over the anterolateral thigh
2. Ischemia to the leg
3. Quadriceps weakness
4. Abductor insufficiency
5. Foot drop

PREFERRED RESPONSE: 3

DISCUSSION: The femoral nerve is the most lateral structure in the anterior neurovascular bundle. The femoral artery and vein lie medial to the nerve. Retractors placed in the anterior acetabular lip should be safe, although neurapraxia of the femoral nerve may occur if retraction is prolonged or forceful leading to quadriceps weakness. The femoral artery and nerve are well protected by the interposed psoas muscle. Damage to the lateral femoral cutaneous nerve, causing numbness over the anterolateral thigh, can occur while developing the interval between the tensor fascia latae and sartorious in the anterior (Smith-Petersen) approach but less likely in the Watson-Jones approach. Superior gluteal injury and accompanying abductor insufficiency may occur during excessive splitting of the glutei during the direct lateral (Hardinge) approach. Foot drop secondary to sciatic injury is more common with a posterior exposure or posterior retractor placement.

REFERENCES: Hoppenfeld S, deBoer P: *Surgical Exposures in Orthopaedics: The Anatomic Approach*. Philadelphia, PA, JB Lippincott, 1984, p 325.

Anderson JE: *Grant's Atlas of Anatomy*, ed 7. Baltimore, MD, Lippincott Williams & Wilkins, 1978, pp 4-17, 4-18.

A-5: A 40-year-old man has had hip pain with increased activity over the past year. Examination reveals restriction of motion and tenderness with combined hip flexion, adduction, and internal rotation. An AP radiograph is shown in Figure 1. What is the most likely diagnosis?

1. Developmental dysplasia of the hip
2. Osteonecrosis
3. Perthes disease
4. Pseudogout
5. Femoral acetabular impingement

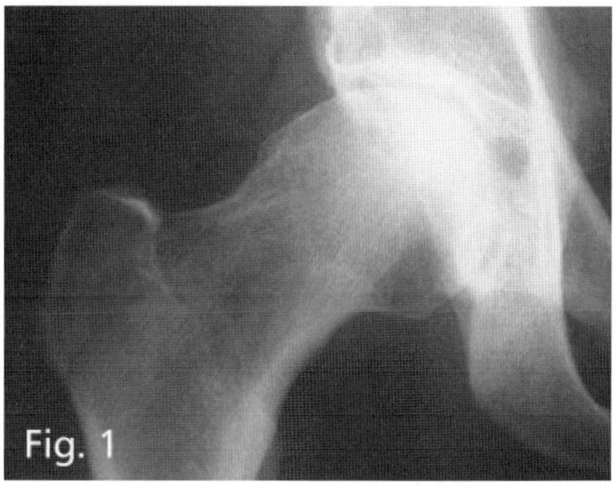
Fig. 1

PREFERRED RESPONSE: 5

DISCUSSION: Femoral acetabular impingement (FAI) is a pathologic entity leading to pain, reduced range of motion in flexion and internal rotation, and development of secondary arthritis of the hip. There are two types of FAI: cam impingement and pincer impingement. Cam impingement is seen when a nonspherical femoral head produces a cam effect when the prominent portion to the femoral head rotates into the joint. This mechanism produces shear forces that damage articular cartilage. Radiographs reveal early joint degeneration and flattening of the head neck junction (pistol grip deformity) as seen in this image. The pincer type of impingement involves abnormal contact between the femoral head neck junction and the acetabulum, in the presence of a spherical femoral head.

REFERENCES: Beall DP, Sweet CF, Martin HD, et al: Imaging findings of femoraoacetabular impingement syndrome. *Skeletal Radiol* 2005;34:691-701.

Mardones RM, Gonzalez C, Chen Q, et al: Surgical treatment of femoroacetabular impingement: Evaluation of the effect of the size of the resection. *J Bone Joint Surg Am* 2006;88:84-91.

A-6: Bleeding is encountered while developing the internervous plane between the tensor fascia lata and the sartorius during the anterior approach to the hip. The most likely cause is injury to what artery?

1. Ascending branch of the lateral femoral circumflex
2. Superior gluteal
3. Femoral
4. Profunda femoris
5. Medial femoral circumflex

PREFERRED RESPONSE: 1

DISCUSSION: The ascending branch of the lateral femoral circumflex artery crosses the gap between the tensor fascia lata and the sartorious and must be identified and ligated or coagulated. The other vessels are out of the field of dissection.

REFERENCES: McGann WA: Surgical approaches, in Barrack RL, Booth RE Jr, Lonner JH, et al, eds: *Orthopaedic Knowledge Update: Hip and Knee Reconstruction*, ed 3. Rosemont, IL, American Academy of Orthopaedic Surgeons, 2006, p 312.

Hoppenfeld S, deBoer P: *Surgical Exposures in Orthopaedics: The Anatomic Approach*. Philadelphia, PA, JB Lippincott, 1984, p 304.

A-7: When using the direct lateral (or Hardinge) approach for hip arthroplasty, three muscles are detached from the femur. In addition to the vastus lateralis, they include the

1. iliopsoas and sartorius.
2. piriformis and obturator internus.
3. gluteus maximus and tensor fascia lata.
4. gluteus minimus and rectus femoris.
5. gluteus medius and gluteus minimus.

PREFERRED RESPONSE: 5

DISCUSSION: This approach is criticized for the episodic limp associated with the muscle detachment and reattachment. Classically, two thirds of the gluteus medius are detached as a sleeve with the vastus lateralis. This exposes the gluteus minimus and the ligament of Bigelow. These must also be detached to allow dislocation of the hip and osteotomy of the femoral neck. The rectus femoris lies medially and anteriorly and does not need to be addressed. The piriformis and obturator internus are exposed during the posterior approach. Neither the gluteus maximus nor tensor fascia lata attach to the anterior femur. The sartorius and iliopsoas are not exposed during this dissection.

REFERENCES: Hoppenfeld S, deBoer P, eds: *Surgical Exposures in Orthopaedics: The Anatomic Approach.* Philadelphia, PA, JB Lippincott, 1984, pp 333-335.

Hardinge K: The direct lateral approach to the hip. *J Bone Joint Surg Br* 1982;64:17-19.

A-8: Figure 2 shows the radiograph of a patient who underwent a total knee revision with a posterior stabilized mobile-bearing prosthesis and who now has recurrent knee dislocations. What is the most likely cause?

1. Loose extension gap
2. Loose flexion gap
3. Malrotation of the tibial component
4. Malrotation of the femoral component
5. Poor prosthetic design

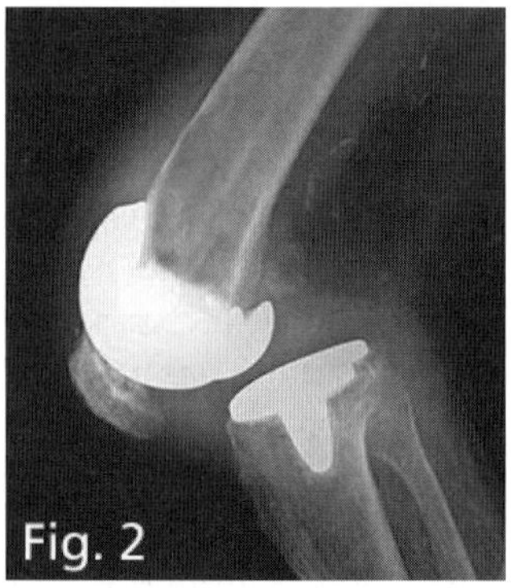
Fig. 2

PREFERRED RESPONSE: 2

DISCUSSION: The patient has a posterior stabilized total knee revision, and the femoral component has dislocated over the tibial polyethylene cam/post. This usually indicates a loose flexion gap, or flexion instability. A loose flexion gap can occur due to undersizing of the femoral component, anteriorization of the femoral component, excessive distal augmentation of the distal femur, or collateral ligament insufficiency, especially if combined with posterior capsular insufficiency. Isolated laxity of the extension gap (with a well-balanced flexion gap) causes varus/valgus instability, but it rarely causes the femoral component to "jump" the tibial cam of a posterior stabilized tibial insert. Malrotation of the components may cause patellar instability or a rotational instability of the tibiofemoral joint but should not cause a frank posterior dislocation of the tibia, unless combined with other errors of balancing. Although a mobile-bearing total knee arthroplasty may be more sensitive to errors in balancing than a fixed-bearing total knee arthroplasty, this complication does not reflect a faulty prosthetic design.

(continued on next page)

(A-8: *continued*)

REFERENCES: Haas SB, Ammeen DJ, Engh GA, et al: Revision total knee replacement, in Pellicci PM, Tria AJ Jr, Garvin KL, eds: *Orthopaedic Knowledge Update: Hip and Knee Reconstruction*, ed 2. Rosemont, IL, American Academy of Orthopaedic Surgeons, 2000, pp 339-365.

Lotke PA, Garino JP: *Revision Total Knee Arthroplasty*. New York, NY, Lippincott-Raven, 1999, pp 173-186, 227-249.

Clarke HD, Scuderi GR: Flexion instability in primary total knee replacement. *J Knee Surg* 2003;16:123-128.

A-9: Figures 3A and 3B show the radiographs of a 72-year-old man with aseptic loosening of the tibial component of his total knee arthroplasty. Optimal management should include

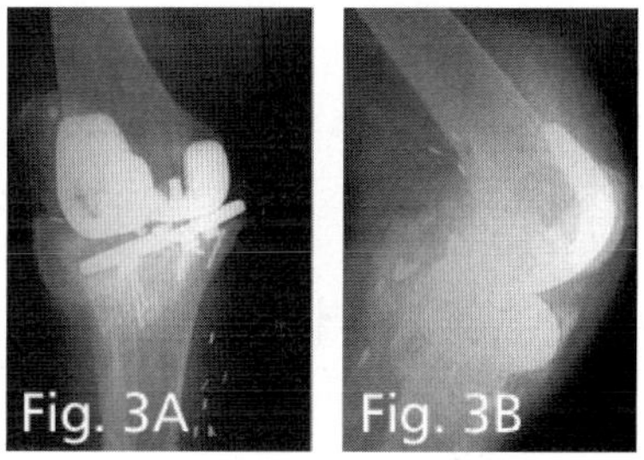

1. tibial revision only, without stems or augmentations.
2. tibial revision only, with stems and augmentations.
3. revision of the tibial and femoral components, without stems or augmentations.
4. revision of the tibial and femoral components, with stems and augmentations.
5. primary arthrodesis.

PREFERRED RESPONSE: 4

DISCUSSION: The radiographs show massive subsidence of the lateral side of the tibia with severe tibial bone loss and a fractured proximal fibula. Reconstruction should consist of a large metal or bony lateral tibial augmentation, and a stem long enough to bypass the defect is required. The femoral and tibial components are articulating without any remaining polyethylene medially; therefore, the femoral component is damaged and needs revision. The insertions of the lateral ligaments are absent, thereby rendering the lateral side of the knee predictably unstable. Also, the large valgus deformity compromises the medial collateral ligament. The posterior cruciate ligament is also likely to be deficient with this much tibial bone destruction. The patient requires a posterior stabilized femoral component at the minimum, and possibly a constrained femoral component. Retention of the femoral component, even though it may be well fixed, jeopardizes the outcome.

REFERENCES: Lotke PA, Garino JP: *Revision Total Knee Arthroplasty*. New York, NY, Lippincott-Raven, 1999, pp 137-250.

Insall JN, Windsor RE, Scott WN, et al, eds: *Surgery of the Knee*, ed 2. New York, NY, Churchill Livingstone, 1993, pp 935-957.

Haas SB, Ameen DJ, Engh GA, et al: Revision total knee replacement, in Pellicci PM, Tria AJ Jr, Garvin KL, eds: *Orthopaedic Knowledge Update: Hip and Knee Reconstruction*, 2. Rosemont, IL, American Academy of Orthopaedic Surgeons, 2000, pp 339-365.

A-10: Figure 4 shows the AP radiograph of a patient with diabetes mellitus who has knee pain. A semiconstrained knee prosthesis was used in this patient to prevent which of the following complications?

1. Infection
2. Instability
3. Stiffness
4. Bone loss
5. Malalignment

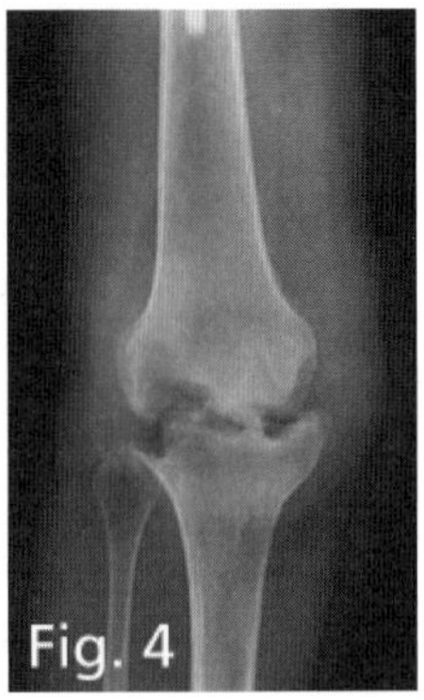

PREFERRED RESPONSE: 2

DISCUSSION: The radiographic appearance of the joint is highly suspicious for neuropathic joint (Charcot joint). Evidence of bone loss on both the tibial and the femoral sides may necessitate the use of metal and/or bone augments. Patients with a neuropathic joint often have excellent range of motion, and postoperative stiffness is not a problem. The main problem with these patients is instability that occurs secondary to ligamentous laxity. Use of a semiconstrained prosthesis prevents the latter complication.

REFERENCES: Parvizi J, Marrs J, Morrey BF: Total knee arthroplasty for neuropathic (Charcot) joints. *Clin Orthop* 2003;416:145-150.

Kim YH, Kim JS, Oh SW: Total knee arthroplasty in neuropathic arthropathy. *J Bone Joint Surg Br* 2002;84:216-219.

A-11: A 75-year-old woman who fell on her right knee now reports pain and is unable to bear weight. History reveals that she underwent total knee arthroplasty on the right knee 6 years ago. Radiographs are shown in Figure 5. Management should now consist of

1. closed reduction and casting for 6 weeks.
2. open reduction and internal fixation, using a locked intramedullary rod.
3. open reduction and internal fixation, using two cancellous screws.
4. open reduction and internal fixation, using a locked plate and screws.
5. open reduction and internal fixation and revision of the femoral component.

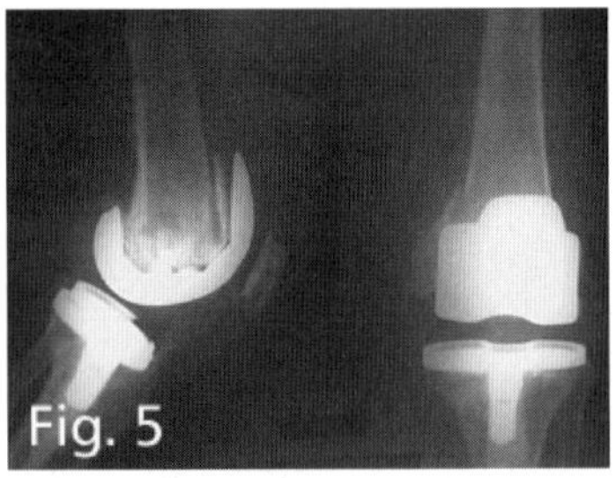

PREFERRED RESPONSE: 5

DISCUSSION: The radiographs show a loose femoral component with an associated medial condyle distal femoral fracture. The treatment of choice is open reduction and internal fixation with revision of the femoral component because of the femoral component loosening.

REFERENCES: Moran MC, Brick GW, Sledge CB, et al: Supracondylar femoral fracture following total knee arthroplasty. *Clin Orthop* 1996;324:196-209.

McLaren AC, DuPont JA, Schroeber DC: Open reduction internal fixation of supracondylar fractures above total knee arthroplasties using the intramedullary supracondylar rod. *Clin Orthop* 1994;302:194-198.

Figgie MP, Goldberg VM, Figgie HE III, et al: The results of treatment of supracondylar fracture above total knee arthroplasty. *J Arthroplasty* 1990;5:267-276.

A-12: A 64-year-old man undergoes a primary total knee arthroplasty. Three months after surgery he reports persistent pain, weakness, and difficulty ambulating. Postoperative radiographs are shown in Figures 6A through 6C. What is the best course of action at this time?

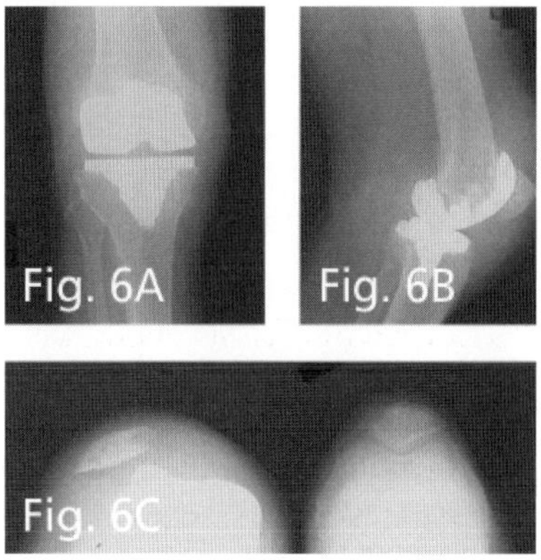
Fig. 6A Fig. 6B Fig. 6C

1. Hinged knee brace
2. Patellar component revision with a tantalum implant and lateralization of the patella
3. Revision knee arthroplasty with greater internal rotation of the tibial component
4. Revision total knee arthroplasty with a lateral release and external rotation of the femoral component
5. Revision total knee arthroplasty with a lateral release and internal rotation of the femoral component

PREFERRED RESPONSE: 4

DISCUSSION: The Merchant view reveals subluxation of the patellar component. The etiology of maltracking of the patella includes internal rotation of the femoral component, internal rotation of the tibial component, excessive patellar height, and lateralization of the patella component. The treatment of choice in this patient is revision total knee arthroplasty with external rotation of the femoral component. Preoperatively the patient also may require a lateral release, revision of the tibial component if it is internally rotated, and possibly a soft-tissue realignment. Component malalignment needs to be addressed first.

REFERENCES: Kelly MA: Extensor mechanism complications in total knee arthroplasty. *Instr Course Lect* 2004;53: 193-199.

Malkani AL, Karandikar N: Complications following total knee arthroplasty. *Sem Arthroplasty* 2003;14:203-214.

Norman AJ, Scott S, David GN, eds: *Master Techniques in Knee Arthroplasty*, ed 2. Philadelphia, PA, Lippincott Williams & Wilkins, 2003.

A-13: Compared to metal-on-polyethylene total hip bearing surfaces, the debris particles generated by metal-on-metal articulations are

1. larger and less numerous.
2. larger and more numerous.
3. smaller and less numerous.
4. smaller and more numerous.
5. not detectable.

PREFERRED RESPONSE: 4

DISCUSSION: Retrieval studies have shown that the debris particles produced by metal-on-metal articulations in total hip arthroplasty are several orders of magnitude smaller and may be up to 100 times more numerous than those found with metal-on-polyethylene articulations.

REFERENCES: Davies AP, Willert HG, Campbell PA, et al: An unusual lymphocytic perivascular infiltration in tissues around contemporary metal-on-metal joint replacements. *J Bone Joint Surg Am* 2005;87:18-27.

(continued on next page)

Preservation, Arthroplasty, and Salvage Surgery of the Hip and Knee: Answers

(A-13: *continued*)

Firkins PJ, Tipper JL, Saadatzadeh MR, et al: Quantitative analysis of wear and wear debris from metal-on-metal hip prostheses tested in a physiological hip joint simulator. *Biomed Mater Eng* 2001;11:143-157.

A-14: A 60-year-old patient had the procedure shown in Figure 7 performed 5 years ago. During transition to a total knee arthroplasty (TKA), what patellar problem is commonly encountered intraoperatively?

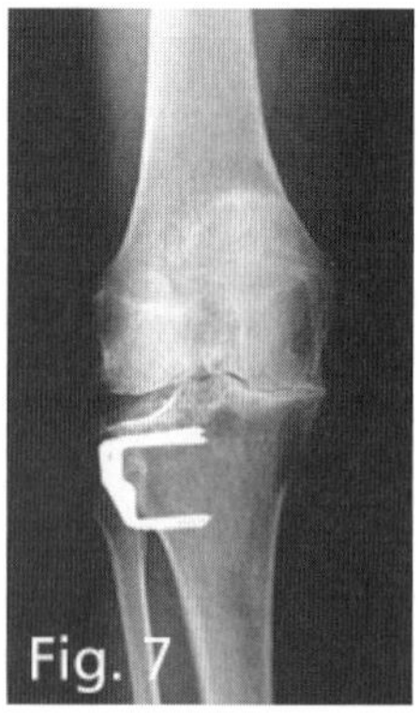
Fig. 7

1. Fracture
2. Patella baja
3. Patella alta
4. Osteonecrosis
5. Maltracking

PREFERRED RESPONSE: 2

DISCUSSION: Patella baja is commonly encountered when converting a high tibial osteotomy (HTO) to a TKA. Patella baja most likely occurs because of scarring. Meding and associates' study did not show an increased rate of lateral release when converting a knee that had undergone a previous HTO.

REFERENCES: Yoshino N, Shinro T: Total knee arthroplasty after failed high tibial osteotomy, in Callaghan JJ, Rosenberg AG, Rubash HE, et al, eds: *The Adult Knee*. Philadelphia, PA, JB Lippincott, 2003, vol 2, pp 1265-1271.

Meding JB, Keating EM, Ritter MA, et al: Total knee arthroplasty after high tibial osteotomy: A comparison study in patients who had bilateral total knee replacement. *J Bone Joint Surg Am* 2000;82:1252-1259.

A-15: Figures 8A and 8B show the radiographs of a 75-year-old man who underwent a revision total knee arthroplasty with a long-stemmed tibial component. In rehabilitation, he reports fullness and tenderness in the proximal medial leg (at the knee). The strategy that would best limit this postoperative problem is use of

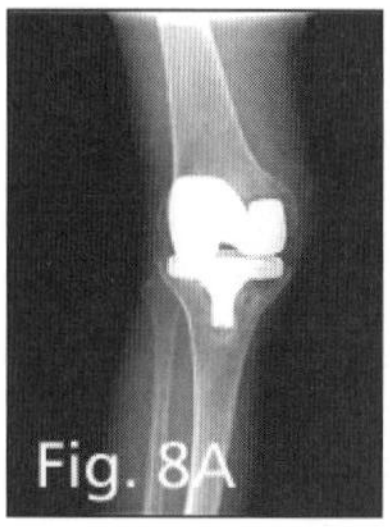
Fig. 8A

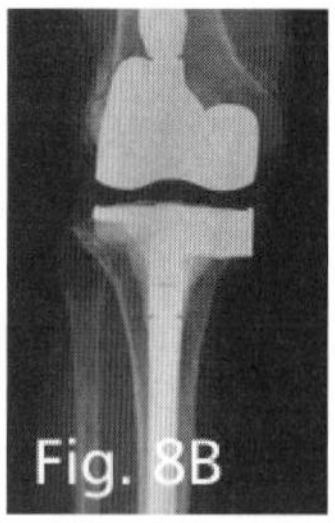
Fig. 8B

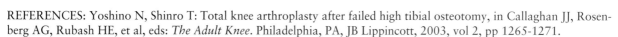

1. a base plate with an offset tibial stem attachment.
2. a bone ingrowth surface on the augment.
3. a nonstemmed tibial base plate.
4. allograft bone instead of metal augments.
5. bone cement to smooth the outline of the proximal medial tibia.

PREFERRED RESPONSE: 1

DISCUSSION: The problem with this reconstruction is the medial protrusion of the base plate. The use of a base plate with an offset stem can prevent the protrusion and thus the impingement and pain. Allograft bone or smoothing the outline with cement would be just as prominent and likely to cause pain. An ingrowth surface may improve soft-tissue attachment but would still leave the implant protruding

(continued on next page)

(A-15: *continued*)

medially and likely to cause pain. A nonstemmed tibial base plate would lead to less medial protrusion but at the expense of a smaller area for load carriage on the proximal tibia.

REFERENCE: Gustke K: Cemented tibial stems are not requisite in revision. *Orthopedics* 2004;27:991-992.

A-16: Figure 9 shows the AP radiograph of an ambulatory 76-year-old patient. What is the most appropriate surgical treatment option for this patient?

1. Revision arthroplasty using a cemented femoral component
2. Impaction allografting of the femoral component
3. Proximal femoral replacement arthroplasty
4. Resection arthroplasty
5. Hip arthrodesis

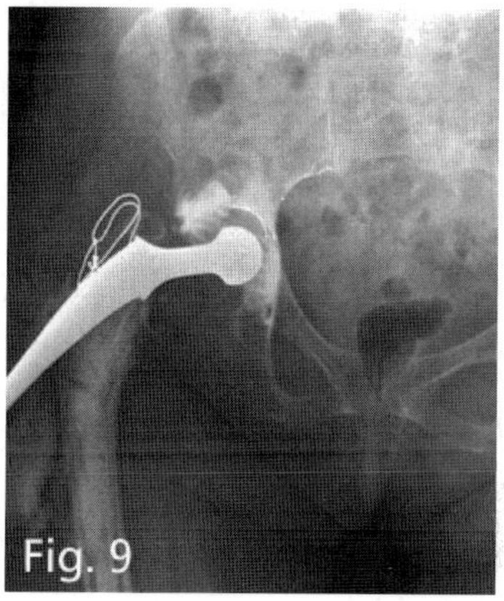

Fig. 9

PREFERRED RESPONSE: 3

DISCUSSION: The patient has a periprosthetic fracture around a loose cemented femoral component. The proximal bone stock is poor; therefore, this fracture may be categorized as Vancouver 3-B. Hip arthrodesis and resection arthroplasty provide suboptimal results, particularly for ambulatory patients. Although impaction allografting may be an option to restore the bone stock in a younger patient, the latter procedure will be very difficult to perform when the proximal bone is poor in quality and fractured. Cementing another component into this wide femur is not an option. The best option for revision of the femoral component in this elderly patient is proximal femoral replacement arthroplasty.

REFERENCES: Malkani AL, Settecerri JJ, Sim FH, et al: Long-term results of proximal femoral replacement for non-neoplastic disorders. *J Bone Joint Surg Br* 1995;77:351-356.

Parvizi J, Sim FH: Proximal femoral replacements with megaprostheses. *Clin Orthop* 2004;420:169-175.

A-17: Increasing articular conformity of the tibial polyethylene insert of a fixed-bearing total knee arthroplasty (TKA) prosthesis will have which of the following biomechanical effects?

1. Decreased contact stress within the polyethylene
2. Decreased risk of patellofemoral instability
3. Decreased risk of mechanical loosening
4. Increased risk of subsurface polyethylene cracking
5. Increased tibial rollback during flexion

PREFERRED RESPONSE: 1

DISCUSSION: Increasing articular conformity increases the surface area for contact between the polyethylene and the femoral component. Advantages of this include lower peak contact stress within the polyethylene and less risk of polyethylene fatigue failure. Patellofemoral tracking is unchanged by increasing conformity unless gross component apposition is present. A potential disadvantage of increasing conformity includes some restriction in tibial rollback. Modest changes in conformity have not been

(continued on next page)

(A-17: *continued*)

shown to alter the rate of mechanical loosening. If conformity was increased to the extent of significant constraint, a potential increased risk of loosening would be expected, not a decrease. Design of modern TKAs includes a compromise in achieving enough constraint to lower polyethylene stress, without providing so much constraint as to limit kinematics and stress the fixation interfaces.

REFERENCES: D'Lima DD, Chen PC, Colwell CW Jr: Polyethylene contact stresses, articular congruity, and knee alignment. *Clin Orthop* 2001;392:232-238.

Wright TM: Biomechanics of total knee design, in Pellicci PM, Tria AJ Jr, Garvin KL, eds: *Orthopaedic Knowledge Update: Hip and Knee Reconstruction*, ed 2. Rosemont, IL, American Academy of Orthopaedic Surgeons, 2000, pp 265-274.

A-18: A 63-year-old woman reports giving way of the knee and pain after undergoing primary total knee arthroplasty (TKA) 1 year ago. Examination reveals that the knee is stable in full extension but has gross anteroposterior instability at 90° of flexion. The patient can fully extend her knee with normal quadriceps strength. Studies for infection are negative. AP and lateral radiographs are shown in Figures 10A and 10B, respectively. What is the appropriate management?

1. Anti-inflammatory drugs
2. Knee brace
3. Physical therapy for quadriceps strengthening
4. Revision to a thicker polyethylene insert
5. Revision to a larger, posterior stabilized implant

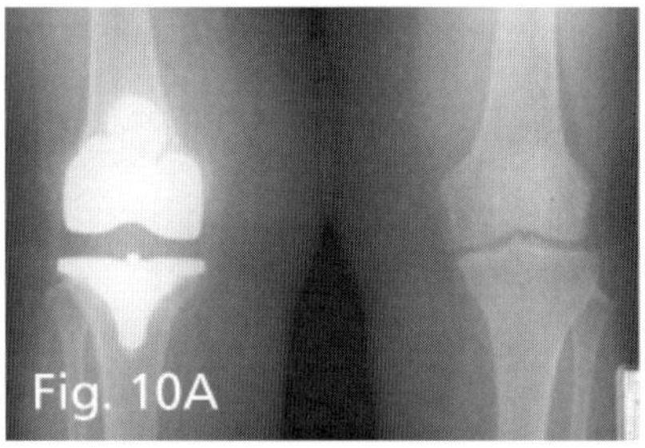
Fig. 10A

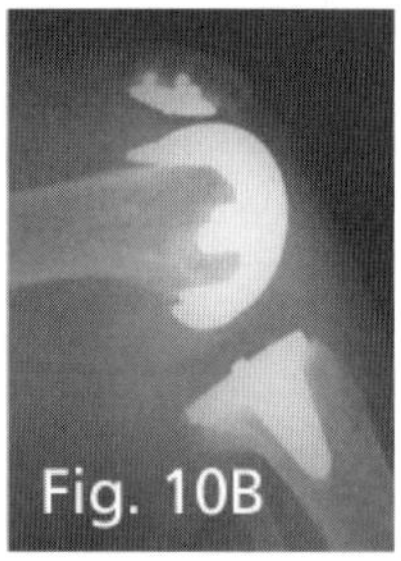
Fig. 10B

PREFERRED RESPONSE: 5

DISCUSSION: The radiographs show posterior flexion instability that is the result of a flexion-extension gap imbalance and posterior cruciate ligament incompetence after a posterior cruciate ligament-retaining TKA. The femur is anteriorly displaced on the tibia, with lift-off of the femoral component from the tibial polyethylene. Revision to a larger femoral component will address the larger flexion gap relative to the extension gap, and a posterior stabilized implant will address the posterior cruciate ligament insufficiency. Pagnano and associates, reporting on a series of painful TKAs previously diagnosed as pain of unknown etiology, showed that the pain was secondary to flexion instability. Pain relief was achieved by revision to a posterior stabilized implant.

REFERENCES: Pagnano MW, Hanssen AD, Lewallen DG, et al: Flexion instability after primary posterior cruciate retaining total knee arthroplasty. *Clin Orthop* 1998;356:39-46.

Fehring TK, Valadie AL: Knee instability after total knee arthroplasty. *Clin Orthop* 1994;299:157-162.

Fehring TK, Odum S, Griffin WL, et al: Early failures in total knee arthroplasty. *Clin Orthop* 2001;392:315-318.

A-19: Stiffness can occur following total knee arthroplasty. What is the most appropriate management for a patient who has deteriorating arc of motion after undergoing a revision knee arthroplasty 9 months ago?

1. Aggressive physical therapy
2. Manipulation under anesthesia
3. Investigation for periprosthetic infection
4. Revision knee arthroplasty
5. Resection arthroplasty

PREFERRED RESPONSE: 3

DISCUSSION: Stiffness following total knee arthroplasty can be a disabling condition. There are many reasons for loss of knee motion following total knee arthroplasty. Technical errors, such as overstuffing of the patella, malpositioning of the components, and ligamentous imbalance, all are known to result in stiffness following total knee arthroplasty. In some patients with a possible genetic predisposition, aggressive arthrofibrosis may develop and result in loss of knee motion. In any patient who has deteriorating knee motion, particularly after revision arthroplasty, deep infection should be ruled out. Although on occasion surgical intervention may be required to address knee stiffness, the outcome of revision surgery is poor if no reason for stiffness can be determined.

REFERENCES: Kim J, Nelson CL, Lotke PA: Stiffness after total knee arthroplasty: Prevalence of the complication and outcomes of revision. *J Bone Joint Surg Am* 2004;86:1479-1484.

Gonzalez MH, Mekhail AO: The failed total knee arthroplasty: Evaluation and etiology. *J Am Acad Orthop Surg* 2004;12:436-446.

A-20: A 59-year-old woman who underwent a total hip arthroplasty 5 years ago now has recurrent dislocation following bariatric surgery and a weight loss of 200 lb. An attempt at conversion to a larger head size and trochanteric advancement has failed. Her components are well aligned. What is the best course of action?

1. Resection arthroplasty
2. Hip abduction brace
3. Constrained acetabular liner
4. Thermal ablation of the posterior capsule
5. Conversion to a bipolar prosthesis

PREFERRED RESPONSE: 3

DISCUSSION: When a patient has well-aligned components and soft-tissue tensioning with a larger femoral head and trochanteric advancement has failed, options are limited. The use of a constrained acetabular liner is the best option in this situation. Goetz and associates and Shrader and associates have demonstrated good results with these implants. Shrader and associates used this device on 109 patients with recurrent instability with a successful outcome in all but 2 patients. Resection arthroplasty is a salvage situation and currently is not the best option. A hip abduction brace does not address the soft-tissue laxity. Conversion to a bipolar arthroplasty, although possibly minimizing the incidence of dislocation, will lead to groin pain and migration of the component with diminished functional results.

(continued on next page)

(A-20: *continued*)

REFERENCES: Goetz DD, Capello WN, Callaghan JJ, et al: Salvage of recurrently dislocating hip prosthesis with use of a constrained acetabular component: A retrospective analysis of fifty-six cases. *J Bone Joint Surg Am* 1998;80:502-509.

Shrader MW, Parvizi J, Lewallen DG: The use of constrained acetabular component to treat instability after total hip arthroplasty. *J Bone Joint Surg Am* 2003;85:2179-2183.

Hamilton WG, McAuley JP: Evaluation of the unstable total hip arthroplasty. *Inst Course Lect* 2004;53:87-92.

A-21: Figure 11 shows the radiograph of an otherwise healthy 62-year-old woman who fell. Management should consist of

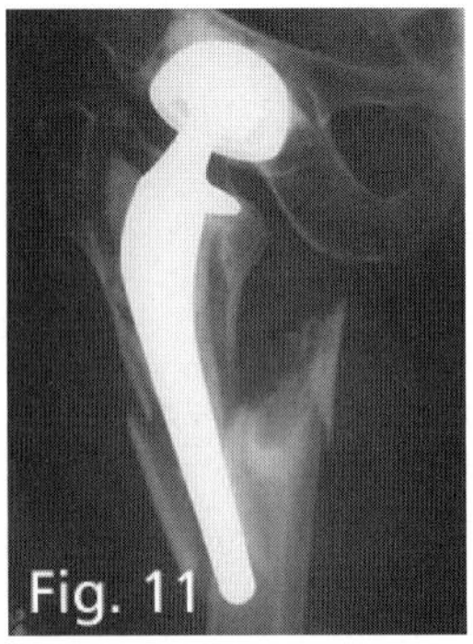
Fig. 11

1. revision total hip arthroplasty with a cemented femoral component and adjuvant fracture fixation.
2. revision total hip arthroplasty with a cementless femoral component and adjuvant fracture fixation.
3. open reduction and internal fixation of the fracture and retention of the original components.
4. removal of the components, open reduction and internal fixation of the fracture, and delayed replantation of the components when the fracture is healed.
5. resection arthroplasty and internal fixation of the fracture.

PREFERRED RESPONSE: 2

DISCUSSION: The radiograph reveals that the femoral component is grossly loose as evidenced by disruption of the cement column; therefore, retention of the original components will not yield a successful outcome. A cementless revision is the procedure of choice. A strut graft and/or plate may be added at the surgeon's discretion. A resection arthroplasty would only be considered in a nonambulatory patient. Cemented fixation of the revision component would be problematic given the numerous fracture fragments and the inability to contain the cement.

REFERENCES: Springer BD, Berry DJ, Lewallen DG: Treatment of periprosthetic fractures following total hip arthroplasty with femoral component revision. *J Bone Joint Surg Am* 2003;85:2156-2162.

Duwelius PJ, Schmidt AH, Kyle RF, et al: A prospective, modernized treatment protocol for periprosthetic femur fractures. *Orthop Clin North Am* 2004;35:485-492.

A-22: A 75-year-old woman undergoes hybrid total hip arthroplasty for osteoarthritis. A postoperative radiograph obtained in the recovery room is shown in Figure 12. Treatment should now consist of

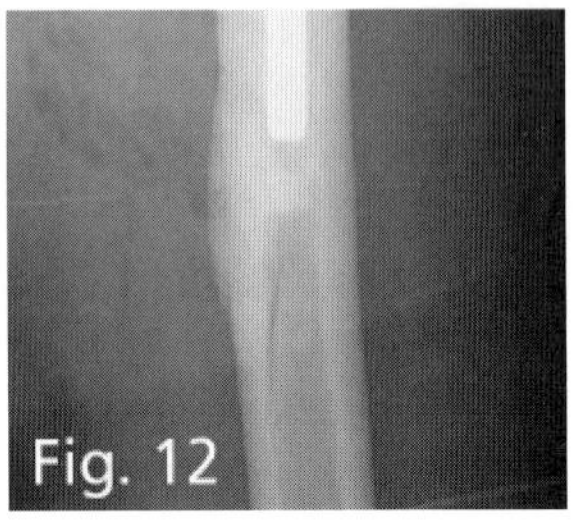
Fig. 12

1. open reduction and internal fixation with strut graft and cerclage wire.
2. open reduction and internal fixation with a plate, screws, and bone graft.
3. exchange of the femoral components with insertion of a long stem cementless implant.
4. cast immobilization.
5. minimal weight bearing and observation.

PREFERRED RESPONSE: 5

(continued on next page)

(A-22: *continued*)

DISCUSSION: Intraoperative femoral fractures can often be avoided by careful preoperative planning to optimize implant design and size. Most fractures occur during implantation of a cementless implant; many can be avoided by careful femoral preparation and component implantation, with particular caution in osteopenic bone. Intraoperative femoral fractures are managed according to fracture severity. Minor cracks that do not affect stability or femoral integrity can often be managed intraoperatively with cerclage fixation, limited weight bearing, and observation. Femoral fractures that compromise implant stability or femoral integrity require fracture fixation with cerclage wires, strut grafts, or plates and may require conversion to a long-stem implant. This patient's fracture is nondisplaced and the implant is well seated; therefore, limited weight bearing is considered appropriate management.

REFERENCES: Lee SR, Bostrom MP: Periprosthetic fractures of the femur after total hip arthroplasty. *Instr Course Lect* 2004;53:111-118.

Kelley SS: Periprosthetic femoral fractures. *J Am Acad Orthop Surg* 1994;2:164-172. Berry DJ: Management of periprosthetic fractures: The hip. *J Arthroplasty* 2002;17:11-13.

A-23: A 58-year-old man reports a 2-month onset of groin pain with no history of trauma. Examination reveals that range of motion of the hip is mildly restricted, and he has pain with both weight bearing and at rest. An MRI scan is shown in Figure 13. Treatment should consist of

1. protected weight bearing and anti-inflammatory drugs.
2. core decompression of the femoral head.
3. vascularized free fibular grafting to the femoral head.
4. bipolar hemiarthroplasty of the hip.
5. total hip arthroplasty.

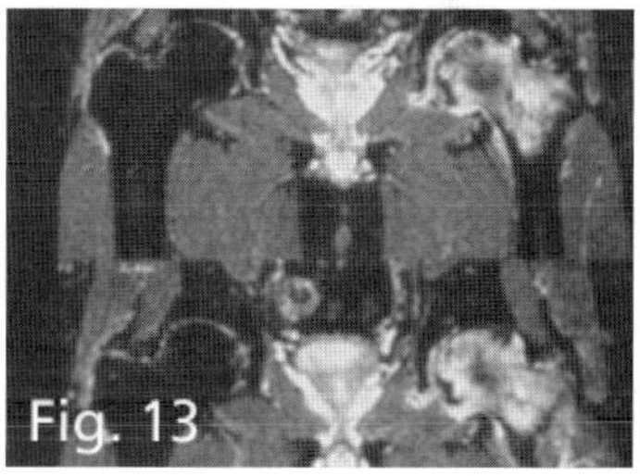
Fig. 13

PREFERRED RESPONSE: 1

DISCUSSION: The MRI findings show highly increased signal through the entire femoral head and neck on short tau inversion recovery imaging, diagnostic of transient osteoporosis of the femoral head. This disease entity can be seen in middle-aged men, and should be treated nonsurgically. The natural history is that of self-resolution.

REFERENCES: Guerra JJ, Steinberg ME: Distinguishing transient osteoporosis from avascular necrosis of the hip. *J Bone Joint Surg Am* 1995;77:616-624.

Urbanski SR, de Lange EE, Eschenroeder HC Jr: Magnetic resonance imaging of transient osteoporosis of the hip: A case report. *J Bone Joint Surg Am* 1991;73:451-455.

A-24: Figure 14 shows the radiograph of a 32-year-old patient with right hip pain that has failed to respond to nonsurgical management. What is the most appropriate surgical treatment at this time?

1. Femoral derotational osteotomy
2. Total hip arthroplasty
3. Arthrodesis
4. Surgical dislocation of the hip
5. Periacetabular osteotomy

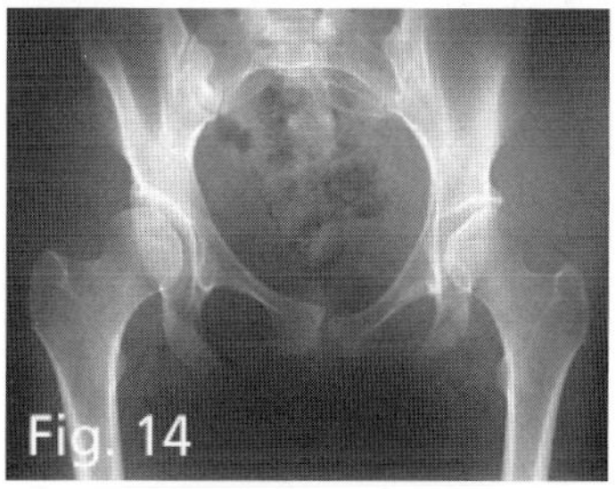
Fig. 14

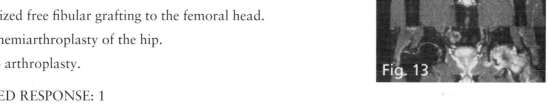

(continued on next page)

Preservation, Arthroplasty, and Salvage Surgery of the Hip and Knee: Answers

(A-24: *continued*)

PREFERRED RESPONSE: 5

DISCUSSION: The radiograph reveals developmental dysplasia of both hips. The patient has classic anterolateral undercoverage of the femoral head on the right side as demonstrated by a high acetabular index (measured at 27°). Anterior undercoverage can be determined by drawing the marking for the anterior wall that fails to overlap the femoral head in this patient. Currently in North America, the most accepted surgical management for symptomatic dysplasia of the hip with good joint space is a Bernese (Ganz) periacetabular osteotomy. Surgical dislocation of the hip and femoroacetabular osteoplasty may be considered for patients with symptomatic femoroacetabular impingement of the hip.

REFERENCES: Ganz R, Klaue K, Vinh TS, et al: A new periacetabular osteotomy for the treatment of hip dysplasias: Technique and preliminary results. *Clin Orthop* 1988;232:26-36.

Trousdale RT, Ekkernkamp A, Ganz R, et al: Periacetabular and intertrochanteric osteotomy for the treatment of osteoarthrosis in dysplastic hips. *J Bone Joint Surg Am* 1995;77:73-85.

A-25: A patient reports pain in the hip with functional positioning. With the patient supine, pain in which of the following positions would be typical for femoral acetabular impingement?

1. Hip is internally rotated, passively flexed to 90°, and adducted
2. Hip is internally rotated, passively flexed to 90°, and abducted
3. Hip is externally rotated, maximally flexed to 90°, and adducted
4. Hip is externally rotated, passively flexed to 90°, and abducted
5. Hip is externally rotated, maximally flexed, and abducted

PREFERRED RESPONSE: 1

DISCUSSION: Patients with dysplasia often have a hypertrophic labrum. Abnormal contact between the femoral neck and the acetabular rim leads to labral injury, especially in the anterior-superior acetabular zone. Typically, young patients with the condition report pain with activity or long periods of sitting or driving. The hips often have limited motion, in particular in internal rotation and flexion. Forceful adduction with the maneuver causes pain.

REFERENCES: Parvizi J, Purtill JJ: Hip, pelvic reconstruction, and arthroplasty, in Vaccaro AR, ed: *Orthopaedic Knowledge Update*, ed 8. Rosemont, IL, American Academy of Orthopaedic Surgeons, 2005, pp 411-424.

Beck M, Leunig M, Parvizi J, et al: Anterior femoroacetabular impingement: Part II. Midterm results of surgical treatment. *Clin Orthop* 2004;418:67-73.

McCarthy JC, Noble PC, Schuck MR, et al: The role of labral lesions to development of early degenerative hip disease. *Clin Orthop* 2001;393:25-37.

A-26: A 38-year-old man who is an avid tennis player has had persistent pain over the medial aspect of his knee for the past 6 years. He notes that the pain occurs on a daily basis with any significant activity. NSAIDs have failed to provide relief. Radiographs are shown in Figures 15A and 15B. What is the best course of action?

1. Total knee arthroplasty
2. Unicompartmental arthroplasty
3. Insertion of a unispacer
4. Tibial osteotomy
5. Knee arthroscopy

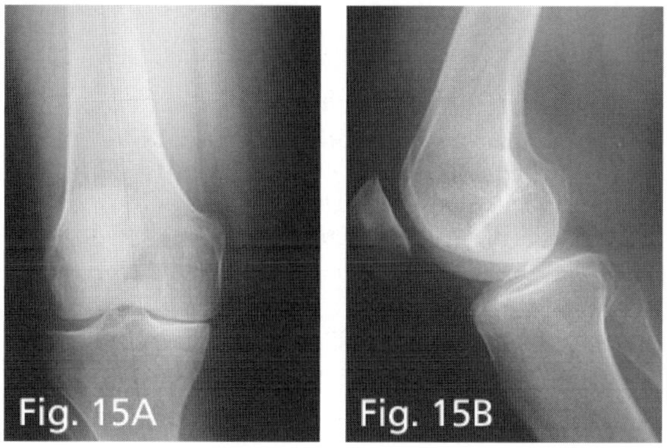

PREFERRED RESPONSE: 4

DISCUSSION: In a relatively young patient who is an avid tennis player, the treatment of choice is a joint-preserving procedure. The radiographs reveal varus alignment with loading of the medial compartment. After all nonsurgical management options have been used, the best treatment option is a medial opening wedge osteotomy. A lateral closing wedge osteotomy of the proximal tibia is also a reasonable option, but it is not one of the choices. A unicompartmental arthroplasty or a total knee arthroplasty would place significant restrictions in this patient. A unispacer may be a temporizing procedure but is controversial and without substantial data in the literature. The knee arthroscopy will not address the medial compartment osteoarthritis.

REFERENCES: Nagel A, Insall JN, Scuderi GR: Proximal tibial osteotomy: A subjective outcome study. *J Bone Joint Surg Am* 1996;78:1353-1358.

Rinonapoli E, Mancini GB, Corvaglia A, et al: Tibial osteotomy for varus gonarthrosis: A 10- to 21-year followup study. *Clin Orthop* 1998;353:185-193.

Manifold SG, Kelly MA, Richardson L, et al: Osteotomies about the knee, in Fitzgerald RH, Kaufer H, Malkani AL, eds: *Orthopaedics*. St Louis, MO, Mosby, 2002, pp 947-961.

A-27: Which of the following statements best describes the outcome of the routine use of continuous passive motion (CPM) machines after total knee arthroplasty (TKA)?

1. CPM is likely to improve early range of motion and final range of motion.
2. CPM may improve early range of motion but is unlikely to improve final range of motion.
3. CPM is likely to decrease postoperative pain.
4. CPM is likely to improve extension but not flexion.
5. CPM is likely to restore quicker ambulatory ability.

PREFERRED RESPONSE: 2

DISCUSSION: Although CPM machines are used widely in the United States for patients undergoing TKA, the benefit, if any, seems to be marginal. Numerous randomized trials have shown that final outcomes after TKA are unaffected by the use of CPM machines postoperatively. Some studies have suggested that use of CPM may improve flexion in the first few weeks, but any short-term benefit from the machine was lost by intermediate-term follow-up. Aside from potential improvement in flexion within the first few postoperative weeks, there does not appear to be any benefit from the machines. There is

(continued on next page)

(A-27: *continued*)

no improvement in pain, ambulation, or extension. The cost-effectiveness of these machines has been questioned by many authors.

REFERENCES: Stern SH: The Knee: Rehabilitation, in Pellicci PM, Tria AJ, Garvin KL, eds: *Orthopaedic Knowledge Update: Hip and Knee Reconstruction*, ed 2. Rosemont, IL, American Academy of Orthopaedic Surgeons, 2000, pp 287-293.

McInnes J, Larson MG, Daltroy LH, et al: A controlled evaluation of continuous passive motion in patients undergoing total knee arthroplasty. *JAMA* 1992;268:1423-1428.

Kumar PJ, McPherson EJ, Dorr LD, et al: Rehabilitation after total knee arthroplasty: A comparison of 2 rehabilitation techniques. *Clin Orthop* 1996;331:93-101.

A-28: When performing knee arthroplasty, which of the following procedures provides the most consistent fixation for the tibial component?

1. Cementless fixation of the tibial component
2. Augmenting cementless fixation of the tibial component with pegs or screws
3. Cementing the metaphyseal portion and press fitting the keel of the tibial component
4. Cementing the metaphyseal and keel portions of the tibial component
5. Cemented fixation of the tibial component with screws

PREFERRED RESPONSE: 4

DISCUSSION: All of the options, except cementing the metaphyseal portion and press fitting the keel of the tibial component, have been shown to create strong and long-lasting constructs; however, cementing of both the platform and the keel offers the most predictable solution. Cementing the platform and not the keel has been shown to have a higher loosening rate than the more traditional methods of fully cementing or using screws to augment fixation.

REFERENCE: Froimson MI: Knee reconstruction and replacement, in Vaccaro AR, ed: *Orthopaedic Knowledge Update*, ed 8. Rosemont, IL, American Academy of Orthopaedic Surgeons, 2005, pp 457-468.

A-29: Figure 16 shows the radiograph of an 84-year-old woman who has pain and is unable to extend her knee. History reveals that she underwent total knee arthroplasty 8 years ago. Aspiration and studies for infection are negative. During revision surgery, management of the tibial bone loss should consist of

1. reconstruction with a metal augmented revision tibial implant.
2. reconstruction with a hinged prosthesis.
3. reconstruction with a structural allograft.
4. reconstruction with iliac crest bone graft.
5. filling the defect with cement.

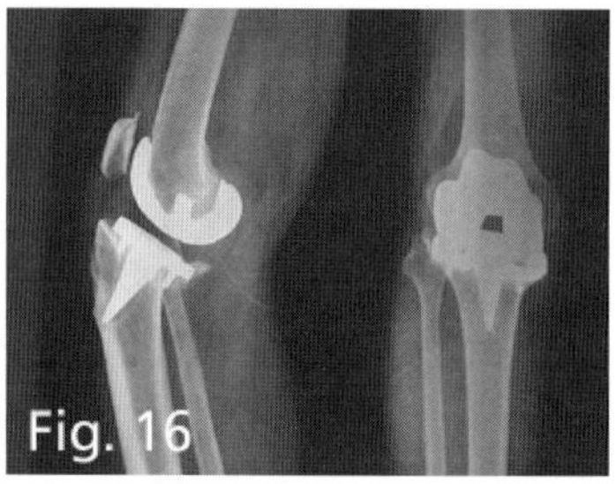
Fig. 16

PREFERRED RESPONSE: 1

DISCUSSION: Massive bone loss encountered in revision total knee arthroplasty remains a significant challenge. Recent reports have shown high success rates using structural allograft to reconstruct large

(continued on next page)

(A-29: *continued*)

structural bone defects. A hinged prosthesis is not required in this setting. In this patient, a large amount of posterior cortex has been lost, making the area too large to fill with cement or iliac crest bone graft. Because of the patient's age, the treatment of choice is a revision tibial implant and metal augments. Structural allograft would be suitable in a younger patient.

REFERENCES: Mow CS, Wiedel JD: Structural allografting in revision total knee arthroplasty. *J Arthroplasty* 1996;11:235-241.

Engh GA, Herzwurm PJ, Parks NL: Treatment of major defects of bone with bulk allografts and stemmed components during total knee arthroplasty. *J Bone Joint Surg Am* 1997;79:1030-1039.

Clatworthy MG, Ballance J, Brick GW, et al: The use of structural allograft for uncontained defects in revision total knee arthroplasty: A minimum five-year review. *J Bone Joint Surg Am* 2001;83:404-411.

A-30: A 62-year-old woman with a bone mineral density (BMD) T-score of -2.0 sustained a subcapital fracture of her hip. She is an avid tennis player, and history reveals no previous fractures. What is the most appropriate follow-up care?

1. Antiresorptive bisphosphonate medication
2. A repeat dual-energy x-ray absorptiometry scan (DEXA) and treatment if the T-score is less than −2.5
3. A repeat DEXA scan and treatment if the T-score is greater than −1.5
4. No treatment since the BMD is not in osteoporotic range
5. Parathyroid hormone followed by surgery

PREFERRED RESPONSE: 1

DISCUSSION: A DEXA scan is most appropriately used to establish a baseline score. Even if the BMD is not within the osteoporotic range (T-score less than -2.5), a prior fragility fracture is a strong risk factor for a second fracture as a result of factors other than bone density, such as worsening vision or balance, confusion, or other predispositions to falls. The guidelines of the National Osteoporosis Foundation indicate that, following a fragility hip fracture, active antiosteoporotic medication should be initiated, whether or not a DEXA scan is performed. A recent study showed that antiresorptive therapy following a hip fracture reduces not only the risk of a second fracture but also overall mortality.

REFERENCE: Gardner MJ, Brophy RH, Demetrakopoulos D, et al: Interventions to improve osteoporosis treatment following hip fracture: A prospective, randomized trial. *J Bone Joint Surg Am* 2005;87:3-7.

A-31: A 58-year-old patient who underwent bilateral hip arthroplasty 12 years ago now reports pain in his hips and difficulty with ambulation to the point where he now uses crutches. A radiograph of the hip and pelvis is shown in Figure 17. What is the best treatment option for this patient?

1. Revision hip arthroplasty with a bipolar implant
2. Revision hip arthroplasty with impaction grafting on the femoral and acetabular side
3. Revision hip arthroplasty with a cemented jumbo acetabular component
4. Revision hip arthroplasty with a cementless acetabular component
5. Acetabular component revision with a tri-flange protrusio ring

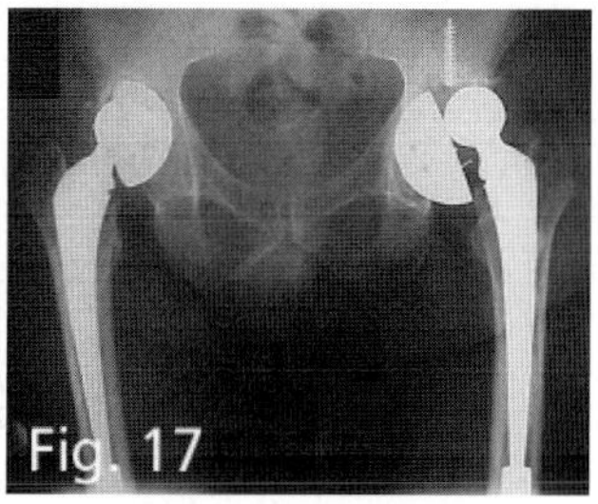

(A-31: *continued*)

PREFERRED RESPONSE: 4

DISCUSSION: The radiographs reveal acetabular component failure with bone loss. There are several treatment options available. The best option for survivorship is a cementless porous-coated acetabular component. This patient may or may not require structural bone graft, which may need to be determined at the time of surgery. Bipolar implants and cemented acetabular components for revision surgery have not demonstrated long-term success. The use of a protrusio ring is reserved primarily for massive bone loss such as Paprosky type III bone loss with significant superior migration of the acetabular component. The best clinical results for acetabular component revision have been achieved with cementless porous-coated implants.

REFERENCES: Haddad FS, Masri BA, Garbuz DS, et al: Acetabulum, in Fitzgerald RH, Kaufer H, Malkani AL, eds: *Orthopaedics*. St Louis, MO, Mosby, 2002, pp 923-936.

D'Antonio JA: Periprosthetic bone loss of the acetabulum: Classification and management. *Orthop Clin North Am* 1992;23:279-290.

Rubash HE, Sinha RK, Paprosky W, et al: A new classification system for the management of acetabular osteolysis after total hip arthroplasty. *Instr Course Lect* 1999;48:37-42.

A-32: Embolic material (shown in Figure 18) generated during total knee arthroplasty (TKA) is composed of which of the following substances?

1. Fat only
2. Fat and air
3. Fat and marrow
4. Fat and cement
5. Fat and bone

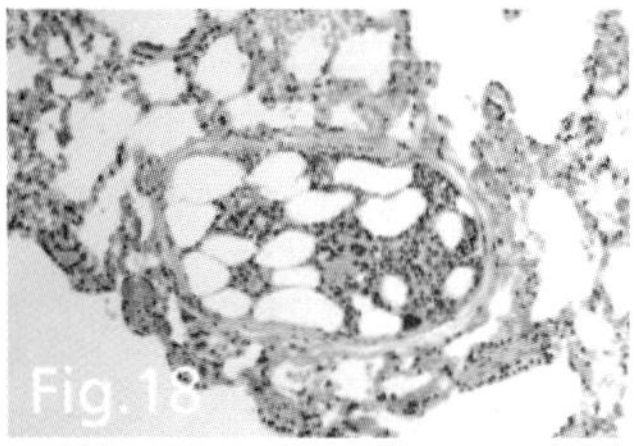

Fig. 18

PREFERRED RESPONSE: 3

DISCUSSION: Emboli are created during TKA. Usually there is an increased incidence with the use of intramedullary rods that disrupt the marrow contents. These are not fat emboli per se. They are material composed of fat cells and marrow that act like pulmonary emboli to obstruct small arterioles in the lung. They are different from free fat emboli that are seen in fractures and that lead to chemical injury to the lung rather than obstructive injury.

REFERENCES: Markel DC, Femino JE, Farkas P, et al: Analysis of lower extremity embolic material after total knee arthroplasty in a canine model. *J Arthroplasty* 1999;14:227-232.

Pell AC, Christie J, Keating JF, et al: The detection of fat embolism by transoesophageal echocardiography during reamed intramedullary nailing: A study of 24 patients with femoral and tibial fractures. *J Bone Joint Surg Br* 1993;75:921-925.

McGrath BJ, Hsia J, Boyd A, et al: Venous embolization after deflation of lower extremity tourniquets. *Anesth Analg* 1994;78:349-353.

A-33: A 30-year-old patient has had severe left hip pain and difficulty ambulating, necessitating the use of a cane, for the past 6 months. A photomicrograph of the femoral head sectioned at the time of surgery is shown in Figure 19. What is the most likely diagnosis?

1. Renal osteodystrophy
2. Pyogenic osteomyelitis
3. Osteoarthritis
4. Osteonecrosis
5. Tuberculosis osteomyelitis

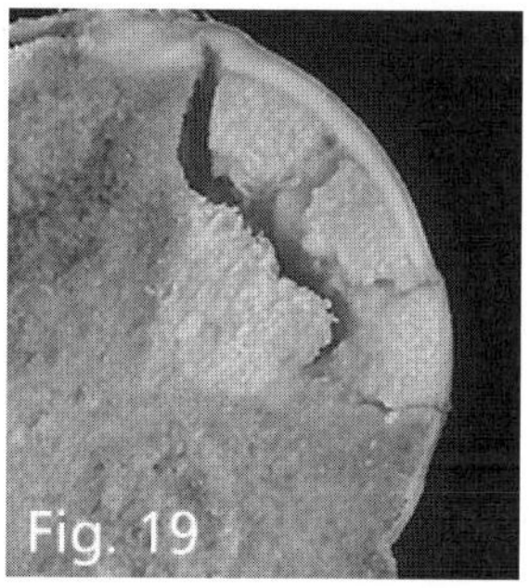
Fig. 19

PREFERRED RESPONSE: 4

DISCUSSION: The photomicrograph demonstrates a wedge-shaped infarct with femoral head collapse; therefore, the diagnosis is osteonecrosis of the femoral head. Perthes disease and osteoarthritis do not involve a wedge-shaped defect. Tuberculosis of the hip joint results in greater destruction of the articular cartilage.

REFERENCES: Basset LW, Mirra JM, Cracchiolo A III: Ischemic necrosis of the femoral head: Correlation between magnetic resonance imaging and histologic sections. *Clin Orthop* 1987;223:181-187.

Sugano N: Osteonecrosis, in Fitzgerald RH, Kaufer H, Malkani AL, eds: *Orthopedics*. St Louis, MO, Mosby, 2002, pp 878-887.

A-34: When comparing mobile-bearing total knee arthroplasty (TKA) to fixed-bearing total condylar arthroplasty, the mobile-bearing procedure provides

1. no improvement in survivorship.
2. approximately 15° greater flexion.
3. appreciable reduction in wear rates.
4. a faster recovery profile.
5. better quadriceps strength.

PREFERRED RESPONSE: 1

DISCUSSION: Survivorship is similar in the two groups. In a recent study, mobile-bearing TKAs showed a slightly higher maximum flexion than the total condylar fixed-bearing-type designs (112° versus 108° with no difference in recovery rate). Using a fixed-bearing or a mobile-bearing design did not seem to influence the recovery rate in early results after knee arthroplasty. Mobile-bearing arthroplasties are suggested, in theory, to offer a reduction in polyethylene wear; however, clinical studies have not yet proven this. Recovery rates have yet to be statistically seen as improved with either method. Differences in strength have not been shown.

REFERENCES: Aglietti P, Baldini A, Buzzi R, et al: Comparison of mobile-bearing and fixed-bearing total knee arthroplasty: A prospective randomized study. *J Arthroplasty* 2005;20:145-153.

Sorrells RB: The rotating platform mobile bearing TKA. *Orthopedics* 1996;19:793-796.

Dennis DA, Komistek RD: Kinematics of mobile-bearing total knee arthroplasty. *Instr Course Lect* 2005;54:207-220.

A-35: Based on the type of articulation shown in Figure 20, wear is not affected by which of the following factors?

1. Radial mismatch of the femoral head to the acetabular component
2. Sphericity of the bearings
3. Surface finish of the articulation
4. Carbon content of the metal-on-metal bearing
5. Head-to-neck ratio

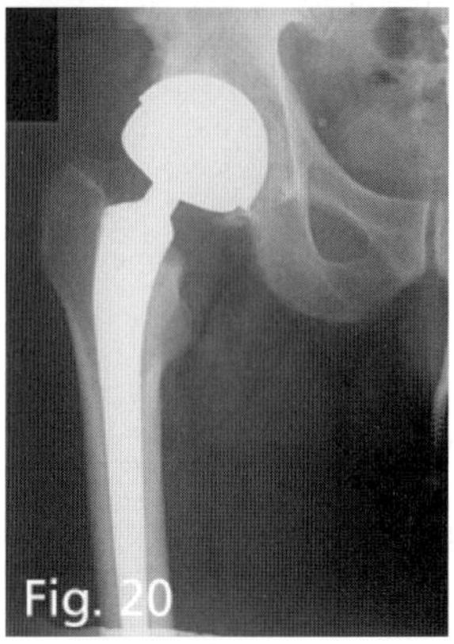

PREFERRED RESPONSE: 5

DISCUSSION: Wear in total hip arthroplasty is a very complex phenomenon. The radial mismatch of the femoral head to the acetabular component has been shown in multiple studies to be a significant factor in wear. The mismatch can neither be too small nor too large. When the mismatch is too small, seizing of the implants can occur. When the mismatch is too large, contact stresses increase and produce exceptionally high wear. The ideal radial mismatch should be approximately 50 microns. Surface roughness and ball sphericity are two items that are extremely important with respect to wear. High carbon content has been shown to decrease wear. This device has a very large head-to-neck ratio, so impingement-related wear is unlikely.

REFERENCES: Amstutz HC, Grigoris P: Metal on metal bearings in hip arthroplasty. *Clin Orthop* 1996;329:S11-S34.

Amstutz HC, Campbell P, McKellop H, et al: Metal on metal total hip replacement workshop consensus document. *Clin Orthop* 1996;329:S297-S303.

McKellop H, Park SH, Chiesa R, et al: In vivo wear of three types of metal on metal hip prostheses during two decades of use. *Clin Orthop* 1996;329:S128-S140.

A-36: A 78-year-old patient undergoing revision total knee arthroplasty has bone loss throughout the knee at the time of revision. A distal femoral augment is used to restore the joint line. One month after surgery, the patient reports pain and is unable to ambulate. A lateral radiograph is shown in Figure 21. What is the most likely etiology of this problem?

1. Inadequate restoration of the joint line
2. Patellar tendon rupture
3. Excessive internal rotation of the tibial component
4. Flexion gap instability
5. Hyperextension of the femoral component

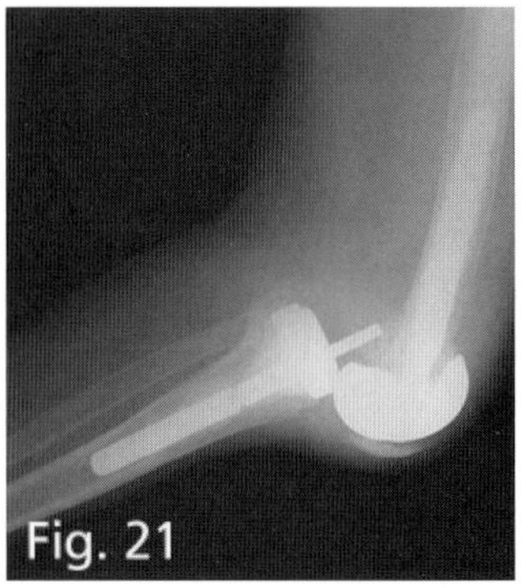

PREFERRED RESPONSE: 4

DISCUSSION: Instability is a leading cause of failure following total knee arthroplasty. Instability can present as global instability, extension gap (varus/valgus) instability, or flexion gap (anterior/posterior) instability. Treatment options are numerous based on the exact pathology. The radiograph reveals anterior/posterior instability with dislocation consistent with flexion gap instability. A loose flexion gap can allow the femoral component to ride above the tibial cam post mechanism, resulting in dislocation. Distal femoral augments treat extension gap instability, whereas tibial augments can treat both flexion and extension

(continued on next page)

(A-36: *continued*)

gap instability. Posterior condyle augments at the distal femur can also be used to treat flexion gap instability. Flexion gap instability is further aggravated by extension mechanism incompetence. Note the excessively thin patella on the lateral radiograph.

REFERENCES: Pagnano MW, Hanssen AD, Lewallen DG, et al: Flexion instability after primary cruciate retaining total knee arthroplasty. *Clin Orthop* 1998;356:39-46.

McAuley J, Engh GA, Ammeen DJ: Treatment of the unstable total knee arthroplasty. *Inst Course Lect* 2004;53:237-241.

Naudie DD, Rorabeck CH: Managing instability in total knee arthroplasty with constrained and linked implants. *Instr Course Lect* 2004;53:207-215.

A-37: Figure 22 reveals a periprosthetic fracture around a cemented femoral stem in an 81-year-old patient with Paget disease and mild coagulopathy. What is the most appropriate reconstructive management on the femoral side?

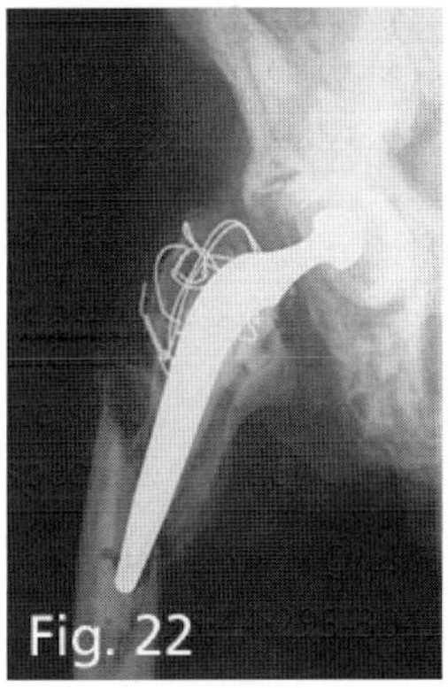
Fig. 22

1. Open reduction and internal fixation
2. Impaction allografting
3. Proximally coated femoral stem
4. Allograft prosthetic composite (APC)
5. Proximal femoral replacement (PFR)

PREFERRED RESPONSE: 5

DISCUSSION: This is an example of a Vancouver B3 periprosthetic fracture that consists of a fracture around a loose femoral stem with poor proximal bone support. Therefore, open reduction and internal fixation is not an option. PFR is an excellent choice for elderly inactive patients with poor femoral bone stock. The surgery can be performed in an expeditious manner, which is very important in a patient with mild coagulopathy. Impaction allografting and APC are both options for younger patients who have bone stock that needs to be restored. The results of revision arthroplasty using proximally coated stems, especially under these circumstances, are poor.

REFERENCES: Duncan CP, Masri BA: Fractures of the femur after hip replacement. *Instr Course Lect* 1995;44:293-304.

Parvizi J, Sim FH: Proximal femoral replacements with megaprostheses. *Clin Orthop* 2004;420:169-175.

Klein GR, Parvizi J, Rapuri V, et al: Proximal femoral replacement for treatment of periprosthetic fractures. *J Bone Joint Surg Am* 2005;87:1777-1781.

A-38: A patient with a documented allergy to nickel requires a total knee arthroplasty. Which of the following prostheses is most likely to provide long-term success in this individual?

1. All-polyethylene tibial component and pure titanium femoral component
2. All-polyethylene tibial component and cobalt-chromium alloy femoral component
3. Cobalt-chromium alloy tibial component and cobalt-chromium alloy femoral component
4. Modular titanium tibial component and pure titanium femoral component
5. Modular titanium tibial component and oxidized zirconium femoral component

PREFERRED RESPONSE: 5

DISCUSSION: Nickel allergy is not an infrequent preoperative finding. The ramifications of such allergies in arthroplasty patients are poorly understood at this time. Stainless steel and cobalt-chromium alloys contain relatively high concentrations of nickel. Titanium, oxidized zirconium, and polyethylene do not contain significant amounts of nickel. Titanium is not a good surface for the articulating portion of the femoral component because of its propensity for metallosis. Oxidized zirconium is the only suitable femoral component for patients allergic to nickel. A modular titanium tibial component or an all-polyethylene tibial component would be satisfactory for these patients.

REFERENCES: Laskin RS: An oxidized Zr ceramic surfaced femoral component for total knee arthroplasty. *Clin Orthop* 2003;416:191-196.

Nasser S, Campbell PA, Kilgus D, et al: Cementless total joint arthroplasty prostheses with titanium-alloy articular surfaces: A human retrieval analysis. *Clin Orthop* 1990;261:171-185.

A-39: A 42-year-old man reports the recent onset of right hip pain. A radiograph and MRI scan are shown in Figures 23A and 23B. White blood cell count, erythrocyte sedimentation rate, and hip aspiration results are within normal limits. Management should now consist of

1. core decompression.
2. biopsy of the femoral head.
3. protected weight bearing and observation.
4. total hip arthroplasty.
5. percutaneous cannulated pin fixation of the femoral neck.

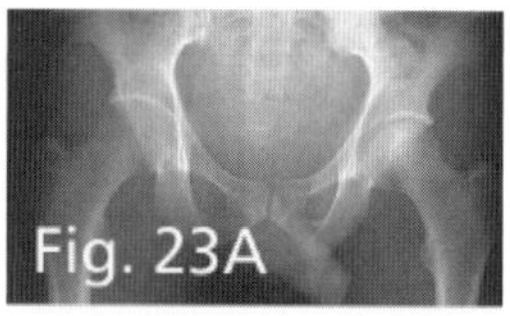
Fig. 23A

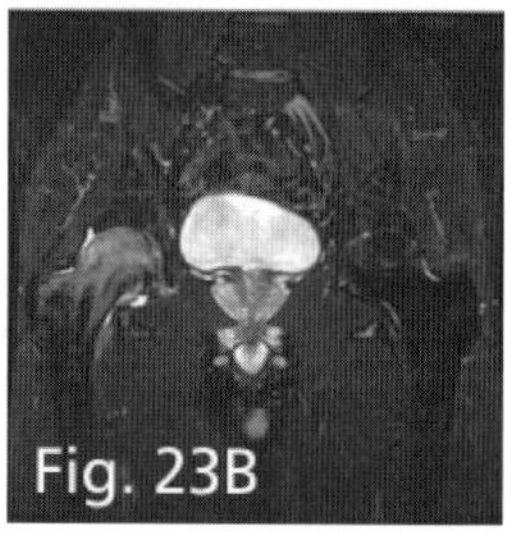
Fig. 23B

PREFERRED RESPONSE: 3

DISCUSSION: Transient osteoporosis of the hip is an uncommon problem, usually affecting women in the last trimester of pregnancy and middle-aged men. Symptoms include pain in the involved hip with temporary osteopenia; however, there is no joint space involvement. In this patient, the imaging findings are consistent with transient osteoporosis. Short repetition time/echo time images reveal diffusely decreased signal intensity in the femoral head and intracapsular region of the femoral neck. Increased signal intensity is seen with increased T2-weighting. Within a few months, the pain, as well as the imaging findings, will completely resolve without intervention. Distinguishing the diffuse features of transient osteoporosis of the hip from the segmental findings of osteonecrosis is essential. Unlike transient osteoporosis of the hip, osteonecrosis will have a double-density signal on MRI and may progress radiographically. Surgical intervention and oral corticosteriods are not indicated for treatment. Protected weight bearing until the pain resolves may decrease symptoms while the transient osteoporosis resolves.

(continued on next page)

(A-39: *continued*)

REFERENCES: Potter H, Moran M, Scheider R, et al: Magnetic resonance imaging in diagnosis of transient osteoporosis of the hip. *Clin Orthop* 1992;280:223-229.

Bijl M, van Leeuwen MA, van Rijswijk MH: Transient osteoporosis of the hip: Presentation of typical cases for review of the literature. *Clin Exp Rheumatol* 1999;17:601-604.

Montella BJ; Nunley JA, Urbaniak JR: Osteonecrosis of the femoral head associated with pregnancy: A preliminary report. *J Bone Joint Surg Am* 1999;81:790-798.

A-40: During cemented total hip arthroplasty, peak pulmonary embolization of marrow contents occurs when the

1. hip is dislocated.
2. femoral neck is osteotomized.
3. acetabulum is prepared.
4. acetabular component is inserted.
5. femoral stem is inserted.

PREFERRED RESPONSE: 5

DISCUSSION: Peak embolization is observed during femoral stem insertion. Embolization is also observed during acetabular preparation and hip reduction.

REFERENCES: Lewallen DG, Parvizi J, Ereth MH: Perioperative mortality associated with hip and knee arthroplasty, in Morrey BF, ed: *Joint Replacement Arthroplasty*, ed 3. Philadelphia, PA, Churchill-Livingstone, 2003, pp 119-127.

Ereth MH, Weber JG, Abel MD, et al: Cemented versus noncemented total hip arthroplasty: Embolism, hemodynamics, and intrapulmonary shunting. *Mayo Clin Proc* 1992;67:1066-1074.

A-41: What are the optimal conditions for leaving the acetabular shell in place, replacing the acetabular liner, and grafting the osteolytic defect shown in Figure 24?

1. Nonmodular implant
2. Instability
3. Well-designed, well-fixed modular implant
4. Complete radiolucency of the acetabular component
5. Migration of the acetabular component

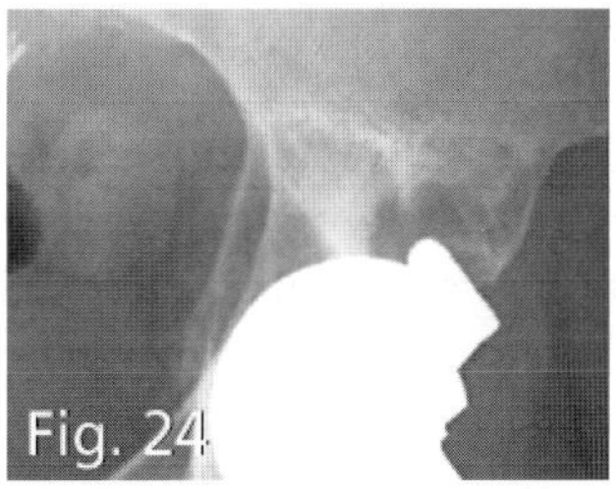

PREFERRED RESPONSE: 3

DISCUSSION: Dense pods of ingrowth into the porous coating of cementless ingrowth sockets are seen. Channels through the noningrown portion allow access to the trabecular bone of the ilium. Polyethylene wear debris can enter these areas through screw holes. Expansile, lytic lesions can result, which can become large without compromising implant fixation. Loosening is late and results from catastrophic loss

(continued on next page)

(A-41: *continued*)

of bone. A well-fixed acetabular component with a modular design, a well-designed locking mechanism, and a good survivorship history is a candidate for exchange of the liner and grafting of the osteolytic lesion.

REFERENCES: Ries MD: Complications in primary total hip arthroplasty: Avoidance and management. Wear. *Instr Course Lect* 2003;52:257-265.

Dumbleton JH, Manley MT, Edidin AA: A literature review of the association between wear rate and osteolysis in total hip arthroplasty. *J Arthroplasty* 2002;17:649-661.

Maloney WJ: Osteolysis, in Pellicci PM, Tria AJ Jr, Garvin KL, eds: *Orthopaedic Knowledge Update: Hip and Knee Reconstruction*, ed 2. Rosemont, IL, American Academy of Orthopaedic Surgeons, 2000, pp 175-180.

A-42: A 53-year-old patient is seen in the emergency department after sustaining a fall onto her left hip. A current radiograph is shown in Figure 25. What is the best treatment option?

1. Bed rest and no weight bearing for 6 to 8 weeks
2. Component retention and open reduction and internal fixation
3. Proximal femoral replacement prosthesis
4. Revision arthroplasty with a long cemented stem
5. Revision arthroplasty with a long porous-coated cylindrical stem

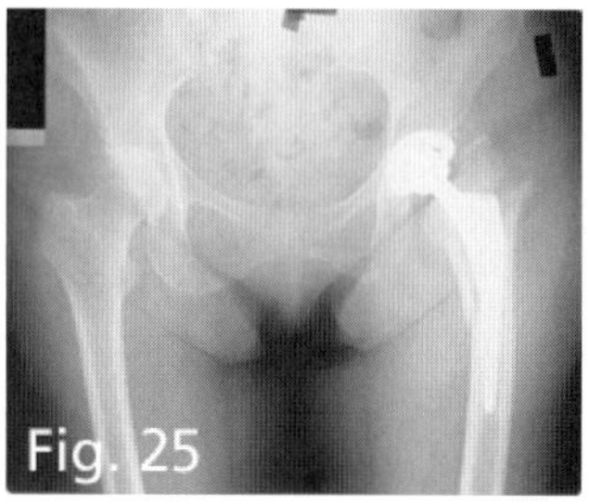
Fig. 25

PREFERRED RESPONSE: 5

DISCUSSION: The patient has sustained a Vancouver B2 periprosthetic femoral fracture (a femoral fracture that occurs around or just distal to a loose stem, with adequate proximal bone stock). The stem is no longer fixed to proximal bone; therefore, retention of the femoral component is not recommended. Nonsurgical management is contraindicated because of the high risk of nonunion and malunion with significant component settling in the distal fragment and leg shortening. Revision femoral arthroplasty must attain distal fixation in adequate host bone, which is usually successful with a porous-coated cylindrical stem.

REFERENCES: Parvizi J, Rapuri VR, Purtill JJ, et al: Treatment protocol for proximal femoral periprosthetic fractures. *J Bone Joint Surg Am* 2004;86:8-16.

Springer BD, Berry DJ, Lewallen DG: Treatment of periprosthetic femoral fractures following total hip arthroplasty with femoral component revision. *J Bone Joint Surg Am* 2003;85:2156-2162.

A-43: Figure 26 shows the radiograph of a 65-year-old man who underwent a revision arthroplasty to remove a loose, cemented femoral stem. When planning the postoperative restrictions, the surgeon should be aware that

1. the approach used reduces the torque-to-failure (fracture) of the construct to less than 50% of the intact femur.
2. the technique of repair can return the reconstructed prosthesis/bone composite to nearly the strength of the intact femur.
3. there is no relationship between the density of the native bone and the strength of the prosthesis/bone composite.

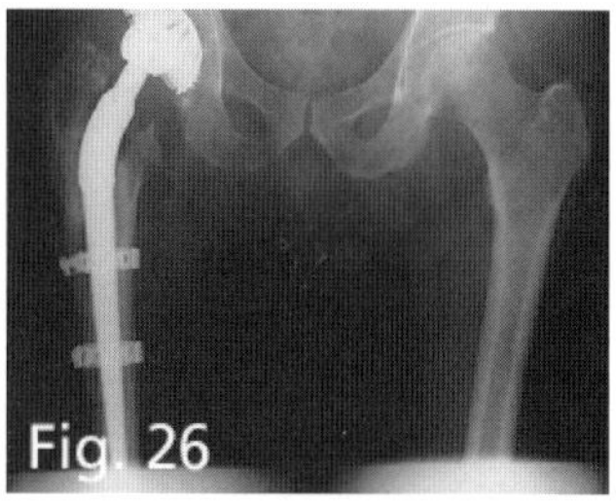
Fig. 26

(continued on next page)

(A-43: *continued*)

4. the addition of bone graft substitute or autograft has been shown to lessen the time to complete healing.
5. there is a one in five chance of fracture with this technique; therefore, the surgeon must carefully weigh the potential benefits versus this risk.

PREFERRED RESPONSE: 1

DISCUSSION: The transfemoral approach, also known as the extended trochanteric osteotomy, is an important technique to master for revision hip surgery. When performed correctly, it allows excellent exposure of the femoral canal and aids in exposure of the acetabulum. As demonstrated in the study cited, however, it markedly reduces the torque that the composite can withstand without failure. This type of basic science study is important to guide postoperative rehabilitation.

REFERENCE: Noble AR, Branham D, Willis M, et al: Mechanical effects of the extended trochanteric osteotomy. *J Bone Joint Surg Am* 2005;87:521-529.

A-44: A 37-year-old man who works in a factory has isolated, lateral unicompartmental pain about his knee with activities. Nonsurgical management has failed to provide relief. The radiograph shown in Figure 27 reveals a tibiofemoral angle of approximately 15° that is clinically correctable to neutral. What is the best surgical option in this patient?

1. Unicompartmental arthroplasty
2. Total knee arthroplasty
3. Lateral closing wedge proximal tibial osteotomy
4. Medial opening wedge proximal tibial osteotomy
5. Medial closing wedge supracondylar femoral osteotomy

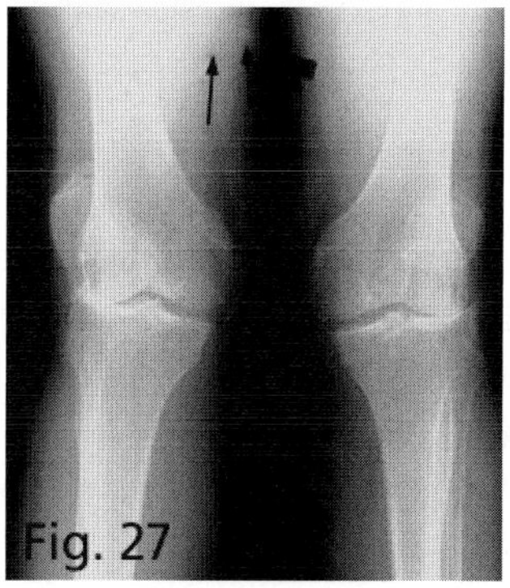

PREFERRED RESPONSE: 5

DISCUSSION: Patients with a valgus alignment about the knee can have lateral compartment arthritis. Similar to a high tibial osteotomy, a supracondylar femoral osteotomy is indicated in younger patients who have a more active lifestyle and isolated unicompartmental disease. In this young patient who works in a factory and has a valgus knee, a medial closing wedge supracondylar femoral osteotomy is the treatment of choice. The role of arthroplasty is limited in younger patients.

REFERENCES: Mathews J, Cobb AG, Richardson S, et al: Distal femoral osteotomy for lateral compartment osteoarthritis of the knee. *Orthopedics* 1998;21:437-440.

Cameron HU, Botsford DJ, Park YS: Prognostic factors in the outcome of supracondylar femoral osteotomy for lateral compartment osteoarthritis of the knee. *Can J Surg* 1997;40:114-118.

A-45: Figure 28 shows the AP radiograph of an active 80-year-old patient with an acetabular fracture. The fracture was initially managed nonsurgically; however, the patient is now scheduled to undergo total hip arthroplasty. What is the treatment of choice for the contained acetabular bone defect?

1. Bipolar femoral component
2. Acetabular cage
3. Large structural allograft
4. Use of the femoral head
5. Double-bubble acetabular cup

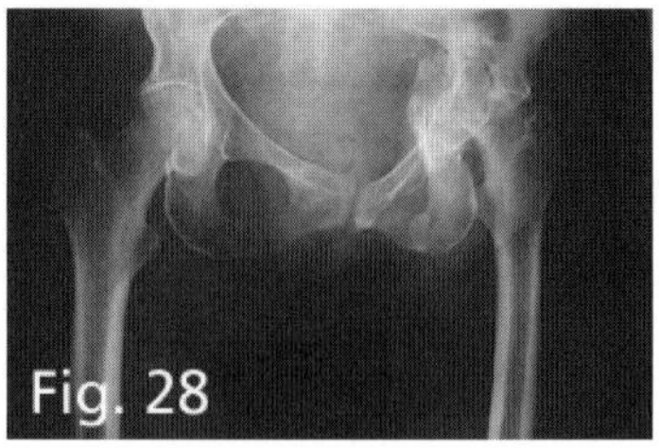
Fig. 28

PREFERRED RESPONSE: 4

DISCUSSION: Acetabular fractures can result in a relative or actual acetabular bone defect. The medial blowout fracture of the acetabulum has united well in this patient. It is likely that a medial shell of bone will be present during hip arthroplasty. The femoral head may be used as morcellized or structural bone to augment the medial defect and is preferred to structural allograft. Bipolar hip arthroplasty is notorious for medial migration in patients without a medial bone defect; therefore, it will not be a good choice in this patient. Filling the defect with methylmethacrylate cement, though an option, is not the best option in this active patient with an extensive medial defect. A double-bubble acetabular cup is used for patients with deficiency of the bone in the dome region.

REFERENCES: Mears DC: Surgical treatment of acetabular fractures in elderly patients with osteoporotic bone. *J Am Acad Orthop Surg* 1999;7:128-141.

Bellabarba C, Berger RA, Bentley CD, et al: Cementless acetabular reconstruction after acetabular fracture. *J Bone Joint Surg Am* 2001;83:868-876.

A-46: After trial placement of components in a primary total knee arthroplasty, the knee is unable to come to full extension, but the flexion gap is appropriately balanced. After adequate soft-tissue releases have been performed, what is the most appropriate next action to balance the reconstruction?

1. Use a larger femoral component
2. Use a thinner polyethylene insert
3. Add posterior femoral augments
4. Resect more proximal tibia
5. Resect additional distal femur

PREFERRED RESPONSE: 5

DISCUSSION: The reconstruction requires additional resection of the distal femur to allow increased extension while maintaining the current flexion gap tension. Resecting more proximal tibia or decreasing the tibial polyethylene thickness will decrease flexion tension as well as extension tension. Adding posterior femoral augments and using a larger femoral component will increase flexion tension.

REFERENCES: Ayers DC, Dennis DA, Johanson NA, et al: Common complications of total knee arthroplasty. *J Bone Joint Surg Am* 1997;79:278-311.

Carey CT, Tria AJ Jr: Surgical principles of total knee replacement: Incisions, extensor mechanism, ligament balancing, in Pellicci PM, Tria AJ Jr, Garvin KL, eds: *Orthopaedic Knowledge Update: Hip and Knee Reconstruction*, ed 2. Rosemont, IL, American Academy of Orthopaedic Surgeons, 2000, pp 281-286.

A-47: During total knee arthroplasty, the patella is noted to subluxate laterally despite a lateral retinacular release. Which of the following methods is most likely to improve patellar stability?

1. Slight external rotation of the tibial component
2. Slight internal rotation of the femoral component
3. Slight anterior translation of the tibial component
4. Use of a fixed-bearing knee as opposed to a mobile-bearing knee
5. Use of a thicker patellar component

PREFERRED RESPONSE: 1

DISCUSSION: Slight external rotation of the tibial component will cause a net medialization of the tibial tubercle during knee articulation. This will help centralize the extensor mechanism over the trochlear groove and minimize the tendency for lateral subluxation. Internal rotation of the femoral component increases the risk of patellar instability. Anterior translation of the tibial component moves the patellar tendon insertion posteriorly, and may increase force on the patella but should not substantially alter patellar tracking. Clinical studies have shown no patellofemoral benefits to the use of fixed- or mobile-bearing designs. Thicker patellar components will not improve tracking, and may compound the problem.

REFERENCES: Nelson C, Lombardi PM, Pellicci PM: Hybrid total hip replacement, in Pellicci PM, Tria AJ Jr, Garvin KL, eds: *Orthopaedic Knowledge Update: Hip and Knee Reconstruction*, ed 2. Rosemont, IL, American Academy of Orthopaedic Surgeons, 2000, p 207.

Pagnano MW, Trousdale RT, Stuart MJ, et al: Rotating platform knees did not improve patellar tracking: A prospective, randomized study of 240 primary total knee arthroplasties. *Clin Orthop* 2004;428:221-227.

Lotke PA, Garino JP, eds: *Revision Total Knee Arthroplasty*. Philadelphia PA, Lippincott-Raven, 1999, pp 427-435.

Mulvey TJ, Thornhill TS, Kelly MA, Healy WL: Complications associated with total knee arthroplasty, in Pellicci PM, Tria AJ Jr, Garvin KL, eds: *Orthopaedic Knowledge Update: Hip and Knee Reconstruction*, ed 2. Rosemont, IL, American Academy of Orthopaedic Surgeons, 2000, pp 323-337.

A-48: A 73-year-old man has stiffness after undergoing primary posterior cruciate ligament-retaining total knee arthroplasty 18 months ago. Extensive physiotherapy, dynamic splinting, and manipulations under anesthesia have failed to result in improvement. Examination reveals range of motion from 30° to 60° of flexion. The components are well fixed, and the evaluation for infection is negative. In discussing the possibility of revision arthroplasty, the patient should be advised that

1. the success of improving range of motion to a functional range of 0° to 90° in the literature is between 75% to 80%.
2. the preoperative arc of motion will not influence the ultimate range of motion after formal component revision.
3. change from a posterior cruciate ligament-retaining to a posterior cruciate ligament-substituting design has a much greater chance of success.
4. manipulation under anesthesia will effectively improve range of motion if postoperative stiffness develops following revision.
5. the major postoperative focus will be to regain near-full extension.

PREFERRED RESPONSE: 5

(continued on next page)

(A-47: *continued*)

DISCUSSION: Stiffness following primary total knee arthroplasty remains a vexing problem. Treatment options have included extensive physical therapy, dynamic splinting, manipulation under anesthesia, arthroscopic arthrolysis, open arthrolysis with polyethylene exchange, and ultimately revision arthroplasty. Results are not as gratifying as would be expected. Babis and associates performed an open arthrolysis and polyethylene exchange on seven patients who were followed for a mean of 4.2 months. The results were poor. The mean improvement in arc of motion was only 20°. Nicholls and Dorr treated 13 patients for stiffness. Only 40% of those patients obtained good to excellent results. Four patients (30%) required manipulation because of recurrent stiffness postoperatively. They noted they could not predictably improve the arc of motion with a revision operation. Haidukewych and associates reported on 15 patients who underwent revision of well-fixed components after total knee arthroplasty for stiffness. Of the 15 patients, 10 (66%) were satisfied with the outcome revision. Interestingly, they noted that in patients for whom the total arc of motion did not improve but who regained near-full extension, there was a greater amount of satisfaction with the procedure than for those who did not regain full extension.

REFERENCES: Babis GC, Trousdale RT, Pagnano MW, et al: Poor outcomes of isolated tibial insert exchange and arthrolysis for the management of stiffness following total knee arthroplasty. *J Bone Joint Surg Am* 2001;83:1534-1536.

Nicholls DW, Dorr LD: Revision surgery for stiff total knee arthroplasty. *J Arthroplasty* 1990;5:S73-S77.

Haidukewych GJ, Jacofsky DJ, Pagnano MW, et al: Functional results after revision of well-fixed components for stiffness after primary total knee arthroplasty. *J Arthroplasty* 2005;20:133-138.

A-49: A 62-year-old patient is seen for routine follow-up after undergoing cementless total hip arthroplasty 2 years ago. The patient reports limited range of motion that severely affects daily activities. A radiograph is shown in Figure 29. Management should now consist of

1. observation only.
2. NSAIDs and protected weight bearing.
3. irradiation to the affected area.
4. surgical excision.
5. surgical excision and postoperative irradiation.

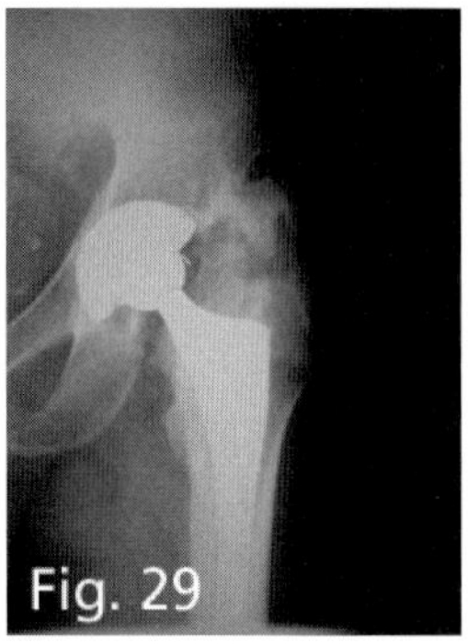

Fig. 29

PREFERRED RESPONSE: 5

DISCUSSION: The patient has symptomatic postoperative heterotopic ossification after total hip arthroplasty. Postoperative prophylactic treatments include NSAIDs (usually indomethacin) or low-dose irradiation. The heterotopic ossification shown here is quite mature; therefore, nonsurgical management will not be successful. Surgical excision of grade III or IV heterotopic ossification should be followed with postoperative irradiation to minimize the chances of recurrence.

REFERENCES: Ayers DC, Evarts CM, Parkinson JR: The prevention of heterotopic ossification in high-risk patients by low-dose radiation therapy after total hip arthroplasty. *J Bone Joint Surg Am* 1986;68:1423-1430.

Healy WL, Lo TC, DeSimone AA, et al: Single-dose irradiation for the prevention of heterotopic ossification after total hip arthroplasty: A comparison of doses of five hundred and fifty and seven hundred centigray. *J Bone Joint Surg Am* 1995;77:590-595.

A-50: What bilateral surgical intervention is considered inappropriate based on the findings shown in the radiograph in Figure 30?

1. Vascularized fibular graft
2. Proximal femoral osteotomy
3. Core decompression
4. Hip arthrodesis
5. Femoral resurfacing

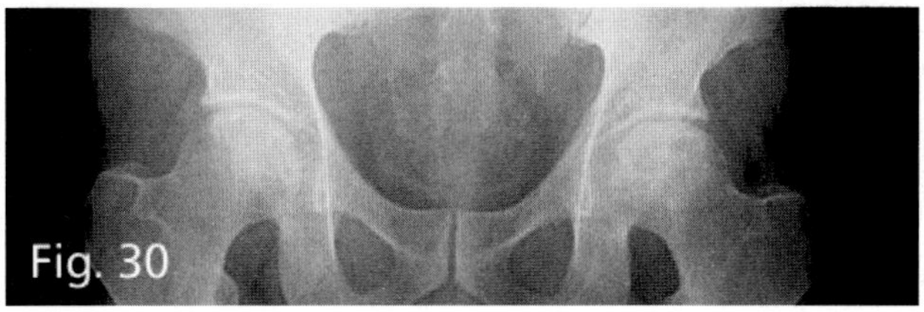

PREFERRED RESPONSE: 4

DISCUSSION: The radiograph reveals osteonecrosis of both femoral heads with reasonably maintained joint surfaces. There may be some slight flattening of the femoral heads. Hip arthrodesis is difficult to perform because of the necrotic bone. Its use in patients with osteonecrotic hips is limited because of the 80% bilaterality; therefore, it is not an acceptable alternative. All the other options are acceptable interventions.

REFERENCES: Mont MA, Jones LC, Sotereanos DG, et al: Understanding and treating osteonecrosis of the femoral head. *Instr Course Lect* 2000;49:169-185.

Barrack R, Berry D, Burak C, et al: Hip and pelvis reconstruction, in Koval KJ, ed: *Orthopaedic Knowledge Update*, ed 7. Rosemont, IL, American Academy of Orthopaedic Surgeons, 2002, pp 417-451.

Sports Injuries of the Knee and Sports Medicine

Q-1: Figure 1 shows a sagittal oblique MRI scan. The arrow is pointing to what structure?

1. Bucket-handle tear of the medial meniscus
2. Ligament of Humphrey
3. Ligament of Wrisberg
4. Posterior intermeniscal ligament
5. Partial tear of the posterior cruciate ligament

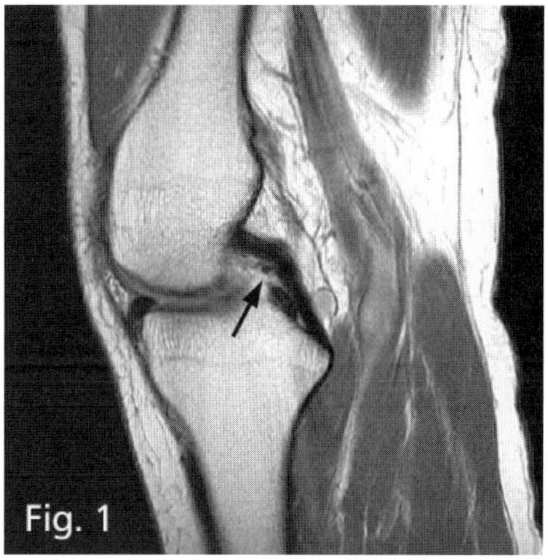

Fig. 1

Q-2: An 18-year-old woman sustains a twisting injury of the knee while skiing. Figures 2A and 2B show the radiograph and coronal MRI scan of the knee. In addition to the injury shown, what is the most likely associated injury?

1. Medial collateral ligament rupture
2. Patellar dislocation
3. Patellar tendon rupture
4. Anterior cruciate ligament rupture
5. Posterior cruciate ligament rupture

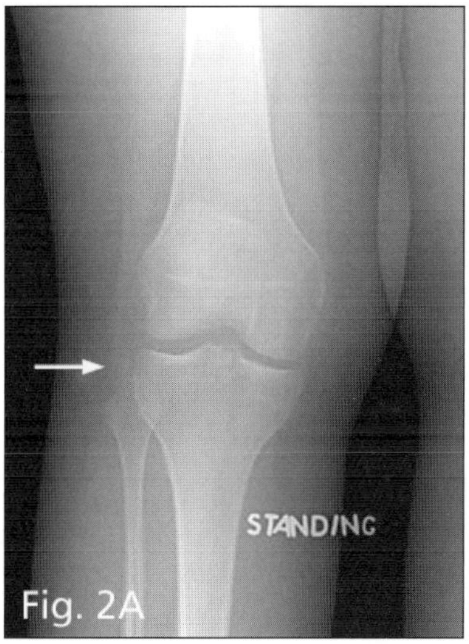

Fig. 2A

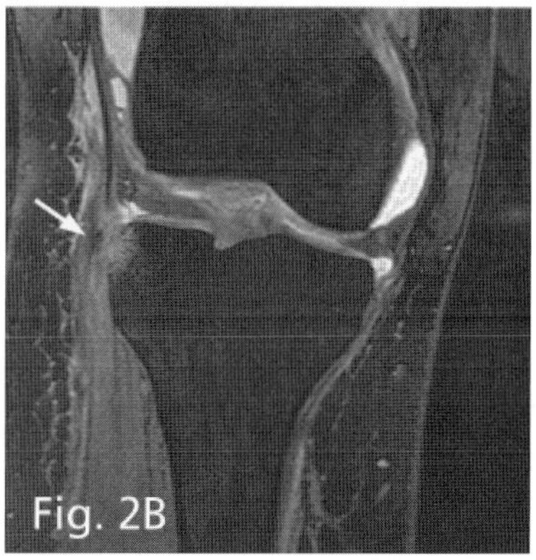

Fig. 2B

Q-3: A 23-year-old woman falls from a bicycle and sustains a right knee injury. Figures 3A through 3D show radiographs and MRI scans of the knee. What is the most likely diagnosis?

1. Posterior cruciate ligament avulsion from the tibia
2. Anterior cruciate ligament avulsion from the tibia
3. Avulsion of the lateral meniscus anterior horn
4. Midsubstance posterior cruciate ligament rupture
5. Midsubstance anterior cruciate ligament rupture

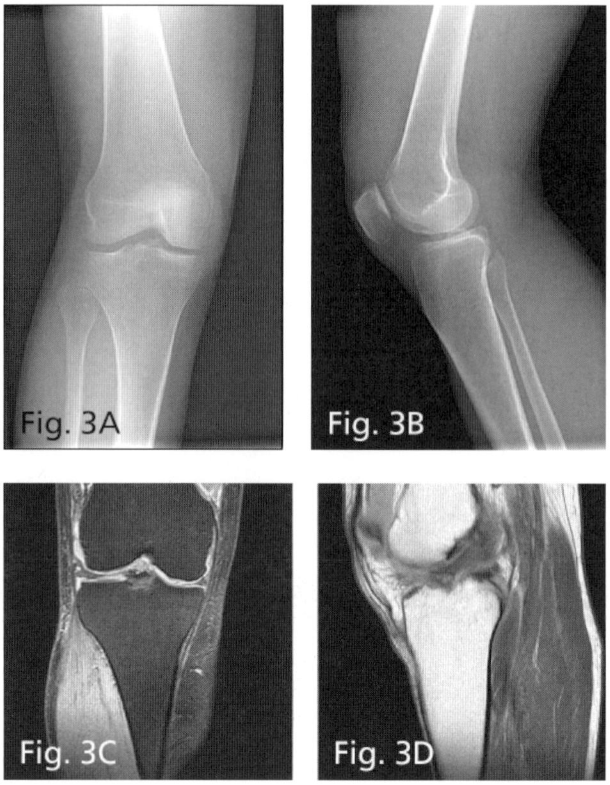
Fig. 3A Fig. 3B Fig. 3C Fig. 3D

Q-4: A 16-year-old boy sustains a twisting injury to the left knee while wrestling. MRI scans are shown in Figures 4A through 4C. What is the most likely diagnosis?

1. Anterior cruciate ligament rupture
2. Posterior cruciate ligament rupture
3. Bucket-handle medial meniscus tear
4. Lateral meniscus tear
5. Osteochondral lesion

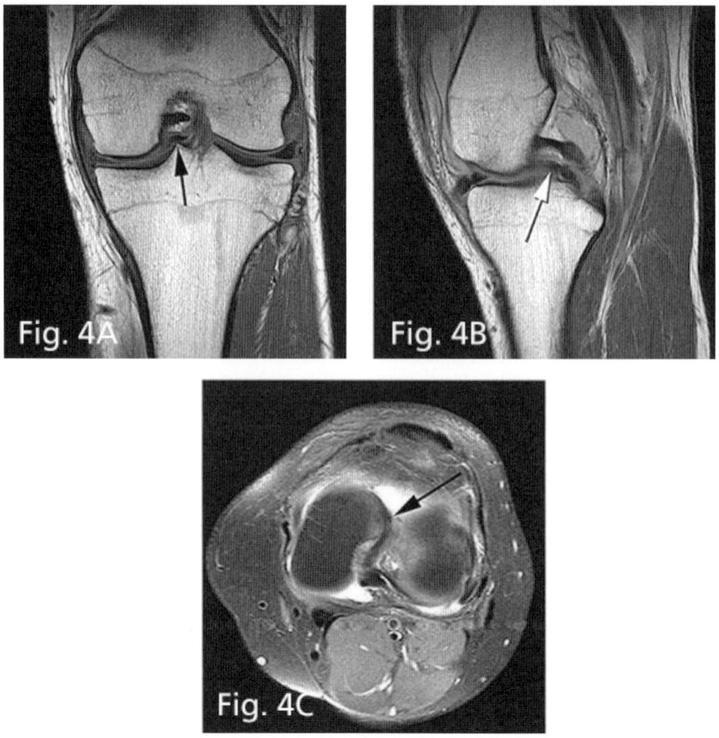
Fig. 4A Fig. 4B Fig. 4C

Q-5: The posterior horn of the medial meniscus receives its primary blood supply from what artery?

1. Middle genicular
2. Medial inferior genicular
3. Medial superior genicular
4. Lateral superior genicular
5. Inferior lateral genicular

Q-6: Figure 5 shows an acute axial MRI scan of a left knee. What is the most likely diagnosis?

1. Patellar tendon rupture
2. Lateral dislocation of the patella
3. Quadriceps tendon rupture
4. Anterior cruciate ligament rupture
5. Posterior cruciate ligament rupture

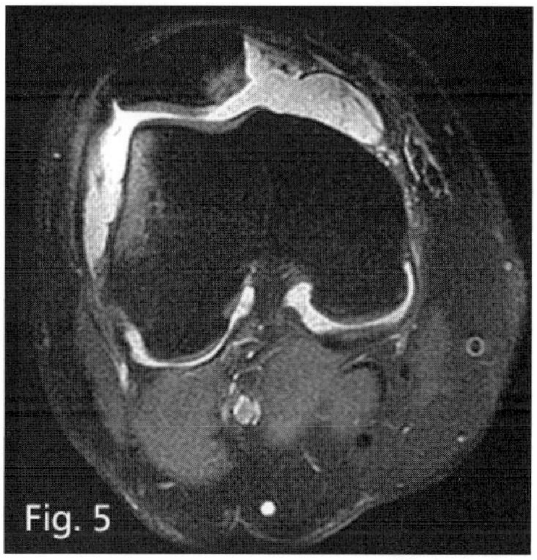

Fig. 5

Q-7: Figure 6 shows an arthroscopic view of the patellofemoral joint from an inferolateral portal. The arrow points to which of the following structures?

1. Loose body
2. Plica
3. Displaced meniscus tear
4. Torn retinaculum
5. Osteochondral defect

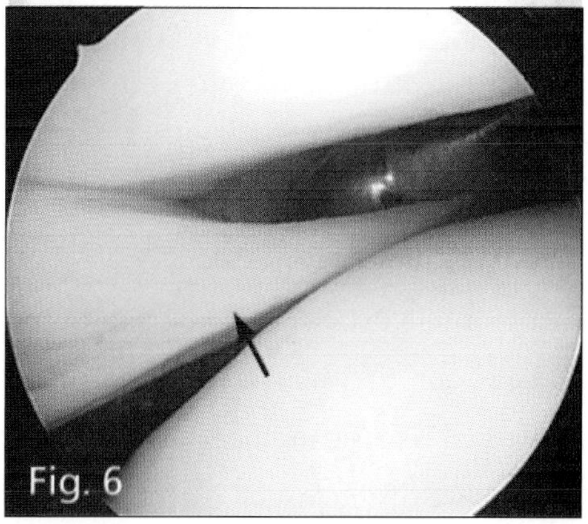

Fig. 6

Q-8: The force generated by a muscle is most highly dependent on its

1. cross-sectional area.
2. fiber type.
3. length.
4. morphology.
5. level of conditioning.

Q-9: A 31-year-old woman has increasing pain and tightness in her right knee, with occasional stiffness and recurrent hemorrhagic effusions. MRI scans are shown in Figures 7A and 7B. What is the most likely diagnosis?

1. Rheumatoid arthritis
2. Pigmented villonodular synovitis (PVNS)
3. Synovial sarcoma
4. Synovial chondromatosis
5. Fibromatosis

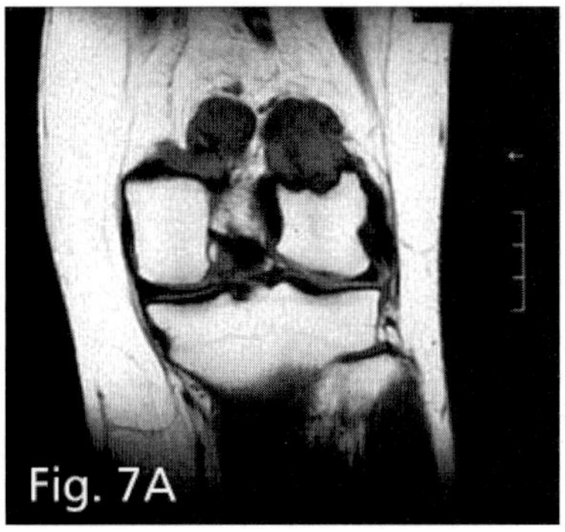
Fig. 7A

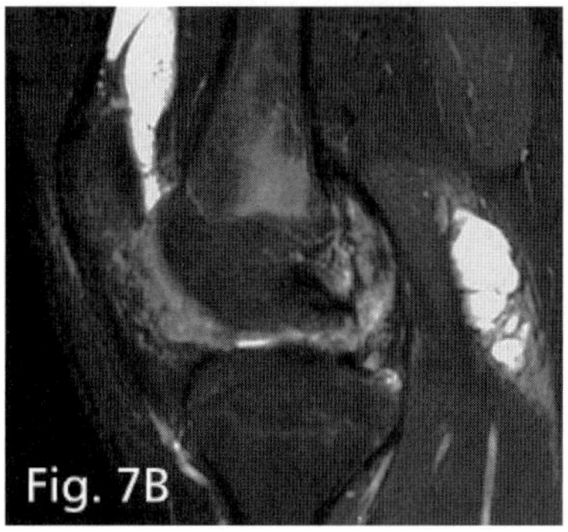
Fig. 7B

Q-10: A 30-year-old patient who is an elite marathon runner reports chronic pain over the lateral aspect of the distal right leg and dysesthesia over the dorsum of the foot with active plantar flexion and inversion of the foot. Examination reveals a tender soft-tissue fullness approximately 10 cm proximal to the lateral malleolus. The pain is exacerbated by passive plantar flexion and inversion of the ankle. There is also a positive Tinel sign over the site of maximal tenderness. There is no motor weakness, and deep tendon reflexes are normal. Radiographs and MRI of the leg are normal. What is the most appropriate next step in management?

1. Biopsy of the soft-tissue mass
2. Epidural corticosteroid injection into the lumbar spine
3. Four-compartment fasciotomy of the leg
4. Fascial release and neurolysis of the superficial peroneal nerve
5. Closure of the fascial defect of the superficial peroneal nerve

Q-11: A 21-year-old patient who is a soccer player reports pain and is unable to straighten his knee following an acute injury during a game. He is unable to continue to play. An MRI scan is shown in Figure 8. What is the most appropriate next step in management?

1. No weight bearing
2. Cortisone injection
3. Physical therapy
4. Arthroscopic meniscectomy or repair
5. Anterior cruciate ligament reconstruction

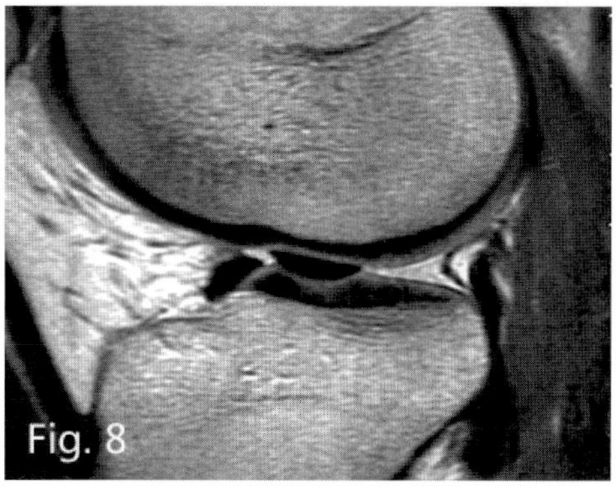
Fig. 8

Q-12: When performing an inside-out lateral meniscal repair, capsule exposure is provided by developing the

1. iliotibial band and biceps tendon interval, then retracting the lateral head of the gastrocnemius anteriorly.
2. iliotibial band and biceps tendon interval, then retracting the lateral head of the gastrocnemius posteriorly.
3. iliotibial band and biceps tendon interval, then retracting the lateral collateral ligament posteriorly.
4. iliotibial band and biceps tendon interval, then splitting the lateral head of the gastrocnemius.
5. lateral head of the gastrocnemius and biceps tendon interval, then retracting the biceps tendon anteriorly.

Q-13: A 15-year-old girl who plays field hockey sustains a blow to the mouth from a hockey stick. Three front teeth are knocked out and shown in Figure 9. In addition to calling a dentist immediately, what is the next best step in management?

1. Place the teeth in an ice water bath.
2. Pour normal saline solution on the teeth and then place them in milk.
3. Have the player gargle with mouthwash and place the teeth in water.
4. Clean the teeth with a toothbrush and then reimplant them.
5. Clean the teeth with a toothbrush and place them on ice.

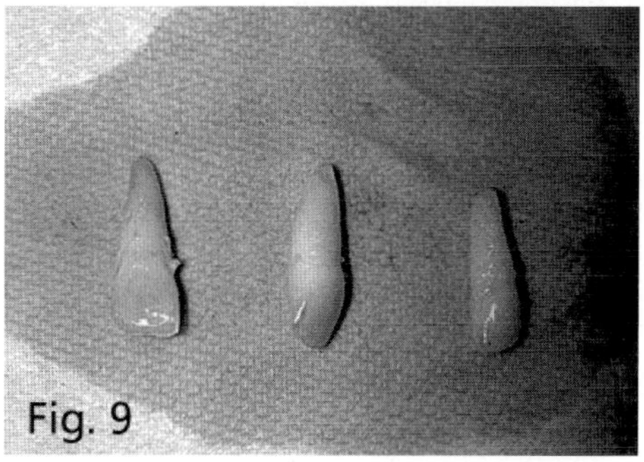
Fig. 9

Sports Injuries of the Knee and Sports Medicine: Questions

Q-14: Commotio cordis is best treated with

1. immediate cardiac defibrillation.
2. the chest thump maneuver.
3. intravenous fluids and hydration.
4. epinephrine.
5. albuterol inhalers.

Q-15: A 40-year-old woman reports the atraumatic onset of severe knee pain and swelling after undergoing an uncomplicated elective cholecystectomy 1 week ago. She denies any history of diabetes mellitus or HIV but has had occasional episodes of mild knee pain and swelling that have always responded to NSAIDs. Radiographs are shown in Figures 10A and 10B. A knee aspiration yields a white blood cell count of 35,000/mm^3. The aspirate should also yield which of the following findings?

1. Strongly negative needle-shaped crystals
2. Weakly positive birefringent rhomboid-shaped crystals
3. Gross blood
4. Gram-positive cocci
5. Gram-negative rods

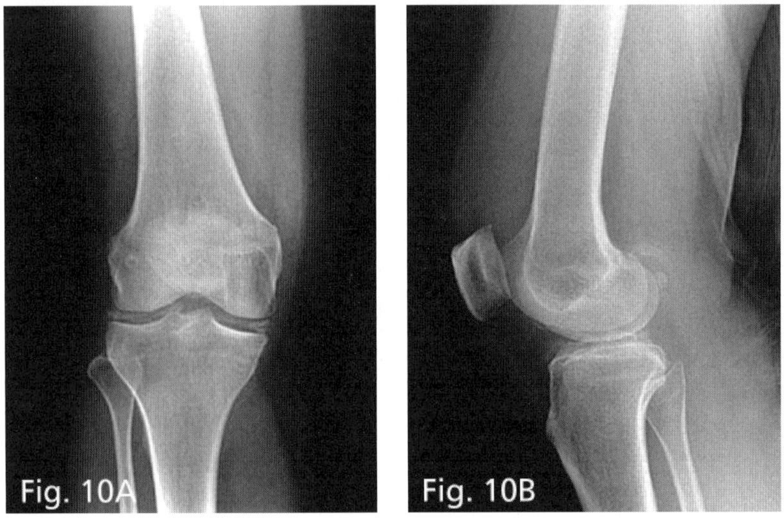

Q-16: What is the maximum acceptable amount of divergence of the interference screw in the femoral tunnel from the bone plug of a bone-patellar tendon-bone graft in anterior cruciate ligament (ACL) reconstruction before pull-out strength is statistically decreased?

1. 0°
2. 10°
3. 15°
4. 30°
5. 45°

Q-17: Use of prophylactic knee bracing in contact sports participants results in which of the following?

1. Decreased incidence of anterior cruciate ligament injuries
2. Decreased incidence of posterior cruciate ligament injuries
3. Decreased incidence of medial collateral ligament injuries
4. Decreased incidence of meniscal tears
5. Decreased incidence of ankle injuries

Q-18: A 22-year-old patient who plays college football reports shortness of breath and dyspnea after a tackle. Examination reveals tachypnea and tachycardia, the trachea is shifted to the right, and there are decreased breath sounds on the left lung fields. The first line of treatment on the field should be

1. placement of a chest tube.
2. insertion of a large-gauge needle into the second intercostal space.
3. cardiopulmonary resuscitation.
4. administration of adrenaline.
5. immediate transfer to the emergency department.

Q-19: Anabolic steroid use has which of the following effects on serum lipoprotein levels?

1. Decrease in low-density lipoprotein only
2. Decrease in high-density lipoprotein only
3. Increase in high-density lipoprotein only
4. Increase in low-density lipoprotein only
5. Increase in both high- and low-density lipoproteins

Q-20: A 20-year-old woman who is a professional jockey is thrown from her horse while wearing a helmet. What is the most likely location of her injury?

1. Face
2. Head
3. Neck
4. Lower back
5. Leg

Q-21: Which of the following complications is more likely with an inside-out repair technique compared to an all-inside techniques for a medial meniscus tear?

1. Failure
2. Intra-articular synovitis
3. Peroneal nerve injury
4. Saphenous nerve injury
5. Arthrofibrosis

Q-22: A 17-year-old boy who plays football is injured during a play and reports abdominal pain that is soon followed by nausea and vomiting. What organ has most likely been injured?

1. Liver
2. Pancreas
3. Spleen
4. Kidney
5. Large intestine

Q-23: Which of the following cardiac conditions is considered an absolute contraindication to vigorous exercise?

1. Hypertrophic cardiomyopathy (HCM)
2. Sclerosis of the aortic valve without stenosis
3. Mild mitral valve regurgitation
4. Left ventricular hypertrophy (LVH)
5. Functional murmurs

Q-24: An 18-year-old woman who plays lacrosse has infectious mononucleosis. What is the recommendation for return to play?

1. Full participation once symptoms resolve
2. Full participation once the splenomegaly resolves
3. Full participation 4 weeks after the onset of symptoms regardless of the size of the spleen
4. Full participation 4 weeks after both the onset of illness and findings of a normal-sized spleen
5. No participation for 8 weeks

Q-25: A 30-year-old patient reports chronic medial knee pain and swelling. Figure 11A shows an articular cartilage lesion observed during arthroscopy. The surgeon decides to treat the lesion with the microfracture technique seen in Figure 11B. A biopsy of the repaired tissue 1 year after treatment is likely to show which of the following findings?

1. Fibrous tissue
2. Bone
3. Articular cartilage
4. Fibrocartilage
5. Type II collagen

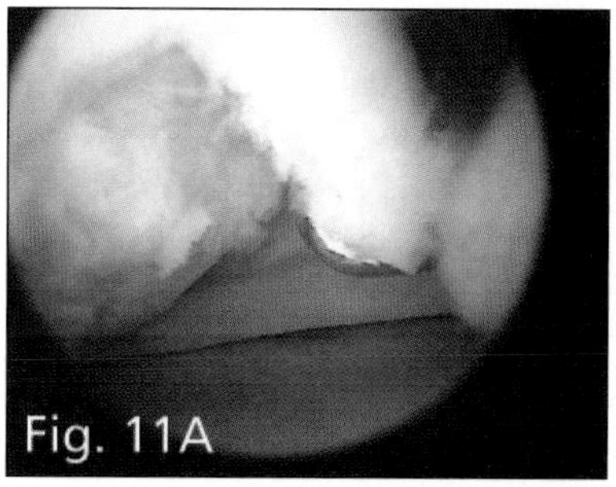
Fig. 11A

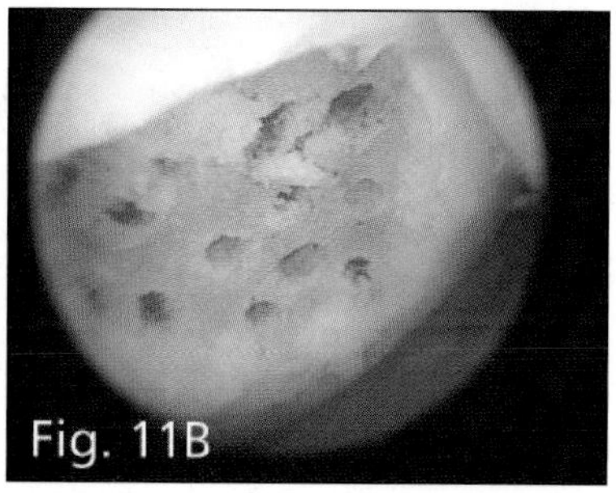
Fig. 11B

Q-26: Kinematic analysis of the medial and lateral menisci has demonstrated that the lateral meniscus has which of the following characteristics compared with the medial meniscus?

1. More soft-tissue attachments/restraints
2. More mobility
3. Less mobility
4. No posterior movement with flexion
5. No anterior movement with extension

Q-27: Which of the following is the most relevant clinical factor in the maturation assessment of an adolescent female athlete contemplating anterior cruciate ligament (ACL) reconstruction?

1. Parental height
2. Height of older male sibling
3. Age of menarche
4. Recent change in shoe size
5. Presence of breast buds

Q-28: Which of the following best describes heat stroke?

1. Transient loss of consciousness with peripheral vasodilation and decreased cardiac output with normal body temperature
2. A condition involving painful contractions of large muscle groups because of decreased hydration and a decrease of serum sodium and chloride
3. Hypernatremia in poorly conditioned athletes, manifested by thirst and oliguria with a core temperature of less than 102.2°F (39°C)
4. Hyperthermia, central nervous system dysfunction, and loss of thermoregulatory function
5. A transient condition that responds to glucose administration

Q-29: Which of the following factors is most critical to the success of a meniscal allograft transplantation?

1. Accurate graft size
2. Donor cell viability
3. Reestablishment of the central meniscal blood supply
4. Suppression of the immune response
5. Cryopreservation of the donor graft

Q-30: What is the most common behavioral effect of anabolic steroid use in athletes?

1. Increased aggression
2. Psychosis
3. Drug dependence
4. Depression
5. Mania

Q-31: What is the effect on knee kinematics following placement of an anterior cruciate ligament (ACL) graft at the 12 o'clock position?

1. Decreased rotational stability
2. Decreased anterior-posterior stability
3. Decreased flexion
4. Decreased extension
5. Graft failure secondary to impingement

Q-32: Which of the following knee ligament injury patterns is most associated with an increase in external tibial rotation with the knee at 90° of flexion?

1. Isolated tear of the posterior cruciate ligament
2. Isolated tear of the lateral collateral ligament
3. Combined tears of the posterior cruciate and lateral collateral ligaments
4. Combined tears of the anterior cruciate and lateral collateral ligaments
5. Combined tears of the lateral collateral and medial collateral ligaments

Q-33: Which of the following statements correctly describes the results of gamma irradiation of musculoskeletal allograft?

1. Exposure to 1.5 Mrad effectively eliminates HIV.
2. Exposure to 4 Mrad does not affect graft mechanical properties.
3. Gamma irradiation has been associated with chronic inflammation after implantation.
4. Gamma irradiation is commonly used alone for sterilization.
5. HIV cannot be eliminated with gamma irradiation alone without compromising the mechanical properties of the graft.

Q-34: A 35-year-old woman who is a recreational runner reports posterior knee pain and tightness in the knee with flexion during running. She denies any history of trauma. Examination reveals normal patellar glide and tilt and no patellar apprehension. Range of motion is 5° to 120°, and quadriceps function and knee ligamentous examination are normal. Radiographs are normal. An MRI scan is shown Figure 12. What is the most likely diagnosis?

1. Baker cyst
2. Torn medial meniscus
3. Patellofemoral pain syndrome
4. Lipoma
5. Ganglion cyst of the cruciates

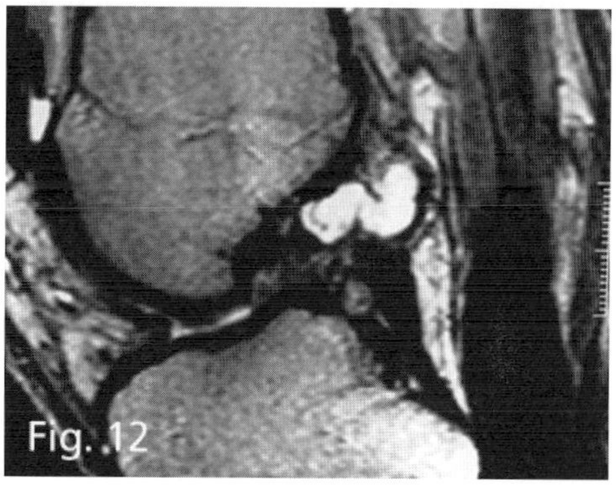

Fig. 12

Q-35: An 18-year-old man underwent open reduction and internal fixation of a tibial spine avulsion and a posterolateral corner repair. Two years later, he underwent lateral collateral ligament (LCL) and posterolateral corner reconstruction because of instability. Examination reveals a pronounced lateral varus knee thrust when ambulating. Varus stress in 30° of flexion produces a 10-mm opening that is eliminated in extension. The Lachman test is 2 mm with a firm end point, and the posterior drawer test is negative. Standing radiographs show widening of the lateral joint space and a 5° mechanical varus alignment. What is the most effective course of treatment?

1. Physical therapy for quadriceps strengthening
2. Functional bracing
3. Anterior cruciate ligament (ACL) reconstruction
4. Revision reconstruction of the LCL and posterolateral corner
5. Valgus-producing high tibial osteotomy (HTO)

Q-36: A favorable outcome following nonsurgical management of a partial tear of the posterior cruciate ligament (PCL) is best associated with

1. hamstring strength.
2. quadriceps strength.
3. a body mass index of less than 30.
4. anterior cruciate ligament stability.
5. compliance with brace use.

Q-37: A player on a professional football team sustains a knee injury and an anterior cruciate ligament rupture is diagnosed. When employed as the team physician, your ethical obligation is to inform

1. the player but not the team.
2. the team but not the player.
3. neither the team nor the player.
4. both the team and the player.
5. the team, the player, and the media.

Q-38: A 20-year-old man who plays soccer collapses after a goal kick and reports weakness and nausea. He appears slightly confused. Examination reveals that he is not sweating. His skin is warm and dry. The outdoor temperature is 80°F (26.6°C) with a relative humidity of 80%. Management should consist of

1. a drink of water.
2. a sports drink with electrolytes.
3. placement in the reverse Trendelenburg position in a shaded area.
4. immersion in a warm water bath.
5. transportation to the emergency department.

Q-39: What is the most accurate description of the relationship between sex and knee loading during landing while playing basketball?

1. Males have greater total valgus knee loading.
2. Females have greater total valgus knee loading.
3. Males have greater total varus knee loading.
4. Females have greater total varus knee loading.
5. There is no sex difference in total varus or valgus knee loading.

Q-40: What is the most common cause of the new onset of amenorrhea in a female endurance athlete who is not sexually active?

1. Insufficient caloric intake
2. Physical stress
3. Use of oral contraceptives
4. Diabetes mellitus
5. Chromosomal abnormalities

Q-41: A 29-year-old man who is an ultramarathoner is halfway into a 50-mile race and begins sweating profusely. He suddenly collapses, is unresponsive, and has violent muscle contractions. Prior to these symptoms, he had been drinking water at every water stop (every 1 mile). What is the most likely diagnosis?

1. Hypernatremia
2. Hyponatremia
3. Hyperkalemia
4. Hypokalemia
5. Hyperuremia

Q-42: Tension force in the anterior cruciate ligament during passive range of motion is highest at

1. full extension.
2. 30° of flexion.
3. 60° of flexion.
4. 90° of flexion.
5. 120° of flexion.

Q-43: Compared to eumenorrheic athletes, amenorrheic athletes have more frequent occurrences of

1. stress fractures.
2. scoliosis.
3. pes planus.
4. meniscal tears.
5. ankle sprains.

Q-44: Figure 13 shows the postoperative radiograph of a patient who underwent an anterior cruciate ligament (ACL) reconstruction (with bone–patellar tendon–bone autograft) that failed. He initially had loss of flexion postoperatively. What is the most likely cause of this failure?

1. Fixation in the tibial tunnel
2. Fixation in the femoral tunnel
3. Posterior placement of the tibial tunnel
4. Anterior placement of the femoral tunnel
5. Size of the patellar autograft

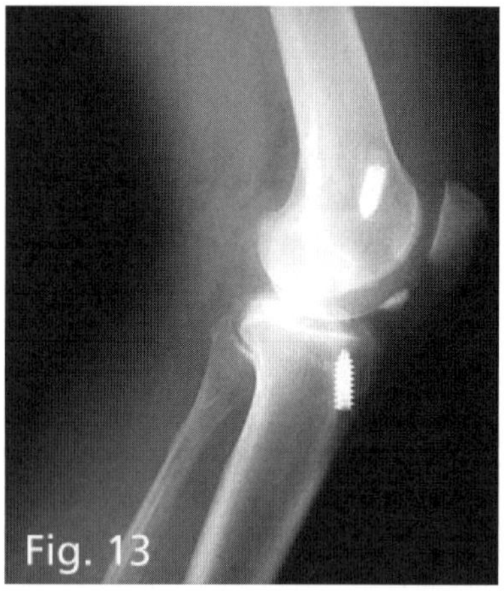
Fig. 13

Q-45: A 22-year-old man reports anterior knee pain, swelling, and inability to perform a straight leg raise after undergoing endoscopic anterior cruciate ligament (ACL) reconstruction with a bone-patellar tendon-bone autograft 1 week ago. He is afebrile. Examination reveals a clean incision, moderate effusion, a weak isometric quadriceps contraction, active knee range of motion of 5° to 45°, and the patella is ballottable. Knee radiographs show postoperative changes with good femoral and tibial tunnel placements, and normal patellar height. What is the next most appropriate step in management?

1. Electromyography (EMG) and nerve conduction velocity studies (NCVS)
2. Diagnostic ultrasonography of the patellar tendon
3. MRI
4. Continuous passive motion
5. Knee aspiration

Q-46: The use of knee arthroscopy following total knee arthroplasty is most effective in treating which of the following conditions?

1. Patellar clunk syndrome
2. Septic arthritis
3. Nonspecific pain
4. Improper tracking of the patellar component
5. Synovitis secondary to polyethylene wear

Q-47: Significant anterior tibial translation occurs during which of the following rehabilitation exercises?

1. Terminal weight-bearing knee extension
2. Terminal non-weight-bearing knee extension
3. Terminal weight-bearing knee flexion
4. Terminal non-weight-bearing knee flexion
5. Midrange weight-bearing knee flexion

Q-48: A 43-year-old man who plays soccer had knee pain following a twisting injury and underwent an arthroscopic meniscectomy 6 months ago. He continues to report posterior knee pain. Examination reveals soft-tissue fullness and tenderness just above the popliteal fossa, trace knee effusion, full range of knee motion, no instability, and negative meniscal signs. Radiographs show some mild medial joint space narrowing but no other bony changes. What is the most appropriate next step in management?

1. Corticosteroid injection
2. MRI
3. Bone scan
4. Unloader brace
5. NSAIDs

Q-49: Storage of musculoskeletal allografts by cryopreservation is achieved by

1. replacing water in the tissue with alcohol to a moisture level of 5% and then using a vacuum process to remove the alcohol from the tissue.
2. maintaining maximum cellular viability of fresh tissue without long-term storage.
3. using chemicals to remove cellular water and controlled rate freezing to prevent ice crystal formation.
4. freezing the graft twice and packaging the tissue without solution at −80°C.
5. freezing the graft in water without an antibiotic solution soak during quarantine, with final storage in liquid nitrogen.

Q-50: Second-impact syndrome (SIS) after head injury is characterized by which of the following?

1. Gradual progression of neurologic symptoms
2. Preventable by restricting return to play until symptom-free
3. Excellent prognosis for full recovery
4. Rarely involves brain stem compromise
5. CT rarely shows brain edema

A-1: Figure 1 shows a sagittal oblique MRI scan. The arrow is pointing to what structure?

1. Bucket-handle tear of the medial meniscus
2. Ligament of Humphrey
3. Ligament of Wrisberg
4. Posterior intermeniscal ligament
5. Partial tear of the posterior cruciate ligament

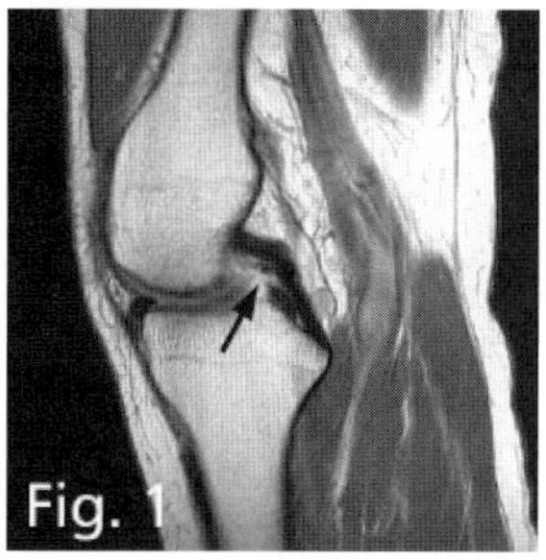
Fig. 1

PREFERRED RESPONSE: 2

DISCUSSION: The meniscofemoral ligaments connect the posterior horn of the lateral meniscus to the intercondylar wall of the medial femoral condyle. The ligament of Humphrey (arrow) passes anterior to the posterior cruciate ligament, whereas the ligament of Wrisberg passes posterior to the posterior cruciate ligament. One or the other has been identified in 71% to 100% of cadaver knees, with the ligament of Wrisberg being more common.

REFERENCES: Clarke HD, Scott WN, Insall JN, et al: Anatomy, in Insall JN, Scott WN, eds: *Surgery of the Knee*, ed 4. Philadelphia, PA, Churchill Livingstone, 2006, vol 1, pp 3-66.

Miller TT: Magnetic resonance imaging of the knee, in Insall JN, Scott WN, eds: *Surgery of the Knee*, ed 4. Philadelphia, PA, Churchill Livingstone, 2006, vol 1, pp 201-224.

A-2: An 18-year-old woman sustains a twisting injury of the knee while skiing. Figures 2A and 2B show the radiograph and coronal MRI scan of the knee. In addition to the injury shown, what is the most likely associated injury?

1. Medial collateral ligament rupture
2. Patellar dislocation
3. Patellar tendon rupture
4. Anterior cruciate ligament rupture
5. Posterior cruciate ligament rupture

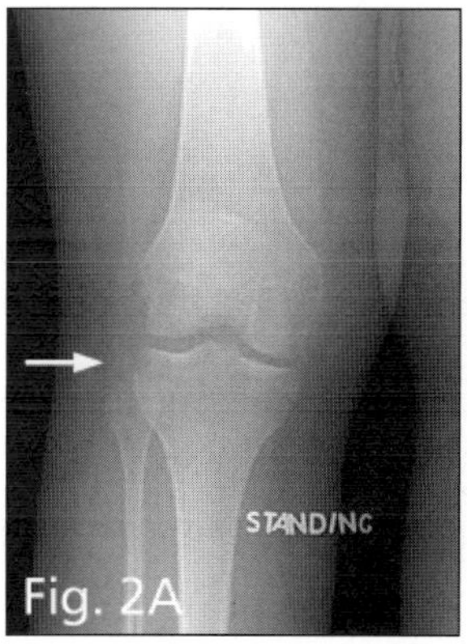

Fig. 2A

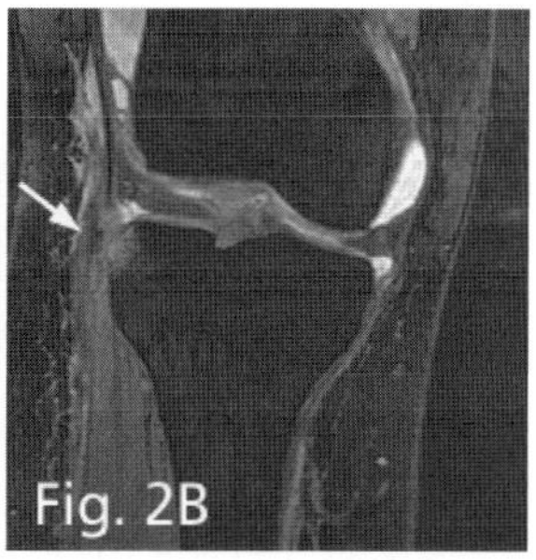
Fig. 2B

PREFERRED RESPONSE: 4

DISCUSSION: The MRI scan shows a Segond fracture, which is a small avulsion of the lateral joint capsule from the anterolateral aspect of the proximal tibia. It is almost always associated with anterior cruciate ligament rupture and often with a tear of either the medial or lateral meniscus.

REFERENCES: Goldman AB, Pavlov H, Rubenstein D: The Segond fracture of the proximal tibia: A small avulsion that reflects major ligamentous damage. *Am J Roentgenol* 1988;151:1163-1167.

Sanders TG, Miller MD: A systematic approach to magnetic resonance imaging interpretation of sports medicine injuries of the knee. *Am J Sports Med* 2005;33:131-148.

Miller TT: Magnetic resonance imaging of the knee, in Insall JN, Scott WN, eds: *Surgery of the Knee*, ed 4. Philadelphia, PA, Churchill Livingstone, 2006, vol 1, pp 201-224.

A-3: A 23-year-old woman falls from a bicycle and sustains a right knee injury. Figures 3A through 3D show radiographs and MRI scans of the knee. What is the most likely diagnosis?

1. Posterior cruciate ligament avulsion from the tibia
2. Anterior cruciate ligament avulsion from the tibia
3. Avulsion of the lateral meniscus anterior horn
4. Midsubstance posterior cruciate ligament rupture
5. Midsubstance anterior cruciate ligament rupture

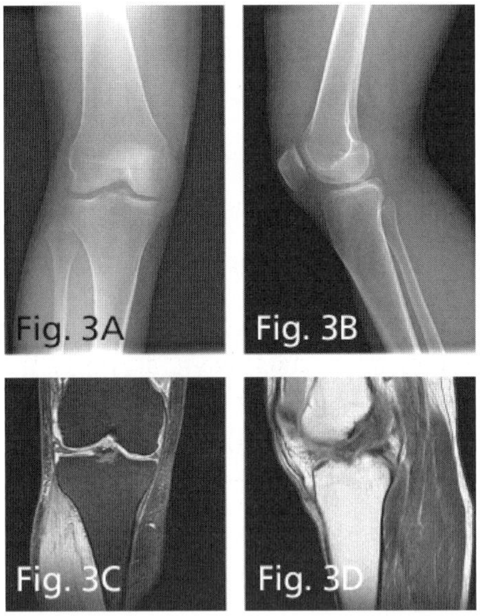

PREFERRED RESPONSE: 2

DISCUSSION: The radiographs and MRI scans both show an avulsion of the anterior cruciate ligament, which has been described by Meyers and McKeever in three different fracture patterns. Type I fractures are nondisplaced or have minimal displacement of the anterior margin. Type II fractures have superior displacement of their anterior aspect with an intact posterior hinge. Type III fractures are completely displaced. Although the injury is visible on the radiographs, it is more subtle in adults than children. Thus, MRI is helpful in clarifying this injury in adults. Open or arthroscopic reduction and internal fixation is recommended for type II and type III fractures that do not respond to closed reduction.

REFERENCES: Meyers MH, McKeever FM: Fracture of the intercondylar eminence of the tibia. *J Bone Joint Surg Am* 1970;52:1677-1684.

Wiss DA, Watson JT: Fractures of the tibial plateau, in Rockwood CA, Green DP, Bucholz RW, et al, eds: *Rockwood and Green's Fractures in Adults*. Philadelphia, PA, Lippincott-Raven, 1996, pp 1920-1953.

Lubowitz JH, Elson WS, Guttmann D: Arthroscopic treatment of tibial plateau fractures: Intercondylar eminence avulsion fractures. *Arthroscopy* 2005;21:86-92.

A-4: A 16-year-old boy sustains a twisting injury to the left knee while wrestling. MRI scans are shown in Figures 4A through 4C. What is the most likely diagnosis?

1. Anterior cruciate ligament rupture
2. Posterior cruciate ligament rupture
3. Bucket-handle medial meniscus tear
4. Lateral meniscus tear
5. Osteochondral lesion

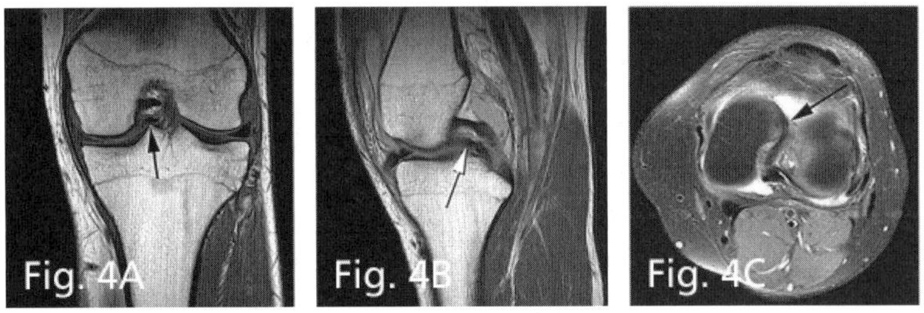

PREFERRED RESPONSE: 3

DISCUSSION: The MRI scans show a displaced bucket-handle medial meniscus tear that can be visualized on coronal, sagittal, and axial views. The sagittal view shows the typical double posterior cruciate ligament sign, in which the low-signal bucket-handle fragment parallels the normal low-signal posterior cruciate ligament. The coronal and axial images both show the displaced medial meniscus in the notch.

REFERENCES: Sanders TG, Miller MD: A systematic approach to magnetic resonance imaging interpretation of sports medicine injuries of the knee. *Am J Sports Med* 2005;33:131-148.

Miller TT: Magnetic resonance imaging of the knee, in Insall JN, Scott WN, eds: *Surgery of the Knee*, ed 4. Philadelphia, PA, Churchill Livingstone, 2006, vol 1, pp 201-224.

A-5: The posterior horn of the medial meniscus receives its primary blood supply from what artery?

1. Middle genicular
2. Medial inferior genicular
3. Medial superior genicular
4. Lateral superior genicular
5. Inferior lateral genicular

PREFERRED RESPONSE: 1

DISCUSSION: The middle genicular artery supplies the posterior capsule and intracapsular structures (anterior cruciate ligament, posterior cruciate ligament, posterior horns of the meniscus). The medial and lateral inferior geniculates anastomose anteriorly to form a capillary network to supply the fat pad, synovial cavity, and patellar tendon. The lateral superior and inferior genicular arteries supply the lateral retinaculum.

REFERENCES: Insall J, Scott WN: Anatomy, in *Surgery of the Knee*, ed 3. Philadelphia, PA, Churchill Livingstone, 2001, pp 64-70.

Scapinelli R: Vascular anatomy of the human cruciate ligaments and surrounding structures. *Clin Anat* 1997;10:151-162.

A-6: Figure 5 shows an acute axial MRI scan of a left knee. What is the most likely diagnosis?

1. Patellar tendon rupture
2. Lateral dislocation of the patella
3. Quadriceps tendon rupture
4. Anterior cruciate ligament rupture
5. Posterior cruciate ligament rupture

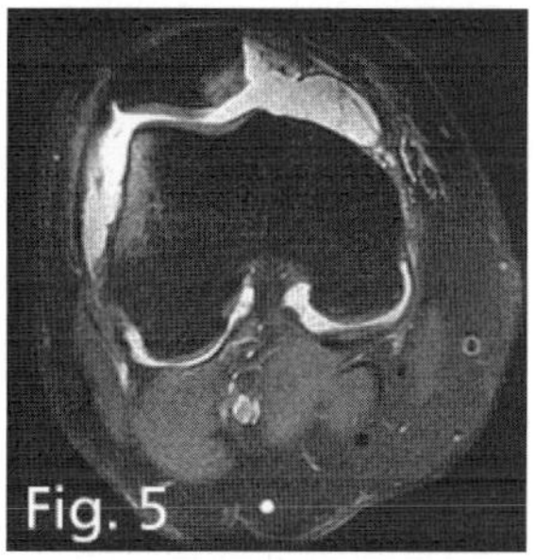

PREFERRED RESPONSE: 2

DISCUSSION: The MRI scan shows bone bruises in the medial aspect of the patella and the lateral aspect of the lateral femoral condyle. Both of these signs are typical for a lateral dislocation of the patella with spontaneous reduction. In addition, there may be associated tearing of the medial retinaculum or distal aspect of the vastus medialis.

REFERENCES: Elias DA, White LM, Fithian DC: Acute lateral patellar dislocation at MR imaging: Injury patterns of medial patellar soft-tissue restraints and osteochondral injuries of the inferomedial patella. *Radiology* 2002;225:736-743.

Sanders TG, Miller MD: A systematic approach to magnetic resonance imaging interpretation of sports medicine injuries of the knee. *Am J Sports Med* 2005;33:131-148.

Miller TT: Magnetic resonance imaging of the knee, in Insall JN, Scott WN, eds: *Surgery of the Knee*, ed 4. Philadelphia, PA, Churchill Livingstone, 2006, vol 1, pp 201-224.

A-7: Figure 6 shows an arthroscopic view of the patellofemoral joint from an inferolateral portal. The arrow points to which of the following structures?

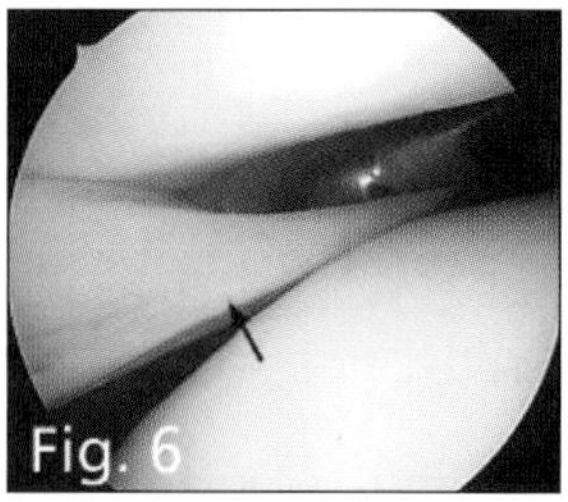

1. Loose body
2. Plica
3. Displaced meniscus tear
4. Torn retinaculum
5. Osteochondral defect

PREFERRED RESPONSE: 2

DISCUSSION: Synovial folds or plicae are the result of incomplete or partial resorption of the synovial membranes during fetal development of the knee. The arthroscopic view shows a medial patellar plica, which has been noted in 5% to 55% of all individuals but becomes symptomatic in only a small number of patients. Symptoms may include crepitus, pain, snapping, and swelling and often respond to nonsurgical management.

REFERENCES: Clarke HD, Scott WN, Insall JN: Anatomic aberrations, in Insall JN, Scott WN, eds: *Surgery of the Knee*, ed 4. Philadelphia, PA, Churchill Livingstone, 2006, vol 1, pp 67-85.

Patel D: Plica as a cause of anterior knee pain. *Orthop Clin North Am* 1986;17:273-277.

A-8: The force generated by a muscle is most highly dependent on its

1. cross-sectional area.
2. fiber type.
3. length.
4. morphology.
5. level of conditioning.

PREFERRED RESPONSE: 1

DISCUSSION: The cross-sectional area of a muscle determines to a great extent the force generated by the muscle. The force of a muscle contraction is controlled by the amount of myofibrils that contract; the greater the amount of contracting myofibrils, the greater the force of contraction. Fiber types have less to do with the force of contraction and more to do with the duration and speed of contraction. Muscle length affects contraction force through the Blix curve. The morphology of a muscle can affect the cross-sectional area by varying the angle of the fibers in relation to the force vector. Conditioning mostly affects duration and fatigability.

REFERENCES: Buckwalter JA, Mow VC, Ratcliffe A: Restoration of injured or degenerated articular cartilage. *J Am Acad Orthop Surg* 1994;2:192-201.

Garrett WE Jr, Best TM: Anatomy, physiology, and mechanics of skeletal muscle, in Buckwalter JA, Einhorn TA, Simon SR, eds: *Orthopaedic Basic Science: Biology and Biomechanics of the Musculoskeletal System*, ed 2. Rosemont, IL, American Academy of Orthopaedic Surgeons, 2000, pp 683-716.

A-9: A 31-year-old woman has increasing pain and tightness in her right knee, with occasional stiffness and recurrent hemorrhagic effusions. MRI scans are shown in Figures 7A and 7B. What is the most likely diagnosis?

1. Rheumatoid arthritis
2. Pigmented villonodular synovitis (PVNS)
3. Synovial sarcoma
4. Synovial chondromatosis
5. Fibromatosis

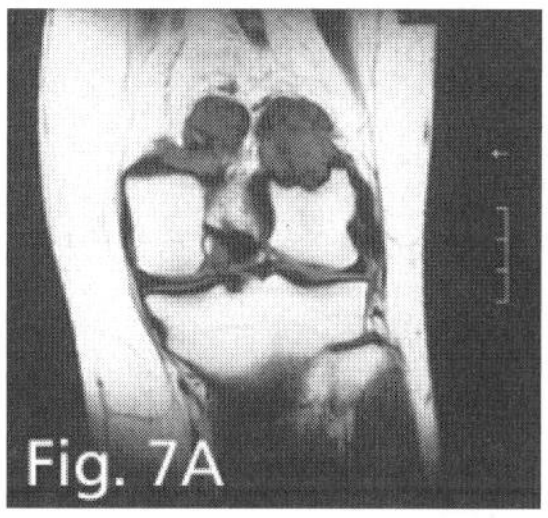
Fig. 7A

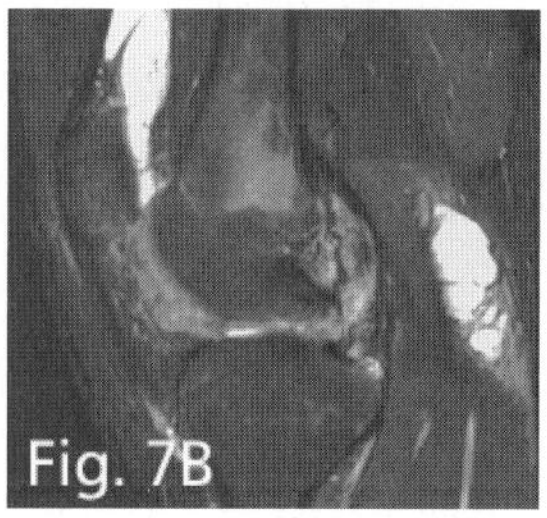
Fig. 7B

PREFERRED RESPONSE: 2

DISCUSSION: PVNS is a rare inflammatory granulomatous condition of unknown etiology, and causes proliferation of the synovium of joints, tendon sheaths, or bursa. The disorder occurs most commonly in the third and fourth decades but can occur at any age. MRI provides excellent delineation of the synovial disease. Characteristic features of PVNS on MRI include the presence of intra-articular nodular masses of low signal intensity on T1- and T2-weighted images and proton density-weighted images. Synovial biopsy should be performed if there is any doubt of the diagnosis. Total synovectomy (open or arthroscopic) is required for the diffuse form, although recurrence is common. Rheumatoid arthritis and synovial chondromatosis are not typically associated with hemorrhagic effusions.

REFERENCES: De Ponti A, Sansone V, Malchere M: Result of arthroscopic treatment of pigmented villonodular synovitis of the knee. *Arthroscopy* 2003;19:602-607.

Chin KR, Barr SJ, Winalski C, et al: Treatment of advanced primary and recurrent diffuse pigmented villonodular synovitis of the knee. *J Bone Joint Surg Am* 2002;84:2192-2202.

Bhimani MA, Wenz JF, Frassica FJ: Pigmented villonodular synovitis: Keys to early diagnosis. *Clin Orthop* 2001;386:197-202.

A-10: A 30-year-old patient who is an elite marathon runner reports chronic pain over the lateral aspect of the distal right leg and dysesthesia over the dorsum of the foot with active plantar flexion and inversion of the foot. Examination reveals a tender soft-tissue fullness approximately 10 cm proximal to the lateral malleolus. The pain is exacerbated by passive plantar flexion and inversion of the ankle. There is also a positive Tinel sign over the site of maximal tenderness. There is no motor weakness, and deep tendon reflexes are normal. Radiographs and MRI of the leg are normal. What is the most appropriate next step in management?

1. Biopsy of the soft-tissue mass
2. Epidural corticosteroid injection into the lumbar spine
3. Four-compartment fasciotomy of the leg
4. Fascial release and neurolysis of the superficial peroneal nerve
5. Closure of the fascial defect of the superficial peroneal nerve

PREFERRED RESPONSE: 4

(continued on next page)

(A-10: *continued*)

DISCUSSION: The patient has entrapment of the superficial peroneal nerve against its fascial opening in the distal leg. It is typically exacerbated by passive or active plantar flexion and inversion of the foot, which leads to traction of the nerve as it exits this opening. Treatment involves release of the fascial opening to reduce this traction phenomenon. Closure of the defect will only aggravate the condition and potentially result in an exertional compartment syndrome. A four-compartment fasciotomy is only indicated for an established compartment syndrome of the leg.

REFERENCES: Styf J: Diagnosis of exercise-induced pain in the anterior aspect of the lower leg. *Am J Sports Med* 1988;16:165-169.

Sridhara CR, Izzo KL: Terminal sensory branches of the superficial peroneal nerve: An entrapment syndrome. *Arch Phys Med Rehabil* 1985;66:789-791.

Styf J: Entrapment of the superficial peroneal nerve: Diagnosis and results of decompression. *J Bone Joint Surg Br* 1989;71:131-135.

A-11: A 21-year-old patient who is a soccer player reports pain and is unable to straighten his knee following an acute injury during a game. He is unable to continue to play. An MRI scan is shown in Figure 8. What is the most appropriate next step in management?

1. No weight bearing
2. Cortisone injection
3. Physical therapy
4. Arthroscopic meniscectomy or repair
5. Anterior cruciate ligament reconstruction

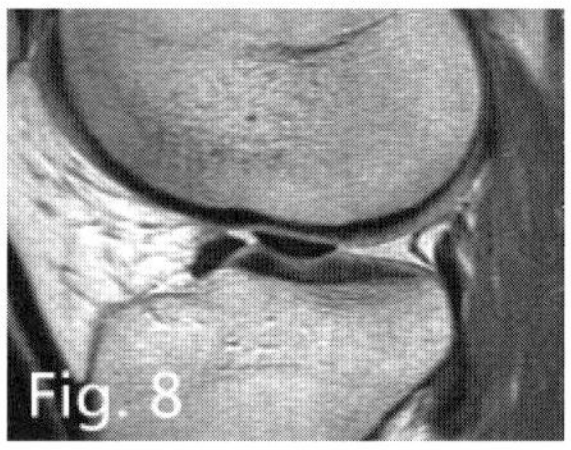
Fig. 8

PREFERRED RESPONSE: 4

DISCUSSION: The patient has a locked knee that cannot be fully extended. This is most likely the result of the mechanical block of a bucket-handle tear that has flipped into the notch. Also, the pain may be so severe that the muscle spasm prevents the knee from straightening out. When the patient is anesthetized, the muscle spasm relaxes and the meniscus can be reduced out of the notch. Arthroscopy is the treatment of choice. A meniscal repair is usually possible in large bucket-handle tears because the meniscus is torn in the red-red zone where most of the vascular supply is located. If the handle portion is badly frayed or damaged, a partial meniscectomy should be performed. The classic finding on MRI is a double PCL sign. This is due to the flipped portion of the meniscus in the notch.

REFERENCES: Critchley IJ, Bracey DJ: The acutely locked knee: Is manipulation worthwhile? *Injury* 1985;16:281-283.

Bansal P, Deehan DJ, Gregory RJ: Diagnosing the acutely locked knee. *Injury* 2002;33:495-498.

A-12: When performing an inside-out lateral meniscal repair, capsule exposure is provided by developing the

1. iliotibial band and biceps tendon interval, then retracting the lateral head of the gastrocnemius anteriorly.
2. iliotibial band and biceps tendon interval, then retracting the lateral head of the gastrocnemius posteriorly.

(continued on next page)

(A-12: *continued*)

3. iliotibial band and biceps tendon interval, then retracting the lateral collateral ligament posteriorly.
4. iliotibial band and biceps tendon interval, then splitting the lateral head of the gastrocnemius.
5. lateral head of the gastrocnemius and biceps tendon interval, then retracting the biceps tendon anteriorly.

PREFERRED RESPONSE: 2

DISCUSSION: Capsular exposure for an inside-out lateral meniscal repair is performed by developing the interval between the iliotibial band and biceps tendon. Posterior retraction of the biceps tendon exposes the lateral head of the gastrocnemius. Posterior retraction of the gastrocnemius provides access to the posterolateral capsule.

REFERENCES: Miller DB Jr: Arthroscopic meniscus repair. *Am J Sports Med* 1988;16:315-320.

Nawab A, Hester PW, Caborn DN: Arthroscopic meniscus repair, in Miller MD, Cole BJ, eds: *Textbook of Arthroscopy*. Philadelphia, PA, WB Saunders, 2004, pp 517-537.

A-13: A 15-year-old girl who plays field hockey sustains a blow to the mouth from a hockey stick. Three front teeth are knocked out and shown in Figure 9. In addition to calling a dentist immediately, what is the next best step in management?

1. Place the teeth in an ice water bath.
2. Pour normal saline solution on the teeth and then place them in milk.
3. Have the player gargle with mouthwash and place the teeth in water.
4. Clean the teeth with a toothbrush and then reimplant them.
5. Clean the teeth with a toothbrush and place them on ice.

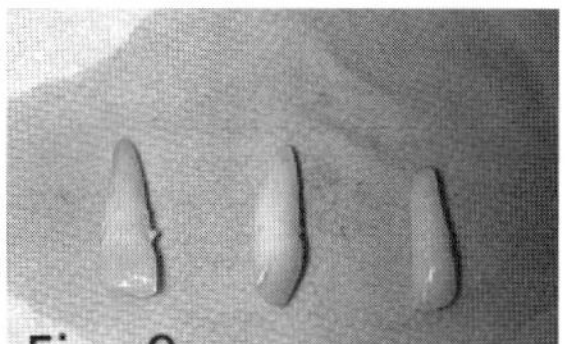
Fig. 9

PREFERRED RESPONSE: 2

DISCUSSION: Tooth avulsions can occur in contact or collision sports. An avulsed tooth is a medical emergency. The likelihood of survival of the tooth depends on the length of time that the tooth is out of the socket and the degree to which the periodontal ligament is damaged. The tooth should be handled only by the crown end and not the root end. It can be rinsed of debris with water or normal saline solution. The tooth should not be brushed or cleaned otherwise. During transport, the tooth must be kept moist. An avulsed tooth can be transported in whole milk, saliva, sterile saline solution, or commercially available kits with physiologic buffer solutions. The tooth and the athlete should be transported to the dentist for reinsertion as soon as possible and preferably within an hour.

REFERENCES: Krasner P: Management of sports-related tooth displacements and avulsions. *Dent Clin North Am* 2000;44:111-135.

Sullivan JA, Anderson SJ, eds: *Care of the Young Athlete*. Rosemont IL, American Academy of Orthopaedic Surgeons, 2000, p 190.

Galante A: Facial trauma, in Baker CL, ed: *The Hughston Clinic Sports Medicine Book*. Baltimore, MD, Williams & Wilkins, 1995, p 121.

A-14: Commotio cordis is best treated with

1. immediate cardiac defibrillation.
2. the chest thump maneuver.
3. IV fluids and hydration.
4. epinephrine.
5. albuterol inhalers.

PREFERRED RESPONSE: 1

DISCUSSION: Commotio cordis is a rare but catastrophic condition that is caused by blunt chest trauma. It results in cardiac fibrillation and is universally fatal unless immediate defibrillation is performed. Although case reports of successful use of the chest thump maneuver exist, the best method of treatment is cardiac defibrillation. Intravenous fluids, epinephrine, and albuterol inhalers are used to treat dehydration, anaphylactic shock, and bronchospasm, respectively, and are not effective in the treatment of commotio cordis.

REFERENCES: McCrory P: Commotio cordis. *Br J Sports Med* 2002;36:236-237.

Boden BP, Tacchetti R, Mueller FO: Catastrophic injuries in high school and college baseball players. *Am J Sports Med* 2004;32:1189-1196.

A-15: A 40-year-old woman reports the atraumatic onset of severe knee pain and swelling after undergoing an uncomplicated elective cholecystectomy 1 week ago. She denies any history of diabetes mellitus or HIV but has had occasional episodes of mild knee pain and swelling that have always responded to NSAIDs. Radiographs are shown in Figures 10A and 10B. A knee aspiration yields a white blood cell count of 35,000/mm^3. The aspirate should also yield which of the following findings?

1. Strongly negative needle-shaped crystals
2. Weakly positive birefringent rhomboid-shaped crystals
3. Gross blood
4. Gram-positive cocci
5. Gram-negative rods

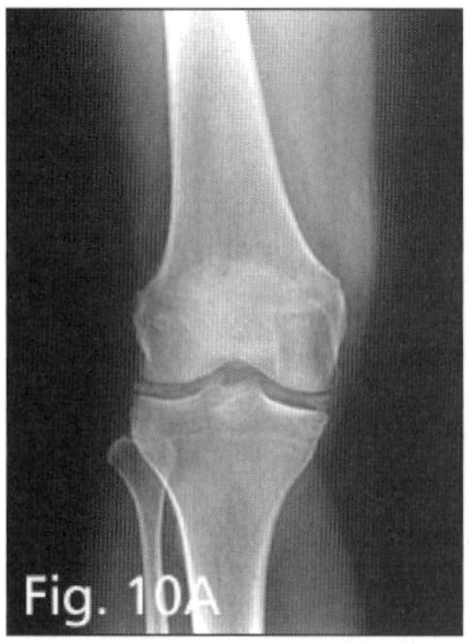

Fig. 10A

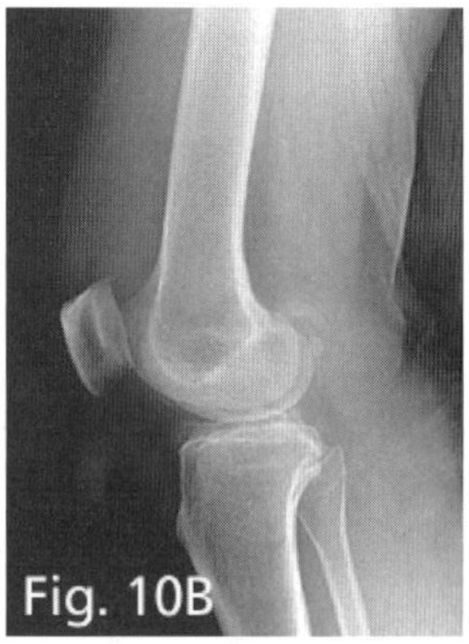

Fig. 10B

PREFERRED RESPONSE: 2

DISCUSSION: The radiographs reveal chondrocalcinosis of the menisci. This is caused by calcium pyrophosphate crystals, which are weakly positive birefringent rhomboid-shaped crystals. Frequently, this condition is asymptomatic; however, routine abdominal surgery may cause precipitation of these crystals and pain. Gout, which is caused by strongly negative birefringent needle-shaped sodium urate crystals, is not associated with chondrocalcinosis and is rare in younger women. Gross blood is uncommon without trauma. Infection is not likely in a healthy patient who underwent uncomplicated surgery.

REFERENCES: Fisseler-Eckhoff A, Muller KM: Arthroscopy and chondrocalcinosis. *Arthroscopy* 1992;8:98-104.

Hough AJ Jr, Webber RJ: Pathology of the meniscus. *Clin Orthop* 1990;252:32-40.

A-16: What is the maximum acceptable amount of divergence of the interference screw in the femoral tunnel from the bone plug of a bone-patellar tendon-bone graft in anterior cruciate ligament (ACL) reconstruction before pull-out strength is statistically decreased?

1. 0°
2. 10°
3. 15°
4. 30°
5. 45°

PREFERRED RESPONSE: 3

DISCUSSION: In the early 1990s, a transition was made from a two-incision ACL reconstruction to a single-incision ACL reconstruction, and there was concern over divergence of the femoral screws. It was shown radiographically that approximately 5% of the time, divergence of the screw was greater than 15° from the bone plug. In a bovine model, there was significant loss of pull-out strength with an increase in divergence from 15° to 30°. Therefore, attempts should be made to minimize divergence to 15° or less.

REFERENCES: Lemos MJ, Jackson DW, Lee TO, et al: Assessment of initial fixation of endoscopic interference femoral screws with divergent and parallel placement. *Arthroscopy* 1995;11:37-41.

Lemos MJ, Albert J, Simon T, et al: Radiographic analysis of femoral interference screw placement during ACL reconstruction: Endoscopic versus open technique. *Arthroscopy* 1993;9:154-158.

A-17: Use of prophylactic knee bracing in contact sports participants results in which of the following?

1. Decreased incidence of anterior cruciate ligament injuries
2. Decreased incidence of posterior cruciate ligament injuries
3. Decreased incidence of medial collateral ligament injuries
4. Decreased incidence of meniscal tears
5. Decreased incidence of ankle injuries

PREFERRED RESPONSE: 3

DISCUSSION: Several studies have looked at the effects of knee bracing, and it appears to be effective in prophylactically decreasing the incidence of medial collateral ligament sprains. Najibi and Albright reported that although evidence is not conclusive, bracing appears to help decrease the incidence of medial collateral ligament injuries. Albright and associates showed similar findings. Prophylactic knee braces have been associated with an increased incidence of ankle injuries.

REFERENCES: Albright JP, Powell JW, Smith W, et al: Medial collateral ligament knee sprains in college football: Effectiveness of preventive braces. *Am J Sports Med* 1994;22:12-18.

Najibi S, Albright JP: The use of knee braces: Part 1. Prophylactic knee braces in contact sports. *Am J Sports Med* 2005;33:602-611.

A-18: A 22-year-old patient who plays college football player reports shortness of breath and dyspnea after a tackle. Examination reveals tachypnea and tachycardia, the trachea is shifted to the right, and there are decreased breath sounds on the left lung fields. The first line of treatment on the field should be

1. placement of a chest tube.
2. insertion of a large gauge needle into the second intercostal space.
3. cardiopulmonary resuscitation.
4. administration of adrenaline.
5. immediate transfer to the emergency department.

PREFERRED RESPONSE: 2

DISCUSSION: The patient has a tension pneumothorax. This is a life-threatening emergency where air is trapped between the pleura and the lung, which prevents expansion of the lung. This causes hypoxia and cardiopulmonary compromise. The first line of treatment is to place a needle into the second intercostal space in the midclavicular line. The athlete should then be transported to the emergency department for chest tube placement. The athlete cannot return to play, and resuscitation is not necessary because he has not gone into cardiopulmonary arrest.

REFERENCES: Amaral JF: Thoracoabdominal injuries in the athlete. *Clin Sports Med* 1997;16:739-753.

Perron AD: Chest pain in athletes. *Clin Sports Med* 2003;22:37-50.

A-19: Anabolic steroid use has which of the following effects on serum lipoprotein levels?

1. Decrease in low-density lipoprotein only
2. Decrease in high-density lipoprotein only
3. Increase in high-density lipoprotein only
4. Increase in low-density lipoprotein only
5. Increase in both high- and low-density lipoproteins

PREFERRED RESPONSE: 2

DISCUSSION: The use of anabolic steroids causes a decrease in high-density lipoprotein levels but has no effect on low-density lipoprotein levels. An abnormally low high-density lipoprotein level should alert the physician to the possibility of steroid use in an athlete.

REFERENCES: Hartgens F, Rietjens G, Keizer HA, et al: Effects of androgenic-anabolic steroids on polipoproteins and lipoprotein (a). *Br J Sports Med* 2004;38:253-259.

Blue JG, Lombardo JA: Steroids and steroid-like compounds. *Clin Sports Med* 1999;18:667-689.

A-20: A 20-year-old woman who is a professional jockey is thrown from her horse while wearing a helmet. What is the most likely location of her injury?

1. Face
2. Head
3. Neck
4. Lower back
5. Leg

PREFERRED RESPONSE: 5

DISCUSSION: The incidence of injury associated with horseback rising is estimated to be 1 per 350 riding hours to 1 per 1,000 riding hours. Of these injuries, approximately 15% to 27% are severe enough to warrant hospital admission. Significant and serious injuries in equestrian activities are associated with recreational riders and those not wearing a helmet. Head and spine injuries are more common in recreational and nonhelmeted riders. Extremity injuries are more common in professional and helmeted riders. Professional riders are less likely to be admitted to the hospital than recreational riders, and are about half as likely to be disabled at 6 months after injury as recreational riders.

REFERENCES: Lim J, Puttaswamy V, Gizzi M, et al: Pattern of equestrian injuries presenting to a Sydney teaching hospital. *ANZ J Surg* 2003;73:567-571.

Petridou E, Kediloglou S, Belechri M, et al: The mosaic of equestrian-related injuries in Greece. *J Trauma* 2004;56:643-647.

A-21: Which of the following complications is more likely with an inside-out repair technique compared to an all-inside techniques for a medial meniscus tear?

1. Failure
2. Intra-articular synovitis
3. Peroneal nerve injury
4. Saphenous nerve injury
5. Arthrofibrosis

PREFERRED RESPONSE: 4

DISCUSSION: All of the answers are possible complications of meniscal repair. There are large volumes of literature evaluating the results of meniscal repair, both for the all-inside technique, as well as the inside-out technique. Failure rates are similar. Intra-articular synovitis occurs with absorbable sutures and absorbable implants. Peroneal nerve injuries are more common with the lateral-sided repairs. Saphenous nerve injuries are more common with medial-sided tears. Because of the incision required and the technique of tying over soft tissue, the risk of a saphenous nerve injury is greater with an inside-out technique than with an all-inside technique.

REFERENCES: Farng E, Sherman O: Meniscal repair devices: A clinical and biomechanical literature review. *Arthroscopy* 2004;20:273-286.

Jones HP, Lemos MJ, Wilk RM, et al: Two-year follow-up of meniscal repair using a bioabsorbable arrow. *Arthroscopy* 2002;18:64-69.

A-22: A 17-year-old boy who plays football is injured during a play and reports abdominal pain that is soon followed by nausea and vomiting. What organ has most likely been injured?

1. Liver
2. Pancreas
3. Spleen
4. Kidney
5. Large intestine

PREFERRED RESPONSE: 3

DISCUSSION: The spleen is the most common organ injured in the abdomen as the result of blunt trauma. It is also the most common cause of death because of an abdominal injury. The liver is the second most commonly injured organ. Injury to the other organs is rare. The diagnosis can be made with CT. Treatment ranges from observation to splenectomy, depending on the severity of injury.

REFERENCES: Green GA: Gastrointestinal disorders in the athlete. *Clin Sports Med* 1992;11:453-470.

Kibler WB, ed: *ACSM's Handbook for Team Physician*. Philadelphia, PA, Williams & Wilkins, 1996, p 151.

A-23: Which of the following cardiac conditions is considered an absolute contraindication to vigorous exercise?

1. Hypertrophic cardiomyopathy (HCM)
2. Sclerosis of the aortic valve without stenosis
3. Mild mitral valve regurgitation
4. Left ventricular hypertrophy (LVH)
5. Functional murmurs

PREFERRED RESPONSE: 1

DISCUSSION: Hypertrophic cardiomyopathy (HCM) accounts for up to 50% of cases of sudden death in young athletes. HCM phenotype becomes evident by age 13 to 14 years. Those at higher risk include individuals with cardiac symptoms, a family history of inherited cardiac disease, and those with a family history of premature sudden death. Echocardiography is useful for detecting structural heart disease, including the cardiomyopathies and valvular abnormalities. Trained adolescent athletes demonstrated greater absolute left ventricular wall thickness (LVWT) compared to controls. HCM should be considered in any trained adolescent male athlete with a LVWT of more than 12 mm (more than 11 mm in female athletes) and a nondilated ventricle. Adolescent and adult athletes differ with respect to the range of LVWT measurements, as a manifestation of left ventricular hypertrophy (LVH). Differentiating LVH ("athlete's heart") from HCM involves looking at additional echocardiographic features. Sharma and associates reported that adolescents with HCM had a small or normal-sized left ventricle (less than 48 mm) chamber size, whereas those with LVH had a chamber size at the upper limits of normal (52 to 60 mm).

(continued on next page)

(A-23: *continued*)

REFERENCES: Sharma S, Maron BJ, Whyte G, et al: Physiologic limits of left ventricular hypertrophy in elite junior athletes: Relevance to differential diagnosis of athlete's heart and hypertrophic cardiomyopathy. *J Am College Cardiol* 2002;40:1431-1436.

Maron BJ, Spirito P, Wesley Y, et al: Development and progression of left ventricular hypertrophy in children with hypertrophic cardiomyopathy. *N Engl J Med* 1986;315:610-614.

Pelliccia A, Culasso F, Di Paolo FM, et al: Physiologic left ventricular cavity dilatation in elite athletes. *Ann Intern Med* 1999;130:23-31.

A-24: An 18-year-old woman who plays lacrosse has infectious mononucleosis. What is the recommendation for return to play?

1. Full participation once symptoms resolve
2. Full participation once the splenomegaly resolves
3. Full participation 4 weeks after the onset of symptoms regardless of the size of the spleen
4. Full participation 4 weeks after both the onset of illness and findings of a normal-sized spleen
5. No participation for 8 weeks

PREFERRED RESPONSE: 4

DISCUSSION: Infectious mononucleosis commonly affects adolescents and young adults. It is a febrile illness accompanied by acute pharyngitis. Splenomegaly may occur and predispose the athlete to splenic rupture. Splenic rupture has been reported in nonathletes as well as in patients with normal-sized spleens. Clinical evidence supports a return to all sports 4 weeks after the onset of symptoms provided that the spleen has returned to normal size.

REFERENCES: Auwaerter PG: Infectious mononucleosis: Return to play. *Clin Sports Med* 2004;23:485-497.

Kinderknecht JJ: Infectious mononucleosis and the spleen. *Curr Sports Med Rep* 2002;1:116-120.

A-25: A 30-year-old patient reports chronic medial knee pain and swelling. Figure 11A shows an articular cartilage lesion observed during arthroscopy. The surgeon decides to treat the lesion with the microfracture technique seen in Figure 11B. A biopsy of the repaired tissue 1 year after treatment is likely to show which of the following findings?

1. Fibrous tissue
2. Bone
3. Articular cartilage
4. Fibrocartilage
5. Type II collagen

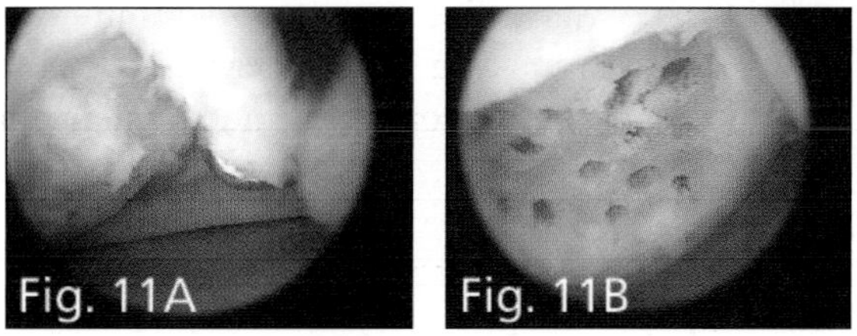

PREFERRED RESPONSE: 4

(continued on next page)

(A-25: *continued*)

DISCUSSION: Microfracture is a marrow stimulation technique where stem cells from the underlying subchondral bone marrow can form at the base of the lesion. The rationale for this technique is based on these cells differentiating into cells that will produce an articular cartilage repair. Biopsy findings in animals and humans have demonstrated primarily a fibrocartilagenous repair tissue and not articular cartilage. The collagen type found in hyaline or articular cartilage is of the type II variety. Fibrocartilage possesses mostly type I and III cartilage.

REFERENCES: Buckwalter JA, Mankin HJ: Articular cartilage: Degeneration and osteoarthritis, repair, regeneration, and transplantation. *Instr Course Lect* 1998;47:487-504.

Mankin HJ, Mow VC, Buckwalter JA: Arthicular cartilage repair and osteoarthritis, in Buckwalter JA, Einhorn TA, Simon SR, eds: *Orthopaedic Basic Science: Biology and Biomechanics of the Musculoskeletal System*, ed 2. Rosemont, IL, American Academy of Orthopaedic Surgeons, 2000, pp 471-488.

A-26: Kinematic analysis of the medial and lateral menisci has demonstrated that the lateral meniscus has which of the following characteristics compared with the medial meniscus?

1. More soft-tissue attachments/restraints
2. More mobility
3. Less mobility
4. No posterior movement with flexion
5. No anterior movement with extension

PREFERRED RESPONSE: 2

DISCUSSION: Kinematic analysis of both menisci demonstrates anterior movement with extension and posterior movement with flexion. The lateral meniscus has more mobility than the medial meniscus because of fewer soft-tissue attachments.

REFERENCES: Insall JN, Scott WN, eds: *Surgery of the Knee*, ed 3. New York, NY, Churchill Livingstone, 2001, vol 1, p 474.

Thompson WO, Thaete FL, Fu FH, et al: Tibial meniscal dynamics using 3D reconstructions of MR images, in *Proceedings of the Orthopaedic Research Society*. 1990;389.

West RV, Fu FH: Soft-tissue physiology and repair, in Vaccaro AR, ed: *Orthopaedic Knowledge Update*, ed 8. Rosemont, IL, American Academy of Orthopaedic Surgeons, 2005, pp 15-28.

A-27: Which of the following is the most relevant clinical factor in the maturation assessment of an adolescent female athlete contemplating anterior cruciate ligament (ACL) reconstruction?

1. Parental height
2. Height of older male sibling
3. Age of menarche
4. Recent change in shoe size
5. Presence of breast buds

(continued on next page)

(A-27: *continued*)

PREFERRED RESPONSE: 3

DISCUSSION: Age of menarche is the most accurate clinical factor to assess the degree of skeletal maturity in the female athlete. Such an assessment is necessary prior to ACL reconstruction in a skeletally immature female because of the risk of damage to the distal femoral and proximal tibial physes. Height of an older male sibling is not relevant to the female athlete. Parental height and recent change in shoe size are only moderately useful in predicting final growth, and hence, skeletal maturity. The presence of breast buds occurs early in adolescent development; therefore, its presence suggests a high likelihood of future growth.

REFERENCES: Micheli LJ, Foster TE: Acute knee injuries in the immature athlete. *Instr Course Lect* 1993;42:473-481.

Stanitski CL: Anterior cruciate ligament injury in the skeletally immature patient: Diagnosis and treatment. *J Am Acad Orthop Surg* 1995;3:146-158.

Fowler PJ: Anterior cruciate ligament injuries in the child, in Drez D, DeLee JD, Miller MD, eds: *Orthopaedic Sports Medicine Principles and Practice*, ed 2. Philadelphia, PA, WB Saunders, 2003, pp 2067-2074.

A-28: Which of the following best describes heat stroke?

1. Transient loss of consciousness with peripheral vasodilation and decreased cardiac output with normal body temperature
2. A condition involving painful contractions of large muscle groups because of decreased hydration and a decrease of serum sodium and chloride
3. Hypernatremia in poorly conditioned athletes, manifested by thirst and oliguria with a core temperature of less than 102.2°F (39°C)
4. Hyperthermia, central nervous system dysfunction, and loss of thermoregulatory function
5. A transient condition that responds to glucose administration

PREFERRED RESPONSE: 4

DISCUSSION: Heat stroke consists of hyperthermia (greater than 105.8°F [41°C]), central nervous system dysfunction, and cessation of sweating with hot, dry skin. It is a medical emergency that results from failure of the thermoregulatory mechanisms of the body. It has a high death rate and requires rapid reduction in body core temperature. Heat syncope is characterized by a transient loss of consciousness with peripheral vasodilation and decreased cardiac output with normal body temperature. Heat cramps involve painful contractions of large muscle groups because of decreased hydration and a decrease of serum sodium and chloride. Heat exhaustion is distinguished by a core temperature of less than 102.2°F (39°C) an absence of central nervous system dysfunction. Hypernatremic heat exhaustion results from inadequate water replacement.

REFERENCES: Knochel JP: Environmental heat illness: An eclectic review. *Arch Intern Med* 1974;133:841-864.

Hubbard RW, Gaffin SL, Squire DL: Heat related illness, in *Wilderness Medicine*, ed 3. St Louis, MO, Mosby, 1995, p 167.

Khosla R, Guntupalli KK: Heat-related illnesses. *Crit Care Clin* 1999;15:251-263.

A-29: Which of the following factors is most critical to the success of a meniscal allograft transplantation?

1. Accurate graft size
2. Donor cell viability
3. Reestablishment of the central meniscal blood supply
4. Suppression of the immune response
5. Cryopreservation of the donor graft

PREFERRED RESPONSE: 1

DISCUSSION: Success of a meniscal allograft transplantation is strongly dependent on accurate graft sizing, typically within 5% of the native meniscus. Previous studies have established that donor cell viability is not mandatory for the survival of these grafts because they are replaced by the recipient's cells (at least peripherally) within several weeks. Thus, cryopreservation of the graft to ensure cell viability is not necessary. There is a limited immune response to musculoskeletal allografts; therefore, immunosuppression, as is required for visceral organ transplantation, is not indicated.

REFERENCES: Wirth CA, Kohn D: Meniscal transplantation and replacement, in Fu FH, Harner CD, Vince JG, eds: *Knee Surgery*. Baltimore, MD, Williams & Wilkins, 1994, vol 1, pp 631-641.

Brautigan BE, Johnson DL, Caborn DM, et al: Allograft tissues, in Drez D, DeLee JD, Miller MD, eds: *Orthopaedic Sports Medicine: Principles and Practice*, ed 2. Philadelphia, PA, WB Saunders, 2003, pp 205-213.

Shaffer B, Kennedy S, Klimkiewicz J, et al: Preoperative sizing of meniscal allografts in meniscus transplantation. *Am J Sports Med* 2000;28:524-533.

A-30: What is the most common behavioral effect of anabolic steroid use in athletes?

1. Increased aggression
2. Psychosis
3. Drug dependence
4. Depression
5. Mania

PREFERRED RESPONSE: 1

DISCUSSION: Users of anabolic steroids often display increased feelings of hostility and aggression. Although reports of psychotic, depressive, and manic behavior have been reported with the use of steroids, they are rare. Drug dependence, such as seen with narcotics, is not a feature of steroid use.

REFERENCES: Hartgens F, Kuipers H: Effects of androgenic-anabolic steroids in athletes. *Sports Med* 2004;34:513-554.

Blue JG, Lombardo JA: Steroids and steroid-like compounds. *Clin Sports Med* 1999;19:667-689.

A-31: What is the effect on knee kinematics following placement of an anterior cruciate ligament (ACL) graft at the 12 o'clock position?

1. Decreased rotational stability
2. Decreased anterior-posterior stability
3. Decreased flexion
4. Decreased extension
5. Graft failure secondary to impingement

PREFERRED RESPONSE: 1

DISCUSSION: Endoscopic ACL reconstructive techniques may result in a vertical graft placement. The reconstructed ligament will resist anterior translation of the tibia but the graft will not restore rotatory stability. Decreased flexion and extension are caused by placement of the femoral tunnel too anterior and posterior, respectively. Impingement of the graft on the femoral notch is caused by anterior placement of the tibial tunnel or inadequate notchplasty.

REFERENCES: Scopp JM, Jasper LE, Belkoff SM, et al: The effect of oblique femoral tunnel placement on rotational constraint of the knee reconstructed using patellar tendon autografts. *Arthroscopy* 2004;20:294-299.

Carson EW, Simonian PT, Wickiewicz TL, et al: Revision anterior cruciate ligament reconstruction. *Instr Course Lect* 1998;47:361-368.

A-32: Which of the following knee ligament injury patterns is most associated with an increase in external tibial rotation with the knee at 90° of flexion?

1. Isolated tear of the posterior cruciate ligament
2. Isolated tear of the lateral collateral ligament
3. Combined tears of the posterior cruciate and lateral collateral ligaments
4. Combined tears of the anterior cruciate and lateral collateral ligaments
5. Combined tears of the lateral collateral and medial collateral ligaments

PREFERRED RESPONSE: 3

DISCUSSION: Cadaver studies have shown that external rotation of the tibia is most pronounced following transection of the posterior cruciate and lateral collateral ligaments with the knee at 90° of flexion. Isolated release of the lateral collateral ligament results in increased external tibial rotation at 30°.

REFERENCES: Gollehon DL, Torzilli PA, Warren RF: The role of the posterolateral and cruciate ligaments in the stability of the human knee: A biomechanical study. *J Bone Joint Surg Am* 1987;69:233-242.

Cooper DE: Tests for posterolateral instability of the knee in normal subjects: Results of examination under anesthesia. *J Bone Joint Surg Am* 1991;73:30-36.

Veltri DM, Xeng XH, Torzilli PA, et al: The role of the cruciate and posterolateral ligaments in stability of the knee: A biomechanical study. *Am J Sports Med* 1995;23:436-443.

A-33: Which of the following statements correctly describes the results of gamma irradiation of musculoskeletal allograft?

1. Exposure to 1.5 Mrad effectively eliminates HIV.
2. Exposure to 4 Mrad does not affect graft mechanical properties.
3. Gamma irradiation has been associated with chronic inflammation after implantation.
4. Gamma irradiation is commonly used alone for sterilization.
5. HIV cannot be eliminated with gamma irradiation alone without compromising the mechanical properties of the graft.

PREFERRED RESPONSE: 5

DISCUSSION: Low-dose gamma irradiation (less than 3.0 Mrad) with antibiotic soaks is one of the most common techniques for secondary sterilization. Elimination of HIV with gamma irradiation requires doses estimated to be greater than 3.5 Mrad. Gamma irradiation levels of 4 Mrad have been shown to alter the mechanical properties of human infrapatellar tendons. Ethylene oxide, also used for allograft sterilization, has been associated with a chronic inflammatory process that resolved after graft removal.

REFERENCES: Jackson DW, Windler GE, Simon TM: Intraarticular reaction associated with the use of freeze-dried, ethylene oxide-sterilized bone-patella tendon-bone allografts in the reconstruction of the anterior cruciate ligament. *Am J Sports Med* 1990;18:1-10.

Conway B, Tomford W, Mankin HJ, et al: Radiosensitivity of HIV-1: Potential application to sterilization of bone allografts. *AIDS* 1991;5:608-609.

Rasmussen TJ, Feder SM, Butler DL, et al: The effects of 4 Mrad of gamma irradiation on the initial mechanical properties of bone-patellar tendon-bone grafts. *Arthroscopy* 1994;10:188-197.

A-34: A 35-year-old woman who is a recreational runner reports posterior knee pain and tightness in the knee with flexion during running. She denies any history of trauma. Examination reveals normal patellar glide and tilt and no patellar apprehension. Range of motion is 5° to 120°, and quadriceps function and knee ligamentous examination are normal. Radiographs are normal. An MRI scan is shown Figure 12. What is the most likely diagnosis?

1. Baker cyst
2. Torn medial meniscus
3. Patellofemoral pain syndrome
4. Lipoma
5. Ganglion cyst of the cruciates

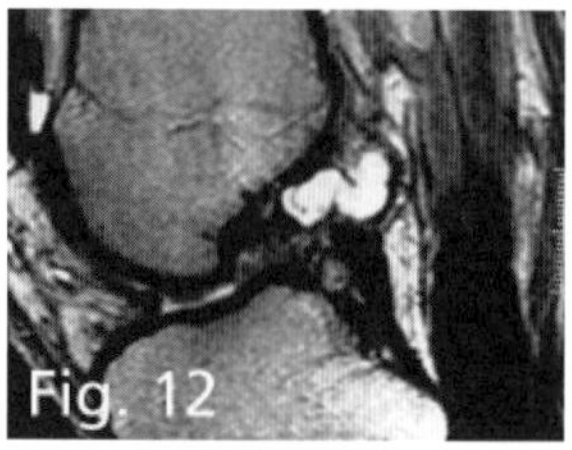

PREFERRED RESPONSE: 5

DISCUSSION: Ganglia involving the cruciate ligaments have been recently reported as a cause of knee pain that interferes with knee flexion and extension. The symptoms are poorly localized in this patient and not along the medial joint line, making the diagnosis of a torn medial meniscus less likely. In addition, the MRI findings do not show a significant medial meniscal lesion. A Baker cyst is usually posteromedial and extends posterior to the interval between the medial head of the gastrocnemius and semimembranosus. MRI scans show a fluid-filled lesion with an increased signal on T1- and T2-weighted images. A lipoma would be bright on the T1-weighted image only.

(continued on next page)

(A-34: *continued*)

REFERENCES: Deutsch A, Veltri DM, Altchek DW, et al: Symptomatic intraarticular ganglia of the cruciate ligaments of the knee. *Arthroscopy* 1994;10:219-223.

Brown MF, Dandy DJ: Intra-articular ganglia of the knee. *Arthroscopy* 1990;6:322-323.

A-35: An 18-year-old man underwent open reduction and internal fixation of a tibial spine avulsion and a posterolateral corner repair. Two years later, he underwent lateral collateral ligament (LCL) and posterolateral corner reconstruction because of instability. Examination reveals a pronounced lateral varus knee thrust when ambulating. Varus stress in 30° of flexion produces a 10-mm opening that is eliminated in extension. The Lachman test is 2 mm with a firm end point, and the posterior drawer test is negative. Standing radiographs show widening of the lateral joint space and a 5° mechanical varus alignment. What is the most effective course of treatment?

1. Physical therapy for quadriceps strengthening
2. Functional bracing
3. Anterior cruciate ligament (ACL) reconstruction
4. Revision reconstruction of the LCL and posterolateral corner
5. Valgus-producing high tibial osteotomy (HTO)

PREFERRED RESPONSE: 5

DISCUSSION: The patient has chronic posterolateral instability with a varus knee alignment; therefore, the most effective treatment is a valgus-producing HTO. A repeat soft-tissue reconstruction without correction of the varus alignment will most likely fail. An ACL reconstruction is not indicated with a normal Lachman test. Physical therapy and bracing will have little effect.

REFERENCES: Naudie DD, Amendola A, Fowler PJ: Opening wedge high tibial osteotomy for symptomatic hyperextension-varus thrust. *Am J Sports Med* 2004;32:60-70.

Covey DC: Injuries of the posterolateral corner of the knee. *J Bone Joint Surg Am* 2001;83:106-118.

A-36: A favorable outcome following nonsurgical management of a partial tear of the posterior cruciate ligament (PCL) is best associated with

1. hamstring strength.
2. quadriceps strength.
3. a body mass index of less than 30.
4. anterior cruciate ligament stability.
5. compliance with brace use.

PREFERRED RESPONSE: 2

DISCUSSION: Rehabilitation of the quadriceps muscle following a partial tear of the PCL has been associated with a favorable outcome. The quadriceps acts as an antagonist to the PCL because its contraction results in anterior tibial translation, which reduces the tensile stress on the injured ligament.

(continued on next page)

(A-36: *continued*)

Strengthening of the hamstring musculature increases posterior tibial translation and is contraindicated during the early rehabilitative phase following a PCL injury. Brace use has not been found to significantly alter the outcome following nonsurgical management of PCL tears.

REFERENCES: Parolie JM, Bergfeld JA: Long-term results of nonoperative treatment of isolated posterior cruciate ligament injuries in the athlete. *Am J Sports Med* 1986;14:35-38.

Griffin JR, Annunziata CC, Harner CD: Posterior cruciate ligament injuries in the adult, in Drez D, DeLee JD, Miller MD, eds: *Orthopaedic Sports Medicine Principles and Practice*, ed 2. Philadelphia, PA, WB Saunders, 2003, pp 2083-2106.

A-37: A player on a professional football team sustains a knee injury and an anterior cruciate ligament rupture is diagnosed. When employed as the team physician, your ethical obligation is to inform

1. the player but not the team.
2. the team but not the player.
3. neither the team nor the player.
4. both the team and the player.
5. the team, the player, and the media.

PREFERRED RESPONSE: 4

DISCUSSION: When you are employed as a team physician, you are obligated to inform the players and the team organization of all athletically relevant medical issues. This differs significantly from the normal rule of patient confidentiality. If the player came to see you and you were not the team physician, you may not inform the team unless the player so desires. As the team physician, you are not obligated to inform the media.

REFERENCES: Tucker AM: Ethics and the professional team physician. *Clin Sports Med* 2004;23:227-241.

Johnson R: The unique ethics of sports medicine. *Clin Sports Med* 2004;23:175-182.

A-38: A 20-year-old man who plays soccer collapses after a goal kick and reports weakness and nausea. He appears slightly confused. Examination reveals that he is not sweating. His skin is warm and dry. The outdoor temperature is 80°F (26.6°C) with a relative humidity of 80%. Management should consist of

1. a drink of water.
2. a sports drink with electrolytes.
3. placement in the reverse Trendelenburg position in a shaded area.
4. immersion in a warm water bath.
5. transportation to the emergency department.

PREFERRED RESPONSE: 5

(continued on next page)

(A-36: *continued*)

DISCUSSION: There is a spectrum of heat-related conditions. Heat cramps are the mildest form of heat illness. In heat exhaustion, cramps are associated with headache and weakness, and the skin is pale and moist. Treatment of heat cramps or heat exhaustion consists of removing and loosening excess clothing, applying ice to the axilla and groin, ingestion of cool water, and cool water sprays. This patient demonstrates symptoms of heat stroke which is a medical emergency. The core body temperature may be as high as 106 to 110°F (41.1 to 43.3°C). In heat stroke, the patient may no longer be sweating, and the skin may be hot and red. The athlete is usually confused, weak, nauseated, and may have seizure activity. Central nervous system depression has been called the most important marker of heat stroke, and progresses from confusion and bizarre behavior to collapse, delirium, and coma. Bizarre behavior is often the first sign of heat stroke. The patient needs to be treated and moved to a medical facility rapidly. During transfer, intravenous fluids and cooling of the athlete should be initiated. The best treatment of heat-related illness appears to be prevention with adequate hydration and monitoring of conditions (temperature and humidity), with cancellation of competition when conditions do not comply with guidelines.

REFERENCES: Griffin LY: Emergency preparedness: Things to consider before the game starts. *J Bone Joint Surg Am* 2005;87:894-902.

Barker TA, Motz HA, Gersoff WK: Environmental factors in athletic performance, in Fu FH, Stone DA, eds: *Sports Injuries*, ed 2. Philadelphia, PA, Lippincott, 2001, pp 67-68.

Roberts WO: Environmental concerns, in Kibler WB, ed: *ACSM's Handbook for the Team Physician*. Baltimore, MD, Williams & Wilkins, 1996, p 172.

A-39: What is the most accurate description of the relationship between sex and knee loading during landing while playing basketball?

1. Males have greater total valgus knee loading.
2. Females have greater total valgus knee loading.
3. Males have greater total varus knee loading.
4. Females have greater total varus knee loading.
5. There is no sex difference in total varus or valgus knee loading.

PREFERRED RESPONSE: 2

DISCUSSION: Ford and associates studied 81 high school basketball players and found that females landed with greater total valgus knee loading and a greater maximum valgus knee angle than male athletes. Hewett and associates reported in a study of 205 female athletes that those with increased dynamic valgus and high abduction loads were at increased risk of anterior cruciate ligament injury.

REFERENCES: Hewett TE, Myer GD, Ford KR, et al: Biomechanical measures of neuromuscular control and valgus loading of the knee predict anterior cruciate ligament injury risk in female athletes: A prospective study. *Am J Sports Med* 2005;33:492-501.

Ford KR, Meyer GD, Hewett TE: Valgus knee motion during landing in high school female and male basketball players. *Med Sci Sports Exer* 2003;35:1745-1750.

A-40: What is the most common cause of the new onset of amenorrhea in a female endurance athlete who is not sexually active?

1. Insufficient caloric intake
2. Physical stress
3. Use of oral contraceptives
4. Diabetes mellitus
5. Chromosomal abnormalities

PREFERRED RESPONSE: 1

DISCUSSION: Insufficient caloric intake caused by either a poor diet or an eating disorder is the most common cause for the loss of menses in a female athlete. In the face of adequate caloric intake, stress is unlikely to cause amenorrhea. Oral contraceptives control menses but do not eliminate it. Diabetes mellitus does not cause the new onset of amenorrhea. Pregnancy can be a cause in a sexually active athlete. Chromosomal abnormalities can result in delayed or absent menarche but not the onset of amenorrhea in a postmenarchal female.

REFERENCES: Constantini NW: Clinical consequences of amenorrhea. *Sports Med* 1994;17:213-223.

Bennell KL, Malcolm SA, Thomas SA, et al: Risk factors for stress fractures in track and field athletes: A twelve-month prospective study. *Am J Sports Med* 1996;24:810-818.

A-41: A 29-year-old man who is an ultramarathoner is halfway into a 50-mile race and begins sweating profusely. He suddenly collapses, is unresponsive, and has violent muscle contractions. Prior to these symptoms, he had been drinking water at every water stop (every 1 mile). What is the most likely diagnosis?

1. Hypernatremia
2. Hyponatremia
3. Hyperkalemia
4. Hypokalemia
5. Hyperuremia

PREFERRED RESPONSE: 2

DISCUSSION: Hyponatremia (water intoxication) can occur in endurance athletes such as ultramarathoners who are sweating profusely and drinking only water as fluid replacement. Sports drinks that contain electrolytes are a better replacement in this group of athletes. Sodium is the mineral most commonly affected by physical exercise. Sodium concentration in sweat depends on diet, hydration, and heat acclimation. In most cases, sodium lost in sweat can be replaced by regular diet. Potassium plays an important role in nerve conduction and muscle contraction but is not lost in excessive amounts in sweat during exercise. The most frequent loss of potassium is through gastrointestinal disorders or excessive loss from the kidneys. Rehrer reported that overhydrating during very long-lasting exercise in the heat with low or negligible sodium intake can result in reduced performance and hyponatremia. With hyponatremia, the serum sodium is abnormally low, resulting in brain swelling, seizures, coma, and potentially death. Interestingly, hyponatremia is rarely seen in adolescent athletes and young children.

REFERENCES: Griffin LY: Emergency preparedness: Things to consider before the game starts. *J Bone Joint Surg Am* 2005;87:894-902.

Rehrer NJ: Fluid and electrolyte balance in ultra-endurance sport. *Sports Med* 2001;31:701-715.

A-42: Tension force in the anterior cruciate ligament during passive range of motion is highest at

1. full extension.
2. 30° of flexion.
3. 60° of flexion.
4. 90° of flexion.
5. 120° of flexion.

PREFERRED RESPONSE: 1

DISCUSSION: Tension forces in the healthy, as well as the reconstructed, anterior cruciate ligament were measured and found to be highest with the knee in full extension and decreased as the flexion increased.

REFERENCES: Markolf KL, Burchfield DM, Shapiro MM, et al: Biomechanical consequences of replacement of the anterior cruciate ligament with a patellar ligament allograft. Part II: Forces in the graft compared with forces in the intact ligament. *J Bone Joint Surg Am* 1996;78:1728-1734.

Beynnon BD, Johnson RJ, Fleming BC, et al: The measurement of elongation of anterior cruciate-ligament grafts in vivo. *J Bone Joint Surg Am* 1994;76:520-531.

A-43: Compared to eumenorrheic athletes, amenorrheic athletes have more frequent occurrences of

1. stress fractures.
2. scoliosis.
3. pes planus.
4. meniscal tears.
5. ankle sprains.

PREFERRED RESPONSE: 1

DISCUSSION: In secondary amenorrhea, women do not receive the estrogen needed to maintain adequate bone mineralization. This hypoestrogenic state affects bone density, and there is evidence that stress fractures are more frequent in amenorrheic than eumenorrheic athletes. The other conditions are not seen with increased frequency in amenorrheic athletes.

REFERENCES: Warren MP: Health issues for women athletes: Exercise-induced amenorrhea. *J Clin Endocrinol Metab* 1999;84:1892-1896.

Rencken ML, Chesnut CH III, Drinkwater BL: Bone density at multiple skeletal sites in amenorrheic athletes. *JAMA* 1996;276:238-240.

A-44: Figure 13 shows the postoperative radiograph of a patient who underwent an anterior cruciate ligament (ACL) reconstruction (with bone–patellar tendon–bone autograft) that failed. He initially had loss of flexion postoperatively. What is the most likely cause of this failure?

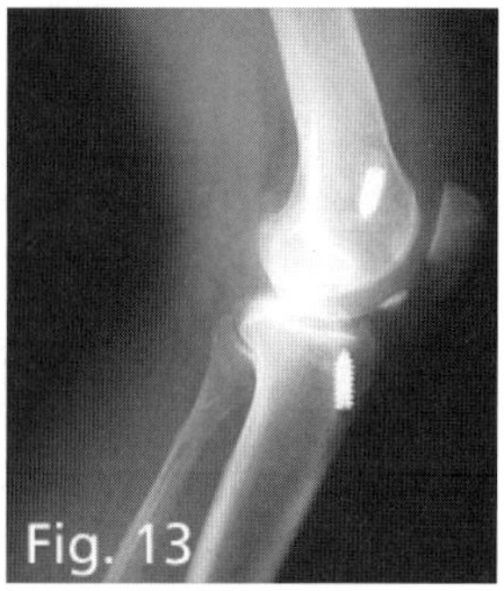

1. Fixation in the tibial tunnel
2. Fixation in the femoral tunnel
3. Posterior placement of the tibial tunnel
4. Anterior placement of the femoral tunnel
5. Size of the patellar autograft

PREFERRED RESPONSE: 4

DISCUSSION: The key to this question is the fact that the patient initially lost flexion postoperatively and this relates to anterior placement of the femoral tunnel, thus capturing the knee. The bone plug seen on the radiograph is actually from the tibial tunnel, but this occurred as the patient forced flexion until failure of the ACL graft and pullout of the plug from the tunnel. Although it could be argued that better tibial fixation would have prevented this failure, poor placement of the femoral tunnel led to the failure of this ACL reconstruction.

REFERENCES: Fu FH, Bennett CH, Latterman C, et al: Current trends in anterior cruciate ligament reconstruction: Part 1. Biology and biomechanics of reconstruction. *Am J Sports Med* 1999;27:821-830.

Fu FH, Bennett CH, Ma CB, et al: Current trends in anterior cruciate ligament reconstruction: Part II. Operative procedures and clinical correlations. *Am J Sports Med* 2000;28:124-130.

A-45: A 22-year-old man reports anterior knee pain, swelling, and inability to perform a straight leg raise after undergoing endoscopic anterior cruciate ligament (ACL) reconstruction with a bone-patellar tendon-bone autograft 1 week ago. He is afebrile. Examination reveals a clean incision, moderate effusion, a weak isometric quadriceps contraction, active knee range of motion of 5° to 45°, and the patella is ballottable. Knee radiographs show postoperative changes with good femoral and tibial tunnel placements, and normal patellar height. What is the next most appropriate step in management?

1. Electromyography (EMG) and nerve conduction velocity studies (NCVS)
2. Diagnostic ultrasonography of the patellar tendon
3. MRI
4. Continuous passive motion
5. Knee aspiration

PREFERRED RESPONSE: 5

DISCUSSION: Knee pain and swelling in the first week after ACL reconstruction is usually related to a postoperative hemarthrosis. A large hemarthrosis creates capsular distension, which inhibits active quadriceps contraction by a neurologic reflex, the H-reflex. Kennedy and associates reported that an experimentally induced knee effusion at 60 mL was found to result in profound inhibition of reflexly evoked quadriceps contraction. Removal of the hemarthrosis by aspiration will improve strength and often instantaneously restore the ability to contract the quadriceps muscle. A large effusion will also limit knee flexion. EMG and NCVS are not necessary unless there is a high index of suspicion of a femoral neuropathy. Diagnostic ultrasonography is not necessary in this patient but can be useful in the assessment of patellar tendon integrity. MRI is not indicated and would most likely be limited by artifact and

(continued on next page)

(A-45: *continued*)

postoperative changes. Continuous passive motion is not indicated and would most likely worsen the patient's symptoms.

REFERENCES: Kennedy JC, Alexander IJ, Hayes KC: Nerve supply of the human knee and its functional importance. *Am J Sports Med* 1982;10:329-335.

Fahrer H, Rentsch HU, Gerber NJ, et al: Knee effusion and reflex inhibition of the quadriceps: A bar to effective retraining. *J Bone Joint Surg Br* 1988;70:635-638.

A-46: The use of knee arthroscopy following total knee arthroplasty is most effective in treating which of the following conditions?

1. Patellar clunk syndrome
2. Septic arthritis
3. Nonspecific pain
4. Improper tracking of the patellar component
5. Synovitis secondary to polyethylene wear

PREFERRED RESPONSE: 1

DISCUSSION: Patellar clunk syndrome is associated with certain types of posterior stabilized knee arthroplasties. Arthroscopic resection of the band of inflammatory tissue inferior to the patellar component is effective in treating this condition. Arthroscopic lavage of infected knee arthroplasties is not associated with an acceptable success rate. Diagnostic arthroscopy for nonspecific pain following arthroplasty is not uniformly successful. Patellar component maltracking is frequently associated with component malposition and is not alleviated by an arthroscopic lateral release. Synovitis secondary to polyethylene wear is best treated by exchange of the polyethylene spacer and not arthroscopic synovectomy.

REFERENCES: Lucas TS, DeLuca PF, Nazarian DG, et al: Arthroscopic treatment of patellar clunk. *Clin Orthop* 1999;367:226-229.

Takahashi M, Miyamoto S, Nagano A: Arthroscopic treatment of soft-tissue impingement under the patella after total knee arthroplasty. *Arthroscopy* 2002;18:E20.

A-47: Significant anterior tibial translation occurs during which of the following rehabilitation exercises?

1. Terminal weight-bearing knee extension
2. Terminal non-weight-bearing knee extension
3. Terminal weight-bearing knee flexion
4. Terminal non-weight-bearing knee flexion
5. Midrange weight-bearing knee flexion

(continued on next page)

(A-47: *continued*)

PREFERRED RESPONSE: 2

DISCUSSION: Terminal non-weight-bearing knee extension exercises from 60° to 0° of flexion increase anterior tibial translation. It is for this reason that this type of exercise should be avoided in the early phase of rehabilitation following anterior cruciate ligament reconstruction so as not to place a tensile strain on the graft. The other rehabilitation exercises either lead to posterior tibial translation in relation to the femur or have no significant effect on tibial translation.

REFERENCES: Grood ES, Suntay WJ, Noyes FR, et al: Biomechanics of the knee extension exercise: Effect of cutting the anterior cruciate ligament. *J Bone Joint Surg Am* 1984;66:725-734.

Lutz GE, Palmitier RA, An KN: Comparison of tibiofemoral joint forces during open-kinetic-chain and closed-kinetic-chain exercises. *J Bone Joint Surg Am* 1993;75:732-739.

Wilk KE, Escamilla RF, Fleisig GS, et al: A comparison of tibiofemoral joint forces and electromyographic activity during open and closed kinetic chain exercises. *Am J Sports Med* 1996;24:518-527.

A-48: A 43-year-old man who plays soccer had knee pain following a twisting injury and underwent an arthroscopic meniscectomy 6 months ago. He continues to report posterior knee pain. Examination reveals soft-tissue fullness and tenderness just above the popliteal fossa, trace knee effusion, full range of knee motion, no instability, and negative meniscal signs. Radiographs show some mild medial joint space narrowing but no other bony changes. What is the most appropriate next step in management?

1. Corticosteroid injection
2. MRI
3. Bone scan
4. Unloader brace
5. NSAIDs

PREFERRED RESPONSE: 2

DISCUSSION: The phenomenon of tumors misdiagnosed as athletic injuries has been termed sports tumors. Lewis and Reilly presented a series of 36 patients who initially were thought to have a sports-related injury but ultimately the diagnosis of primary bone tumor, soft-tissue tumor, or tumor-like condition was made. Muscolo and associates presented a series of 25 tumors that had been previously treated with an intra-articular procedure as a result of a misdiagnosis of an athletic injury. Initial diagnoses included 21 meniscal lesions, one traumatic synovial cyst, one patellofemoral subluxation, one anterior cruciate ligament tear, and one case of nonspecific synovitis. The final diagnoses were a malignant tumor in 14 patients and a benign tumor in 11 patients. The authors noted that oncologic surgical treatment was affected in 15 of the 25 patients. The most frequent causes of erroneous diagnosis were initial poor-quality radiographs and an unquestioned original diagnosis despite persistent symptoms. Persistent symptoms warrant further diagnostic studies, not additional treatment such as physical therapy, corticosteroid injection, or an unloader brace. Although a bone scan may be helpful in this case and confirm arthrosis of the medial compartment, the suspicion of a soft-tissue mass makes MRI the imaging modality of choice.

REFERENCES: Muscolo DL, Ayerza MA, Makino A, et al: Tumors about the knee misdiagnosed as athletic injuries. *J Bone Joint Surg Am* 2003;85:1209-1214.

Lewis MM, Reilly JF: Sports tumors. *Am J Sports Med* 1987;15:362-365.

A-49: Storage of musculoskeletal allografts by cryopreservation is achieved by

1. replacing water in the tissue with alcohol to a moisture level of 5% and then using a vacuum process to remove the alcohol from the tissue.
2. maintaining maximum cellular viability of fresh tissue without long-term storage.
3. using chemicals to remove cellular water and controlled rate freezing to prevent ice crystal formation.
4. freezing the graft twice and packaging the tissue without solution at −80°C.
5. freezing the graft in water without an antibiotic solution soak during quarantine, with final storage in liquid nitrogen.

PREFERRED RESPONSE: 3

DISCUSSION: Cryopreservation uses chemicals to remove cellular water and controlled rate freezing to prevent ice crystal formation. The tissue is procured, cooled to wet ice temperature for quarantine, and then stored in a container with cryoprotectant solution of dimethyl sulfoxide or glycerol, which displaces the cellular water. The controlled rate freezing is then done to prevent ice crystal formation. Fresh allografts are not frozen in order to maintain maximum cellular viability, and this process limits the shelf life of osteochondral allografts. Freeze-drying involves replacement of water in the tissue with alcohol to a moisture level of 5% and then uses a vacuum process to remove the alcohol from the tissue. Preparation of fresh frozen grafts involves freezing the graft twice and packaging the tissue without solution at −80°C.

REFERENCES: American Association of Tissue Banks: *Standards for Tissue Banking*. MacLean, VA, American Association of Tissue Banks, 1999.

Vangsness CT Jr, Triffon MJ, Joyce MJ, et al: Soft tissue allograft reconstruction of the human knee: A survey of the American Association of Tissue Banks. *Am J Sports Med* 1996;24:230-234.

Brautigan BE, Johnson DL, Caborn DM, et al: Allograft tissues, in DeLee JC, Drez D Jr, eds: *Orthopaedic Sports Medicine: Principles and Practice*. Philadelphia, PA, WB Saunders, 2003, pp 205-213.

A-50: Second-impact syndrome (SIS) after head injury is characterized by which of the following?

1. Gradual progression of neurologic symptoms
2. Preventable by restricting return to play until symptom-free
3. Excellent prognosis for full recovery
4. Rarely involves brain stem compromise
5. CT rarely shows brain edema

PREFERRED RESPONSE: 2

DISCUSSION: SIS is a devastating but preventable complication of head injury. It occurs when return to activities is allowed prior to complete resolution of the symptoms of the first head injury. A second, sometimes trivial, head injury can lead to a devastating series of events that can result in sudden death. The symptoms tend to progress rapidly and often involve the brain stem. The prognosis is poor.

REFERENCES: Cantu RC: Second-impact syndrome. *Clin Sports Med* 1998;17:37-44.

Saunders RL, Harbaugh RE: Second impact in catastrophic contact-sports head trauma. *JAMA* 1984;252:538-539.

Stevenson KL, Adelson PD: Pediatric sports-related head injuries, in Delee JC, Drez D, eds: *Orthopaedic Sports Medicine: Principles and Practice*, ed 2. Philadelphia, PA, WB Saunders, 2003, vol 1, p 781.

Foot and Ankle

Q-1: A 42-year-old man who works as an athletic trainer has a persistent popping sensation about the lateral ankle associated with weakness and pain following a remote injury. Deficiency in what structure directly leads to this pathology?

1. Lateral talar process
2. Superior peroneal retinaculum
3. Inferior peroneal retinaculum
4. Extensor retinaculum
5. Crural fascia

Q-2: Which of the following structures is most vulnerable during a medial sesamoidectomy of the hallux?

1. Abductor hallucis tendon
2. Intermetatarsal ligament
3. Plantar-medial cutaneous nerve of the hallux
4. Dorsomedial cutaneous nerve of the hallux
5. Crista

Q-3: A 30-year-old man who sustained a tibial fracture with a peroneal nerve palsy 2 years ago now has footdrop and weak eversion of the foot. He reports success with stretching exercises, but he catches his toes when his foot tires. Examination reveals that the foot is plantigrade and supple. What is the most appropriate next step in management?

1. Posterior tibial tendon transfer to the cuboid
2. Anterior tibial tendon transfer to the cuboid
3. Achilles tendon lengthening
4. Ankle-foot orthosis with dorsiflexion assist
5. Nerve grafting

Q-4: Removal of both hallucal sesamoids should be reserved as a salvage procedure because of the high incidence of which of the following postoperative complications?

1. Hallux rigidus
2. Hallux varus
3. Flexion contracture of the hallux metatarsophalangeal joint
4. Persistent neuritic pain
5. Cock-up deformity of the great toe and hallux valgus

Q-5: A 63-year-old woman with a history of poliomyelitis has a fixed 30° equinus contracture of the ankle, rigid hindfoot valgus, and normal knee strength and stability. She reports persistent pain and has had several medial forefoot ulcerations despite a program of stretching, bracing, and custom footwear. What is the most appropriate next step in management?

1. Charcot restraint orthotic walker
2. Hyperbaric oxygen treatment
3. Triple arthrodesis with Achilles tendon lengthening
4. Transtibial amputation
5. Ankle arthrodesis

Q-6: What is the most common foot deformity associated with myelomeningocele?

1. Talipes equinovarus
2. Congenital vertical talus
3. Calcaneus valgus
4. Calcaneus varus
5. Cavus

Q-7: Where is the watershed zone for tarsal navicular vascularity?

1. Medial one third
2. Central one third
3. Lateral one third
4. Tuberosity
5. Inferior pole

Q-8: A 37-year-old woman has had intermittent paresthesias and numbness in the plantar foot for the past 6 months. She reports that the symptoms are worse with activity, and the paresthesias are beginning to awaken her at night. MRI scans are shown in Figures 1A and 1B. What is the most likely diagnosis?

1. Lipoma
2. Giant cell tumor of the tendon sheath
3. Synovial sarcoma
4. Metastatic adenocarcinoma
5. Ganglion cyst

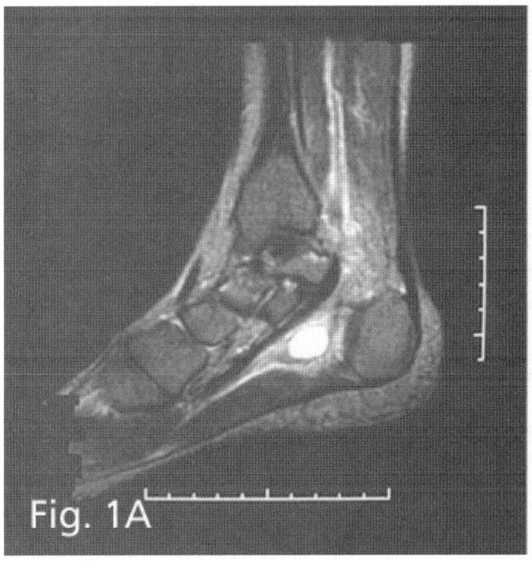

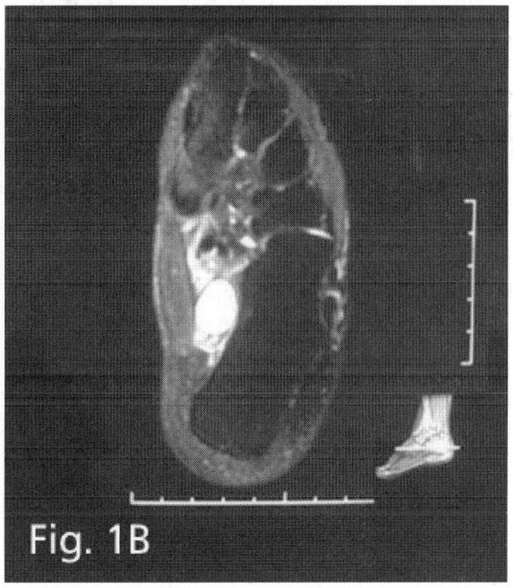

Q-9: Figure 2 shows the CT scan of a 25-year-old man who plays soccer who has had posterior ankle pain with plantar flexion for the past 2 years. Immobilization has failed to provide relief. He is ambulatory. Management should consist of

1. a local steroid injection into the flexor hallucis longus tendon sheath.
2. range-of-motion exercises.
3. open reduction and internal fixation.
4. NSAIDs.
5. excision of the fragment.

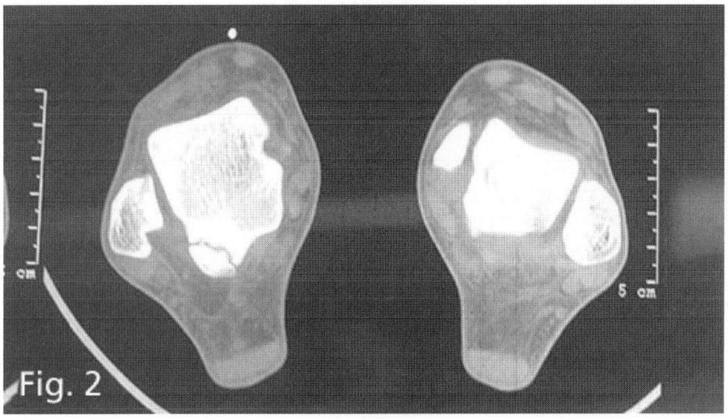

Q-10: Figure 3 shows the CT scan of an 11-year-old boy who has had a 1-year history of worsening painful flatfeet. He reports pain associated with physical education at school, especially with running and jumping. Management consisting of activity restriction, anti-inflammatory drugs, and casting has failed to provide relief. Treatment should now consist of

1. a subtalar arthroereisis with a titanium implant.
2. triple arthrodesis.
3. resection of the accessory navicular and advancement of the posterior tibial tendon bilaterally.
4. resection of the talocalcaneal middle facet coalition in each foot.
5. resection of the calcaneonavicular coalition in both feet.

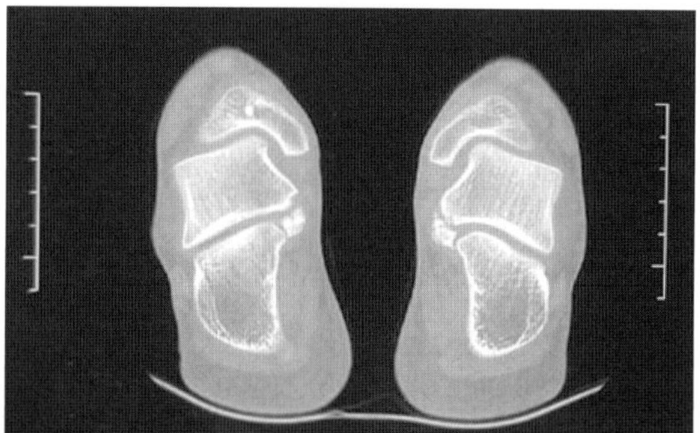

Fig. 3

Q-11: What is the optimum position of immobilization of the foot and ankle immediately after Achilles tendon repair to maximize skin perfusion?

1. 10° of dorsiflexion
2. 10° of plantar flexion
3. 20° of plantar flexion
4. Neutral
5. Resting equinus

Q-12: A 32-year-old man who sustained a tarsometatarsal (Lisfranc) injury 3 years ago now reports increasing pain in the left foot. Orthotics, NSAIDs, and injections have provided only temporary relief. Examination reveals swelling and tenderness over the tarsometatarsal joints. Radiographs show advanced arthrosis of the first and second tarsometatarsal joints. Management should now include

1. midfoot arthrodesis.
2. a rocker sole shoe with orthotic inserts.
3. shock wave therapy or orthotripsy.
4. an ankle-foot orthosis.
5. triple arthrodesis.

Q-13: An 11-year-old girl has had pain in the medial arch of her foot for the past 3 months. She reports that pain is present even with daily activities such as walking to class at school, and ibuprofen provides some relief. She denies any history of trauma. Examination reveals a flexible pes planus with focal tenderness over a prominent tarsal navicular tuberosity. Radiographs show a prominent accessory navicular. Management should consist of

1. cast immobilization for 4 to 6 weeks.
2. posterior tibial tendon advancement and repair (Kidner procedure).
3. corticosteroid injection of the posterior tibial tendon insertion.
4. triple arthrodesis.
5. needle biopsy of the trochar.

Q-14: Figures 4A and 4B show the radiographs of a 28-year-old woman who sustained a head injury and a closed injury, without soft-tissue compromise, to her right lower extremity in a motor vehicle accident. Appropriate management of the foot injury should include

1. external fixation with a circular frame.
2. open reduction and internal fixation with screws.
3. closed reduction and percutaneous pinning.
4. closed reduction and cast immobilization.
5. amputation.

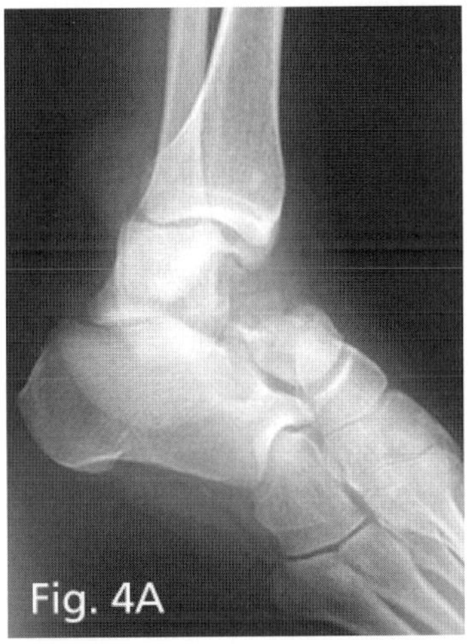
Fig. 4A

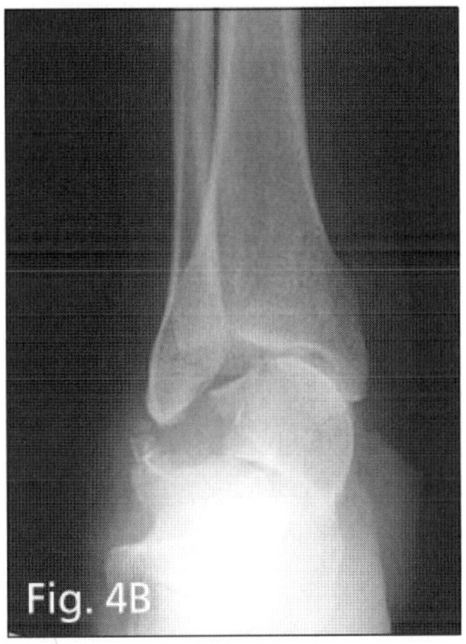
Fig. 4B

Q-15: An active 47-year-old woman with rheumatoid arthritis reports forefoot pain and deformity and has difficulty with shoe wear. Examination reveals hallux valgus and claw toes. A radiograph is shown in Figure 5. What is the most appropriate surgical treatment?

1. Distal chevron osteotomy bunionectomy with lesser metatarsal head resections
2. Proximal first metatarsal osteotomy with flexor-to-extensor tendon transfer for the lesser toes
3. First metatarsophalangeal arthrodesis with lesser metatarsal head resections
4. First tarsometatarsal realignment arthrodesis (Lapidus procedure) with flexor-to-extensor tendon transfer for the lesser toes
5. Resection of the base of the hallux proximal phalanx (Keller procedure) with flexor-to-extensor tendon transfer for the lesser toes

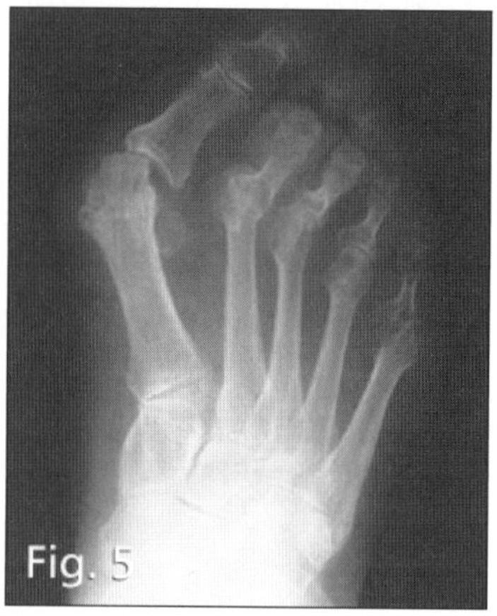

Fig. 5

Q-16: A 32-year-old woman has left second toe dactylitis (sausage toe). Radiographs show a "pencil in cup" distal interphalangeal joint deformity. Examination reveals that subtalar motion is markedly reduced. What is the most likely diagnosis?

1. Rheumatoid arthritis
2. Lyme disease
3. Psoriatic arthritis
4. Crohn disease arthropathy
5. Gout

Q-17: Which of the following is considered the most common infectious organism causing osteochondritis in pediatric puncture wounds of the foot?

1. *Eikenella corrodens*
2. *Pseudomonas aeruginosa*
3. *Pasteurella multocida*
4. *Serratia marcescens*
5. *Proteus mirabilis*

Q-18: Figure 6 shows the clinical photograph of a 66-year-old man who has had an increasingly painful right foot deformity for the past 3 years. Examination reveals that the subtalar joint is fixed in 15° of valgus, and forefoot supination can be corrected to 10° from neutral. Nonsurgical management has failed to provide relief. Treatment should now consist of

1. medial sliding calcaneal osteotomy with flexor digitorum longus (FDL) transfer.
2. isolated subtalar arthrodesis.
3. isolated talonavicular arthrodesis.
4. triple arthrodesis.
5. subtalar arthroereisis.

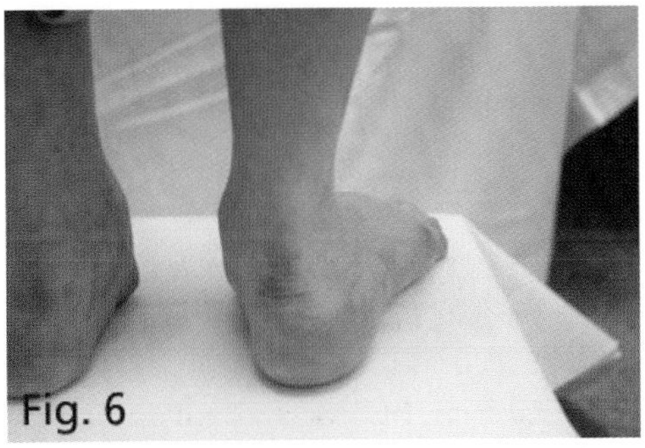

Fig. 6

Q-19: When evaluating a patient with hallux rigidus, what is the most important clinical factor indicating the need for an arthrodesis as opposed to a cheilectomy?

1. Dorsal foot pain with shoe wear
2. Pronounced limited motion in the first metatarsophalangeal joint
3. Pain at the midrange of motion in the first metatarsophalangeal joint
4. Large dorsal osteophytes clinically and radiographically
5. Flattened first metatarsal head with periarticular sclerosis

Q-20: A patient who has recalcitrant medial plantar heel pain and pain directly over the medial side of the heel undergoes open release of the plantar fascia. After releasing a portion of the plantar fascia, the deep fascia of the abductor hallucis muscle is released to relieve pressure on which of the following structures?

1. Lateral plantar artery
2. Tibial nerve
3. First branch of the lateral plantar nerve
4. Sural nerve
5. Flexor hallucis brevis muscle

Q-21: A 47-year-old woman has a painful bunion of the right foot, and shoe wear modifications have failed to provide relief. Examination reveals a severe hallux valgus with dorsal subluxation of the second toe. Radiographs are shown in Figures 7A and 7B. The most appropriate management should include

1. hallux metatarsophalangeal arthrodesis.
2. custom orthotics.
3. chevron osteotomy with second toe correction.
4. Keller resection arthroplasty with second toe correction.
5. proximal metatarsal osteotomy with second toe correction.

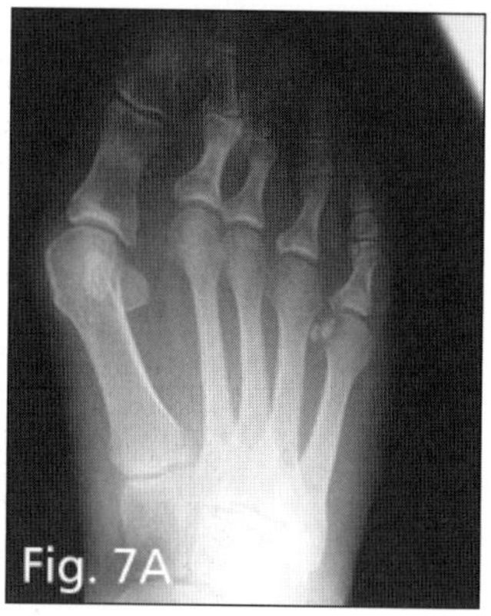
Fig. 7A

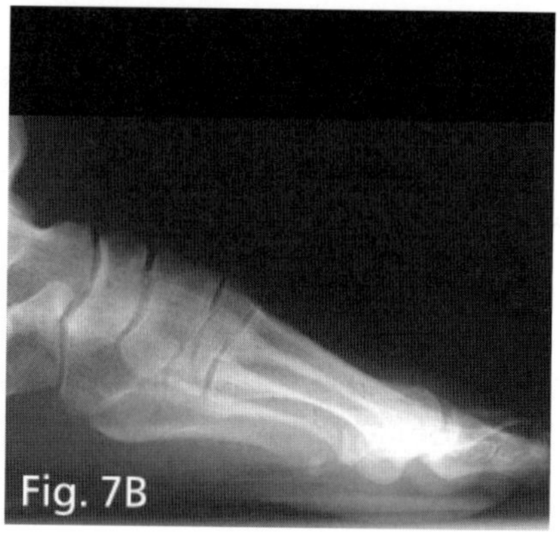
Fig. 7B

Q-22: What is the most appropriate orthosis for hallux rigidus?

1. Morton extension
2. Metatarsal arch pad
3. Full-length semirigid longitudinal arch support
4. Full-length semirigid longitudinal arch support with medial hindfoot posting
5. Full-length semirigid longitudinal arch support with lateral forefoot posting

Q-23: Figures 8A through 8C show the radiographs of a 23-year-old man who plays football and who was injured when another player fell on his flexed and planted foot. He reports severe pain in the midfoot with a feeling of numbness on the dorsum of the foot, and he is unable to bear weight on the limb. Examination reveals mild swelling. Management should consist of

1. casting.
2. closed reduction, casting, and no weight bearing for 6 weeks.
3. open reduction and internal fixation.
4. closed reduction and percutaneous Kirschner wire fixation.
5. closed reduction and percutaneous screw fixation.

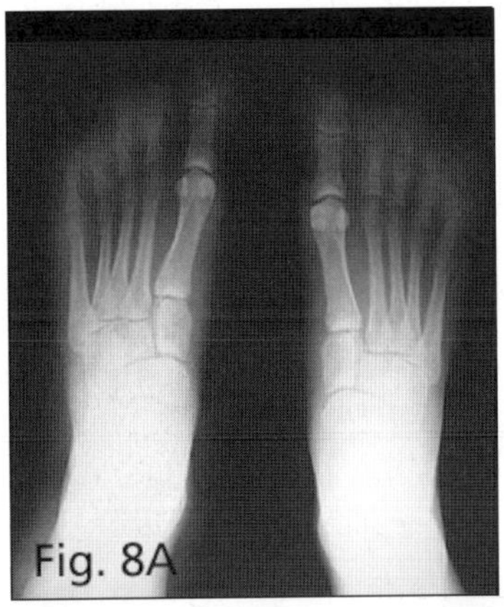
Fig. 8A

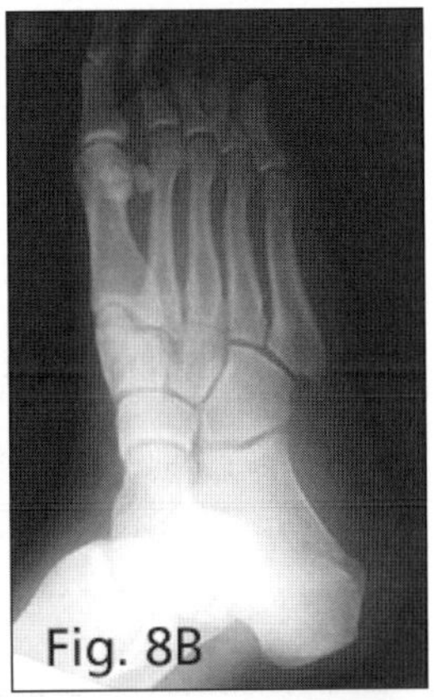
Fig. 8B

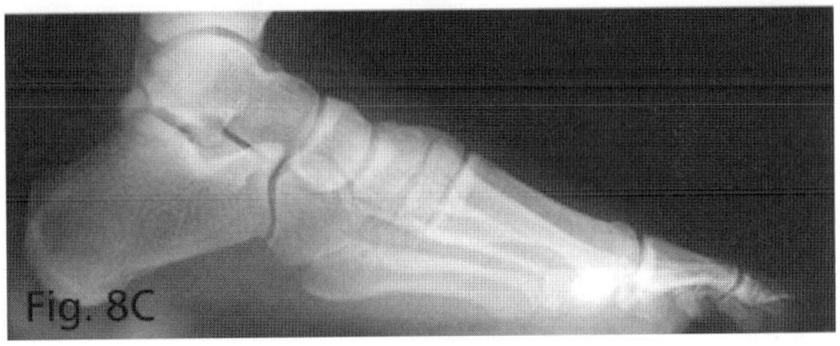
Fig. 8C

Q-24: Which of the following methods best aids in diagnosis of an interdigital neuroma?

1. Ultrasound
2. MRI
3. Web space injection
4. Electromyography and nerve conduction velocity studies
5. History and physical examination

Q-25: A 58-year-old man has had a 3-year history of recurrent ulcerations of the left ankle and instability despite multiple attempts at custom bracing, contact casting, and surgical débridement. He has an ankle-brachial index of 0.76. A clinical photograph and radiographs are shown in Figures 9A through 9C. Treatment should now consist of

1. transtibial amputation.
2. a double upright brace.
3. dressing changes with platelet-derived growth factor.
4. tibiocalcaneal arthrodesis.
5. total ankle arthroplasty.

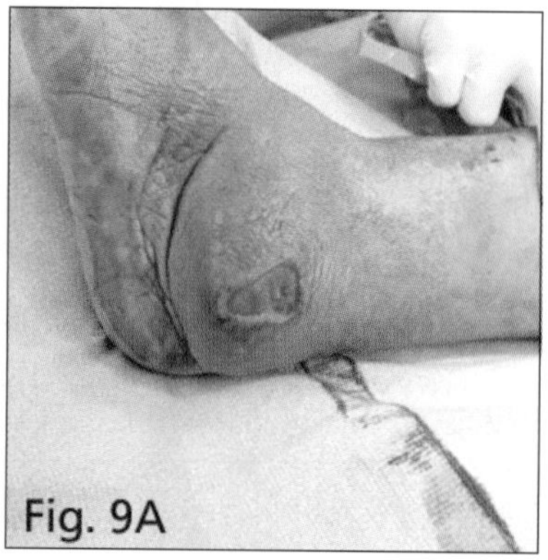
Fig. 9A

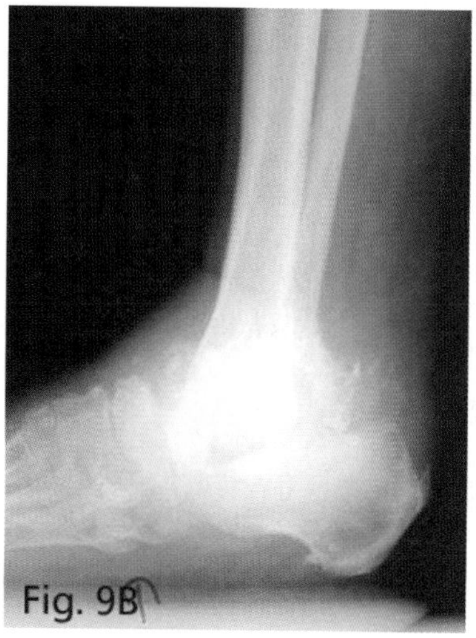
Fig. 9B

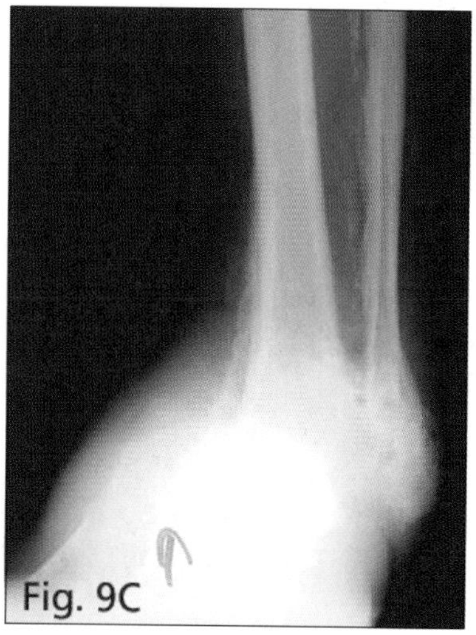
Fig. 9C

Q-26: Figures 10A and 10B show the radiographs of a 32-year-old patient who is a professional athlete and who sustained an injury to the first metatarsal. A view of the opposite noninjured side is shown in Figure 10C. Management of the fracture should consist of

1. open reduction and internal fixation.
2. a postoperative stiff-soled shoe with weight bearing as tolerated.
3. a postoperative shoe with no weight bearing for 3 weeks.
4. a short leg cast with no weight bearing.
5. percutaneous pinning.

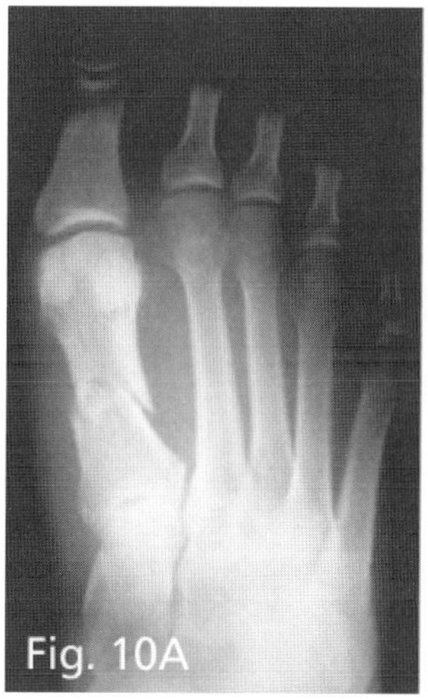

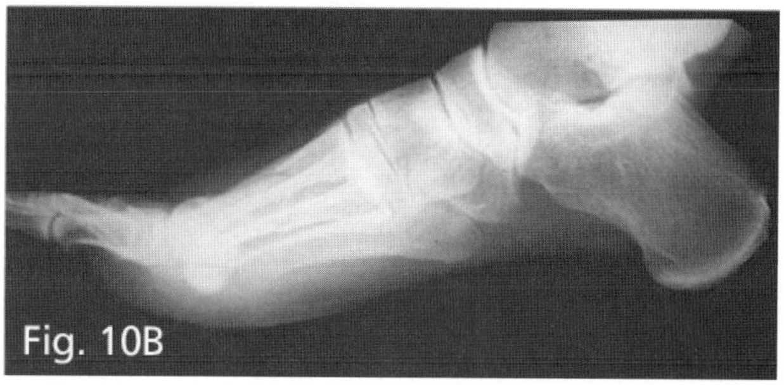

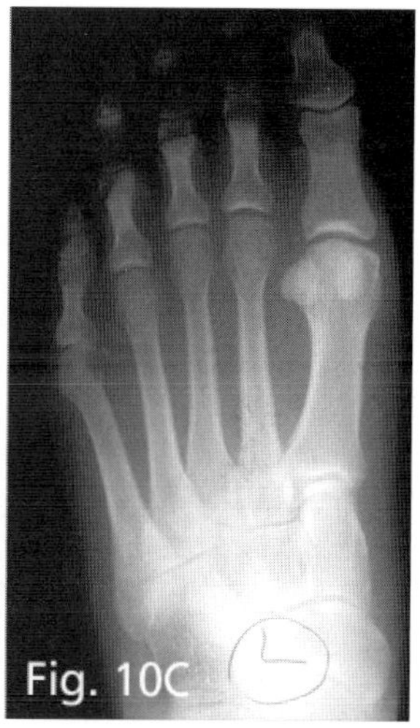

Q-27: Which of the following are considered appropriate nonsurgical bracing/orthotic options for a supple adult-acquired flatfoot deformity with forefoot abduction, secondary to posterior tibial tendon insufficiency?

1. Rigid orthotic with a lateral post
2. Custom-molded leather and polypropylene orthosis (Arizona brace)
3. UCBL orthosis with lateral posting
4. One quarter-inch lateral heel and sole wedge applied to the shoe
5. Three-quarter heel lift

Q-28: A 28-year-old man underwent open reduction and internal fixation of a closed, displaced, intra-articular calcaneal fracture 8 weeks ago. Examination now reveals that the lateral wound is red and draining purulent material. Cultures obtained from the wound grow out *Staphylococcus aureus*. Radiographs show early healing of the fracture. What is the most appropriate next step in management?

1. Intravenous antibiotics
2. Débridement of the wound without hardware removal
3. Débridement of the wound with hardware removal
4. Vacuum-assisted closure (VAC) and negative pressure therapy
5. Total calcanectomy

Q-29: A 37-year-old man with a history of congenital flatfoot reports worsening pain on the medial aspect of his ankle for the past year. The pain is worse with weight bearing and is better with rest and the use of an ankle brace. What findings are shown on the MRI scans in Figures 11A through 11C?

1. The flexor digitorum longus tendon is ruptured.
2. The posterior tibial tendon has a normal appearance.
3. The posterior tibial tendon has a physiologic amount of fluid in its sheath.
4. The posterior tibial tendon is completely ruptured and retracted (type III tear).
5. The posterior tibial tendon has a chronic longitudinal split with enlargement (type II tear).

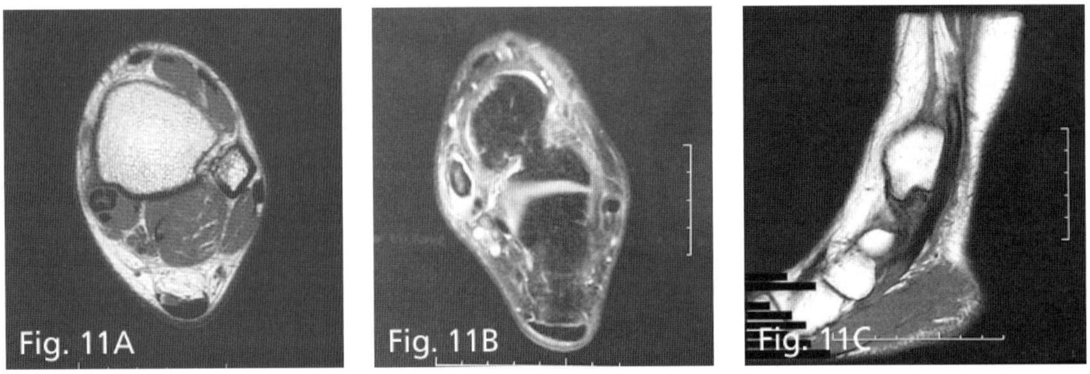

Fig. 11A Fig. 11B Fig. 11C

Q-30: A 60-year-old man reports increasing pain in his right foot with limited ankle dorsiflexion and anterior ankle pain after sustaining a fracture of the calcaneus during a fall several years ago. Bracing, NSAIDs, and cortisone injections have failed to provide significant relief. Radiographs are shown in Figures 12A and 12B. What is the most appropriate next step in management?

1. Subtalar distraction arthrodesis
2. Subtalar arthroscopy with débridement
3. Custom orthotics
4. Ankle arthrodesis
5. Calcaneal osteotomy

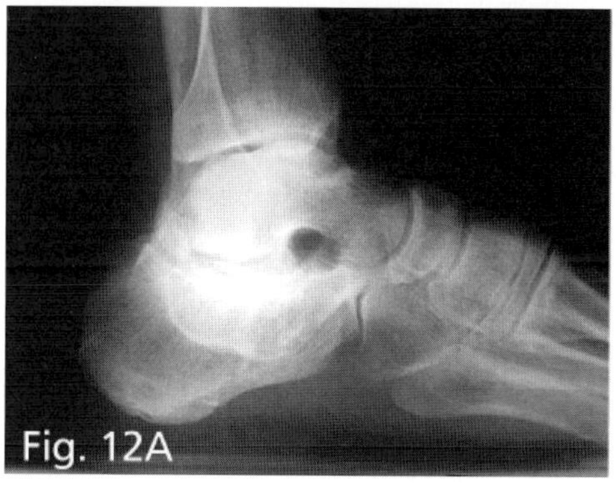

Fig. 12A

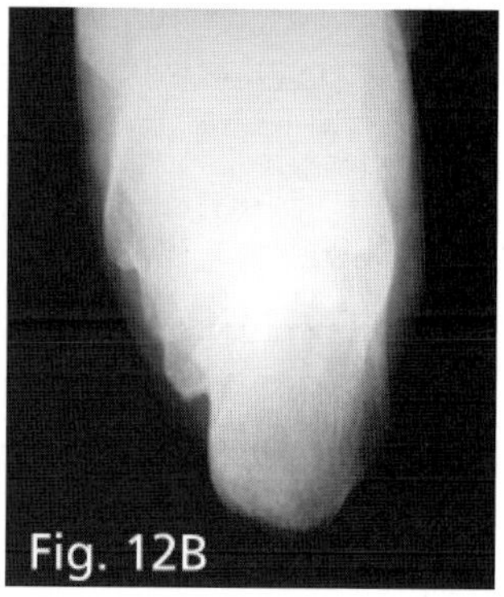

Fig. 12B

Q-31: A 58-year-old woman sustained a ruptured Achilles tendon 1 year ago, and management consisted of an ankle-foot orthosis. She now reports increasing difficulty with ambulation and increasing pain. An MRI scan shows a 6-cm defect in the right Achilles tendon. Management should now consist of

1. continued use of an ankle-foot orthosis.
2. direct repair of the Achilles tendon.
3. V-Y repair of the Achilles tendon.
4. transfer of the plantaris tendon.
5. Achilles tendon turndown with flexor hallucis longus tendon transfer.

Q-32: A 29-year-old woman reports dysesthesias and burning after undergoing bunion surgery that consisted of a proximal crescentic first metatarsal osteotomy 6 months ago. Examination reveals a positive Tinel sign at the proximal aspect of the healed incision. What injured nerve is responsible for the patient's continued symptoms?

1. Recurrent branch of the deep peroneal
2. Recurrent branch of the sural
3. Terminal cutaneous branch of the saphenous
4. Dorsomedial cutaneous branch of the superficial peroneal
5. Medial plantar

Q-33: Figure 13 shows the clinical photograph of the foot of a man who has had diabetes mellitus controlled with oral medication for the past 10 years. He wears soft-soled shoes and only uses leather-soled shoes for important business meetings. Examination reveals palpable dorsalis pedis and posterior tibial pulses, although they are somewhat diminished. He is insensate to pressure with the 5.07 Semmes-Weinstein monofilament. The ulcer heals after treatment with a full contact cast. What is the best course of action at this time?

1. Referral to his primary care physician
2. Foot-specific patient education, depth-inlay shoes, custom accommodative foot orthoses, and follow-up observation
3. Dorsiflexion osteotomy of the first and third metatarsals
4. Excision of the second and third metatarsal heads
5. Achilles tendon lengthening and dorsiflexion osteotomy of the first and third metatarsals

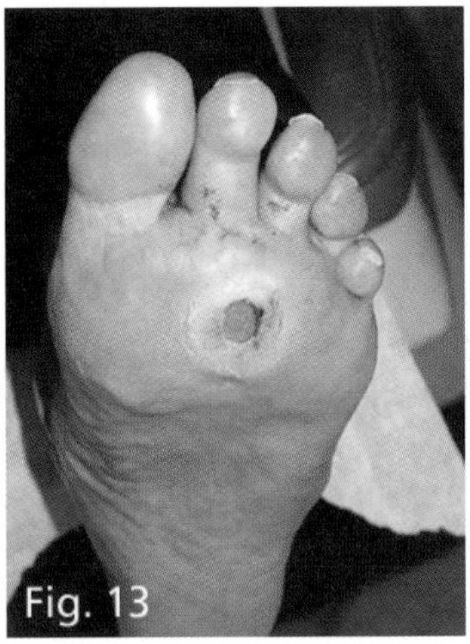
Fig. 13

Q-34: Figures 14A and 14B show the clinical photograph and radiograph of a 15-year-old girl who has a deformity of her feet. Her parents are concerned because there is a family history of Charcot-Marie-Tooth disease. The patient reports some mild instability of the ankle and has noticed mild early callosities; however, she is not having any significant pain. Coleman block testing reveals a forefoot valgus and supple hindfoot. She has weakness to eversion and dorsiflexion. Initial management should consist of

1. dorsiflexion osteotomy of the first metatarsal with peroneus longus to brevis transfer.
2. plantar fasciotomy with dorsiflexion osteotomy of the first metatarsal and calcaneal osteotomy.
3. a stretching and strengthening physical therapy program and accommodative inserts.
4. observation.
5. calcaneal osteotomy, dorsiflexion osteotomy of the first metatarsal, peroneus longus to brevis transfer, plantar fascia release, Achilles tendon lengthening, and midfoot osteotomy.

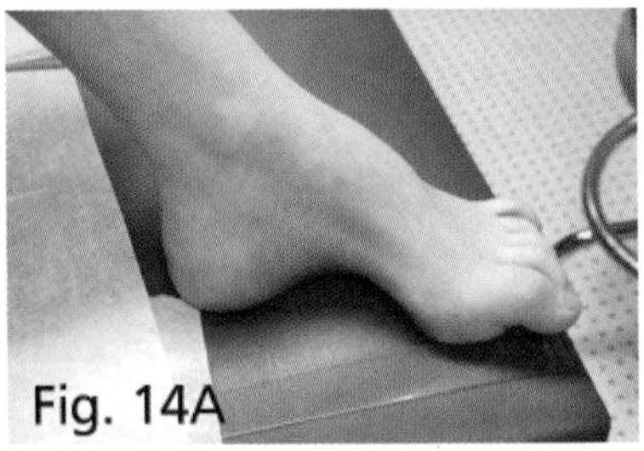
Fig. 14A

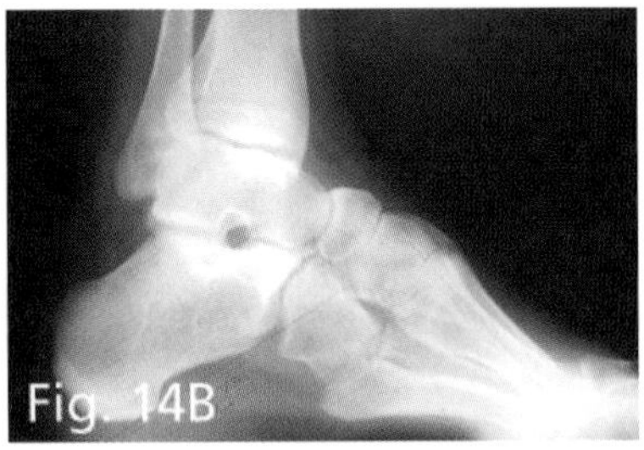
Fig. 14B

Q-35: A 64-year-old man with a history of diabetes mellitus underwent open reduction and internal fixation of a displaced ankle fracture 8 weeks ago. Examination now reveals recent onset erythema, warmth, and swelling of the midfoot. Radiographs are shown in Figures 15A through 15D. What is the most likely reason for the swelling of the foot?

1. Infection
2. Charcot arthropathy
3. Delayed compartment syndrome
4. Deep venous thrombosis
5. Gout

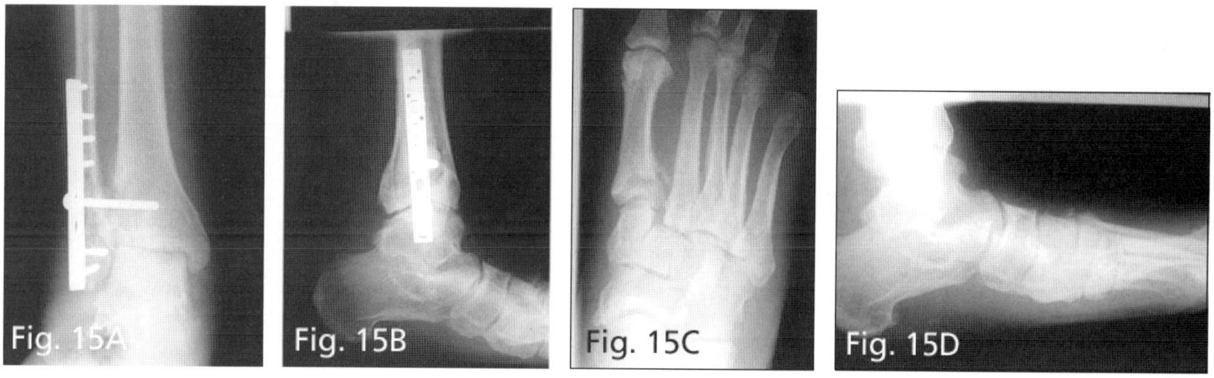

Q-36: What complication is frequently associated with the Weil lesser metatarsal osteotomy (distal, oblique) in the treatment of claw toe deformities?

1. Floating toe
2. Nonunion
3. Osteonecrosis
4. Inadequate shortening
5. Dorsal displacement

Q-37: A 77-year-old man with diabetes mellitus has had a nonhealing Wagner grade I ulcer under the medial sesamoid for the past 3 months. He smokes tobacco regularly. He has undergone several débridements and total contact casting. Examination reveals no palpable pulses. He has no erythema or purulence, and he is afebrile. Radiographs reveal no abnormalities. What is the best initial diagnostic test to help determine why the ulcer has failed to heal?

1. 5.07 Semmes-Weinstein monofilament
2. Bone scan
3. Thompson test
4. CT
5. Noninvasive vascular studies

Q-38: A 28-year-old man who sustained an ankle fracture in a motor vehicle accident underwent open reduction and internal fixation 3 months ago. He continues to report significant ankle pain with ambulation. Radiographs are shown in Figure 16. What is the next most appropriate step in management?

1. Articulated ankle-foot orthosis
2. Revision open reduction and internal fixation of the syndesmosis with débridement of the medial gutter
3. Ankle arthrodesis
4. Syndesmosis arthrodesis
5. Ankle arthroscopy and débridement

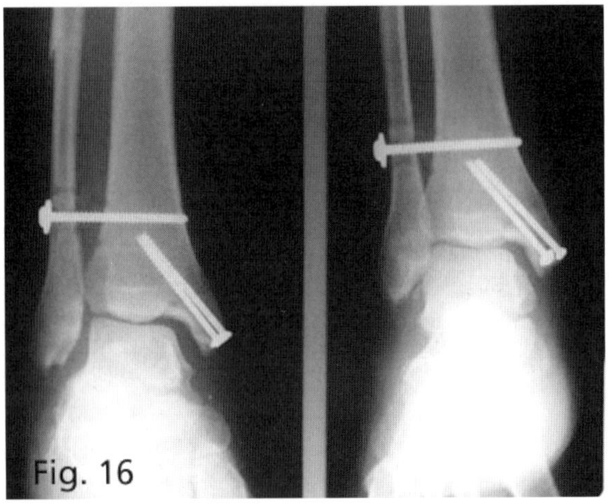
Fig. 16

Q-39: The radiograph shown in Figure 17 shows measurement of what angle?

1. Hallux valgus
2. Distal metatarsal articular
3. Intermetatarsal
4. Sesamoid divergence
5. Angle of joint congruence

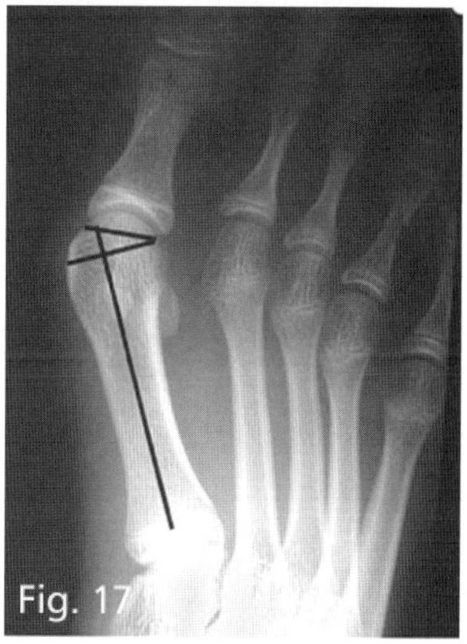

Fig. 17

Q-40: A 5-year-old boy has had midfoot pain with activity for the past 3 months. He has no pain at rest. Radiographs are shown in Figures 18A and 18B. Management should consist of

1. a vascularized pedicle bone graft.
2. a short leg walking cast.
3. a custom-molded orthotic.
4. surgical débridement followed by antibiotics.
5. a bone stimulator.

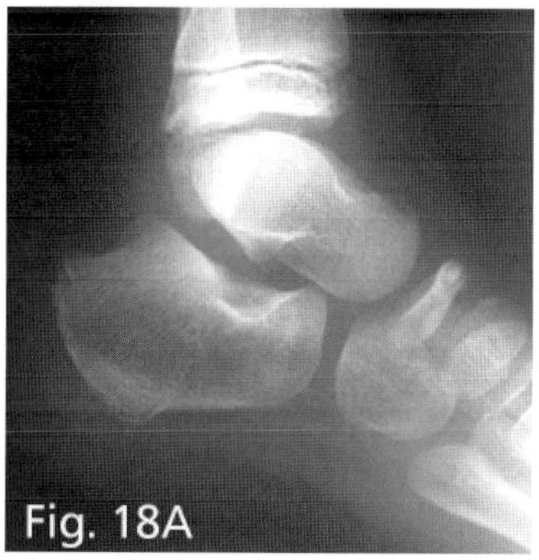

Fig. 18A

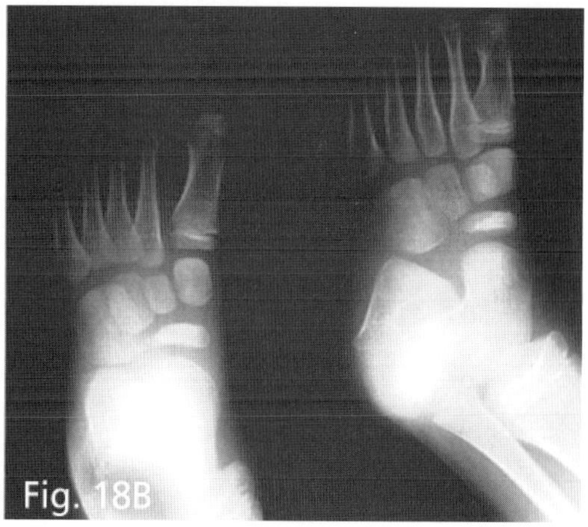

Fig. 18B

Q-41: A 62-year-old man with diabetes mellitus has had a persistent 2-cm ulcer under the third metatarsal head for the past 4 months. He reports that he has had similar ulcers twice before, and both healed with nonsurgical management. He has used multiple types of commercial walking braces, shoes, and commercial dressings without resolution. He is insensate to the 5.07 Semmes-Weinstein monofilament. When the wound is probed with culture swab, there is no communication with the metatarsal head. Radiographs, bone scans, and laboratory studies reveal no evidence of osteomyelitis. What is the most predictable method of accomplishing wound healing without recurrence?

1. Transmetatarsal amputation
2. Excision of the third metatarsal head
3. Percutaneous Achilles tendon lengthening and a total contact cast
4. Viral recombitant growth factor and a commercial removeable walking boot
5. A non–weight-bearing total contact cast that is changed every week until the ulcer is healed

Q-42: An 11-year-old boy stepped on a nail and sustained a puncture to the right forefoot 6 days ago. He was wearing tennis shoes at the time of injury. Treatment in the emergency department consisted of local débridement and tetanus prophylaxis; a radiograph was negative for foreign body, chondral defect, or fracture. He was discharged with a 3-day prescription of amoxicillin and clavulanate. The patient now has increasing pain and tenderness at the puncture site. What is the best course of action?

1. Change the antibiotic to ciprofloxacin
2. Initiate gentamicin
3. Resume the prescription for amoxicillin and clavulanate
4. Observation and follow-up in 48 hours
5. Surgical débridement

Q-43: A 20-year-old man who is an elite college football player has ecchymosis, swelling, and pain on the lateral side of his foot after a game. Radiographs are shown in Figures 19A through 19C. Management should consist of

1. open reduction and internal fixation with a plate and screws.
2. open treatment with calcaneal bone graft.
3. percutaneous screw fixation with a 4.5-mm screw.
4. weight-bearing cast for 8 weeks.
5. spanning external fixation.

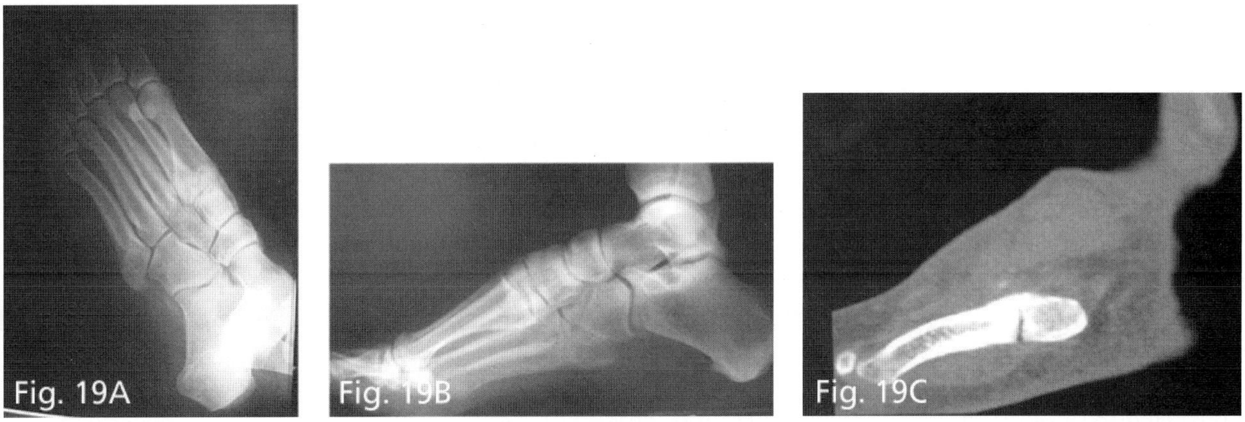

Fig. 19A Fig. 19B Fig. 19C

Q-44: A 55-year-old man who runs on the weekends reports a 1-year history of continued pain directly posteriorly in the heel. Management consisting of anti-inflammatory drugs, icing techniques, a heel-counter in his shoe split, and physical therapy consisting of stretching, contrast baths, custom orthotics, and iontophoresis has failed to provide relief. Not only is his lifestyle disrupted with respect to running, but he now has pain with normal ambulation with all forms of shoe wear. He is not necessarily concerned with returning to running; he is primarily seeking pain relief. A lateral radiograph and clinical photograph are shown in Figures 20A and 20B. Treatment should now consist of

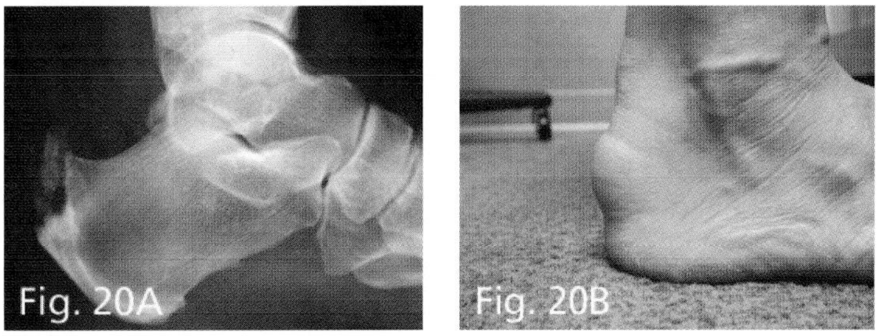

Fig. 20A Fig. 20B

1. injection directly into the tendon with triamcinolone or methylprednisolone.
2. shock wave therapy to the posterior heel to break up calcific deposits.
3. brisement.
4. a simple lateral surgical approach to the posterior heel, with resection of the Haglund exostosis.
5. a central-splitting surgical approach through the tendon, excision of the Haglund exostosis and the insertional calcifications, bursectomy, flexor hallucis longus tendon transfer to the posterior tuberosity, and attachment of the tendon to the calcaneus.

Q-45: Figures 21A and 21B show the clinical photographs of a 46-year-old woman who has a painful deformity of the second toe. Surgical treatment consisting of metatarsophalangeal capsulotomy and proximal interphalangeal joint resection arthroplasty resulted in satisfactory correction, but the toe remains unstable at the metatarsophalangeal joint. What is the most appropriate next step?

1. Flexor digitorum longus tenotomy
2. Resection of the metatarsal head and pin fixation
3. Transfer of the flexor digitorum longus to the extensor tendon
4. Excision at the base of the proximal phalanx and syndactyly with the third toe
5. Arthrodesis of the second metatarsophalangeal joint

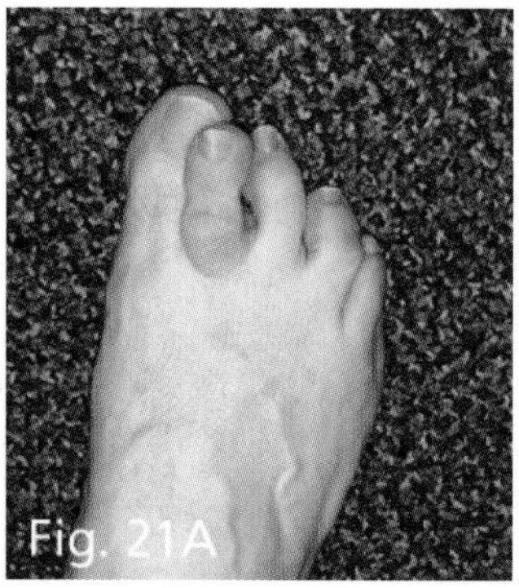
Fig. 21A

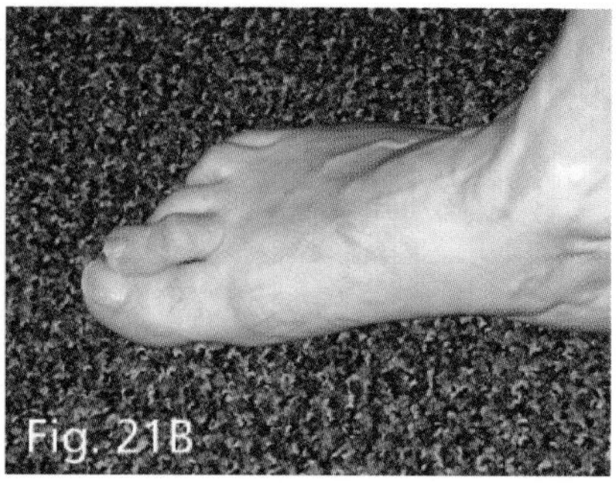
Fig. 21B

Q-46: A 40-year-old man fell 10 feet from a tree and sustained the closed isolated injury shown in Figures 22A and 22B. Management consists of splinting. At his 2-week follow-up visit, the patient clinically passes the wrinkle test. He agrees to open reduction and internal fixation. What is the best surgical approach to obtain anatomic reduction and limit wound dehiscence?

1. Closed reduction and percutaneous pinning
2. Open reduction and internal fixation with a lateral approach, extensile right-angled lateral incision, vertical limb 0.5 cm anterior to the Achilles tendon, and horizontal limb at the junction of the lateral skin and the plantar glabrous skin
3. Open reduction and internal fixation with a lateral approach, extensile right-angled lateral incision, vertical limb 2.0 cm anterior to the Achilles tendon, and horizontal limb 2.0 cm proximal to the line marking the plantar glabrous skin
4. Sinus tarsi approach
5. Ollier approach

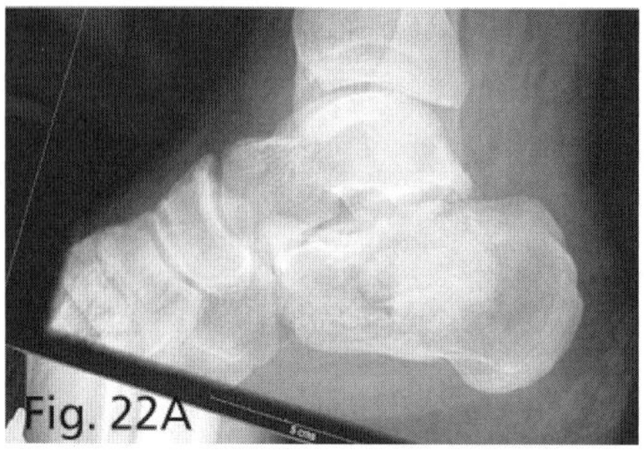
Fig. 22A

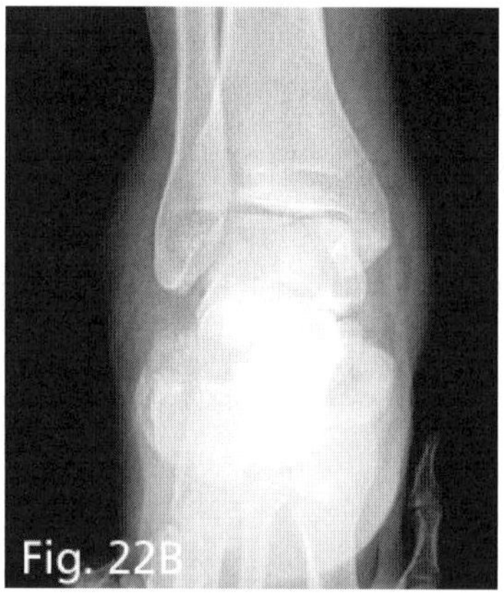
Fig. 22B

Q-47: A 17-year-old patient sustained a closed calcaneal fracture when he jumped off of a roof 2 years ago, and he underwent nonsurgical management at the time of injury. The patient now reports lateral hindfoot pain that is worse with weight-bearing activities. Anti-inflammatory drugs and orthoses have failed to provide relief. Coronal and sagittal CT scans are shown in Figures 23A and 23B. What is the best course of action?

1. In situ subtalar arthrodesis
2. Cortisone injection in the subtalar joint followed by casting for 4 to 6 weeks
3. UCBL insert
4. Lateral wall exostectomy
5. Bone block arthrodesis of the subtalar joint

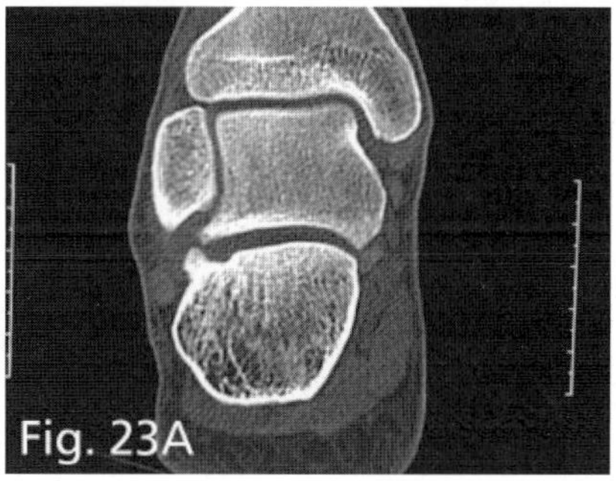

Fig. 23A

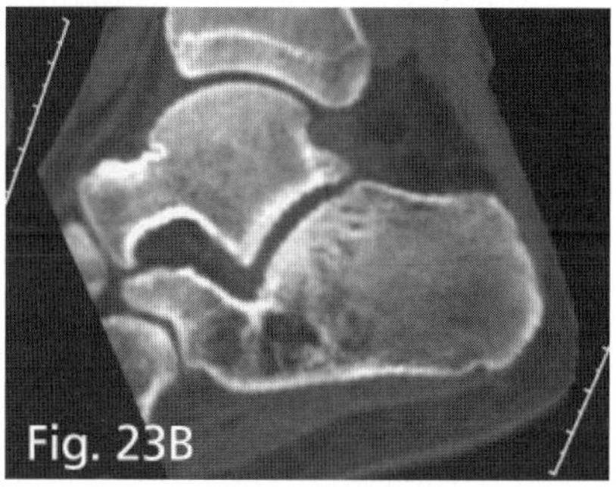

Fig. 23B

Q-48: Figures 24A and 24B show the clinical photographs of a 43-year-old patient with type I diabetes mellitus who has a stump ulcer after undergoing successful transtibial amputation 1 year ago. Which of the following is considered the most predictable method of healing the ulcer and preventing recurrent ulceration?

1. Refrain from using the prosthesis until the ulcer heals.
2. Refrain from using the prosthesis and apply platelet-derived growth factor daily until the ulcer heals.
3. Have a prosthetist relieve the area of the anterior-distal tibia to eliminate pressure and allow the ulcer to heal.
4. Replace the prosthetic socket liner with a thick silicone liner.
5. Perform a wedge resection of the infected tissue, create a soft-tissue envelope with muscle covering the bone, and allow primary healing of the skin.

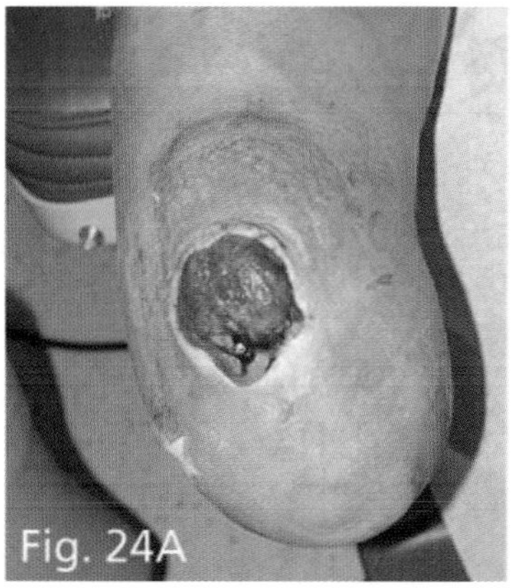

Fig. 24A

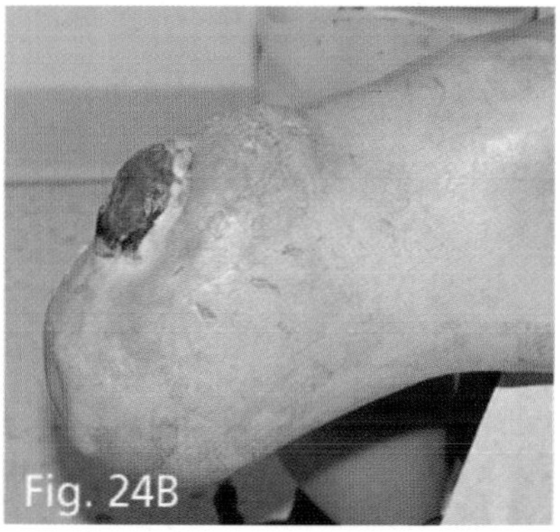

Fig. 24B

Q-49: The Coleman block test is used to evaluate the cavovarus foot. What is the most important information obtained from this test?

1. Determines the patient's ability to balance
2. Determines hindfoot flexibility
3. Determines forefoot flexibility
4. Assesses the patient for Achilles tendon contractures
5. Evaluates peroneus longus strength

Q-50: A 35-year-old woman has had significant pain and swelling in the left medial ankle inferior to the medial malleolus for the past 8 months. Physical therapy, brace and orthotic management, and immobilization have failed to provide relief. She is now requesting a more aggressive option to assist in pain relief. Clinical photographs and radiographs are seen in Figures 25A through 25F. Following exposure, a complete rupture of the posterior tibial tendon is visible. What is the most appropriate surgical reconstruction?

1. Subtalar arthrodesis
2. Flexor digitorum longus transfer
3. Flexor digitorum longus tendon transfer, medial slide calcaneal osteotomy, and spring ligament repair
4. Primary repair of the posterior tibial tendon
5. Talonavicular arthrodesis

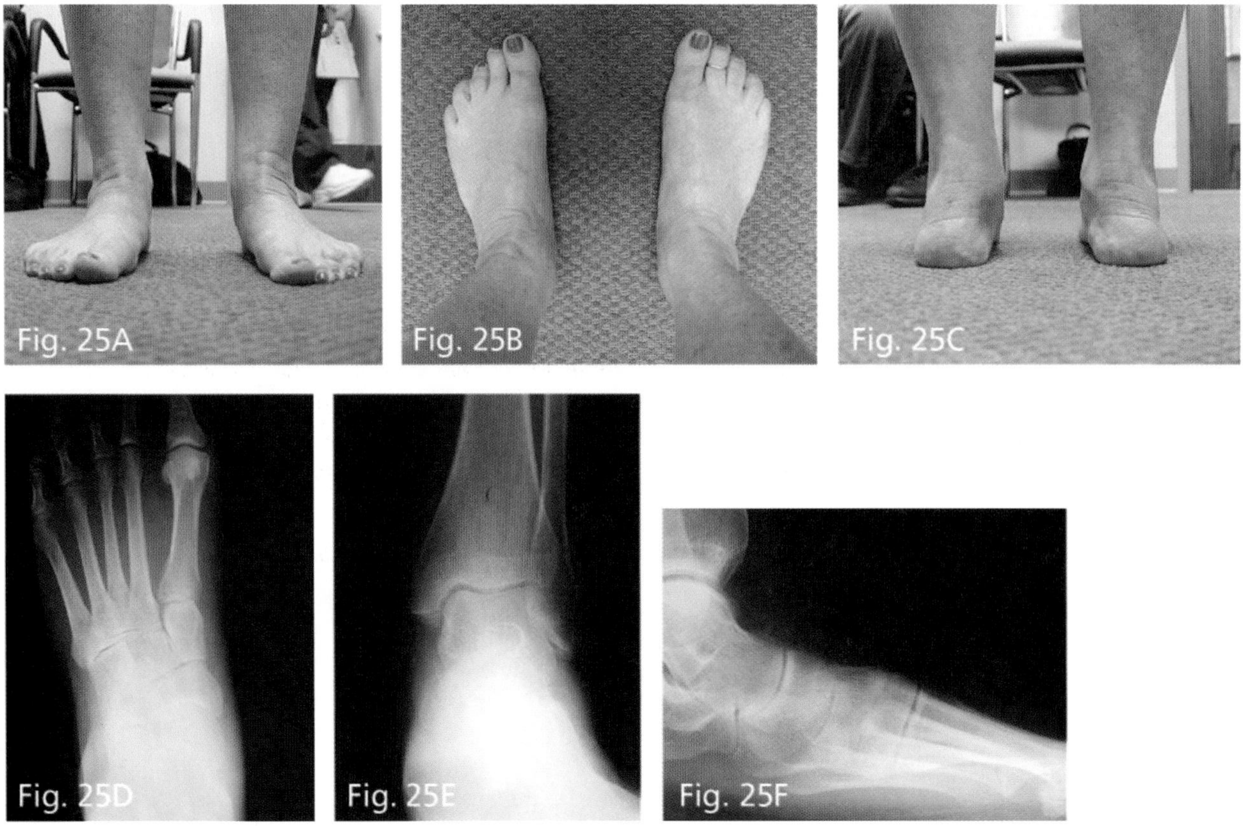

Fig. 25A Fig. 25B Fig. 25C

Fig. 25D Fig. 25E Fig. 25F

A-1: A 42-year-old man who works as an athletic trainer has a persistent popping sensation about the lateral ankle associated with weakness and pain following a remote injury. Deficiency in what structure directly leads to this pathology?

1. Lateral talar process
2. Superior peroneal retinaculum
3. Inferior peroneal retinaculum
4. Extensor retinaculum
5. Crural fascia

PREFERRED RESPONSE: 2

DISCUSSION: The patient has instability of the peroneal tendon. The superior peroneal retinaculum is the primary retaining structure preventing peroneal subluxation. It is a thickening of fascia that arises off the posterior margin of the distal 1 to 2 cm of the fibula and runs posteriorly to blend with the Achilles tendon sheath. The inferior peroneal retinaculum attaches to the peroneal tubercle of the calcaneus and is not involved in this pathology. A deficient groove in the posterior distal fibula may also be a contributing factor in the development of the condition.

REFERENCE: Maffuli N, Ferran NA, Oliva F, et al: Recurrent subluxation of the peroneal tendons. *Am J Sports Med* 2006;34:986-992.

A-2: Which of the following structures is most vulnerable during a medial sesamoidectomy of the hallux?

1. Abductor hallucis tendon
2. Intermetatarsal ligament
3. Plantar-medial cutaneous nerve of the hallux
4. Dorsomedial cutaneous nerve of the hallux
5. Crista

PREFERRED RESPONSE: 3

DISCUSSION: The plantar-medial cutaneous nerve is at risk with the surgical approach to the medial sesamoid. It is found directly underlying an incision made at the junction of the glabrous skin of the hallux and must be identified before the approach can proceed. Transection will result in a painful neuroma that impinges on the plantar-medial surface of the toe and cause problems with shoe wear. The only other structure that lies near the surgical field is the abductor hallucis tendon which lies dorsal to the incision.

REFERENCE: Sarrafian SK: *Anatomy of the Foot and Ankle, Descriptive, Topographic, Functional*, ed 2. Philadelphia, PA, JB Lippincott, 1993, p 377.

A-3: A 30-year-old man who sustained a tibial fracture with a peroneal nerve palsy 2 years ago now has footdrop and weak eversion of the foot. He reports success with stretching exercises, but he catches his toes when his foot tires. Examination reveals that the foot is plantigrade and supple. What is the most appropriate next step in management?

1. Posterior tibial tendon transfer to the cuboid
2. Anterior tibial tendon transfer to the cuboid
3. Achilles tendon lengthening
4. Ankle-foot orthosis with dorsiflexion assist
5. Nerve grafting

PREFERRED RESPONSE: 4

DISCUSSION: The patient has a supple plantigrade foot that would benefit from a footdrop brace to prevent catching of the toes. Tendon transfer should not be considered until the patient has undergone bracing. Achilles tendon lengthening is not necessary because the foot is plantigrade and flexible. Nerve grafting is not indicated because of the length of time the peroneal nerve palsy has been present.

REFERENCES: Dehne R: Congenital and acquired neurologic disorders, in Mann RA, Coughlin MJ, eds: *Surgery of the Foot and Ankle*, ed 7. St. Louis, MO, Mosby, 1999, vol 1, pp 552-553.

Santi MD, Botte MJ: Nerve injury and repair in the foot and ankle. *Foot Ankle Int* 1996;17:425-439.

A-4: Removal of both hallucal sesamoids should be reserved as a salvage procedure because of the high incidence of which of the following postoperative complications?

1. Hallux rigidus
2. Hallux varus
3. Flexion contracture of the hallux metatarsophalangeal joint
4. Persistent neuritic pain
5. Cock-up deformity of the great toe and hallux valgus

PREFERRED RESPONSE: 5

DISCUSSION: Removal of both sesamoids is associated with a high incidence of postoperative hallux valgus and cock-up deformity of the great toe because of weakening of the flexor hallucis brevis tendon. The sesamoids lie within these tendons and require meticulous repair following excision.

REFERENCES: Padanilam TG: Disorders of the first ray, in Richardson EG, ed: *Orthopaedic Knowledge Update: Foot and Ankle*, ed 3. Rosemont, IL, American Academy of Orthopaedic Surgeons, 2003, pp 17-25.

Richardson EG: Hallucal sesamoid pain: Causes and surgical treatment. *J Am Acad Orthop Surg* 1999;7:270-278.

A-5: A 63-year-old woman with a history of poliomyelitis has a fixed 30° equinus contracture of the ankle, rigid hindfoot valgus, and normal knee strength and stability. She reports persistent pain and has had several medial forefoot ulcerations despite a program of stretching, bracing, and custom footwear. What is the most appropriate next step in management?

1. Charcot restraint orthotic walker
2. Hyperbaric oxygen treatment
3. Triple arthrodesis with Achilles tendon lengthening
4. Transtibial amputation
5. Ankle arthrodesis

PREFERRED RESPONSE: 3

DISCUSSION: The patient has a fixed deformity of the hindfoot and an Achilles tendon contracture; therefore, the treatment of choice is triple arthrodesis with Achilles tendon lengthening. Further bracing will not be helpful. Amputation is not indicated, and ankle arthrodesis will not address the hindfoot deformity. Palliative management would be more appropriate if the knee was unstable or the quadriceps were weak, because the equinus balances the ground reaction force across the knee.

REFERENCES: Perry J, Fontaine JD, Mulroy S: Findings in post-poliomyelitis syndrome: Weakness of muscles of the calf as a source of late pain and fatigue of muscles of the thigh after poliomyelitis. *J Bone Joint Surg Am* 1995;77:1148-1153.

Dehne R: Congenital and acquired neurologic disorders, in Mann RA, Coughlin MJ, eds: *Surgery of the Foot and Ankle*, ed 7. St. Louis, MO, Mosby, 1999, vol 1, pp 552-553.

A-6: What is the most common foot deformity associated with myelomeningocele?

1. Talipes equinovarus
2. Congenital vertical talus
3. Calcaneus valgus
4. Calcaneus varus
5. Cavus

PREFERRED RESPONSE: 1

DISCUSSION: All of the above conditions can be associated with myelomeningocele, but talipes equinovarus occurs in 50% to 90% of patients with myelomeningocele. Congenital vertical talus is rarely associated with any neuromuscular diseases other than myelomeningocele but is not the most common deformity in myelomeningocele.

REFERENCES: Stans AA, Kehl DK: The pediatric foot, in Baratz ME, Watson AD, Imbriglia JE, eds: *Orthopaedic Surgery: The Essentials*. New York, NY, Thieme, 1999, pp 702-703.

Lindseth RE: Myelomeningocele, in Morrissy RT, Weinstein SL, eds: *Lovell and Winter's Pediatric Orthopaedics*, ed 5. Philadelphia, PA, Lippincott, Williams & Wilkins, 2001, pp 622-628.

A-7: Where is the watershed zone for tarsal navicular vascularity?

1. Medial one third
2. Central one third
3. Lateral one third
4. Tuberosity
5. Inferior pole

PREFERRED RESPONSE: 2

DISCUSSION: The central one third has been established as the watershed zone by angiographic studies, and has been borne out in clinical conditions involving the navicular, such as stress fractures and osteonecrosis. These findings account for the susceptibility to injury at this level.

REFERENCES: Haidukewych GJ: Osteonecrosis of the navicular, in Nunley JA, Pfeffer GB, Sanders RW, Trepman E, eds: *Advanced Reconstruction: Foot and Ankle.* Rosemont, IL, American Academy of Orthopaedic Surgeons, 2004, pp 239-242.

Sarrafian SK: *Anatomy of the Foot and Ankle.* Philadelphia, PA, JB Lippincott, 1983, pp 299-302.

A-8: A 37-year-old woman has had intermittent paresthesias and numbness in the plantar foot for the past 6 months. She reports that the symptoms are worse with activity, and the paresthesias are beginning to awaken her at night. MRI scans are shown in Figures 1A and 1B. What is the most likely diagnosis?

1. Lipoma
2. Giant cell tumor of the tendon sheath
3. Synovial sarcoma
4. Metastatic adenocarcinoma
5. Ganglion cyst

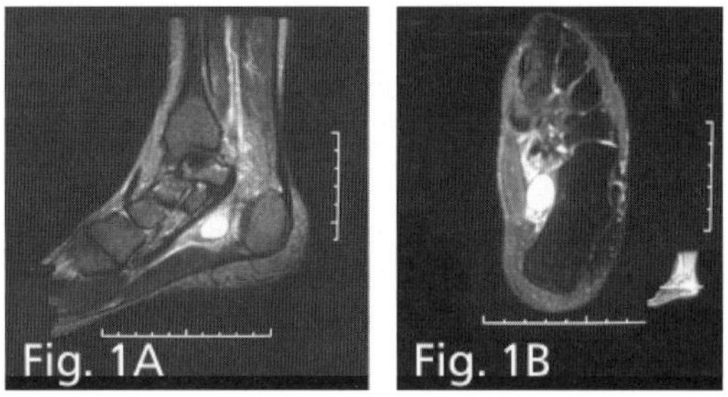

Fig. 1A Fig. 1B

PREFERRED RESPONSE: 5

DISCUSSION: The symptoms are consistent with tarsal tunnel syndrome. Ganglion cysts are a well-known cause of tarsal tunnel syndrome. The MRI scans show a high intensity, well-circumscribed mass in the tarsal tunnel that is consistent with a fluid-filled cyst. Patients usually respond well to excision of the ganglion and resolution of the tarsal tunnel symptoms. The surrounding fat is a different signal intensity on the MRI scans, which rules out a lipoma. Synovial cell sarcoma has a heterogeneous appearance on an MRI scan. Metastatic tumors are most commonly found in the osseous structures of the foot, not the soft tissues.

REFERENCES: Rozbruch SR, Chang V, Bohne WH, et al: Ganglion cysts of the lower extremity: An analysis of 54 cases and review of the literature. *Orthopedics* 1998;21:141-148.

Llauger J, Palmer J, Monill JM, et al: MR imaging of benign soft-tissue masses of the foot and ankle. *Radiographics* 1998;18:1481-1498.

Takakura Y, Kitada C, Sugimoto K, et al: Tarsal tunnel syndrome: Causes and results of operative treatment. *J Bone Joint Surg Br* 1991;73:125-128.

A-9: Figure 2 shows the CT scan of a 25-year-old man who plays soccer who has had posterior ankle pain with plantar flexion for the past 2 years. Immobilization has failed to provide relief. He is ambulatory. Management should consist of

1. a local steroid injection into the flexor hallucis longus tendon sheath.
2. range-of-motion exercises.
3. open reduction and internal fixation.
4. NSAIDs.
5. excision of the fragment.

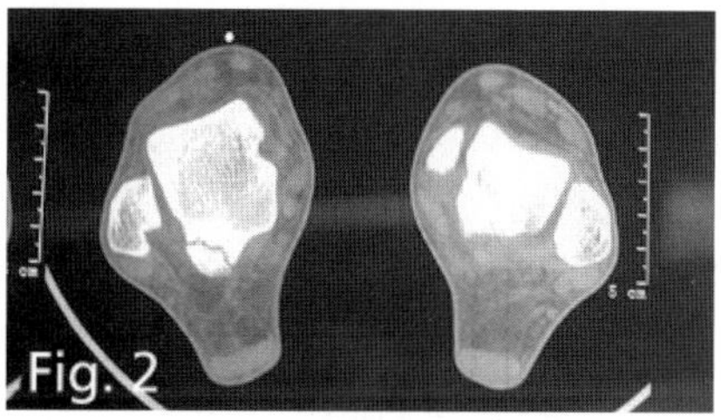
Fig. 2

PREFERRED RESPONSE: 5

DISCUSSION: An os trigonum is usually asymptomatic, but this accessory bone has been associated with persistent posterior ankle pain, which has been described as os trigonum syndrome. This usually affects athletes and ballerinas. Forced plantar flexion leads to impingement of the os trigonum against the posterior tibial plafond, and flexor hallucis tendinitis may develop. It may be difficult to differentiate a fractured trigonal process from the os trigonum. MRI may reveal bone marrow edema that may aid in the diagnosis of os trigonum syndrome. Steroid injections may lead to tendon rupture. The results of excision of a symptomatic os trigonum through a posteromedial or lateral approach are favorable, with a rapid return to full function. The main complication of this procedure is sural nerve injury with a lateral approach.

REFERENCES: Hedrick MR, McBryde AM: Posterior ankle impingement. *Foot Ankle Int* 1994;15:2-8.

Abramowitz Y, Wollstein R, Barzilay Y, et al: Outcome of resection of a symptomatic os trigonum. *J Bone Joint Surg Am* 2003;85:1051-1057.

A-10: Figure 3 shows the CT scan of an 11-year-old boy who has had a 1-year history of worsening painful flatfeet. He reports pain associated with physical education at school, especially with running and jumping. Management consisting of activity restriction, anti-inflammatory drugs, and casting has failed to provide relief. Treatment should now consist of

1. a subtalar arthroereisis with a titanium implant.
2. triple arthrodesis.
3. resection of the accessory navicular and advancement of the posterior tibial tendon bilaterally.
4. resection of the talocalcaneal middle facet coalition in each foot.
5. resection of the calcaneonavicular coalition in both feet.

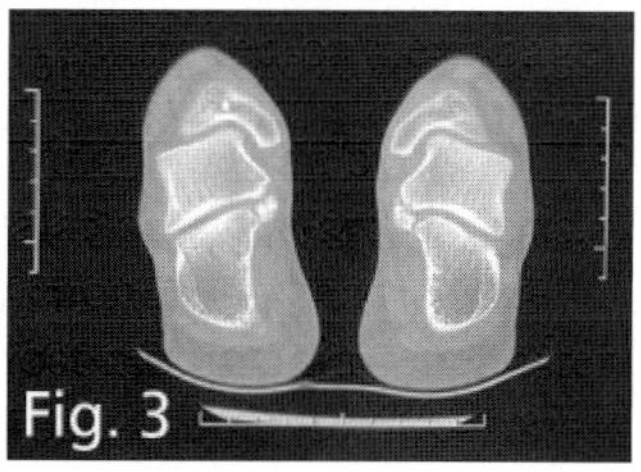
Fig. 3

PREFERRED RESPONSE: 4

DISCUSSION: In most patients with symptomatic talocalcaneal coalition involving less than 50% of the subtalar joint, resection with fat graft interposition is preferred over a subtalar or triple arthrodesis, especially if reasonable range of motion can be achieved. This patient has a synchondrosis that is partially cartilaginous. Although patients may have a residual gait abnormality, most report pain relief after surgery.

(continued on next page)

(A-10: *continued*)

REFERENCES: Scranton PE Jr: Treatment of symptomatic talocalcaneal coalition. *J Bone Joint Surg Am* 1987;69: 533-539.

Kitaoka HB, Wikenheiser MA, Schaughnessy WJ, et al: Gait abnormalities following resection of talocalcaneal coalition. *J Bone Joint Surg Am* 1997;79:369-374.

Vincent KA: Tarsal coalition and painful flatfoot. *J Am Acad Orthop Surg* 1998;6:274-281.

A-11: What is the optimum position of immobilization of the foot and ankle immediately after Achilles tendon repair to maximize skin perfusion?

1. 10° of dorsiflexion
2. 10° of plantar flexion
3. 20° of plantar flexion
4. Neutral
5. Resting equinus

PREFERRED RESPONSE: 3

DISCUSSION: Achilles tendon tension is not affected by knee position when the ankle is in 20° to 25° of plantar flexion. Skin perfusion overlying the Achilles tendon is maximal in 20° of plantar flexion and is reduced beyond 20° of plantar flexion. Neutral flexion or any amount of dorsiflexion compromises the repair.

REFERENCE: Poynton AR, O'Rourke K: An analysis of skin perfusion over the Achilles tendon in varying degrees of plantar flexion. *Foot Ankle Int* 2001;22:572-574.

A-12: A 32-year-old man who sustained a tarsometatarsal (Lisfranc) injury 3 years ago now reports increasing pain in the left foot. Orthotics, NSAIDs, and injections have provided only temporary relief. Examination reveals swelling and tenderness over the tarsometatarsal joints. Radiographs show advanced arthrosis of the first and second tarsometatarsal joints. Management should now include

1. midfoot arthrodesis.
2. a rocker sole shoe with orthotic inserts.
3. shock wave therapy or orthotripsy.
4. an ankle-foot orthosis.
5. triple arthrodesis.

PREFERRED RESPONSE: 1

DISCUSSION: The patient has advanced arthrosis of the midfoot, and orthotic management has failed to provide relief. Therefore, the treatment of choice is midfoot arthrodesis. Shock wave therapy has not been shown to be beneficial for arthritis. An ankle-foot orthosis would not be appropriate based on findings of a normal ankle joint. Triple arthrodesis would not be helpful because the hindfoot joint is not affected in a Lisfranc injury.

(continued on next page)

(A-12: *continued*)

REFERENCES: Sangeorzan BJ, Veith GR, Hansen ST Jr: Salvage of Lisfranc's tarsometatarsal joints by arthrodesis. *Foot Ankle* 1990;10:193-200.

Komenda GA, Myerson MS, Biddinger KR: Results of arthrodesis of the tarsometatarsal joints after traumatic injury. *J Bone Joint Surg Am* 1996;78:1665-1676.

A-13: An 11-year-old girl has had pain in the medial arch of her foot for the past 3 months. She reports that pain is present even with daily activities such as walking to class at school, and ibuprofen provides some relief. She denies any history of trauma. Examination reveals a flexible pes planus with focal tenderness over a prominent tarsal navicular tuberosity. Radiographs show a prominent accessory navicular. Management should consist of

1. cast immobilization for 4 to 6 weeks.
2. posterior tibial tendon advancement and repair (Kidner procedure).
3. corticosteroid injection of the posterior tibial tendon insertion.
4. triple arthrodesis.
5. needle biopsy of the trochar.

PREFERRED RESPONSE: 1

DISCUSSION: The patient has the classic symptoms, examination findings, and radiographs for a painful accessory navicular. Initial treatment should always be nonsurgical, specifically cast immobilization. Surgery should be reserved for those patients in whom nonsurgical management has failed. Corticosteroids should not be injected into a posterior tibial tendon or insertion point because they can weaken the tendon and possibly cause tendon rupture. Triple arthrodesis and biopsy have no role in the management of a painful accessory navicular.

REFERENCE: Bordelon RL: Flatfoot in children and young adults, in Coughlin MJ, Mann RA, eds: *Surgery of the Foot and Ankle*, ed 6. St. Louis, MO, Mosby, 1993, pp 717-756.

A-14: Figures 4A and 4B show the radiographs of a 28-year-old woman who sustained a head injury and a closed injury, without soft-tissue compromise, to her right lower extremity in a motor vehicle accident. Appropriate management of the foot injury should include

1. external fixation with a circular frame.
2. open reduction and internal fixation with screws.
3. closed reduction and percutaneous pinning.
4. closed reduction and cast immobilization.
5. amputation.

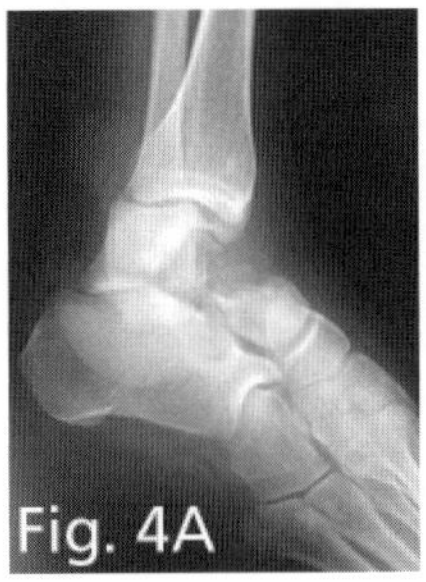
Fig. 4A

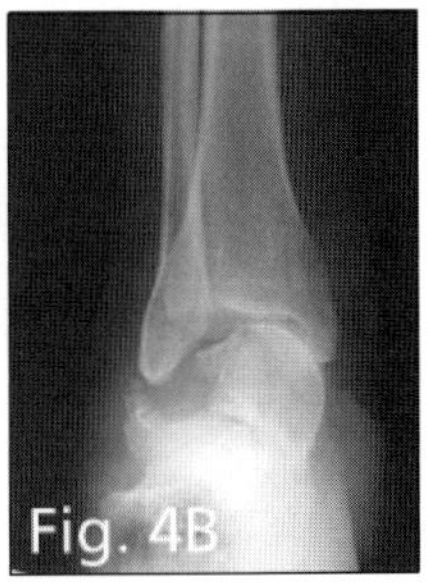
Fig. 4B

PREFERRED RESPONSE: 2

DISCUSSION: The displaced talar neck fracture should be treated with open reduction and internal fixation using screws. Closed reduction and casting will not maintain position, and percutaneous pinning is not able to maintain reduction to allow union. External fixation and amputation are not necessary for this injury unless there is severe soft-tissue loss.

REFERENCE: Adelaar RS: Fractures of the talus. *Instr Course Lect* 1990;39:147-156.

A-15: An active 47-year-old woman with rheumatoid arthritis reports forefoot pain and deformity and has difficulty with shoe wear. Examination reveals hallux valgus and claw toes. A radiograph is shown in Figure 5. What is the most appropriate surgical treatment?

1. Distal chevron osteotomy bunionectomy with lesser metatarsal head resections
2. Proximal first metatarsal osteotomy with flexor-to-extensor tendon transfer for the lesser toes
3. First metatarsophalangeal arthrodesis with lesser metatarsal head resections
4. First tarsometatarsal realignment arthrodesis (Lapidus procedure) with flexor-to-extensor tendon transfer for the lesser toes
5. Resection of the base of the hallux proximal phalanx (Keller procedure) with flexor-to-extensor tendon transfer for the lesser toes

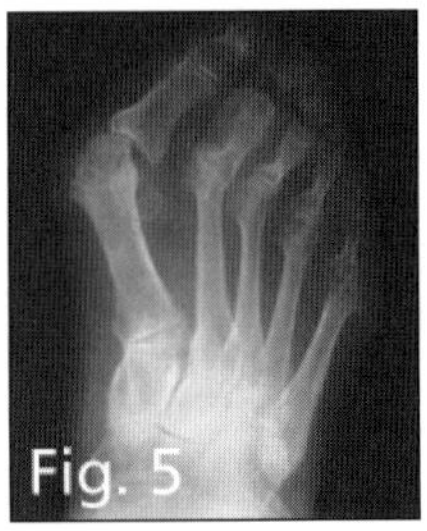
Fig. 5

PREFERRED RESPONSE: 3

DISCUSSION: Rheumatoid arthritis commonly affects the metatarsophalangeal joints, which become destabilized with time resulting in hallux valgus and dislocated lesser claw toes. The result is metatarsalgia as the dislocated claw toes "pull" the fat pad distally. Severe hallux valgus reduces first ray load, which compounds the metatarsalgia because the load is transferred to the lesser metatarsal heads. First metatarsophalangeal arthrodesis restores weight bearing medially and corrects the painful bunion. Metatarsal head resection slackens the toe tendons to allow correction of the claw toes by whatever means necessary and decreases plantar load over the forefoot. Rheumatoid arthritis in the first metatarsophalangeal joint will continue to progress if osteotomies or a Lapidus procedure are performed. Keller resection arthroplasty increases transfer metatarsalgia and reduces push-off power during gait. Flexor-to-extensor tendon transfer of the lesser toes does not address the metatarsalgia and does not correct the dislocation of the metatarsophalangeal joint.

REFERENCES: Coughlin MJ: Arthritides, in Coughlin MJ, Mann RA, eds: *Surgery of the Foot and Ankle*, ed 7. St. Louis, MO, Mosby, 1999, p 572.

Abdo RV, Iorio LJ: Rheumatoid arthritis of the foot and ankle. *J Am Acad Orthop Surg* 1994;2:326-332.

A-16: A 32-year-old woman has left second toe dactylitis (sausage toe). Radiographs show a "pencil in cup" distal interphalangeal joint deformity. Examination reveals that subtalar motion is markedly reduced. What is the most likely diagnosis?

1. Rheumatoid arthritis
2. Lyme disease
3. Psoriatic arthritis
4. Crohn disease arthropathy
5. Gout

PREFERRED RESPONSE: 3

DISCUSSION: The patient's clinical picture is considered the classic presentation for psoriatic arthritis. The other answers are not applicable for the constellation of findings.

REFERENCES: Jahss MH: *Disorders of the Foot and Ankle*, ed 2. Philadelphia, PA, WB Saunders, 1991, pp 1691-1693.

Juliano PJ: Arthritis of the midfoot and forefoot, in Richardson EG, ed: *Orthopaedic Knowledge Update: Foot and Ankle*, ed 3. Rosemont, IL, American Academy of Orthopaedic Surgeons, 2004, pp 172-173.

A-17: Which of the following is considered the most common infectious organism causing osteochondritis in pediatric puncture wounds of the foot?

1. *Eikenella corrodens*
2. *Pseudomonas aeruginosa*
3. *Pasteurella multocida*
4. *Serratia marcescens*
5. *Proteus mirabilis*

PREFERRED RESPONSE: 2

DISCUSSION: Pseudomonas aeruginosa is the most common infectious organism causing osteochondritis in pediatric puncture wounds of the foot. Eikenella corrodens is found in human bites, and Pasteurella multocida is characteristically seen with animal bites. Serratia marcescens and Proteus mirabilis have been reported but are much less likely.

REFERENCES: Jacobs RF, Adelman L, Sack CM, et al: Management of pseudomonas osteochondritis complicating puncture wounds of the foot. *Pediatrics* 1982;69:432-435.

Donati NL Jr: Deformities of the lesser toes and metatarsophalangeal joint disorders, in Mizel MS, Miller RA, Scioli MW, eds: *Orthopaedic Knowledge Update: Foot and Ankle*, ed 2. Rosemont, IL, American Academy of Orthopaedic Surgeons, 1998, pp 171-172.

A-18: Figure 6 shows the clinical photograph of a 66-year-old man who has had an increasingly painful right foot deformity for the past 3 years. Examination reveals that the subtalar joint is fixed in 15° of valgus, and forefoot supination can be corrected to 10° from neutral. Nonsurgical management has failed to provide relief. Treatment should now consist of

1. medial sliding calcaneal osteotomy with flexor digitorum longus (FDL) transfer.
2. isolated subtalar arthrodesis.
3. isolated talonavicular arthrodesis.
4. triple arthrodesis.
5. subtalar arthroereisis.

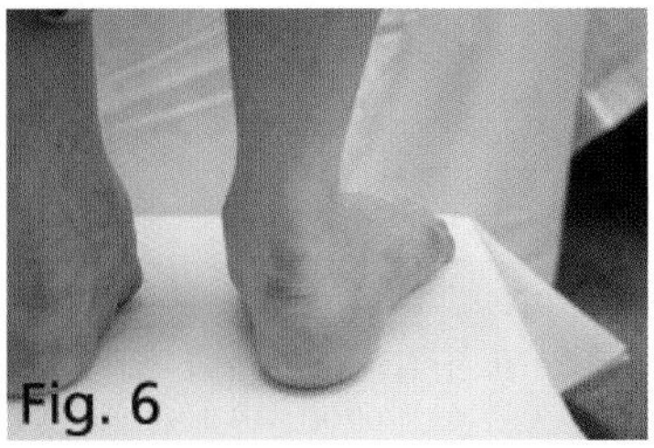
Fig. 6

PREFERRED RESPONSE: 4

DISCUSSION: The most important determining factor for correction of an adult flatfoot without an arthrodesis is the flexibility of the subtalar and transverse tarsal joints. Rigid deformities cannot be corrected with a medial sliding calcaneal osteotomy with FDL transfer or a subtalar arthroereisis. Isolated subtalar or talonavicular arthrodesis does not correct the deformities entirely. If the patient has forefoot supination that can be corrected to less than 7°, an isolated subtalar fusion is a possible alternative.

REFERENCE: Mann RA: Flatfoot in adults, in Coughlin MJ, Mann RA, eds: *Surgery of the Foot and Ankle*, ed 6. St. Louis, MO, Mosby, 1993, pp 757-784.

A-19: When evaluating a patient with hallux rigidus, what is the most important clinical factor indicating the need for an arthrodesis as opposed to a cheilectomy?

1. Dorsal foot pain with shoe wear
2. Pronounced limited motion in the first metatarsophalangeal joint
3. Pain at the midrange of motion in the first metatarsophalangeal joint
4. Large dorsal osteophytes clinically and radiographically
5. Flattened first metatarsal head with periarticular sclerosis

PREFERRED RESPONSE: 3

DISCUSSION: Cheilectomy has been shown to provide satisfactory pain relief and improved function in long-term studies. It is important to select patients appropriately when choosing a cheilectomy versus an arthrodesis. Pain at the midrange of motion and loss of more than 50% of the metatarsal head cartilage are predictors of a poor outcome following cheilectomy, and these patients should receive an arthrodesis.

REFERENCES: Coughlin MJ, Shurnas PS: Hallux rigidus: Grading and long-term results of operative treatment. *J Bone Joint Surg Am* 2003;85:2072-2088.

Easley ME, Davis WH, Anderson RB: Intermediate to long-term follow-up of medial-approach dorsal cheilectomy for hallux rigidus. *Foot Ankle Int* 1999;20:147-152.

A-20: A patient who has recalcitrant medial plantar heel pain and pain directly over the medial side of the heel undergoes open release of the plantar fascia. After releasing a portion of the plantar fascia, the deep fascia of the abductor hallucis muscle is released to relieve pressure on which of the following structures?

1. Lateral plantar artery
2. Tibial nerve
3. First branch of the lateral plantar nerve
4. Sural nerve
5. Flexor hallucis brevis muscle

PREFERRED RESPONSE: 3

DISCUSSION: The deep fascia of the abductor hallucis muscle is released to relieve pressure on the first branch of the lateral plantar nerve. The tibial nerve lies more proximal to this area. The medial plantar nerve has already passed dorsally and medially, whereas the sural nerve lies on the lateral side of the foot. The flexor hallucis brevis muscle lies deep to the plantar fascia, not the abductor fascia.

REFERENCES: Baxter DE, Pfeffer GB: Treatment of chronic heel pain by surgical release of the first branch of the lateral plantar nerve. *Clin Orthop* 1992;279:229-236.

Davies MS, Weiss GA, Saxby TS: Plantar fasciitis: How successful is surgical intervention? *Foot Ankle Int* 1999;20: 803-807.

A-21: A 47-year-old woman has a painful bunion of the right foot, and shoe wear modifications have failed to provide relief. Examination reveals a severe hallux valgus with dorsal subluxation of the second toe. Radiographs are shown in Figures 7A and 7B. The most appropriate management should include

1. hallux metatarsophalangeal arthrodesis.
2. custom orthotics.
3. chevron osteotomy with second toe correction.
4. Keller resection arthroplasty with second toe correction.
5. proximal metatarsal osteotomy with second toe correction.

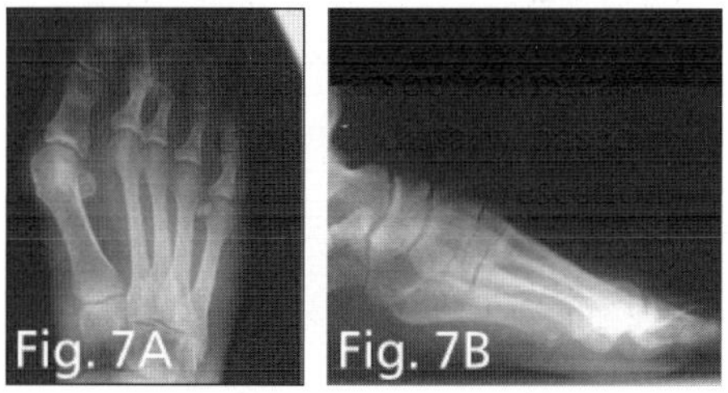

Fig. 7A Fig. 7B

PREFERRED RESPONSE: 5

DISCUSSION: The radiographs do not show significant arthrosis of the hallux metatarsophalangeal joint; therefore, arthrodesis is unnecessary. Orthotics will not correct the deformity. A distally based osteotomy will not achieve sufficient correction of the incongruity of deformity, and a Keller resection is not indicated in the younger population. The treatment of choice is a proximal metatarsal osteotomy with second toe correction.

REFERENCE: Mann RA, Rudicel S, Graves SC: Repair of hallux valgus with a distal soft-tissue procedure and proximal metatarsal osteotomy: A long-term follow-up. *J Bone Joint Surg Am* 1992;74:124-129.

A-22: What is the most appropriate orthosis for hallux rigidus?

1. Morton extension
2. Metatarsal arch pad
3. Full-length semirigid longitudinal arch support
4. Full-length semirigid longitudinal arch support with medial hindfoot posting
5. Full-length semirigid longitudinal arch support with lateral forefoot posting

PREFERRED RESPONSE: 1

DISCUSSION: A Morton extension limits excursion of the first metatarsophalangeal joint. It also functions as a ground reaction stabilizer during the toe-off phase of gait and thus reduces torque and joint reaction force at the first metatarsophalangeal joint. The metatarsal arch pad and full-length semirigid longitudinal arch support may help by dorsiflexing the first metatarsal relative to the phalanx and thus decompress the first metatarsophalangeal joint. However, they are not as biomechanically effective as the Morton extension. Both medial hindfoot and lateral forefoot posting are contraindicated because they increase ground reaction at the first metatarsophalangeal joint.

REFERENCES: Coughlin MJ: Arthritides, in Coughlin MJ, Mann RA, eds: *Surgery of the Foot and Ankle*, ed 7. St. Louis, MO, Mosby, 1999, p 611.

Watson AD, Wapner KL: Foot and ankle reconstruction, in Baratz ME, Watson AD, Imbriglia JE, eds: *Orthopaedic Surgery: The Essentials*. New York, NY, Thieme, 1999, p 635.

A-23: Figures 8A through 8C show the radiographs of a 23-year-old man who plays football and who was injured when another player fell on his flexed and planted foot. He reports severe pain in the midfoot with a feeling of numbness on the dorsum of the foot, and he is unable to bear weight on the limb. Examination reveals mild swelling. Management should consist of

1. casting.
2. closed reduction, casting, and no weight bearing for 6 weeks.
3. open reduction and internal fixation.
4. closed reduction and percutaneous Kirschner wire fixation.
5. closed reduction and percutaneous screw fixation.

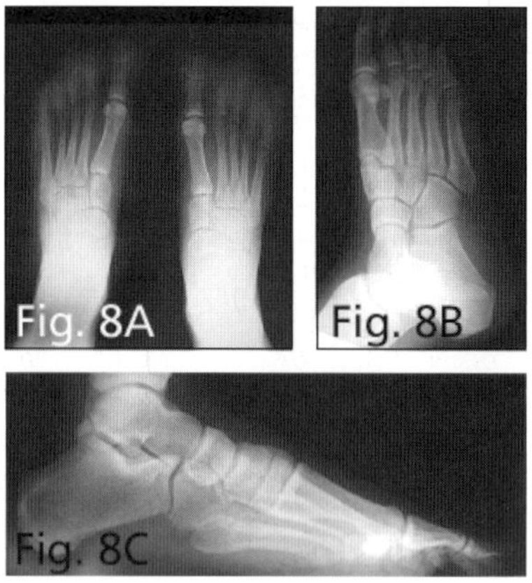

PREFERRED RESPONSE: 3

DISCUSSION: Myerson and associates studied the outcomes of 19 patients with tarsometatarsal joint injuries during athletic activity. Injuries were classified as first- or second-degree sprains of the tarsometatarsal joint or a third-degree sprain with diastasis between the metatarsals or cuneiforms. Poor functional results were seen in those with a delay in diagnosis and with inadequate treatment. For patients with third-degree sprains, poor results were obtained with nonsurgical management. These patients required open reduction and internal fixation for optimal return to function. The anatomic reduction is critical to the outcome; therefore, open reduction is preferred.

REFERENCES: Baxter DE: *The Foot and Ankle in Sport*. St. Louis, MO, Mosby, 1995, pp 107-123.

Curtis MJ, Myerson M, Szura B: Tarsometatarsal joint injuries in the athlete. *Am J Sports Med* 1993;21:497-502.
Kuo RS, Tejwani NC, DiGiovanni CW, et al: Outcome after open reduction and internal fixation of Lisfranc joint injuries. *J Bone Joint Surg Am* 2000;82:1609-1618.

Thompson MC, Mormino MA: Injury to the tarsometatarsal joint complex. *J Am Acad Orthop Surg* 2003;11:260-267.

A-24: Which of the following methods best aids in diagnosis of an interdigital neuroma?

1. Ultrasound
2. MRI
3. Web space injection
4. Electromyography and nerve conduction velocity studies
5. History and physical examination

PREFERRED RESPONSE: 5

DISCUSSION: History and physical examination are still the gold standard for diagnosis of an interdigital neuroma. Ultrasound and MRI may be helpful adjuncts but are dependent on equipment and operator expertise. Web space injection may be helpful for diagnostic and therapeutic purposes. Electromyography and nerve conduction velocity studies are of little benefit for distal lesions.

REFERENCES: Chao W: Interdigital neuroma and tarsal tunnel syndrome, in Richardson EG, ed: *Orthopaedic Knowledge Update: Foot and Ankle*, ed 3. Rosemont, IL, American Academy of Orthopaedic Surgeons, 2004, pp 145-147.

Bennett GL, Graham CE, Mauldin DM: Morton's interdigital neuroma: A comprehensive treatment protocol. *Foot Ankle Int* 1995;16:760-763.

A-25: A 58-year-old man has had a 3-year history of recurrent ulcerations of the left ankle and instability despite multiple attempts at custom bracing, contact casting, and surgical débridement. He has an ankle-brachial index of 0.76. A clinical photograph and radiographs are shown in Figures 9A through 9C. Treatment should now consist of

1. transtibial amputation.
2. a double upright brace.
3. dressing changes with platelet-derived growth factor.
4. tibiocalcaneal arthrodesis.
5. total ankle arthroplasty.

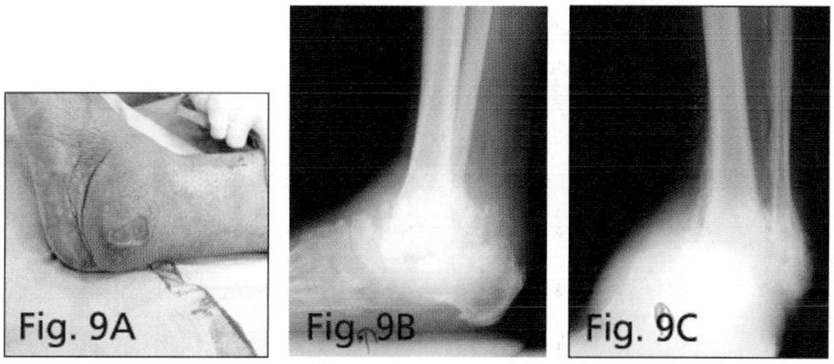

PREFERRED RESPONSE: 4

DISCUSSION: Nonsurgical management has failed to provide relief; therefore, the treatment of choice is arthrodesis with an intramedullary nail. Amputation may be indicated if the arthrodesis fails. The patient does have adequate circulation for an attempt at salvage. Total ankle arthroplasty is not indicated in a neuropathic patient.

REFERENCES: Pinzur MS, Kelikian A: Charcot ankle fusion with a retrograde locked intramedullary nail. *Foot Ankle Int* 1997;18:699-704.

Herbst SA: External fixation of Charcot arthropathy. *Foot Ankle Clin* 2004;9:595-609.

A-26: Figures 10A and 10B show the radiographs of a 32-year-old patient who is a professional athlete and who sustained an injury to the first metatarsal. A view of the opposite noninjured side is shown in Figure 10C. Management of the fracture should consist of

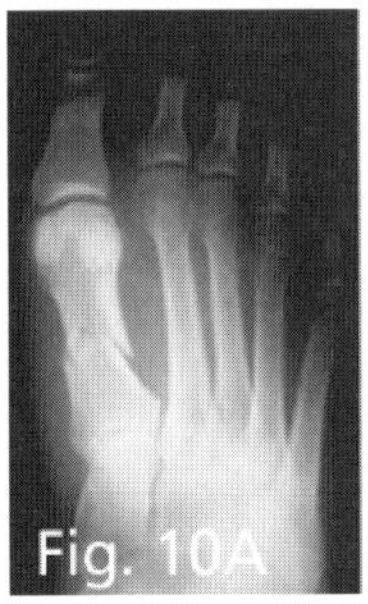
Fig. 10A

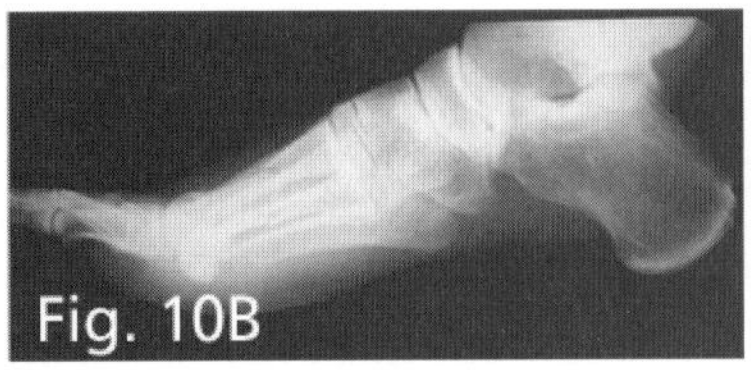
Fig. 10B

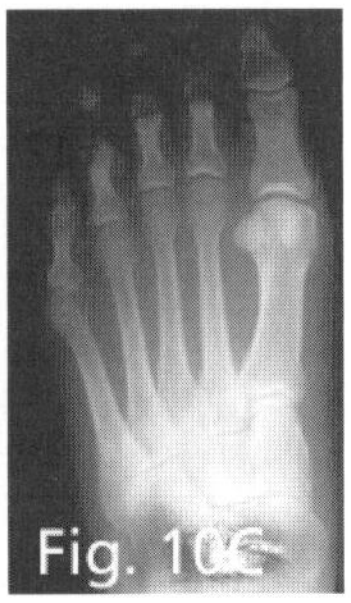
Fig. 10C

1. open reduction and internal fixation.
2. a postoperative stiff-soled shoe with weight bearing as tolerated.
3. a postoperative shoe with no weight bearing for 3 weeks.
4. a short leg cast with no weight bearing.
5. percutaneous pinning.

PREFERRED RESPONSE: 1

DISCUSSION: Parameters for first metatarsal fracture management are different than for shaft fractures of the central second, third, and fourth metatarsals. The first metatarsal carries a greater load and if malunited, can create transfer lesions by virtue of uneven weight distribution; therefore, nonsurgical management is not indicated for this patient. Percutaneous pinning is not as likely to result in an anatomic reduction as open reduction and internal fixation. Because the patient's livelihood depends on an expeditious return to function, the choice of open reduction and internal fixation allows for earlier motion and rehabilitation.

REFERENCES: Stroud CC: Fractures of the midtarsals, metatarsals, and phalanges, in Richardson EG, ed: *Orthopaedic Knowledge Update: Foot and Ankle*, 3. Rosemont, IL, American Academy of Orthopaedic Surgeons, 2004, pp 64-65.

Shereff MJ: Compartment syndromes of the foot. *Instr Course Lect* 1990;39:127-132.

A-27: Which of the following are considered appropriate nonsurgical bracing/orthotic options for a supple adult-acquired flatfoot deformity with forefoot abduction, secondary to posterior tibial tendon insufficiency?

1. Rigid orthotic with a lateral post
2. Custom-molded leather and polypropylene orthosis (Arizona brace)
3. UCBL orthosis with lateral posting
4. One quarter-inch lateral heel and sole wedge applied to the shoe
5. Three-quarter heel lift

PREFERRED RESPONSE: 2

DISCUSSION: The initial stages of posterior tibial tendon insufficiency, where the deformity remains supple, may be treated with bracing or an orthotic for pain relief. The Arizona brace was introduced in 1988, and assists in pain relief and deformity correction by minimizing hindfoot valgus alignment, lateral calcaneal displacement, and medial ankle collapse. It is particularly helpful in those patients with advanced disease that cannot tolerate an ankle-foot orthosis. All other choices are incorrect because of

(continued on next page)

(A-27: *continued*)

the addition of lateral posting, which is not advantageous in valgus deformities. The addition of medial posting to any of the above choices would render them correct alternatives. A heel lift is applicable in Achilles tendon disorders, not posterior tibial tendon disorders.

REFERENCES: Chao W, Wapner KL, Lee TH, et al: Nonoperative management of posterior tibial tendon dysfunction. *Foot Ankle Int* 1996;17:736-741.

Imhauser CW, Abidi NA, Frankel DZ, et al: Biomechanical evaluation of the efficacy of external stabilizers in conservative treatment of acquired flat foot deformity. *Foot Ankle Int* 2002;23:727-737.

A-28: A 28-year-old man underwent open reduction and internal fixation of a closed, displaced, intra-articular calcaneal fracture 8 weeks ago. Examination now reveals that the lateral wound is red and draining purulent material. Cultures obtained from the wound grow out *Staphylococcus aureus*. Radiographs show early healing of the fracture. What is the most appropriate next step in management?

1. Intravenous antibiotics
2. Débridement of the wound without hardware removal
3. Débridement of the wound with hardware removal
4. Vacuum-assisted closure (VAC) and negative pressure therapy
5. Total calcanectomy

PREFERRED RESPONSE: 3

DISCUSSION: Intravenous antibiotics alone will not adequately treat this infection. At 8 weeks after surgery, the hardware must be removed because *Staphylococcus aureus* is a virulent microbe. VAC therapy alone is not adequate without débridement and hardware removal, but it may play a role in postoperative wound care. Calcanectomy is a salvage procedure for calcaneal osteomyelitis or recalcitrant heel ulceration.

REFERENCES: Benirschke SK, Kramer PA: Wound healing complications in closed and open calcaneal fractures. *J Orthop Trauma* 2004;18:1-6.

Lim EV, Leung JP: Complications of intra-articular calcaneal fractures. *Clin Orthop* 2001;391:7-16.

Folk JW, Starr AJ, Early JS: Early wound complications of operative treatment of calcaneus fractures: Analysis of 190 fractures. *J Orthop Trauma* 1999;13:369-372.

A-29: A 37-year-old man with a history of congenital flatfoot reports worsening pain on the medial aspect of his ankle for the past year. The pain is worse with weight bearing and is better with rest and the use of an ankle brace. What findings are shown on the MRI scans in Figures 11A through 11C?

1. The flexor digitorum longus tendon is ruptured.
2. The posterior tibial tendon has a normal appearance.
3. The posterior tibial tendon has a physiologic amount of fluid in its sheath.
4. The posterior tibial tendon is completely ruptured and retracted (type III tear).
5. The posterior tibial tendon has a chronic longitudinal split with enlargement (type II tear).

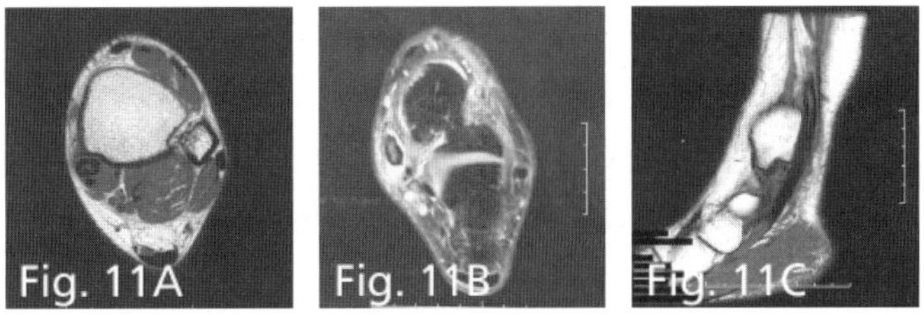
Fig. 11A Fig. 11B Fig. 11C

PREFERRED RESPONSE: 5

DISCUSSION: The MRI scans reveal an enlarged posterior tibial tendon, with degenerative signal within the tendon and an excessive amount of fluid in its sheath. This is a type II tear, as noted by Conti and associates, which is the most commonly seen tear.

REFERENCES: Slovenkai MP: Clinical and radiographic evaluation (Adult flatfoot: Posterior tibial tendon dysfunction). *Foot Ankle Clin* 1997;2:241-260.

Conti S, Michelson J, Jahss M: Clinical significance of magnetic resonance imaging in preoperative planning for reconstruction of posterior tibial tendon ruptures. *Foot Ankle* 1992;13:208-214.

A-30: A 60-year-old man reports increasing pain in his right foot with limited ankle dorsiflexion and anterior ankle pain after sustaining a fracture of the calcaneus during a fall several years ago. Bracing, NSAIDs, and cortisone injections have failed to provide significant relief. Radiographs are shown in Figures 12A and 12B. What is the most appropriate next step in management?

1. Subtalar distraction arthrodesis
2. Subtalar arthroscopy with débridement
3. Custom orthotics
4. Ankle arthrodesis
5. Calcaneal osteotomy

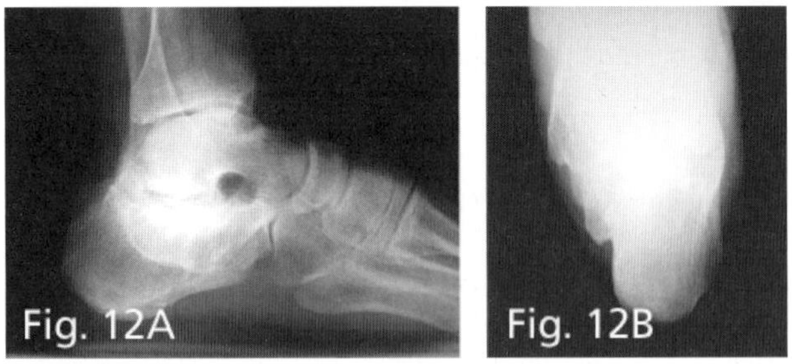
Fig. 12A Fig. 12B

PREFERRED RESPONSE: 1

DISCUSSION: Following a calcaneal fracture, the patient has severe subtalar arthritis with loss of talar declination and shortening of the heel; therefore, the treatment of choice is subtalar distraction arthrodesis. Orthotics will not provide significant relief as bracing has failed. Ankle arthrodesis will not be beneficial because the arthritis is in the subtalar joint. Subtalar arthroscopy would only be helpful for a small area of arthrosis, and calcaneal osteotomy would not be beneficial given the extent of the arthritis of the subtalar joint.

REFERENCE: Robinson TF, Murphy GA: Arthrodesis as salvage for calcaneal avulsions. *Foot Ankle Clin* 2002;7:107-120.

A-31: A 58-year-old woman sustained a ruptured Achilles tendon 1 year ago, and management consisted of an ankle-foot orthosis. She now reports increasing difficulty with ambulation and increasing pain. An MRI scan shows a 6-cm defect in the right Achilles tendon. Management should now consist of

1. continued use of an ankle-foot orthosis.
2. direct repair of the Achilles tendon.
3. V-Y repair of the Achilles tendon.
4. transfer of the plantaris tendon.
5. Achilles tendon turndown with flexor hallucis longus tendon transfer.

PREFERRED RESPONSE: 5

DISCUSSION: With a gap of less than 4 cm, a V-Y repair would be appropriate without a tendon transfer. For gaps greater than 5 cm, a lengthening with augmentation is the most appropriate treatment. Therefore, the treatment of choice is an Achilles tendon turndown with flexor hallucis longus tendon transfer. The plantaris tendon is not a strong enough repair, and direct repair is not possible given the large defect in the Achilles tendon. Continued use of the ankle-foot orthosis will not provide adequate relief for this patient.

REFERENCE: Myerson MS: Achilles tendon ruptures. *Instr Course Lect* 1999;48:219-230.

A-32: A 29-year-old woman reports dysesthesias and burning after undergoing bunion surgery that consisted of a proximal crescentic first metatarsal osteotomy 6 months ago. Examination reveals a positive Tinel sign at the proximal aspect of the healed incision. What injured nerve is responsible for the patient's continued symptoms?

1. Recurrent branch of the deep peroneal
2. Recurrent branch of the sural
3. Terminal cutaneous branch of the saphenous
4. Dorsomedial cutaneous branch of the superficial peroneal
5. Medial plantar

PREFERRED RESPONSE: 4

DISCUSSION: Painful incisional neuromas after bunion surgery frequently involve the dorsomedial cutaneous branch of the superficial peroneal nerve. This is the medial branch of the superficial peroneal nerve that terminates as the dorsomedial cutaneous nerve to the hallux. Branches of the deep peroneal nerve to this area are rare, and no branches to this area exist from the sural nerve. The saphenous nerve branches are generally more proximal, and the medial plantar nerve lies plantarly.

REFERENCES: Kenzora JE: Sensory nerve neuromas: Leading to failed foot surgery. *Foot Ankle* 1986;7:110-117.

Sarrafian SK: *Anatomy of the Foot and Ankle: Descriptive, Topographic, Functional*, ed 2. Philadelphia, PA, JB Lippincott, 1993.

A-33: Figure 13 shows the clinical photograph of a man who has had diabetes mellitus controlled with oral medication for the past 10 years. He wears soft-soled shoes and only uses leather-soled shoes for important business meetings. Examination reveals palpable dorsalis pedis and posterior tibial pulses, although they are somewhat diminished. He is insensate to pressure with the 5.07 Semmes-Weinstein monofilament. The ulcer heals after treatment with a full contact cast. What is the best course of action at this time?

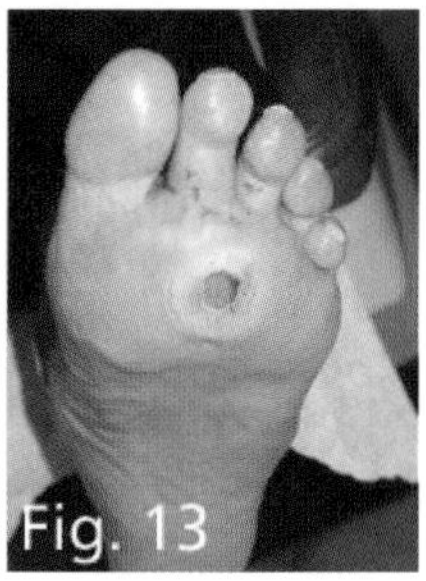
Fig. 13

1. Referral to his primary care physician
2. Foot-specific patient education, depth-inlay shoes, custom accommodative foot orthoses, and follow-up observation
3. Dorsiflexion osteotomy of the first and third metatarsals
4. Excision of the second and third metatarsal heads
5. Achilles tendon lengthening and dorsiflexion osteotomy of the first and third metatarsals

PREFERRED RESPONSE: 2

DISCUSSION: The patient has not undergone a trial of foot-specific patient education and accommodative/therapeutic shoe wear. He must wear therapeutic shoes at all times, as even the occasional use of pressure-concentrating shoes has a high likelihood of leading to the development of a diabetic foot ulcer.

REFERENCES: Pinzur MS, Kernan-Schroeder D, Emmanuele NV, et al: Development of a nurse-provided health system strategy for diabetic foot care. *Foot Ank Int* 2001;22:744-746.

Pinzur MS, Shields N, Goelitz B, et al: American Orthopaedic Foot and Ankle Society shoe survey of diabetic patients. *Foot Ankle Int* 1999;20:703-707.

Reiber GE, Smith DG, Wallace CM, et al: Effect of therapeutic footwear on foot reulceration in patients with diabetes: A randomized controlled trial. *JAMA* 2002;287:2552-2558.

A-34: Figures 14A and 14B show the clinical photograph and radiograph of a 15-year-old girl who has a deformity of her feet. Her parents are concerned because there is a family history of Charcot-Marie-Tooth disease. The patient reports some mild instability of the ankle and has noticed mild early callosities; however, she is not having any significant pain. Coleman block testing reveals a forefoot valgus and supple hindfoot. She has weakness to eversion and dorsiflexion. Initial management should consist of

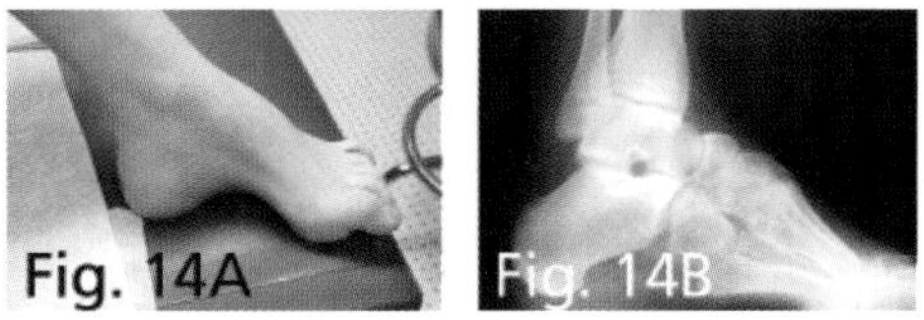

Fig. 14A Fig. 14B

1. dorsiflexion osteotomy of the first metatarsal with peroneus longus to brevis transfer.
2. plantar fasciotomy with dorsiflexion osteotomy of the first metatarsal and calcaneal osteotomy.
3. a stretching and strengthening physical therapy program and accommodative inserts.
4. observation.
5. calcaneal osteotomy, dorsiflexion osteotomy of the first metatarsal, peroneus longus to brevis transfer, plantar fascia release, Achilles tendon lengthening, and midfoot osteotomy.

PREFERRED RESPONSE: 3

DISCUSSION: Initial management of a young patient with a cavovarus deformity of the foot and a family history of Charcot-Marie-Tooth disease should focus on mobilization and strengthening of the weakening muscular units and an accommodative insert. Surgical intervention should be delayed until progression of the deformity begins to cause symptoms and/or weakness of the muscular units, resulting in contractures of the antagonistic muscle units.

REFERENCES: Pinzur MS: Charcot's foot. *Foot Ankle Clin* 2000;5:897-912.

Holmes JR, Hansen ST Jr: Foot and ankle manifestations of Charcot-Marie-Tooth disease. *Foot Ankle* 1993;14:476-486.

Thometz JG, Gould JS: Cavus deformity, in *The Child's Foot and Ankle*. New York, NY, Raven Press, 1992, pp 343-353.

A-35: A 64-year-old man with a history of diabetes mellitus underwent open reduction and internal fixation of a displaced ankle fracture 8 weeks ago. Examination now reveals recent onset erythema, warmth, and swelling of the midfoot. Radiographs are shown in Figures 15A through 15D. What is the most likely reason for the swelling of the foot?

1. Infection
2. Charcot arthropathy
3. Delayed compartment syndrome
4. Deep venous thrombosis
5. Gout

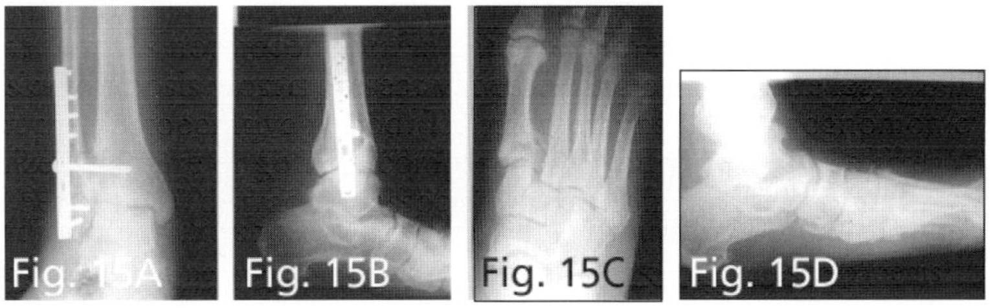

Fig. 15A Fig. 15B Fig. 15C Fig. 15D

PREFERRED RESPONSE: 2

DISCUSSION: A Charcot flare in adjacent joints is not uncommon in patients with neuropathy who undergo surgery or other trauma. Venous thrombosis would present with swelling of the entire leg, whereas infection would present earlier in the postoperative period. The radiographs are pathognomonic of Charcot arthropathy, not an unrecognized fracture or gout. A compartment syndrome this late after injury is extremely rare, and there would be no bony distraction associated with compartment syndrome.

REFERENCE: Connolly JF, Csencsitz TA: Limb threatening neuropathic complications from ankle fractures in patients with diabetes. *Clin Orthop* 1998;348:212-219.

Foot and Ankle: Answers

A-36: What complication is frequently associated with the Weil lesser metatarsal osteotomy (distal, oblique) in the treatment of claw toe deformities?

1. Floating toe
2. Nonunion
3. Osteonecrosis
4. Inadequate shortening
5. Dorsal displacement

PREFERRED RESPONSE: 1

DISCUSSION: Weil osteotomies are useful in achieving shortening of a lesser metatarsal with preservation of the distal articular surface. The osteotomy is oriented from distal-dorsal to proximal-plantar; therefore, proximal displacement of the distal fragment is associated with plantar (not dorsal) displacement as well. Plantar displacement can result in the intrinsics acting dorsal to the center of the metatarsophalangeal joint and the development of an extended or "floating" toe. Nonunion, osteonecrosis, and inadequate shortening are infrequent complications associated with the Weil lesser metatarsal osteotomy.

REFERENCES: Trnka HJ, Nyska M, Parks BG, et al: Dorsiflexion contracture after the Weil osteotomy: Results of cadaver study and three-dimensional analysis. *Foot Ankle Int* 2001;22:47-50.

Trnka HJ, Muhlbauer M, Zettl R, et al: Comparison of the results of the Weil and Helal osteotomies for the treatment of metatarsalgia secondary to dislocation of the lesser metatarsophalangeal joints. *Foot Ankle Int* 1999;20:72-79.

A-37: A 77-year-old man with diabetes mellitus has had a nonhealing Wagner grade I ulcer under the medial sesamoid for the past 3 months. He smokes tobacco regularly. He has undergone several débridements and total contact casting. Examination reveals no palpable pulses. He has no erythema or purulence, and he is afebrile. Radiographs reveal no abnormalities. What is the best initial diagnostic test to help determine why the ulcer has failed to heal?

1. 5.07 Semmes-Weinstein monofilament
2. Bone scan
3. Thompson test
4. CT
5. Noninvasive vascular studies

PREFERRED RESPONSE: 5

DISCUSSION: The best initial test for this patient is to assess the vascular supply to the foot. An elderly smoker with diabetes mellitus has a high risk of peripheral vascular disease. Decreased weight bearing has not been successful. Although a bone scan might be helpful, it would take secondary consideration to the patient's vascular supply, especially in the absence of any acute infection. Monofilament testing would help diagnosis neuropathy, which is a root cause behind the ulcer forming, but does not prevent it from healing. The Thompson test is used to diagnosis an Achilles tendon rupture.

REFERENCE: Brodsky JW: Evaluation of the diabetic foot. *Instr Course Lect* 1999;48:289-303.

A-38: A 28-year-old man who sustained an ankle fracture in a motor vehicle accident underwent open reduction and internal fixation 3 months ago. He continues to report significant ankle pain with ambulation. Radiographs are shown in Figure 16. What is the next most appropriate step in management?

1. Articulated ankle-foot orthosis
2. Revision open reduction and internal fixation of the syndesmosis with débridement of the medial gutter
3. Ankle arthrodesis
4. Syndesmosis arthrodesis
5. Ankle arthroscopy and debridement

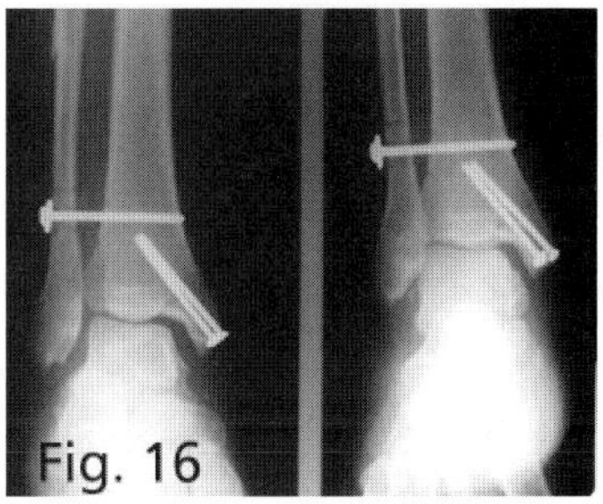

PREFERRED RESPONSE: 2

DISCUSSION: The patient sustained a bimalleolar ankle fracture with a syndesmosis disruption. The initial open reduction and internal fixation did not successfully reduce the distal tibiofibular joint. The patient may need a derotational distraction osteotomy of the fibula to reduce the syndesmosis. The other procedures do not address the primary problem of the fibular malunion and syndesmosis malreduction. There is no radiographic evidence of significant arthritis; therefore, ankle arthrodesis is not indicated.

REFERENCE: Heier KA, Walling AK: Treatment of ankle fractures. *Foot Ankle Clin* 1999;4:521-534.

A-39: The radiograph shown in Figure 17 shows measurement of what angle?

1. Hallux valgus
2. Distal metatarsal articular
3. Intermetatarsal
4. Sesamoid divergence
5. Angle of joint congruence

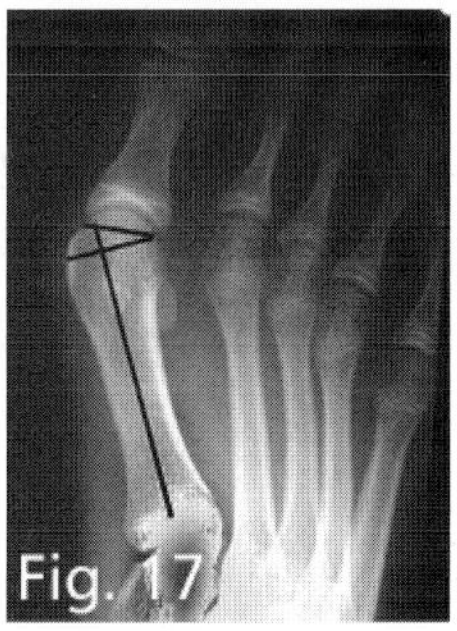

PREFERRED RESPONSE: 2

DISCUSSION: The relationship between the distal articular surface of the first metatarsal head and the long axis of the first metatarsal is called the distal metatarsal articular angle. This angle has been validated by Richardson and associates to measure and determine the congruence of the first metatarsophalangeal joint. This angle is critical in determining the appropriate surgical procedure to perform on a patient with a bunion deformity because a congruent joint requires a procedure to maintain congruence of the articular surfaces following osteotomy. Therefore, a chevron becomes a biplanar chevron, and a Lapidus procedure adds a second osteotomy of the distal metatarsal to tilt the metatarsal head into a congruent location.

REFERENCES: Coughlin MJ: Juvenile hallux valgus: Etiology and treatment. *Foot Ankle Int* 1995;16:682-697.

Steel MW III, Johnson KA, DeWitz MA, et al: Radiographic measurements of the normal foot. *Foot Ankle* 1980;1:151-158.

Richardson EG, Graves SC, McClure JT, et al: First metatarsal head-shaft angle: A method of determination. *Foot Ankle* 1993;14:181-185.

Foot and Ankle: Answers

A-40: A 5-year-old boy has had midfoot pain with activity for the past 3 months. He has no pain at rest. Radiographs are shown in Figures 18A and 18B. Management should consist of

1. a vascularized pedicle bone graft.
2. a short leg walking cast.
3. a custom-molded orthotic.
4. surgical débridement followed by antibiotics.
5. a bone stimulator.

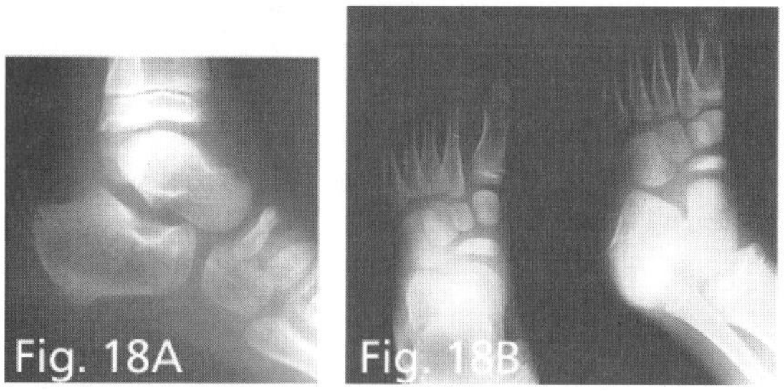
Fig. 18A Fig. 18B

PREFERRED RESPONSE: 2

DISCUSSION: The radiographs show classic findings for Koehler disease (osteochondrosis of the navicular). The patient's age and clinical history are typical for this self-limiting condition. Patients will improve with time, but the duration of symptoms is much shorter if the patient is placed in a cast. There is no role for surgery in this disease.

REFERENCE: Williams GA, Cowell HR: Koehler's disease of the tarsal navicular. *Clin Orthop* 1981;158:53-58.

A-41: A 62-year-old man with diabetes mellitus has had a persistent 2-cm ulcer under the third metatarsal head for the past 4 months. He reports that he has had similar ulcers twice before, and both healed with nonsurgical management. He has used multiple types of commercial walking braces, shoes, and commercial dressings without resolution. He is insensate to the 5.07 Semmes-Weinstein monofilament. When the wound is probed with culture swab, there is no communication with the metatarsal head. Radiographs, bone scans, and laboratory studies reveal no evidence of osteomyelitis. What is the most predictable method of accomplishing wound healing without recurrence?

1. Transmetatarsal amputation
2. Excision of the third metatarsal head
3. Percutaneous Achilles tendon lengthening and a total contact cast
4. Viral recombitant growth factor and a commercial removeable walking boot
5. A non–weight-bearing total contact cast that is changed every week until the ulcer is healed

PREFERRED RESPONSE: 3

DISCUSSION: The patient has a persistent diabetic foot ulcer without evidence of osteomyelitis. He has evidence of a sensory peripheral neuropathy and a concomitant motor neuropathy, leading to a dynamic motor imbalance. Use of a total contact cast would offer a high probability of healing the resistant ulcer but with a high potential for recurrence. Combining the total contact cast with Achilles tendon lengthening allows wound healing without a high risk for recurrence. Excision of the noninfected metatarsal head would make the patient vulnerable to the development of a transfer lesion under one of the remaining metatarsal heads.

REFERENCES: Robertson DD, Mueller MJ, Smith KE, et al: Structural changes in the forefoot of individuals with diabetes and a prior plantar ulcer. *J Bone Joint Surg Am* 2002;84:1395-1404.

Mueller MJ, Sinacore DR, Hastings MK, et al: Effect of Achilles tendon lengthening on neuropathic plantar ulcers. *J Bone Joint Surg Am* 2003;85:1436-1445.

A-42: An 11-year-old boy stepped on a nail and sustained a puncture to the right forefoot 6 days ago. He was wearing tennis shoes at the time of injury. Treatment in the emergency department consisted of local débridement and tetanus prophylaxis; a radiograph was negative for foreign body, chondral defect, or fracture. He was discharged with a 3-day prescription of amoxicillin and clavulanate. The patient now has increasing pain and tenderness at the puncture site. What is the best course of action?

1. Change the antibiotic to ciprofloxacin
2. Initiate gentamicin
3. Resume the prescription for amoxicillin and clavulanate
4. Observation and follow-up in 48 hours
5. Surgical débridement

PREFERRED RESPONSE: 5

DISCUSSION: The initial treatment consisting of oral antibiotics was appropriate but with progressive symptoms, surgical débridement is necessary. Ciprofloxacin is contraindicated in children, and at this stage, oral antibiotics are inadequate. Intravenous antibiotics may be necessary, but surgical débridement is paramount. Failure to respond to the initial management precludes further observation.

REFERENCES: Riegler HP, Routson T: Complications of deep puncture wounds of the foot. *J Trauma* 1979;19:18-22.

Green NE: Musculoskeletal infections in children: Part IV. Pseudomonas infections of the foot following puncture wounds. *Instr Course Lect* 1983;32:43-46.

A-43: A 20-year-old man who is an elite college football player has ecchymosis, swelling, and pain on the lateral side of his foot after a game. Radiographs are shown in Figures 19A through 19C. Management should consist of

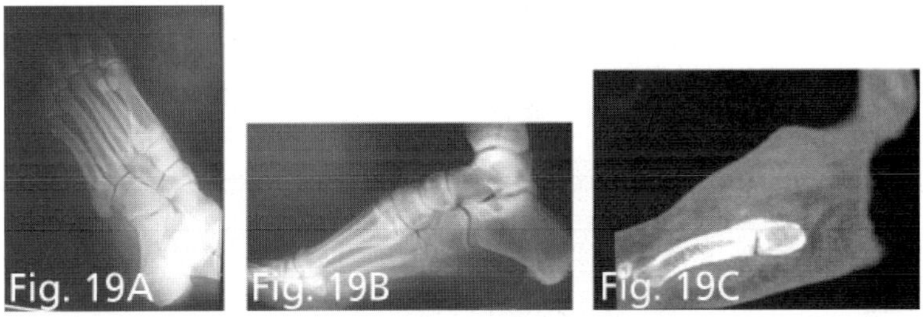

1. open reduction and internal fixation with a plate and screws.
2. open treatment with calcaneal bone graft.
3. percutaneous screw fixation with a 4.5-mm screw.
4. weight-bearing cast for 8 weeks.
5. spanning external fixation.

PREFERRED RESPONSE: 3

DISCUSSION: Metaphyseal-diaphyseal junction fractures of the fifth metatarsal require careful evaluation. In athletes, early intervention with a 4.5-mm intramedullary screw correlates with an earlier return to activity. One study examining the failure of surgically managed Jones fractures revealed that use of anything other than a 4.5-mm malleolar screw for internal fixation correlated with failure.

REFERENCES: Glasgow MT, Naranja RJ Jr, Glasgow SG, et al: Analysis of failed surgical management of fractures of the base of the fifth metatarsal distal to the tuberosity: The Jones fracture. *Foot Ankle Int* 1996;17:449-457.

Beskin JL: Injuries to the midfoot and forefoot, in Mizel MS, Miller RA, Scioli MW, eds: *Orthopaedic Knowledge Update: Foot and Ankle*, ed 2. Rosemont, IL, American Academy of Orthopaedic Surgeons, 1998, pp 243-252.

A-44: A 55-year-old man who runs on the weekends reports a 1-year history of continued pain directly posteriorly in the heel. Management consisting of anti-inflammatory drugs, icing techniques, a heel-counter in his shoe split, and physical therapy consisting of stretching, contrast baths, custom orthotics, and iontophoresis has failed to provide relief. Not only is his lifestyle disrupted with respect to running, but he now has pain with normal ambulation with all forms of shoe wear. He is not necessarily concerned with returning to running; he is primarily seeking pain relief. A lateral radiograph and clinical photograph are shown in Figures 20A and 20B. Treatment should now consist of

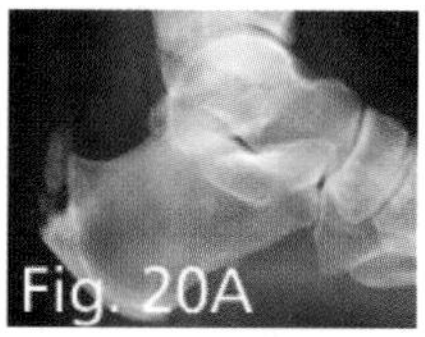
Fig. 20A

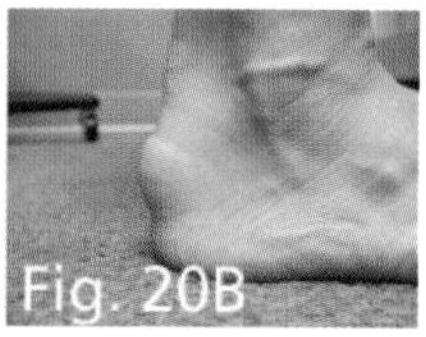
Fig. 20B

1. injection directly into the tendon with triamcinolone or methylprednisolone.
2. shock wave therapy to the posterior heel to break up calcific deposits.
3. brisement.
4. a simple lateral surgical approach to the posterior heel, with resection of the Haglund exostosis.
5. a central-splitting surgical approach through the tendon, excision of the Haglund exostosis and the insertional calcifications, bursectomy, flexor hallucis longus tendon transfer to the posterior tuberosity, and attachment of the tendon to the calcaneus.

PREFERRED RESPONSE: 5

DISCUSSION: The patient has severe calcifications at the insertion of the Achilles tendon. Failure to address the Haglund exostosis and the calcifications will leave the patient with persistent pain. Steroids should not be injected directly into the tendon because of the increased risk of tendon rupture. Shock wave therapy may have some value in treating plantar fasciitis, but its efficacy has not been documented with insertional calcifications and Haglund exostosis treatment. Brisement is injection of saline solution around the Achilles tendon in an attempt to decompress the peritenon. This may be valuable in intrasubstance Achilles tendinosis or peritendinitis but has no value with insertional disease. Symptoms persisting beyond 6 months are difficult to treat nonsurgically; therefore, the appropriate treatment protocol is aggressive and must address all pathology. The patient may not be able to run at the level achieved prior to surgery, but the goal of the surgery is pain relief.

REFERENCES: Clain M, Baxter D: Achilles tendinitis. *Foot Ankle* 1992;13:482-487.

Schepsis A, Wagner C, Leach R: Surgical management of Achilles tendon overuse injuries: A long-term follow-up study. *Am J Sports Med* 1994;22:611-619.

Schepsis A, Leach R: Surgical management of Achilles tendinitis. *Am J Sports Med* 1987;15:308-315.

Keck S, Kelly P: Bursitis of the posterior part of the heel: Evaluation of surgical treatment of eighteen patients. *J Bone Joint Surg Am* 1965;47:267-273.

A-45: Figures 21A and 21B show the clinical photographs of a 46-year-old woman who has a painful deformity of the second toe. Surgical treatment consisting of metatarsophalangeal capsulotomy and proximal interphalangeal joint resection arthroplasty resulted in satisfactory correction, but the toe remains unstable at the metatarsophalangeal joint. What is the most appropriate next step?

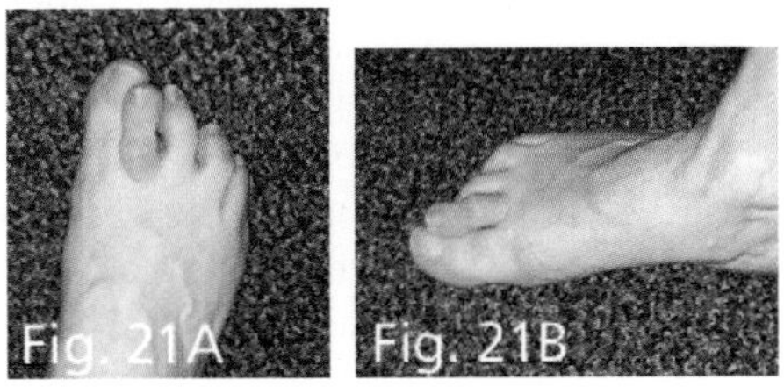

1. Flexor digitorum longus tenotomy
2. Resection of the metatarsal head and pin fixation
3. Transfer of the flexor digitorum longus to the extensor tendon
4. Excision at the base of the proximal phalanx and syndactyly with the third toe
5. Arthrodesis of the second metatarsophalangeal joint

PREFERRED RESPONSE: 3

DISCUSSION: Crossover second toes are attributed to attenuation or rupture of the plantar plate and lateral collateral ligament and are associated with varying degrees of instability. Flexor-to-extensor transfer (Girdlestone-Taylor procedure) can provide intrinsic stability to the toe. Although plantar metatarsal head condylectomy can increase stability by resulting in scarring of the plantar plate, excision of the entire second metatarsal head carries a high risk of transfer metatarsalgia. Removal of the base of the proximal phalanx destabilizes the toe and should be reserved as a salvage procedure. Simple flexor tenotomy alone will not improve stability, and arthrodesis of the second metatarsophalangeal joint will limit motion and impair function.

REFERENCES: Coughlin MJ: Crossover second toe deformity. *Foot Ankle* 1987;8:29-39.

Thompson FM, Deland JT: Flexor tendon transfer for metatarsophalangeal instability of the second toe. *Foot Ankle* 1993;14:385-388.

Foot and Ankle: Answers

A-46: A 40-year-old man fell 10 feet from a tree and sustained the closed isolated injury shown in Figures 22A and 22B. Management consists of splinting. At his 2-week follow-up visit, the patient clinically passes the wrinkle test. He agrees to open reduction and internal fixation. What is the best surgical approach to obtain anatomic reduction and limit wound dehiscence?

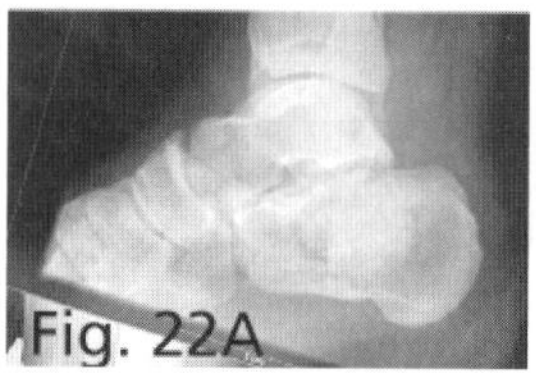

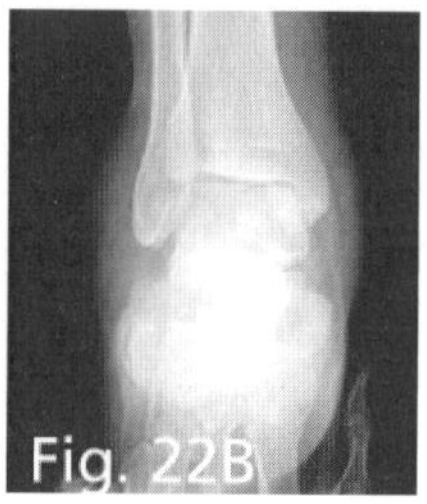

1. Closed reduction and percutaneous pinning
2. Open reduction and internal fixation with a lateral approach, extensile right-angled lateral incision, vertical limb 0.5 cm anterior to the Achilles tendon, and horizontal limb at the junction of the lateral skin and the plantar glabrous skin
3. Open reduction and internal fixation with a lateral approach, extensile right-angled lateral incision, vertical limb 2.0 cm anterior to the Achilles tendon, and horizontal limb 2.0 cm proximal to the line marking the plantar glabrous skin
4. Sinus tarsi approach
5. Ollier approach

PREFERRED RESPONSE: 2

DISCUSSION: The approach to the calcaneus has evolved from several different patterns, driven by a high wound complication rate of 10%. The current extensile lateral approach was described by Zwipp and associates in 1988. The surgical exposure uses an L-shaped incision, with the vertical component positioned one half a finger's breath anterior to the Achilles tendon and extending distally to the junction of the lateral skin and the plantar skin. Borrelli and Lashgari mapped the angiosome of the lateral calcaneal flap and found that the major arterial blood supply to this flap consisted of three arteries: the lateral calcaneal artery, the lateral malleolar artery, and the lateral tarsal artery. The lateral calcaneal artery appeared to be responsible for most of the blood supply to the corner of the flap. This was found 1.5 cm anterior to the Achilles tendon. Division of this artery with inaccurate placement of the vertical limb of the incision can cause ischemia of the lateral skin flap.

REFERENCES: Borrelli J Jr, Lashgari C: Vascularity of the lateral calcaneal flap: A cadaveric injection study. *J Orthop Trauma* 1999;13:73-77.

Freeman BJC, Duff S, Allen PE, et al: The extended lateral approach to the hindfoot: An anatomical basis and surgical implications. *J Bone Joint Surg Br* 1998;80:139-142.

Zwipp H, Tscherne H, Wulker N: Osteosynthesis of dislocated intra-articular calcaneus fractures. *Unfallchirurg* 1988;91:507-515.

A-47: A 17-year-old patient sustained a closed calcaneal fracture when he jumped off of a roof 2 years ago, and he underwent nonsurgical management at the time of injury. The patient now reports lateral hindfoot pain that is worse with weight-bearing activities. Anti-inflammatory drugs and orthoses have failed to provide relief. Coronal and sagittal CT scans are shown in Figures 23A and 23B. What is the best course of action?

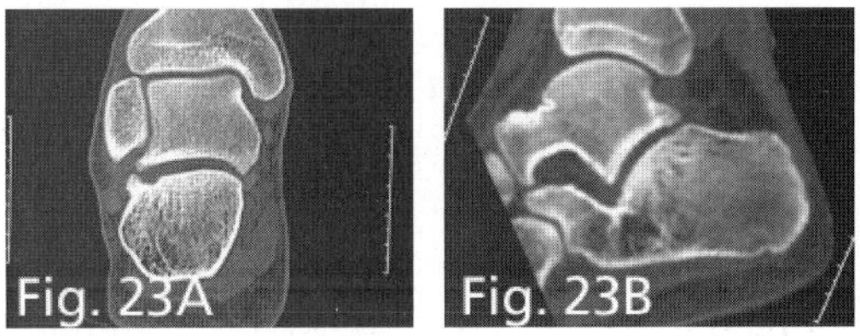
Fig. 23A Fig. 23B

1. In situ subtalar arthrodesis
2. Cortisone injection in the subtalar joint followed by casting for 4 to 6 weeks
3. UCBL insert
4. Lateral wall exostectomy
5. Bone block arthrodesis of the subtalar joint

PREFERRED RESPONSE: 4

DISCUSSION: The CT scans show evidence of a lateral wall blowout and malunion without significant arthrosis of the subtalar joint. In a young patient, it is preferable to avoid a fusion and allow residual motion by performing an exostectomy that decompresses the lateral subtalar joint and peroneal tendons.

REFERENCES: Chandler JT, Bonar SK, Anderson RB, et al: Results of in situ subtalar arthrodesis for late sequelae of calcaneus fractures. *Foot Ankle Int* 1999;20:18-24.

Werner MR: Calcaneal fractures, in Richardson EG, ed: *Orthopaedic Knowledge Update: Foot and Ankle*, ed 3. Rosemont, IL, American Academy of Orthopaedic Surgeons, 2003, p 52.

A-48: Figures 24A and 24B show the clinical photographs of a 43-year-old patient with type I diabetes mellitus who has a stump ulcer after undergoing successful transtibial amputation 1 year ago. Which of the following is considered the most predictable method of healing the ulcer and preventing recurrent ulceration?

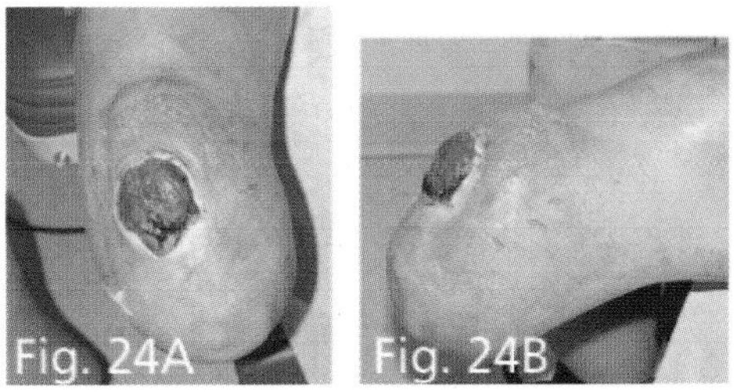
Fig. 24A Fig. 24B

1. Refrain from using the prosthesis until the ulcer heals.
2. Refrain from using the prosthesis and apply platelet-derived growth factor daily until the ulcer heals.
3. Have a prosthetist relieve the area of the anterior-distal tibia to eliminate pressure and allow the ulcer to heal.
4. Replace the prosthetic socket liner with a thick silicone liner.
5. Perform a wedge resection of the infected tissue, create a soft-tissue envelope with muscle covering the bone, and allow primary healing of the skin.

PREFERRED RESPONSE: 5

DISCUSSION: The ulcer occurred as the result of a mismatch between the shape of the residual limb and the prosthetic socket. With the mismatch, the residual limb pistoned and the tissue failed because of the applied shear forces. The most predictable short- and long-term solution is reconstruction of the residual limb. Refraining from use of the prosthesis will prevent the patient from walking for months. It is unlikely that prosthetic socket modification will allow resolution of this large ulcer.

REFERENCE: Hadden W, Marks R, Murdoch G, et al: Wedge resection of amputation stumps: A valuable salvage procedure. *J Bone Joint Surg Br* 1987;69:306-308.

A-49: The Coleman block test is used to evaluate the cavovarus foot. What is the most important information obtained from this test?

1. Determines the patient's ability to balance
2. Determines hindfoot flexibility
3. Determines forefoot flexibility
4. Assesses the patient for Achilles tendon contractures
5. Evaluates peroneus longus strength

PREFERRED RESPONSE: 2

DISCUSSION: Coleman block testing, performed by placing an elevation under the lateral border of the foot, is used to determine if the forefoot and/or plantar flexed first ray is causing a compensatory varus in the hindfoot. The block is placed under the lateral border of the foot, and therefore does not have any relation to the Achilles tendon and suppleness of the hindfoot.

REFERENCES: Holmes JR, Hansen ST Jr: Foot and ankle manifestations of Charcot-Marie-Tooth disease. *Foot Ankle* 1993;14:476-486.

Thometz JG, Gould JS: Cavus deformity, in *The Child's Foot and Ankle*. New York, NY, Raven Press, 1992, pp 343-353.

A-50: A 35-year-old woman has had significant pain and swelling in the left medial ankle inferior to the medial malleolus for the past 8 months. Physical therapy, brace and orthotic management, and immobilization have failed to provide relief. She is now requesting a more aggressive option to assist in pain relief. Clinical photographs and radiographs are seen in Figures 25A through 25F. Following exposure, a complete rupture of the posterior tibial tendon is visible. What is the most appropriate surgical reconstruction?

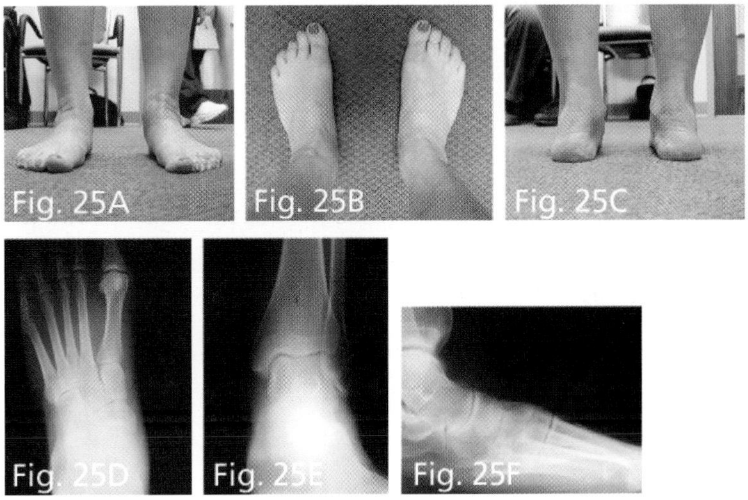

1. Subtalar arthrodesis
2. Flexor digitorum longus transfer
3. Flexor digitorum longus tendon transfer, medial slide calcaneal osteotomy, and spring ligament repair
4. Primary repair of the posterior tibial tendon
5. Talonavicular arthrodesis

PREFERRED RESPONSE: 3

DISCUSSION: The patient has a complete rupture of the posterior tibial tendon with minimal hindfoot valgus deformity. The deformity is supple, and there is no arthritis in the subtalar, talonavicular, or calcaneocuboid joints; therefore, joint-sparing procedures are appropriate in this patient (avoidance of arthrodeses). The treatment of choice is flexor digitorum longus tendon transfer, medial slide calcaneal osteotomy, and spring ligament repair. Primary repair of an incompetent posterior tibial tendon can lead to failure and recurrence of pain and deformity. Talonavicular arthrodesis corrects the forefoot abduction and elevates a plantar flexed talus; however, the patient does not have this deformity; therefore, the procedure is not indicated.

REFERENCES: Myerson MS, Corrigan J, Thompson F, et al: Tendon transfer combined with calcaneal osteotomy for treatment of posterior tibial tendon insufficiency: A radiological investigation. *Foot Ankle Int* 1995;16:712-718.

Trnka HJ, Easley ME, Myerson MS: The role of calcaneal osteotomies for correction of adult flat foot. *Clin Orthop* 1999;365:50-64.

Jahss MH: Spontaneous rupture of the tibialis posterior tendon: Clinical findings, tenographic studies, and a new technique for repair. *Foot Ankle* 1982;3:158-166.

Toolan BC, Sangeorzan BJ, Hansen ST Jr: Complex reconstruction for the treatment of dorsolateral peritalar subluxation of the foot. *J Bone Joint Surg Am* 1999;81:1545-1560.